Management of High-Risk Pregnancy

Management of High-Risk Pregnancy

An Evidence-Based Approach

EDITED BY

John T. Queenan

Professor and Chairman Emeritus
Department of Obstetrics and Gynecology
Georgetown University Medical Center
Washington, DC

Catherine Y. Spong

Bethesda, MD

Charles J. Lockwood

Professor and Chair
Yale University School of Medicine
Department of Obstetrics, Gynecology and Reproductive Sciences
New Haven, CT

FIFTH EDITION

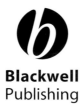

Blackwell
Publishing

© 2007 by Blackwell Publishing Ltd
© 1999 by Blackwell Science Inc
Blackwell Publishing, Inc., 350 Main Street, Malden, Massachusetts 02148-5020, USA
Blackwell Publishing Ltd, 9600 Garsington Road, Oxford OX4 2DQ, UK
Blackwell Publishing Asia Pty Ltd, 550 Swanston Street, Carlton, Victoria 3053, Australia

Fourth edition first published in 1999
Fifth edition 2007

1   2007

Library of Congress Cataloging-in-Publication Data

Management of high-risk pregnancy / edited by John T. Queenan, Catherine Y. Spong, Charles
    J. Lockwood. – 5th ed.
      p.   ;   cm.
    Includes bibliographical references and index.
    ISBN-13: 978-1-4051-2782-0 (alk. paper)
    ISBN-10: 1-4051-2782-1 (alk. paper)
    1. Pregnancy–Complications.   I. Queenan, John T.   II. Spong, Catherine Y.
  III. Lockwood, Charles J.   IV. Title: High-risk pregnancy.
    [DNLM: 1. Pregnancy, High-Risk.   2. Pregnancy Complications.   WQ 240 M266
  2007]
    RG571.M24 2007
    618.3–dc22

2006026263

ISBN-13: 978-1-4051-2782-0

A catalogue record for this title is available from the British Library

Set in 9/12 Palatino by SNP Best-set Typesetter Ltd., Hong Kong
Printed and bound in Singapore by COS Printers Pte Ltd

Commissioning Editor: Stuart Taylor
Editorial Assistant: Jennifer Seward
Development Editor: Adam Gilbert
Production Controller: Debbie Wyer

For further information on Blackwell Publishing, visit our website:
http://www.blackwellpublishing.com

Contents

Contents

List of contributors

Alfred Abuhamad
MD
Eastern Virginia Medical School
Norfolk, Virginia 23507
USA

Robert H. Ball
MD
Department of Obstetrics, Gynecology and
*   Reproductive Sciences*
Fetal Treatment Center
University of California, San Francisco
San Francisco, CA 94143-0132
USA

Ron Beloosesky
MD
Department of Obstetrics and Gynecology
Rambam Medical Center
Haifa, Israel

Vincenzo Berghella
MD
Department of Obstetrics and Gynecology
Division of Maternal-Fetal Medicine
Thomas Jefferson University
Philadelphia, PA 19107
USA

Caterina Bocchi
MD
Department of Pediatrics, Obstetrics and
*   Reproductive Medicine*
University of Siena
Siena, Italy

Catalin S. Buhimschi
MD
Yale University School of Medicine
Department of Obstetrics, Gynecology and
*   Reproductive Sciences*
New Haven, CT 06520-8063
USA

Brian Casey
MD
UT Southwestern Medical Center at Dallas
Department of Obstetrics and Gynecology
Dallas, TX 75390-9032
USA

Nancy C. Chescheir
MD
Vanderbilt University School of Medicine
Department of Obstetrics and Gynecology
R-1127 Medical Center North
Nashville, TN 37232-2521
USA

Erin A. S. Clark
MD
University of Utah Health Sciences Center
Department of Obstetrics and Gynecology
Salt Lake City, UT 84132
USA

Deborah L. Conway
MD
University of Texas Health Science Center—San
*   Antonio*
Department of Obstetrics and Gynecology
San Antonio, TX 78229
USA

Mary E. D'Alton
MD
Columbia University
Department of Obstetrics and Gynecology
New York, NY 10032
USA

Deborah A. Driscoll
MD
Department of Obstetrics and Gynecology
University of Pennsylvania Health System
Philadelphia, PA 19104
USA

Patrick Duff
MD
Department of Obstetrics and Gynecology
University of Florida College of Medicine
Gainesville, Florida 32610-0294
USA

Avroy A. Fanaroff
MD
Department of Pediatrics
Rainbow Babies and Children's Hospital
Cleveland, OH 44106
USA

Michael R. Foley
MD
Department of Obstetrics and Gynecology
University of Arizona School of Medicine
150IN Campbell Avenue
PO Box 245078
Tuscon, AZ 85274
USA

Edmund Funai
MD
Yale University School of Medicine
Department of Obstetrics, Gynecology and
*   Reproductive Sciences*
New Haven, CT 06520-8063
USA

Steven G. Gabbe
MD
Vanderbilt University School of Medicine
Department of Obstetrics and Gynecology
Nashville, TN 37232-2104
USA

Alessandro Ghidini
MD
Inova Alexandria Hospital
Perinatal Diagnostic Center
Alexandria, VA 22304
USA

Labib M. Ghulmiyyah
MD
University of Cincinnati College of Medicine
Department of Obstetrics and Gynecology
Cincinnati, OH 45267-0526
USA

Ronald S. Gibbs
MD
University of Colorado School of Medicine
Department of Obstetrics and Gynecology
Denver, CO 80262
USA

Larry C. Gilstrap
MD
University of Texas Houston Medical School
Department of Obstetrics, Gynecology, and
    Reproductive Sciences
Houston, TX 77030
USA

Laura Goetzl
MD, MPH
Medical University of South Carolina
Obstetrics and Gynecology
Division of Maternal-Fetal Medicine
Charleston, SC 29464
USA

Jane Cleary-Goldman
MD
Division of Maternal-Fetal Medicine
Columbia University Medical Center
New York, NY 10032
USA

Gilbert J. Grant
MD
New York University School of Medicine
Department of Anesthesiology
New York, NY 10016
USA

Benjamin Hamar
MD
Beth Israel Deaconess Medical Center
Department of Obstetrics and Gynecology
Division of Maternal-Fetal Medicine
Boston, MA 02215
USA

Gary D. V. Hankins
MD
Department of Obstetrics and Gynecology
Division of Maternal-Fetal Medicine
The University of Texas Medical Branch
Galveston, Texas 77555-0587
USA

Michael R. Harrison
MD
Department of Obstetrics, Gynecology and
    Reproductive Sciences
Fetal Treatment Center
University of California, San Francisco
San Francisco, CA 94143-0570
USA

John Hayslett
MD
Section of Nephrology
Department of Internal Medicine
Yale School of Medicine
New Haven, CT 06520-8029
USA

C. Kevin Huls
MD
Department of Obstetrics and Gynecology
University of Wisconsin School of Medicine and
    Public Health
Madison, WI 53715
USA

Garrett K. Lam
MD
Phoenix Perinatal Associates
Phoenix, AZ 85006
USA

Mark B. Landon
MD
Division of Maternal-Fetal Medicine
The Ohio State University College of Medicine
Columbus OH 43210-1228
USA

Hanmin Lee
MD
Department of Obstetrics, Gynecology and
    Reproductive Sciences
Division of Pediatric Surgery and the Fetal Treatment
    Center
University of California, San Francisco
San Francisco, CA 94143-0570
USA

Young Mi Lee
MD
Division of Maternal-Fetal Medicine
Department of Obstetrics and Gynecology
Columbia University Medical Center
New York, NY 10032
USA

Monica Longo
MD, PhD
Department of Obstetrics and Gynecology
Division of Maternal-Fetal Medicine
The University of Texas Medical Branch
Galveston, Texas 77555-0587
USA

Fergal D. Malone
MD
Department of Obstetrics and Gynecology
Royal College of Surgeons in Ireland
The Rotunda Hospital
Parnell Square
Dublin 1
IRELAND

Stephanie R. Martin
DO
Department of Obstetrics and Gynecology
Division of Maternal-Fetal Medicine
Banner Good Samaritan Medical Center
Phoenix, AZ
USA

Paul J. Meis
MD
Wake Forest University Medical Center
Department of Obstetrics and Gynecology
Winston-Salem, NC 27157
USA

Brian M. Mercer
MD
Division of Maternal-Fetal Medicine
Department of Obstetrics and Gynecology
MetroHealth Medical Center
Case Western Reserve University
Cleveland, OH 44109-1998
USA

Howard L. Minkoff
MD
Maimonides Medical Center
Department of Obstetrics and Gynecology
Brooklyn, NY 11219
USA

Kenneth J. Moise, Jr
MD
University of North Carolina School of Medicine
Department of Obstetrics and Gynecology
Chapel Hill, NC 27599-7516
USA

Michael Nageotte
MD
Long Beach Memorial Medical Center
Department of Obstetrics and Gynecology
Long Beach, CA 90801
USA

Edward R. Newton
MD
East Carolina School of Medicine
Brody School of Medicine
Greenville, NC 27858
USA

Errol R. Norwitz

MD, PhD
Yale University School of Medicine
Department of Obstetrics, Gynecology &
  Reproductive Sciences
New Haven, CT 06520-8063
USA

David Nyberg

MD
The Fetal and Women's Center of Arizona
9440 E Ironwood Square Drive
Scottsdale, AZ 85255
USA

John Owen

MD, MSPH
University of Alabama at Birmingham
Department of Obstetrics and Gynecology
Division of Maternal-Fetal Medicine
Birmingham, AL 35249-7333
USA

Yinka Oyelese

MD
Division of Maternal Fetal Medicine,
Department of Obstetrics, Gynecology and
  Reproductive Sciences,
UMDNJ-Robert Wood Johnson Medical School
New Brunswick, NJ 08901
USA

Michael J. Paidas

MD
Yale-New Haven Hospital
Obstetrics and Gynecology
New Haven, CT 06520-8063
USA

Julian T. Parer

MD
University of California, San Francisco
Department of Obstetrics, Gynecology, and
  Reproductive Science
San Francisco, CA 94143-0550
USA

Page B. Pennell

MD
Department of Neurology
Emory University School of Medicine
Atlanta, GA 30322
USA

Christian M. Pettker

MD
Yale University School of Medicine
Department of Obstetrics and Gynecology
Division of Maternal-Fetal Medicine
333 Cedar Street
New Haven, CT 06520-8063

USA

Sarah H. Poggi

MD
Inova Alexandria Hospital
Perinatal Diagnostic Center
Alexandria, VA 22304
USA

Nebojsa Radunovic

MD, PhD
Institute of Obstetrics and Gynecology,
Belgrade University School of Medicine
Koste Todorovica 26,
11000 Beograd, Serbia and Montenegro

William F. Rayburn

MD
University of New Mexico
Department of Obstetrics and Gynecology
Albuquerque, NM 87131-0001
USA

Scott Roberts

MD
UT Southwestern Medical Center at Dallas
Department of Obstetrics and Gynecology
Dallas, TX 75390-9032
USA

Michael G. Ross

MD
Harbor-UCLA Medical Center
Department of Obstetrics and Gynecology
Torrance, CA 90509-2910
USA

George Saade

MD
UTMB at Galveston
Department of Obstetrics and Gynecology
Galveston, TX 77555-1062
USA

Michael Schatz

MD, MS
Kaiser-Permanente Medical Center, San Diego
San Diego, CA 92111
USA

James R. Scott

MD
University of Utah
Department of Obstetrics and Gynecology
Salt Lake City, UT 84132
USA

Brian L. Shaffer

MD
Department of Obstetrics, Gynecology and
  Reproductive Sciences
University of California
San Francisco, CA 94143
USA

Dinesh M. Shah

MD
Department of Obstetrics and Gynecology
University of Wisconsin School of Medicine and
  Public Health
Madison, WI 53715
USA

Jeanne S. Sheffield

MD
UT Southwestern Medical Center at Dallas
Department of Obstetrics and Gynecology
Dallas, TX 75390-9032
USA

Baha M. Sibai

MD
University of Cincinnati College of Medicine
Department of Obstetrics and Gynecology
Cincinnati, OH 45267-0526
USA

Robert M. Silver

MD
University of Utah Health Sciences Center
Department of Obstetrics and Gynecology
Salt Lake City, UT 84132
USA

Victoria Snegovskikh

MD
Yale University School of Medicine
Department of Obstetrics, Gynecology & Reproduc-
  tive Sciences
New Haven, CT 06520
USA

Michael W. Varner

MD
University of Utah Health Sciences Center
Department of Obstetrics and Gynecology
Salt Lake City, UT 84132
USA

Ronald J. Wapner

MD
Division of Maternal Fetal Medicine
Department of Obstetrics and Gynecology
Columbia University
New York, NY 10032-3795
USA

Carl P. Weiner

MD
University of Kansas School of Medicine
Department of Obstetrics and Gynecology
Kansas City, Kansas
USA

Edward R. Yeomans

MD
University of Texas Houston Medical School
Department of Obstetrics, Gynecology, and
  Reproductive Sciences
Houston, TX 77030
USA

Foreword

In 1980 the founding Editor of *Contemporary OB/GYN* assembled 67 chapters by 73 authors from the pages of *Contemporary OB/GYN* to create the first edition of the textbook *Management of High-Risk Pregnancy*. This work became a classic and has provided a consistent up to date resource for physicians interested and involved in the management of at risk pregnancies. The fifth edition presents the latest discoveries and advancements in maternal fetal medicine and now has added two eminent co-editors, Dr. Catherine Y. Spong and Dr. Charles J. Lockwood, who bring evidence-based expertise and strong clinical and research experience which will further enhance the national reputation of this publication.

More than 30 years has passed since the first issue of *Contemporary OB/GYN* was published and its success has been reflected by its consistent number one ranking by independent readership polls. The origin and history of *Contemporary OB/GYN* and this textbook are interwoven and that tradition is further cemented in this fifth edition with Dr. Charles Lockwood the current editor of *Contemporary OB/GYN* joining as a co-editor. Credit for this success most deservedly goes to Dr. John Queenan who not only has had the necessary vision but the unique personal qualities that make it difficult for most of the leaders in the field to say no to him!

The book first focuses on factors affecting pregnancy and genetics, and then discusses fetal monitoring. These sections are followed by a review of maternal diseases in pregnancy and obstetric complications, intrapartum complications, a section on diagnostic and therapeutic procedures, and finally chapters on perinatal asphyxia and neonatal considerations.

The fifth edition will be extremely valuable to all physicians caring for pregnancies with risk but particularly for physicians in training because of the clear and concise manner of presentation by recognized leaders in the discipline of maternal fetal medicine, genetics, neonatology, anesthesia, and pediatric surgery.

It is my opinion that this text has never been more necessary. We are witnessing a significant increase in the age of child bearing women in our country and with it an increasing incidence of medical complications. Added to this, are the successes of assisted reproductive technology and the national epidemic of obesity and its co-morbidities. Our ability to perform prenatal screening and diagnosis is reaching heights we did not dream about 20 years ago. Multidisciplinary care provided by obstetricians, maternal fetal medicine physicians, neonatologists, geneticists, pediatric surgeons, anesthesiologists, and nurses is increasingly needed to provide optimal care to patients during pregnancy. Against this background of increasing risk, what is needed is a text with the primary purpose of providing practicing physicians with a "how to" practical up to date reference in maternal fetal medicine. This edition has fulfilled that objective and will serve well the physicians who care for pregnant women at risk for adverse outcome.

Mary E. D'Alton, M.D.
Willard C. Rappleye Professor of Obstetrics and Gynecology
Chair Department of Obstetrics and Gynecology
Director, Obstetric and Gynecologic Services
Columbia University
New York City

Preface

The fifth edition of *Management of High-Risk Pregnancy*, like its predecessors, is directed to all health professionals involved in the care of women with high-risk pregnancies. The book contains clear, concise, practical material presented in an evidence-based manner.

Two series of articles on high-risk pregnancies that appeared in *Contemporary OB/GYN* were the inspiration for the first edition. These predominantly clinical articles provided a comprehensive perspective on high-risk pregnancy.

Now in the fifth edition of *Management of High-Risk Pregnancy,* I am joined by two outstanding authorities as editors. Catherine Y. Spong, MD is the Chief of the Pregnancy and Perinatology Branch, National Institute of Child Health and Human Development of the National Institutes of Health. Charles J. Lockwood, MD is the Anita O'Keefe Young Professor of Women's Health and Chair, Department of Obstetrics, Gynecology and Reproductive Sciences, Yale University School of Medicine. They are both leaders in research and clinical care with national and international reputations. It has been enlightening and rewarding to work with these outstanding colleagues.

The content of the fifth edition was designed to provide the necessary background material for decision-making in this area. The topics were selected and then the foremost authority for each subject was invited to write the chapter. Illustrative clinical cases are presented at the end of each chapter. The book contains evidence-based, practical information from outstanding perinatal experts.

I welcome the comments of readers, both laudatory and critical. These suggestions will help to improve future editions.

John T. Queenan, MD
Professor and Chairman Emeritus
Department of Obstetrics and Gynecology
Georgetown University School of Medicine
Washington, DC

Acknowledgments

We are fortunate to work in cooperation with a superb editorial staff at Blackwell Publishing. Helen Harvey and Adam Gilbert provided guidance and editorial skills which are evident in this edition. Dr. Stuart Taylor, publisher, has been helpful with his wisdom and guidance.

We acknowledge with great appreciation and admiration the authors, experts all. Their contributions to this book will be translated into a considerable decrease in morbidity and mortality for mothers and their infants. Their efforts are in the best traditions of academic medicine, passing on knowledge and expertise to their colleagues.

We wish to thank our editorial assistant Michele Prince who coordinated the assembly of the manuscripts in a professional and efficient manner. Her editorial and managerial skills are in large part responsible for the success of this book.

Use this book to improve the delivery of care to your patients. We hope it brings you the same level of enjoyment that we experienced in preparing it.

John T. Queenan, MD
Catherine Y. Spong, MD
Charles J. Lockwood, MD

Factors of High-Risk Pregnancy

1 Overview of high-risk pregnancy

John T. Queenan, Catherine Y. Spong, and Charles J. Lockwood

Most pregnancies are low risk and have favorable outcomes. Unpleasant symptoms, physical problems, or minor difficulties with labor and delivery may be a part of such gestations, but the mothers usually recover fully and deliver healthy babies. High-risk pregnancies—the subject of this book—are less common and are potentially serious occurrences.

We classify any pregnancy in which there is a maternal or fetal factor that may adversely affect the outcome as high risk. In these cases, the likelihood of a positive outcome is significantly reduced. In order to improve the outcome of a high-risk pregnancy, we must identify risk factors and attempt to mitigate problems in pregnancy and labor.

Many conditions lend themselves to identification and intervention before or early in the perinatal period. When diagnosed through an appropriate work-up before pregnancy, conditions such as Rh immunization, diabetes, and epilepsy can be managed properly during pregnancy so as to minimize the risks of mortality and morbidity to both mother and baby. It is not possible, however, to diagnose other conditions, such as multiple pregnancies, preeclampsia, and premature rupture of membranes prior to pregnancy. To detect and manage these challenging situations, the obstetrician must maintain constant vigilance once pregnancy is established.

In the management of high-risk pregnancy much progress has been made since the 1950s, yet much remains to be accomplished. Fifty years ago, the delivering physician and the nursing staff were responsible for newborn care. The incidence of perinatal mortality and morbidity was high. Pediatricians began appearing in the newborn nursery in the 1950s, taking responsibility for the infant at the moment of birth. This decade of neonatal awareness ushered in advances that greatly improved neonatal outcome.

Many scientific breakthroughs directed toward evaluation of fetal health and disease marked the 1960s, which is considered the decade of fetal medicine. Early in that decade, the identification of patients with the risk factor of Rh immunization led to the prototype for the high-risk pregnancy clinic. Rh-negative patients were screened for antibodies, and if none were detected, these women were managed as normal or "low-risk" cases. Those who developed antibodies were enrolled in a high-risk pregnancy clinic, where they could be carefully followed by specialists with expertise in Rh immunization. With the advent of scientific advances such as amniotic fluid analysis, intrauterine transfusion, and, finally, Rh immune prophylaxis, these high risk pregnancies became success stories.

During the 1970s, the decade of perinatal medicine, pediatricians and obstetricians combined forces to continue improving perinatal survival. Some of the most significant perinatal advances are listed in Table 1.1. Also included are the approximate dates of these milestones and (where appropriate) the names of investigators who are associated with the advances.

Among the advances in perinatal medicine that occurred during the 1980s were the development of comprehensive evaluation of fetal condition with the biophysical profile, the introduction of cordocentesis for diagnosis and therapy, the development of neonatal surfactant therapy, antenatal steroids and major advances in genetics and assisted reproduction. These technologic advances foreshadowed the "high tech" developments of the 1990s. Clearly, the specialty has come to realize that "high tech" must be accompanied by "high touch" to ensure the emotional and developmental well-being of the baby and the parents. This decade has been one of adjusting to the challenges of managed care under the control of "for profit" insurance companies. The new millennium brought the decade of evidence-based perinatology. Clinicians became aware of the value of systematic reviews of the Cochrane Database. Major perinatal research projects by the Maternal Fetal Medicine Units Network of the National Institute of Child Health and Human Development answered many clinical questions.

The future will bring better methods of determining fetal jeopardy and health. Continuous readout of fetal conditions will be possible during labor in high-risk pregnancies. Look for the new advances to be made in immunology and genetics. Immunization against group B streptococcus,

Table 1.1 Milestones in perinatology.

Before 1950s
Neonatal care by obstetricians and nurses

1950s—Decade of Neonatal Awareness
Pediatricians entered nursery

Year	Author	Event	Year	Author	Event
1950	Allen and Diamond	Exchange transfusions	1956	Bevis	Amniocentesis for bilirubin in Rh immunization
1953	du Vigneaud	Oxytocin synthesis	1958	Donald	Obstetric use of ultrasound
1954	Patz	Limitation of O_2 to prevent toxicity	1958	Hon	Electronic fetal heart rate evaluation
1955	Mann	Neonatal hypothermia			
1956	Tjio and Levan	Demonstration of 46 human chromosomes	1959	Burns, Hodgman, and Cass	Gray baby syndrome

1960s—Decade of Fetal Medicine
Prototype of the high-risk pregnancy clinic

Year	Author	Event	Year	Author	Event
1960	Eisen and Hellman	Lumbar epidural anesthesia	1967		Neonatal blood gases
1962	Saling	Fetal scalp blood sampling	1967		Neonatal transport
1963	Liley	Intrauterine transfusion for Rh immunization	1967	Jacobsen	Diagnosis of cytogenetic disorders *in utero*
1964	Wallgren	Neonatal blood pressure	1968	Dudrick	Hyperalimentation
1965	Steele and Breg	Culture of amniotic fluid cells	1968	Nadler	Diagnosis of inborn errors of metabolism *in utero*
1965	Mizrahi, Blanc, and Silverman	Necrotizing enterocolitis	1968	Stern	NICU effectiveness
1966	Parkman and Myer	Rubella immunization	1968	Freda *et al.*	Rh prophylaxis

1970s—Decade of Perinatal Medicine
Refinement of NICU
Regionalization of high-risk perinatal care

Year	Author	Event	Year	Author	Event
1971	Gluck	L : S ratio and respiratory distress syndrome	1973	Sadovsky	Fetal movement
			1973		Real-time ultrasound
1972	Brock and Sutcliffe	Alpha-fetoprotein and neural tube defects	1973	Hobbins and Rodeck	Clinical fetoscopy
			1975	ABP	Neonatology Boards
1972	Liggins and Howie	Betamethasone for induction of fetal lung maturity	1976	Schifrin	Nonstress test
1972		Neonatal temperature control with radiant heat	1977	March of Dimes	Towards Improving the Outcome of Pregnancy I
1972	Quilligan	Fetal heart rate monitoring	1977	Kaback	Heterozygote identification (Tay–Sachs disease)
1972	Dawes	Fetal breathing movements	1978	Bowman	Antepartum Rh prophylaxis
1972	Ray and Freeman	Oxytocin challenge test	1978	Steptoe and Edwards	*In vitro* fertilization
1972	ABOG	Maternal–Fetal Medicine Boards	1979	Boehm	Maternal transport

1980s—Decade of Progress
Technologic progress

Year	Author	Event	Year	Author	Event
1980	Bartlett	ECMO	1985	Daffos	Cordocentesis
1980	Manning and Platt	Biophysical profile	1986		DNA analysis
1981	Fujiwara, Morley, and Jobe	Neonatal surfactant therapy	1986	NICHD	MFMU Network established
1982	Harrison and Golbus	Vesicoamniotic shunt for fetal hydronephrosis	1986	Michaels *et al.*	Cervical ultrasound and preterm delivery
1983	Kazy, Ward, and Brambati	Chorionic villus sampling			

1990s—Decade of Managed Care
Managed care alters practice patterns

Year	Author	Event	Year	Author	Event
1991	Lockwood *et al.*	Fetal fibronectin and preterm delivery	1994	NIH Consensus Conference	Antenatal corticosteroids
1993	March of Dimes	Towards Improving the Outcome of Pregnancy II Fetal therapy Pre-implantation genetics Stem cell research			

2000s—Decade of Evidence-Based Perinatology

Year	Author	Event	Year	Author	Event
2000	Mari	Middle cerebral artery monitoring for Rh disease	2003	MFMU	Progesterone to prevent recurrent prematurity
2002	CDC	Group B streptococcus guidelines	2006	Merck	Immunization against human papillomavirus
	MFMU	Antibiotics for PPROM			

ABOG, American Board of Obstetrics and Gynecology; ABP, American Board of Pediatrics; CDC, Centers for Disease Control; ECMO, extracorporeal membrane oxygenation; L : S, lecithin : sphingomyelin ratio; MFMU, Maternal Fetal Medicine Units; NICU, neonatal intensive care unit; NICHD, National Institute of Child Health and Human Development; NIH, National Institutes of Health; PPROM, preterm premature rupture of membranes.

and eventually human immunodeficiency virus will become available. Preimplantation genetics will continue to provide new ways to prevent disease. Alas, prematurity and pre-eclampsia with their many multiple etiologies may be the last to be conquered.

New technology will increase the demand for trained workers in the health care industry. The perinatal professional team will expand to emphasize the importance of social workers, nutritionists, child development specialists, and psychologists. New developments will create special ethical issues. Finally, education and enlightened attitudes toward reproductive awareness and family planning will help to prevent unwanted pregnancies.

2 Maternal nutrition

Edward R. Newton

The medical profession and the lay public associate maternal nutrition with fetal development and subsequent pregnancy outcome. Classic studies from Holland and Leningrad during World War II [1] suggested that when maternal caloric intake fell acutely to below 800 kcal/day, birth weights were reduced 535 g in Leningrad and 250 g in Holland, the difference perhaps related to the better nutritional status of the Dutch women prior to the famine and the shorter duration of their famine. Exposure to famine conditions during the second half of pregnancy had the greatest adverse effect on birth weight and placental weight and, to a lesser extent, birth length, head circumference, and maternal postpartum weight [2–4].

While these studies are used as prima facie evidence of a link between maternal nutrition and fetal development, a more discerning examination reveals many confounding variables that are common to the investigation of maternal nutrition and fetal development. While the onset of rationing was distinct and the birth weight and other anthropomorphic measurements were recorded reliably, other confounders were not identified. For example, menstrual data were notoriously unreliable, and the problem of poor determination of gestational dates was exacerbated by the disruption and stress of war.

In 2007, many of the most vulnerable mothers have little or no prenatal care (10–30%), often with unreliable menstrual data (15–35%). In Holland and Leningrad, the stress of war may have been associated with both preterm delivery and reduced birth weight. In a modern context, the urban war produces a similar stress through lack of social supports, domestic violence, and drugs. The content of the individual's diet in wartime Europe or the diet of underprivileged women in the USA in 1998 remains largely speculation; perhaps it was not the total number of kilocalories or protein content but an issue of overall quality that leads to decreased birth weights. In 2005, like in 1944–45, the link between maternal nutrition and pregnancy outcome relies on a relatively weak proxy for a woman's nutritional status, body mass index (BMI). A prospective, longitudinal study that follows a sufficiently large cohort of women from preconception through each trimester and into the puerperium (with and without breastfeeding), measures the quality and quantity of women's diet, and correlates the diet with maternal and fetal and neonatal outcomes has not been performed.

Given the latter challenges, the purpose of this chapter is to review the associations between maternal nutrition and perinatal outcome. A complete review must efficiently summarize the data, define the weaknesses of the data, derive reasonable conclusions, and make practical recommendations for the clinician. This chapter briefly summarizes the basic concepts of fetal growth, the multiple predictors of fetal growth, the use of maternal weight gain as a measure of maternal nutrition, adverse pregnancy outcomes as they relate to extremes in maternal weight gain, and the importance or controversy related to specific components of the diet (i.e., iron, calcium, sodium, and prenatal vitamins). While lactation is not an issue of fetal growth, infant development relies on the transfer of nutriments to the infant; maternal diet retains a central role.

Fetal growth

Linear growth of the fetus is continuous, whereas the velocity of growth varies. Multiple researchers have studied linear fetal growth by examining birth weights or estimated fetal weights as determined by ultrasound, and found it to be nearly a straight line until approximately 35 weeks, when the fetus grows 200–225 g/week (Fig. 2.1). Thereafter, the curve falls such that by 40 weeks the weight gain is 135 g/week [5]. Twin pregnancies have a proportionately lower rate of growth, reaching a maximum at 34–35 weeks (monochorionic placentation, 140–160 g/week; dichorionic placentation, 180–200 g/week) [6]. Thereafter, the growth rate slows to 25–30 g/week in both types of placentation. In 20–30% of term twin pregnancies, one or the other twin, or both, will have a birth weight less than the 10th percentile based on singleton growth charts. There is controversy as to whether singleton or separate twin

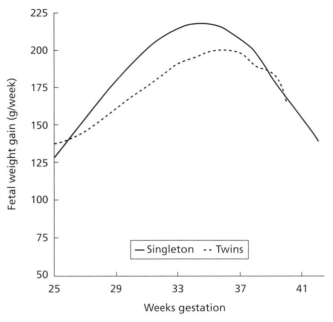

Fig. 2.1 Fetal weight gain in grams among singleton and twin pregnancies.

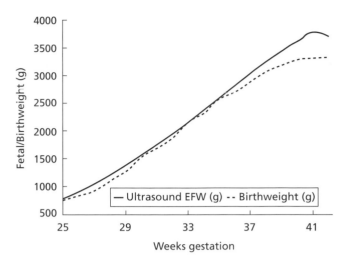

Fig. 2.2 Fetal growth curves by method of estimation: ultrasound or birth weight. EFW, mean estimated fetal weight.

charts should be the comparison resource in an individual pregnancy.

Fetal growth curves are based on two sources for fetal weight: birth weight [7] and estimated fetal weight based on ultrasound findings (Fig. 2.2). Birth weight sources encumber the pathophysiology that led to the preterm birth. A total of 20–25% of preterm births occur as the result of medical intervention in the setting of maternal pathology such as pre-eclampsia. In these cases, the effects of maternal nutrition (BMI) are muted significantly. Fetal growth curves derived by ultrasonographic estimation of fetal weight reflect a more physiologic environment. Unfortunately, the comparison of coincidental estimated fetal weight and birth weight reveals a relatively large error; 20% of estimated fetal weights will differ from the actual weight by one standard deviation or more, 400–600 g at term.

The velocity of fetal growth is more instructive regarding mechanisms of fetal growth restriction [8]. Length peaks earlier than weight, as the fetus stores fat and hepatic glycogen (increasing abdominal circumference) in the third trimester. When an insult occurs early, such as with alcohol exposure, severe starvation, smoking, perinatal infection (cytomegalovirus infection or toxoplasmosis), chromosomal or developmental disorders, or chronic vasculopathies (diabetes, autoimmune disease, chronic hypertension), the result is a symmetrically growth-restricted fetus with similarly reduced growth of its length, head circumference, and abdominal circumference. This pattern is often referred to as *dysgenic growth restriction* and these infants often have persistent handicaps (mental retardation, infectious retinopathy; i.e., toxoplasmosis infection) [9].

When the insult occurs after the peak in the velocity of length growth, the result is a disproportionately reduced body : length ratio (ponderal index), a larger head circumference relative to abdominal circumference. This pattern is often referred to as *nutritional growth restriction* and usually is the result of developing vasculopathy (placental thrombosis/infarcts, pre-eclampsia) or a reduction of the absorptive capacity of the placenta (postdate pregnancy). The obstetrician uses the ultrasonographically defined ratio of head circumference : abdominal circumference as it compares to established nomograms. The pediatrician uses the ponderal index [birth weight (kg)/height (cm) cubed × 100] in a similar fashion. *Abnormality* is defined statistically (i.e., two standard deviations from the mean) rather than as it relates to adverse clinical outcomes. While the risk of adverse outcomes may be considerably higher, most small for gestational age babies (less than the 10th percentile) who are delivered at term have few significant problems. Likewise, the vast majority of term infants whose size is more than the 90th percentile at birth have few perinatal challenges.

Fetal growth requires the transfer of nutriments as building blocks and the transfer of enough oxygen to fuel the machinery to build the fetus. Maternal nutritional and cardiac physiology is changed through placental hormones (i.e., human placental lactogen) to accommodate the fetal–placental needs. The central role of the placenta is the production of pregnancy hormones, the transfer of nutriments, and fetal respiration is demonstrated by the fact that 20% of the oxygen supplied to the fetus is diverted to the metabolic activities of the placenta and placental oxygen consumption at term is approximately 25% higher than the amount consumed by the fetus as a whole. The absorptive surface area of the placenta is strongly associated with fetal growth; the chorionic villus surface area grows from approximately 5 m^2 at 28–30 weeks to 10 m^2 by term.

The measured energy requirement of pregnancy totals 55,000 kcal for an 11.8 kg weight gain [10] or 4.7 kcal/g of weight gain. This value is considerably less than the 8.0 kcal/g required for weight gain in the nonpregnant woman. This discrepancy is likely a result of the poorly understood relationship between pregnancy hormones (i.e., human placental lactogen, corticosteroids, sex steroids) and the pattern of nutriment distribution. Table 2.1 describes the work as measured by weight that must occur to produce a well-grown fetus at term.

Weight gain is essentially linear throughout pregnancy [11]. The mean total weight gain (15–85th percentile) for white, non-Hispanic, married mothers delivering live infants was 13.8 kg (8.6–18.2 kg) for small women (BMI below 19.8); 13.8 kg (7.7–18.6 kg) for average women (BMI of 19.8–26.0); 12.4 kg (6.4–17.3 kg) for large women (BMI of 26.1–29.0); and 8.7 kg (0.5–16.4 kg) for obese women (BMI over 29) [11]. In general, average weight gains (15–85th percentile) per week are 0.15–0.69 kg for gestational ages 13–20 weeks; 0.31–0.65 kg for gestational ages 20–30 weeks; and 0.18–0.61 kg for gestational ages 30–36 weeks. The practical clinical rule of thumb is that a woman with a normal pregnancy should gain approximately 4.5 kg (10 lb) in the first 20 weeks and 9 kg (20 lb) in the second 20 weeks of pregnancy. High-risk thresholds are weight gains less than 6.8 kg (15 lb) and more than 20 kg (45 lb) [11].

Many factors affect the transfer of nutriments and oxygen to the fetus. Table 2.2 lists factors and clinical examples where abnormalities change fetal growth.

Obstetric history reveals a strong tendency to repeat gestational age and birth weight as the result of shared genetic and environmental factors. Bakketeig *et al.* [12] analyzed almost 500,000 consecutive births in Norway over a 7-year period. Table 2.3 depicts the results of their analysis.

In summary, fetal growth is affected by the quantity and quality of maternal diet, the ability of the mother to appropriately absorb and distribute digested micronutriments, maternal cardiorespiratory function, uterine blood flow, placental transfer, placental blood flow, and appropriate distribution and handling of nutriments and oxygen by the fetus. Additionally, genetics and uterine volume characteristics can greatly affect fetal size in the presence of normal physiology; birth size more closely reflects maternal rather than paternal morphometrics, and contractions of uterine volume (i.e., müllerian duct abnormalities or large uterine myomas) are associated with decreased birth size.

Ultimately, any evaluation of the effect of nutrition on fetal outcome must control for these confounders in the analysis. The presence of multiple variables requires large numbers of subjects to be included in the model for the study of main effects alone. As many variables (e.g., parity and preeclampsia) are interactive, the sample size necessarily increases geometrically by the analysis of secondary or higher interactive variables. The resultant complexity and difficulty in obtaining quality data on large numbers of pregnant women has led to

Table 2.1 Weight gain in pregnancy.

Maternal Gains		Fetal Gains	
Blood volume	2 kg (4.4 lb)	Fetus	3.5 kg (7.7 lb)
Uterine size	1 kg (2.2 lb)	Placenta	0.6 kg (0.7 lb)
Breast size	1 kg (2.2 lb)	Amniotic fluid	1.2 kg (2.6 lb)
Fat increase	3 kg (6.6 lb)		
Total weight gain	12.3 kg (27 lb)		

Table 2.2 Factors affecting fetal growth.

Factors	Clinical Examples
Genetics	Parental size Chromosomal disease
Uterine volume	Müllerian duct abnormalities Leiomyomata uteri
Maternal intake	Starvation Fad diets Iron deficiency anemia Neural tube defects (folic acid)
Maternal absorption	Inflammatory bowel disease Gastric bypass
Maternal hypermetabolic states	Hyperthyroidism Adolescent pregnancy Extreme exercise
Maternal cardiorespiratory function	Maternal cardiac disease Sarcoidosis Asthma
Uterine blood flow	Hypertension/preeclampsia Beta-adrenergic blockers Diabetic vasculopathy Autoimmune vasculopathy Smoking (nicotine) Chronic environmental stress
Placental transfer	Infant of a diabetic mother Smoking (carbon monoxide)
Placental absorption	Placental infarcts or thrombosis
Fetal blood flow	Congenital heart disease Increased placental resistance Polycythemia
Fetal metabolic state	Drug effects (amphetamines) Genetic metabolic disease
Reduced fetal cell numbers	Alcohol abuse Chromosomal disease

Table 2.3 Obstetric history and birth weight (BW). (Data from Bakketeig *et al.* [12].)

First Birth	Second Birth	Incidence of Adverse Outcome in Subsequent Birth (Relative Risk*)
Term AGA	—	1.4% (1.0)
Preterm low BW	—	13.1% (4.5)
Term SGA	—	8.2% (5.5)
BW 4500 g	—	22.6% (9.0)
Post-term	—	5.3% (2.2)
Term AGA	Term AGA	1.5% (0.5)
Preterm low BW	Preterm low BW	19.7% (6.8)
Term SGA	Term SGA	29% (19.3)
BW 4500 g	BW 4500 g	45.5% (18.2)
Post-term	Post-term	33.3% (13.9)

AGA, appropriate for gestational age; LGA, large for gestational age (4500 g); Preterm, 36 weeks and 2500 g; Post-term, 44 weeks; SGA, small for gestational age (2500 g).

* The relative risk is the ratio of incidence of "poor" outcomes in the target cohort divided by the incidence of "poor" outcomes in the lowest risk cohort, women in whom all births were normal.

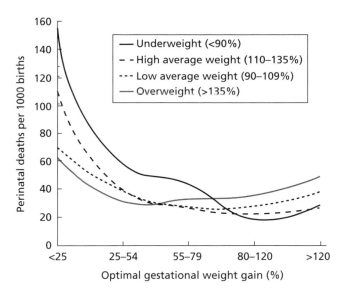

Fig. 2.3 Perinatal mortality rates by prepregnancy weight and height (Metropolitan Life Insurance tables) and the percent of optimal weight gain. (From Naeye [13].)

purposeful exclusion of certain cohorts of women. Exclusions may include women with hypertension or diabetes, poorly dated gestations, or late prenatal care, or middle- and upper-class white Anglo-Americans who seek care from private practitioners. The use of imprecise proxies to control for population differences in nutritional risk, such as educational level, socioeconomic level, age, parity, or ethnicity, adds to the variance. Likewise, determination of the quality and quantity of the maternal diet is severely limited by the time, personnel, and education required to obtain a valid measurement of that diet. As a consequence, most studies of maternal nutrition use the BMI [weight (kg/height in meters)$^2 \times 100$] or maternal weight gain during pregnancy as a proxy for maternal nutrition; the quality and quantity of maternal diet are rarely measured. There is added imprecision with the measurement of weight gain. Most studies rely on reported prepregnancy weight, the accuracy of which is suspect. Additionally, the use of total weight gain in most studies does not account for the variance in the weight of the fetus, amniotic fluid, or placenta. The use of net weight gain (total weight gain – birth weight) is used to reduce the resultant variance.

Body mass index, weight gain, and adverse pregnancy outcomes

Regardless of their imprecise measurement, weight gain and BMI have powerful associations with birth weight and preg-

nancy outcome. Naeye [13] examined the association between weight gain and pregnancy outcome data obtained during the National Collaborative Perinatal Project (1959–65). In this project, approximately 56,000 US women were followed from prenatal enrollment through birth. The infants were followed through the age of 7 years. The National Collaborative Project demonstrated that progressive increases in prepregnancy weight or weight gain, or both, were significantly associated with increases in birth weight. Prepregnancy weight and weight gain appear to act independently of each other and their effects are additive. Increasing prepregnancy weight diminishes the influences of weight gain on birth weight. Among nonsmokers, the difference in birth weight across weight gains (less than 7.25 kg [16 lb] vs. more than 15.8 kg [35 lb] in weight gain) was 556 g (19% difference) for underweight women, 509 g (16.4% difference) for normal-weight women, and 335 g (10% difference) for overweight women. Similarly, among smokers, the difference in birth weight was 683 g (27%) for underweight women, 480 g (16.4%) for normal-weight women, and 261 g (8%) for overweight women [13].

Perinatal mortality rates in underweight women (less than 90% of expected pregnancy weight in the Metropolitan weight-for-height charts) are strongly affected by weight gain (Fig. 2.3). Poor weight gain in underweight women is associated with a fivefold increase in perinatal mortality. Autopsies of fetuses and neonates in the same cohort demonstrated that body and organ size could be predicted by prepregnancy weight and weight gain [14]. Prior to 33 weeks, the relationship is less dramatic and is associated with a smaller liver and adrenals as a result of a reduction in cell numbers in underweight women with poor weight gain. After 33 weeks, when fetal weight gain is expected to be highest, the reduction in organ weights occurs in most organs with a reduction in cell size and numbers.

The Dutch famine during World War II [2–4], during which acute rationing was less than 800 kcal/day, resulted in different reductions in neonatal measurements depending on the gestational age when the rationing was instituted. The greatest adverse effects were seen when the rationing occurred in the last trimester, the parameters most affected being placental weight and birth weight and, to a lesser extent, birth length, head circumference, and maternal postpartum weight. With the progressive loss of calories, maternal weight absorbed the challenge until a critical threshold was met. Then maternal weight loss stabilized and the placental and then fetal weights were reduced. After the rationing was discontinued and intake was increased, maternal weight was the first to recover, followed by placental weight, and, finally, birth weight.

The most representative data on total weight gain in the US population are from the 1980 National Natality Survey [15]. A probability sample of all live births to US women in 1980 was employed. BMI and weight gain were related to the incidence of term growth restricted infants (less than 2500 g and more than 37 weeks' gestation) [16]. The analysis was adjusted for maternal age, parity, height, cigarette smoking, and education level. The relative risk of delivering a term growth restricted infant after a total weight gain of less than the 25th percentile was 2.4 (95% confidence interval [CI], 1.5–4.0) for small women (BMI below 19.8), 3.1 (95% CI, 2.2–4.5) for average women (BMI of 19.8–26.0), and 1.3 (95% CI, 0.6–2.8) for large women (BMI over 26). The effect of low weight gain in large women was not significant. Clinically, the expectation that an obese or large woman who is diagnosed with gestational diabetes should gain 11.3–13.6 kg (25–30 lb) is contrary to the later information. With documentation of a high-quality diet, these large women should gain 4.5–6.8 kg (10–15 lb).

The interaction between weight gain, BMI, and the incidence of preterm delivery (weight less than 2500 g and before 37 weeks) is less clear; women who deliver prematurely have less opportunity to gain weight. The use of total weight gain or net weight gain is inappropriate. Net gain per week of gestation controls for the duration confounder. Subsequent analysis does not define a relationship between net weight gain per week, BMI, and preterm birth. More recently, a maternal prepregnancy weight less than 45 kg (100 lb) has been analyzed as a risk factor for preterm birth; low BMI appears to be a stronger predictor: odds ratio primipara 2.31 (95% CI, 1.37–3.92), multipara 1.76 (95% CI, 1.19–2.61) [17].

An important caveat for any analysis using gestational age as a covariate is the inaccuracy of gestational age estimates. As many as 15–35% of women seeking prenatal care have poor documentation of the first day of their last menstrual period.

If ultrasound dating is used (now in 89% or more of pregnancies), early growth restriction may be obscured; all fetuses are standardized to the size of fetuses in the 50th percentile for that gestational age. The actual error in gestational age may be as high as 1 week by a first trimester ultrasound scan, 2 weeks by a second trimester ultrasound, and 3 weeks or more by a third trimester ultrasound. At term, this systematic error may translate into an 800–1200 g (2–3 lb) discrepancy between estimated fetal weight and actual birth weight. Large epidemiologic studies have not had standard methods of defining gestational age. When patients with poor dates are eliminated, the size of the group most vulnerable for nutritionally related fetal growth restriction is reduced significantly.

Many early studies that examined the relationship between prepregnancy BMI and preterm birth did not adequately control for the decreased exposure necessarily found in a pregnancy of shortened duration [15–20]. However, they found a consistent association in women whose total weight gain was lower with the incidence of preterm birth. The magnitude of the risk varied between a 50% and a 400% increase in preterm births. This variance might be explained by differences in study design. The lower threshold for weight gain varies considerably; 5–9 kg (11–20 lb) of total weight gain. Some studies defined the preterm birth as any birth weight below 2500 g, which included many term, small for gestational age neonates.

The confounding nature of decreased exposure, preterm birth, is illustrated in the analysis of the data from the 1980 National Natality Study [15]. If total weight gain is used, the odds ratio for delivering a preterm infant according to prepregnancy BMI shows a significant relationship between preterm birth and poor weight gain (less than 11 kg): small women, 4.0 (95% CI, 2.7–6.0); average women, 2.8 (95% CI, 2.0–4.0); and large women, 1.6 (95% CI, 0.8–3.2) [15]. However, when the effect of pregnancy duration is controlled by measuring net weight gain per week, the relationship between prepregnancy BMI, poor weight gain, and preterm birth disappears: small women, 1.2 (95% CI, 0.8–1.9); average women, 1.0 (95% CI, 0.7–1.5); and large women, 1.0 (95% CI, 0.5–1.9) [15]. In contrast, two recent studies [21,22] demonstrated a significant risk of preterm birth when weight gain per week was less than 0.23 kg (less than 0.5 lb/week) or less than 0.27 kg (0.6 lb/week). They demonstrated a 40–60% increase in preterm births.

Two recent epidemiologic studies detailed the association between prepregnancy BMI and net weight gain per week, and adverse pregnancy outcomes. Cnattingius *et al.* [21] examined the municipal birth records of 204,555 infants born in Sweden, Denmark, Norway, Finland, and Iceland from 1992 to 1993. The final population included 167,750 women with singleton births for whom prepregnancy BMI data were available. The results were adjusted for maternal age, parity, maternal education, cigarette smoking, and whether the mother was living with the father. Prepregnancy BMI of 20 or greater was associated with a decrease in the incidence of small for gestational age infants [adjusted odds ratio 0.5–0.7 (95% CI, 0.4–0.8)]. Weight gain of less than 0.25 kg/week was associated with an adjusted odds ratio of 3.0 (95% CI, 2.5–3.5) for the incidence of small for gestational age infants. Among low- and normal-weight women there was no association with late fetal death or preterm delivery. Overweight (BMI above 24.9 and less than 30.0) and obese women (BMI over 29.9) were shown to have a risk of late fetal death (after 28 weeks' completed gestation). The adjusted odds ratios for fetal death were 1.7 (95% CI, 1.1–2.4) for overweight women and 2.7 (1.8–4.1) for obese women. In addition, large women have a two- to fourfold increase in diabetes (10–15%).

The failure of prepregnancy BMI to predict preterm birth was confirmed in a 1992–94 study supported by the National Institute of Child Health and Human Development Maternal Fetal Medicine Units (NICHD-MFMU) Network [22]. A cohort of 2929 pregnancies from 11 centers was followed longitudinally through pregnancy. Demographic, social, clinical, and biologic variables were included in the analysis. Subjects were examined at 22–24 weeks and biologic variables including cervical length, fetal fibronectin, bacterial vaginosis, contraction frequency, and the presence of vaginal bleeding were assessed. A positive fetal fibronectin finding and a cervical length below 2.5 cm were associated with spontaneous birth at less than 32, 35, and 37 weeks (adjusted odds ratios of 2.5–10.0). In multiparous women, a history of preterm birth was also associated with preterm birth (adjusted odds ratios of 2.6–5.0). Low prepregnancy BMI was associated with neither early nor late preterm birth. A cautionary note is warranted. The exclusion of net weight gain per week as an intercurrent variable fails to account for the effect of nutrition on outcome. Perhaps poor nutrition has an interactive effect by increasing the likelihood of a positive fetal fibronectin finding or a shortened cervix. The study only examined main effect variables and not interactive variables.

Examination of the effects of nutrition on other adverse pregnancy outcomes is complicated by a paucity of quality research. Nutrition in Western women does not seem to be associated with first or second trimester abortion, congenital abnormalities, or lactational performance. Weight gain during pregnancy can be associated with preeclampsia or diabetes. Very high levels of total weight gain or late-occurring increases in net weight gain per week are quite common in primiparous pregnancies complicated by preeclampsia. If there were any effect from preeclampsia, one would expect a higher rate of fetal growth restriction and spontaneous preterm birth in women who gain excessive weight. The meager amount of existing data seems to support an association, but more research is needed.

Obesity remains a major health issue for developed countries, with obese women at greater risk for hypertension, diabetes, coronary heart disease, and premature death. Retained weight postpartum plays a part. In general, while women with average gestational weight gains retain approximately 1 kg (2.2 lb) postpartum, African-American women tend to retain more weight postpartum regardless of the prepregnancy BMI or prenatal weight gain [23]. African-American women with a normal prepregnancy BMI were twice as likely to retain more than 9 kg (20 lb) as were white women of the same build [23]. Women with high weight gain tend to retain more weight. Researchers [11] reported that retention of more than 2.5 kg (5.5 lb) between the first and second pregnancy was associated with higher weight gain in the last half of pregnancy, 10–20 kg (22–26 lb). In the 1959–65 Collaborative Perinatal Project, women who gained 16.4–18.2 kg (36–40 lb) or gained more than 18.2 kg (more than 40 lb) retained 5 kg (10.9 lb) and 8.0 kg (17.7 lb), respectively [24]. The years when the latter two studies were performed caution interpretation of the data. In 1998, more women gained high amounts of weight during pregnancy; the incidence of excessive weight retention must be higher.

Multifetal pregnancy would be expected to increase the nutritional demand for the mother. Unfortunately, the confounders found in singleton pregnancies are more pronounced in multifetal pregnancy, and the nutritional component of adverse pregnancy outcomes is much harder to delineate. Multifetal pregnancies are associated with higher rates of preterm birth (40–50%), fetal growth restriction (20–40%), more perinatal deaths (four- to sixfold), more preeclampsia, more diabetes, and more frequent "elective" cesarean section. The analysis is complicated further by different fetal growth rates related to differences between like-sex and mixed-sex pregnancies or the differences between monozygotic and heterozygotic gestations.

Most of the published research has focused on weight gain in twin pregnancies. Little research has examined the effects of variation in prepregnancy BMI or net weight gain during pregnancy as a predictor of perinatal death, fetal growth restriction, or preterm birth. Campbell and MacGillivray [25] reviewed and compared weight gain in twin versus singleton pregnancies. Singleton pregnancies gained 0.40–0.47 kg/week while twin pregnancies gained 0.54–0.64 kg/week. In a birth record study of nearly 2000 twin births in Kansas between 1980 and 1986, pregnancies where the infants weighed between 3000 and 3500 g had the lowest perinatal mortality. They were associated with a maternal weight gain of 20.1 kg (44.2 lb) for underweight women, 18.6 kg (40.9 lb) for nomal-weight women, and 13.2 kg (29.2 lb) for very obese women [26].

Nutritional assessment

The strong associations between extremes in prepregnancy BMI, extremes in weight gain, and adverse pregnancy outcome dictate that a basic, patient-centered, individualized nutritional assessment and plan be incorporated in the primary care of women from preconception, throughout pregnancy, and during the postpartum period with special attention for breastfeeding. The nutritional assessment relies on the patient's medical record, history, and physical examination. The main areas of focus are sociodemographic risk (age less than 2 years after menarche, high parity (>4), low socioeconomic status, culture, previous nutritional challenge), obstetric history (small for gestational age and large for gestational age infants, preterm birth), medical history (bowel disease, diabetes, chronic hypertension, hyperthyroid, chronic infection such as tuberculosis or human immunodeficiency virus infection, allergies, autoimmune disease, renal failure), behavioral risks (substance abuse, excessive exercise), nutritional risks (eating disorders, pica, fad diets, strict vegetarian diet, medications), and current diet (deviations in quantity or quality).

In the 24-hour recall method, the patient is asked to recall the type and amount of food and beverages she consumed during the previous day. This technique gives clues to eating behavior rather than providing a quantitative measurement. There is considerable day-to-day variation that relates to issues of memory, lack of knowledge concerning the content of food (i.e., what goes into a beef stew), and inability to estimate correct portion sizes [27–30]. Practical ways to improve reporting include a 3-day or a week of written record on type and amount of food and drinks consumed, discussion with the individual who prepares the food in order to understand the content of mixed food (stew), and education of the patient about portion size. For example, a cup is roughly equal in volume to a clenched fist and an 85-g (3-oz) piece of fish or meat is roughly the size and thickness of the palm of the hand.

Another method uses a standardized survey to identify the usual frequency or dietary history. The accuracy of the survey is improved when portion estimates are included. A major advantage of the survey is the speed at which an assessment can be performed. The precise nature of the data lends itself to population analysis using one of many diet analysis programs available in computer software [31]. When personnel resources are limited, a standardized survey is useful as a screening tool for all pregnant women. The Institute of Medicine developed a standard nutritional survey (Fig. 2.4) [32]. If a high-risk individual is identified by the survey, a more detailed nutritional analysis and intervention are appropriate.

Obstetric care providers and nutritionists would appreciate a memory chip placed in the mouth that could automatically record the type and volume of the consumed food and drink; this will not happen any time soon. We have to rely on simultaneous written records or patient recall. Unfortunately, the accuracy of both the 24-hour recall and the nutritional survey depends on the accuracy of the patient's recall. In general, accuracy is poor and may reflect what the

Table 2.4 Recommended total weight gain during pregnancy.

Prepregnancy Body Mass Index (BMI)	Recommended Total Weight Gain
Underweight (BMI <19.8)	12.5–18.0 kg (28–40 lb)
Normal (BMI 19.8–26.0)	11.5–16.0 kg (25–35 lb)
Overweight (BMI 26.0–29.0)	7.0–11.5 kg (15–25 lb)
Obese (>BMI 29.0)	6.0 kg (15 lb)

provider wishes rather than what was actually consumed [27–30]. The rather large variations in intake, yet the relative lack of demonstrable variation in adverse outcome, except in the extremes, raises concern about the practicality of obtaining a detailed dietary history from every pregnant woman. Because the extremes are important, more detailed nutritional assessment and counseling are needed for populations at high risk for poor dietary practices as defined by 24-hour recall or the standardized survey. Table 2.4 describes the recommended weight gain, stratified by pregnancy BMI [11].

Tables 2.5 (pregnant) and 2.6 (nonsupplemented breastfeeding) compare the average daily intake of nutriments with and without prenatal multivitamins to the 1989 Recommended Dietary Allowances (RDA) [32]. The analysis reveals that the average US woman who is pregnant and taking one tablet daily of the prenatal multivitamins with 0.4–1.0 mg folic acid requires only extra energy (500–600 kcal/day), magnesium (125 mg), and calcium (300–600 mg). Likewise, lactating women who take one tablet daily of prenatal multivitamins and who are not supplementing the infant with artificial milk and solids require the same micronutriments in similar amounts. The reader must keep in mind that the "usual" daily intake that the US medical environment emphasizes includes a higher intake of protein and dairy products during pregnancy and lactation. Recent focus on the fat content of dairy products will lead many women to reduce milk intake. If the liquid need is supplanted by beverages containing caffeine or phosphoric acid (carbonated sodas), the total intake of calcium or protein, or both, may be reduced.

Nutritional interventions

Nutritional intervention beyond prenatal multivitamins is not needed for most pregnant or lactating women who live in the USA. The critical issue is to identify the extremes in amounts: dietary restriction, nonfood competition (pica), or excess metabolic needs (Tables 1.2 & 1.4). It must be remembered that nutritional supplementation most often uses mixed foods (nutritional drink supplying energy, protein, and micronutriments). Mixed food supplementation obscures the benefit of a

What you eat and some of the life-style choices you make can affect your nutrition and health now and in the future. Your nutrition can also have an important effect on your baby's health. Please answer these questions by circling the answers that apply to you.

Eating Behavior

1. Are you frequently bothered by any of the following? (circle all that apply)
   Nausea   Vomiting   Heartburn   Constipation
2. Do you skip meals at least 3 times a week?   No   Yes
3. Do you try to limit the amount or kind of food you eat to control your weight?   No   Yes
4. Are you on a special diet now?   No   Yes
5. Do you avoid any foods for health or religious reasons?   No   Yes

Food Sources

6. Do you have a working stove?   No   Yes
   Do you have a working refrigerator?   No   Yes
7. Do you sometimes run out of food before you are able to buy more?   No   Yes
8. Can you afford to eat the way you should?   No   Yes
9. Are you receiving any food assistance now? (circle all that apply)   No   Yes
   Food stamps   School breakfast   School lunch   WIC
   Donated food   Commodity Supplemental Food Program
   Food from a food pantry, soup kitchen, or food banks
10. Do you feel you need help in obtaining food?   No   Yes

Food and Drink

11. Which of these did you drink yesterday? (circle all that apply)
    Soft drinks   Coffee   Tea   Fruit drink
    Orange juice   Grapefruit juice   Other juices   Milk
    Kool-Aid®   Beer   Wine   Alcoholic drinks
    Water   Other beverages (list) _____
12. Which of these foods did you eat yesterday (circle all that apply):
    Cheese   Pizza   Macaroni and cheese
    Yogurt   Cereal with milk
    Other foods made with cheese (such as tacos, enchiladas, lasagna, cheeseburgers)

Corn	Potatoes	Sweet potatoes	Green salad
Carrots	Collard greens	Spinach	Turnip greens
Broccoli	Green beans	Green peas	Other vegetables
Apples	Bananas	Berries	Grapefruit
Melon	Oranges	Peaches	Other fruit
Meat	Fish	Chicken	Eggs
Peanut butter	Nuts	Seeds	Dried beans
Cold cuts	Hot dog	Bacon	Sausage
Cake	Cookies	Doughnut	Pastry
Chips	French fries	Deep-fried foods, such as fried chicken or egg rolls	
Bread	Rolls	Rice	Cereal
Noodles	Spaghetti	Tortillas	

    Were any of these whole grain?   No   Yes
13. Is the way you ate yesterday the way you usually eat?   No   Yes

Life-style

14. Do you exercise for at least 30 minutes on a regular basis (3 times a week or more?)   No   Yes
15. Do you ever smoke cigarettes or use smokeless tobacco?   No   Yes
16. Do you ever drink beer, wine, liquor, or any other alcoholic beverages?   No   Yes
17. Which of these do you take? (circle all that apply)
    Prescribed drugs or medications
    Any over-the-counter products (such as aspirin, acetaminophen, antacids, or vitamins)
    Street drugs (such as marijuana, speed, downers, crack, or heroin)

Fig. 2.4 Sample of a standard nutrition survey from the Institute of Medicine [11].

specific nutriment. The following section provides a summary of the data concerning interventions related to nutriments.

Multivitamins

Prenatal multivitamins with at least 400 µg of folic acid are recommended for pregnant woman in the USA. In developing countries, the use of multiple micronutriment supplements (prenatal vitamins) have been compared with supplements containing only folic acid and iron, with random assignment of treatment groups [33,34]. The results suggest an increase in birth weight of 50–100 g. Each pack of cigarettes smoked reduces birth weight by 100–150 g. The effect on other adverse outcomes (i.e., small for gestational age neonates, prematurity, perinatal mortality) is less consistent and less clear. The use of prenatal vitamins in developed countries has not been shown to reduce adverse pregnancy outcomes or increase birth weight.

Table 2.5 Usual dietary intake, recommended daily allowance (RDA) and prenatal vitamins (PNV) in pregnant women.

Nutriment	1989 RDA	Usual Intake	PNV	Intake Plus PNV
Total energy (kcal)	2500	1900–2100*	None	2000[†]
Total protein (g)	60	68–91	None	80
Fat-soluble vitamins				
A (μg of RE)	800	1000–1400	450	1650
D (μg)	10	4–6*	10	15
E (mg)	10	3.4–12.0*	22	30
K (μg)	65	300–500	None	465
Water-soluble vitamins				
Folate (μg)	400	168–245*	1000	1207
Thiamine (mg)	1.5	1.2–1.9*	3	8.5
Riboflavin (mg)	1.6	1.7–3.4	3.4	6.0
Pyridoxine (mg)	2.2	0.8–2.2*	10	26
Niacin (mg)	17	17–280	20	42
C (mg)	70	48–1440	100	298
B_{12} (μg)	2.2	2.6–5.70	12	16.5
Minerals				
Calcium (mg)	1200	668–1195*	250	1182[†]
Magnesium (mg)	300	191–269*	25	255[†]
Iron (mg)	30	11.2–17.2*	60	74
Zinc (mg)	15	06.0–12.0*	25	34
Iodine (μg)	175	170	150	320
Selenium (μg)	60	70	None	70

RE, retinol equivalent.

* Deficient without prenatal vitamins or supplement.

[†] Deficient after daily multivitamins.

Energy and protein supplementation

Multiple comparative trials have addressed undernourished (less than 1500 kcal/day) populations in developing countries. When energy (200–800 kcal) and protein (40–60 g) are supplemented in undernourished women, there is a consistent increase in birth weight (100–400 g) and maternal weight gain (0.8–0.9 kg/month). Improvement in infant outcome is less clear; some studies showed a reduction in low birth weight and preterm birth, whereas others did not [11]. Among undernourished pregnant Gambian women, prenatal energy, protein, and micronutriment supplementation resulted in a decrease in the incidence of low birth weight from 23% in the control to 7.5% in the supplemented population [11].

In developing and industrialized countries where the nutrition is better (1600–2100 kcal/day), mixed food supplementation does not result in significant maternal weight gain (20.3–0.1 kg/month) or increases in birth weight (2177–277 g). Few studies have demonstrated differences in perinatal outcomes between supplemented and unsupplemented pregnant women if their intake exceeds 2100–2300 kcal/day. These observations are supported by the systematic review of randomized trials [35,36].

Iron supplementation

Worldwide, iron deficiency anemia complicates the lives of nonpregnant (35%) and pregnant (51%) women. Among nonpregnant (2%) and pregnant (5–10%) women, industrialized countries have much lower incidences of iron deficiency anemia when defined by a low serum ferritin concentration (less than 12 μg/L) and a hemoglobin below 11.0, 10.5, and 11.0 g/dL in the first, second, and third trimesters, respectively (Centers for Disease Control and Prevention definition). Adverse pregnancy outcomes, such as low birth weight, preterm birth, and increased perinatal mortality, are associated with a hemoglobin below 10.4 g/dL before 24 weeks' gestation [11,37,38]. Both the latter study and the National Collaborative Perinatal Project [11,14,16] demonstrated a U-shaped curve when adverse pregnancy outcomes are plotted against hemoglobin concentration. The incidence of poor outcome rises progressively

Table 2.6 Usual dietary intake, recommended daily allowance (RDA), and prenatal vitamins (PNV) in lactating women.

Nutriment	1989 RDA	Usual Intake	PNV	Intake Plus PNV
Total energy (kcal)	2700	1800–2400*	None	2100[‡]
Total protein (g)	62–65	78–115	None	97
Fat-soluble vitamins				
A (µg of RE)	1200	1000–1200*	450	1550
D (µg)	10	136[†]	10	146
E (mg)	12	4.5[†]	22	26.5
K (µg)	NR	NR	None	NR
Water-soluble vitamins				
Folate (µg)	280	169–340*	1000	1255
Thiamine (mg)	1.6	1.39–2.1*	3	1.79
Riboflavin (mg)	1.8	1.87–2.800	3.4	5.7
Pyridoxine (mg)	2.1	1.11–1.690	10	11
Niacin (mg)	20	16.3–70.00	20	63
C (mg)	95	108–1990	100	253
B_{12} (µg)	2.6	2.88–7.960	12	17
Minerals				
Calcium (mg)	1200	1004–1304*	250	1300
Magnesium (mg)	350	221*[†]	25	227[‡]
Iron (mg)	15	12.2–16.2*	60	74
Zinc (mg)	19	09.4–12.2*	25	36
Iodine (µg)	225	NR	150	150[‡]
Selenium (µg)	75	84–870	None	85
Phosphorus (mg)	1200	1350–20050	None	1700

NR, not reported.

* Most studies show deficiency.

[†] One study (Butte NF, Calloway DH, Van Duzen JL. Nutritional assessment of pregnant and lactating Navajo Women. *Am J Clin Nutri* 1981; **34**(10): 2216–28.

[‡] Deficient after daily multivitamins.

when the hemoglobin falls below 10.4 g/dL or rises above 13.2 g/dL.

The pregnant woman has an additional need for iron (3.0 mg/day) above that of a nonpregnant, reproductive-age woman (1.3 mg/day). Her extra needs arise from the 350 mg needed for fetal–placental growth, 250 mg for blood loss at delivery, 450 mg for increases in maternal red cell mass, and a baseline loss of 250 mg. Blood loss at cesarean delivery is two- to threefold higher than blood loss after a vaginal delivery without an episiotomy, an important consideration as 32% of US women have cesarean births. As a fully lactating woman less than 6 months after delivery is usually not menstruating, her needs are considerably lower; 0.3 mg/day (men require 0.9 mg/day).

Luckily, 80% of US women receive daily prenatal multivitamins that contain 30–60 mg iron, and iron absorption is doubled or tripled among pregnant women compared to nonpregnant women [39]. The absorption of iron is affected by many factors. The type of iron supplement is important; the absorption of iron sulfate is 20%; iron gluconate, 12%; and iron fumarate, 32%. Meat sources of iron absorb better than do plant sources (whole grains, legumes) by interaction with phytates, tannins, polyphenols, and plant calcium and phosphate moieties. Between-meal dosing will maximize the absorption of therapeutic iron because of the reduced number of binding compounds in the gastrointestinal tract. There appears to be a threshold for iron absorption; once the dose is increased to above 120 mg/day, the percent absorption falls and the incidence of side-effects increases [39–46]. Orange juice or vitamin C (more than 200 mg) taken at the time of the iron supplement will increase absorption twofold. On the other hand, excessive coffee or tea reduces iron absorption by half.

The prevalence of iron deficiency anemia among nonpregnant women of childbearing age was examined in the Second (1978–80) National Health and Nutrition Survey (NHANES2) [46]. The diagnosis of iron deficiency anemia was based on criteria defined by a mean corpuscular volume (MCV), iron/total iron binding capacity, and erythropoietin (EP) evaluation. The overall baseline incidence of iron deficiency anemia was 2.0% in middle- to upper-class, non-Hispanic, white women. The risk of iron deficiency anemia appears to be greater among the poor (7.8%), those with less than 12 years of education (13.2%), Mexican-Americans (11.2%), African-Americans (5.0%), and adolescents (4.9%), and in women who have given birth to three or four children (11.5%). Multiple pregnancy, maternal bowel disease, chronic infection (tuberculosis, human immunodeficiency virus), chronic aspirin use (0.2–2.0 mg iron loss/day), and persistent vaginal or rectal bleeding (second and third trimester bleeding, placenta previa, hemorrhoids) will increase the likelihood of anemia. In these populations, prophylactic iron therapy (30 mg/day) is warranted.

Clinically, the diagnosis is based on the laboratory findings of anemia with hemoglobin below 10.5 g/dL, a low MCV, and a serum ferritin level below 12 μg/dL. Most studies using random assignment of subjects [11] demonstrated that daily doses of 30–120 mg are equally effective in raising the hemoglobin 0.4–1.7 g/dL by 35–40 weeks' gestation. Unfortunately, the data on improvement in the incidence of adverse pregnancy outcomes are either not reported or obscured by small sample sizes [47].

Calcium and magnesium

Approximately 99% of calcium and magnesium in pregnant women and their fetus or infant is located in their bones and teeth. Pregnancy and lactation are associated with increased bone turnover in order to meet fetal or infant needs for calcium (50 mg/day at 20 weeks, 330 mg/day at 35 weeks, and 300 mg/day during lactation) and increased urinary excretion of calcium (200 mg/day). The fetus actively transports calcium, and fetal levels are higher than maternal calcium levels. The total fetal accretion of calcium is 30 g. The body maintains the serum ionized calcium level within a tight range (4.4–5.2 mg/dL) and if dietary deficiencies occur, maternal bone will supply its calcium to the fetus. While bone turnover is high in pregnant or lactating women, measures of net bone loss during pregnancy and lactation among women in developed countries are inconsistent (24–12%) [11]. One explanation for varied results is increased absorption of dietary calcium related to pregnancy or lactation. Increased absorption is correlated with the highest fetal needs (nonpregnant, 27%; 5–6 months, 54%; and at term, 42%) [11]. Increased absorption is in part caused by progressive increases in 1,25-dihydroxycholecalciferol (the active moiety of vitamin D). On the other hand, a diet high in plant phytates, phosphoric acid (carbonated sodas), aluminum-based antacids, or bismuth-containing over-the-counter medications reduces calcium absorption.

Increased calcium is associated with smooth-muscle relaxation and parathyroid hormone (PTH) has a stimulatory effect on angiotensin II-mediated secretion of aldosterone. Animal and human studies demonstrated a consistent reduction in blood pressure in nonpregnant animals or humans when their dietary calcium is increased. Hypocalciuria is a useful diagnostic tool in the differentiation of preeclampsia from other forms of hypertension in pregnancy [48]. These observations have led to controlled clinical trials to test the hypothesis that calcium supplements during pregnancy reduce the incidence of pregnancy-induced hypertension (and perhaps preterm birth) [49–54]. In these studies, pregnant women were randomly assigned to receive 1500–2000 mg/day calcium or no calcium. The effect on the incidence of pregnancy-induced hypertension has been mixed. The studies that reported a benefit demonstrated a dose–response effect and a reduction of vascular sensitivity to angiotensin II injection. There seemed to be a trend toward a reduction in the incidence of preterm birth. At least two other studies did not demonstrate a benefit from supplemental calcium. The discrepancy between the studies is likely to be related to patient selection and the handling of the analysis when compliance is an issue. Similarly, there does not seem to be a benefit from reduced salt diet in the prevention of preeclampsia [54,55].

At this point, there is no support for the routine supplementation of calcium (2000 mg/day) for all pregnant women. In pregnant women who have a diet deficient in calcium (less than 600 mg/day), prepregnancy hypertension, calcium-losing renal disease, a strong family or personal history of preeclampsia, or chronic use of certain medications (heparin, steroids), may benefit with little risk of toxicity from daily supplemental calcium (2000 mg of elemental calcium or 5000 mg of calcium carbonate). Young women (less than 25 years old) and those women with mild dietary calcium deficiency (600–1200 mg/day) may be treated by extra servings of dairy products; 227 g (8 oz) milk or 28 g (1 oz) hard cheese, which supplies 300 mg of calcium per serving, or supplemental calcium, 600 mg (carbonate).

Calcium metabolism is more complex than the simple percepts outlined earlier indicated. PTH is associated with increased calcium absorption from the intestine and increased bone absorption; a high level in late pregnancy would be expected. Unexpectedly, the biologically active form of PTH is associated with a 40% decrease during pregnancy. Calcitonin acts as a biologic balance to PTH, and as serum calcium levels are maintained within a tight range, higher levels of calcitonin would be expected. The studies that evaluated calcitonin levels during pregnancy had inconsistent results. Magnesium is essential for the release of PTH from the parathyroid and the action of PTH on the intestines, bones, and kidneys. The fetus absorbs 6 mg/day of magnesium. Maternal magnesium levels remain constant during pregnancy despite inadequate intake (Table 2.5). On the other hand, Spatling and Spatling [56] performed a double-blind, placebo-controlled trial where pregnant women (at less than 16 weeks) were assigned randomly to receive magnesium supplementation (360 mg/day) or placebo. Of patients who reported compliance, the magnesium supplement group had 30% fewer hospitalizations, 50% fewer preterm births, and 25% more perinatal hemorrhages compared with the placebo supplement women. The outcomes were not analyzed on an intention-to-treat basis. More study of magnesium supplementation in pregnancy needs to be performed before routine supplementation is recommended.

Vitamin D

Vitamin D is critical in the absorption, distribution, and storage of calcium. Sunlight is the major source of vitamin D, 1,25-hydroxycholecalciferol. Sunlight (ultraviolet light) converts 7-dehydroxycalciferol within the skin to vitamin D. Vitamin D is converted to 25-hydroxycholecalciferol (marker for adequate vitamin D) in the liver and subsequently to 1,25-hydroxycholecalciferol (active form) in the kidney. In latitudes higher than 40° North, especially where clouds obscure sunlight during the winter, the conversion of 7-dehydroxycholecalciferol to 1,25-hydroxycholecalciferol is insufficient to maintain adequate levels of vitamin D. For example, the serum levels of 25-hydroxycholecalciferol vary considerably between fall and spring: from 25 ng/dL in the fall to 17 ng/dL in the spring in England; from 18 ng/dL in the fall to 11 ng/dL in the spring in Finland. While few cases of vitamin D deficiency (less than 5 mg/dL) are encountered in England or the USA, Finland records an incidence of 47% in the spring and 33% in the fall [11].

Relatively few foods are good sources of vitamin D. Vitamin D-fortified milk is the major dietary source in the USA. Fortified milk contains approximately 2.5 µg vitamin D and 120 IU vitamin A. Although vitamin D deficiency is very rare in the USA because of its latitude, propensity toward more exposure of bare skin and the almost uniform vitamin D fortification of milk, selected populations may be at risk for low 25-hydroxycholecalciferol levels. These populations include culturally prescribed full clothing, home-bound, or institutionalized patients who cannot (lactose intolerant) or will not drink milk. In these populations, intervention with vitamin D supplementation (10 µg/day) may be beneficial. No controlled trials have used vitamin D to correct a deficiency and subsequently demonstrate a change in its physiologic actions. In summary, uniform vitamin D supplementation is not recommended [57].

Folate

Folate participates in many bodily processes, especially rapidly growing tissue. Folate functions as a coenzyme in the transfer of single carbon units from one compound to another. This step is essential to the synthesis of nucleic acids and the metabolism of amino acids. As the mother and fetus are rapidly developing new tissue, perturbation in folate intake might be expected to result in adverse pregnancy outcomes. In the last 10 years, a clear and consistent relationship between low folate intake and fetal neural tube defects and, possibly, cleft lip and palate has been identified.

Folate deficiency works with multiple factors to cause birth defects [58]. Genetic factors appear to be a strong cofactor. The population rates of neural tube defects vary considerably: 1 per 1000 births in the USA, 6 per 1000 births in Ireland, and 10 per 1000 births in northern China. Women with a previous child with a neural tube defect have a 1.6–6.0% risk of recurrent neural tube defects. The level of risk is predicted by the frequency of occurrence of neural tube defects in the immediate family. Environmental exposures seem to be an additional cofactor. Preconceptual diabetes or first trimester hyperglycemia is associated with a multiple-fold increase in the incidence of neural tube defects. Drugs such as valproic acid, carbamazepine, folate antagonists, and thalidomide are associated with a 1–4% risk of neural tube defects.

Folate is an essential nutriment for humans, as they cannot manufacture folates and must rely on dietary intake and absorption. Folates are present in leafy green vegetables, fruit, fortified breads and cereals, egg yolks, and yeast. Many multivitamins and fortified cereals contain 350–400 mg folate. Prescription prenatal multivitamins contain 0.8–1.0 mg folic acid. Eighty percent of folate intake in the USA is derived from polyglutamate forms of folate. The absorption of polyglutamate forms is approximately 60%; the absorption of monoglutamate forms is approximately 90%. Multivitamins contain the monoglutamate forms.

The RDA of folate is 3 µg/kg body weight for nonpregnant and nonlactating women. Given a 60–70% absorption rate from their diet, pregnant women should acquire an extra 0.4 mg in their daily diet. Lactating women need an extra 0.2 mg/day. The average daily intake of folate in the USA is 0.20–0.25 mg despite the fact that 20% of US women consume multivitamins containing 0.36 mg or more of folic acid. Dietary deficiency of folic acid is a major public health issue.

There is a progressive pattern of the pathophysiology of folate deficiency with increasing duration and intensity of folate deficiency. At 3 weeks, low serum folate levels (below 3 ng/mL) are manifest. At 5 weeks, neutrophils develop hypersegmentation (more than 3.5 lobes). At 7 weeks, the bone marrow demonstrates megaloblastic changes. At 17 weeks, the erythrocyte folate level is low (below 140 ng/mL). At 20 weeks, a generalized megaloblastic anemia (MCV above 105) is present.

Most interventions with folic acid have focused on the prevention of neural tube defects. In women with a previous history of a child with a neural tube defect, numerous studies involving randomized assignment demonstrated a 75% reduction in the frequency of recurrent neural tube defects when 4–5 mg/day folic acid was taken for 1–2 months preconceptually and through the first trimester [11,59–61]. The current standard of care requires documentation that the benefits of folic acid supplementation in preventing recurrent neural tube defects have been explained and that the supplement has been prescribed to the patient. The recommendation is to supplement with 4 mg/day folic acid from 1 to 3 months preconceptually and through the first trimester.

More recently, daily multivitamins that contain 0.4–0.8 mg folic acid have been shown to decrease the incidence of neural tube defects in low-risk women (no previous pregnancy or family history of neural tube defects). One study [59,60] randomly assigned women to receive either a placebo plus trace elements or a multivitamin that contained 0.8 mg folic acid. Of 2104 women who received folic acid, no neural tube defects occurred and in 2065 women who received the placebo, six pregnancies were complicated by neural tube defects ($P < 0.029$). Women who are at mild risk (distant family history of neural tube defect, inadequate intake, multiple pregnancy [undergoing assisted reproductive technology]) and who are attempting pregnancy should have documentation of adequate dietary folate consumption or daily prescription multivitamins that contain at least 0.8 mg folic acid from 1 to 3 months preconceptually and through the first trimester.

Other nutriments

The benefits of supplementing other specific nutriments in pregnant women have not been confirmed by blinded, placebo-controlled trials with random assignment of subjects, or the studies that do exist have major methodologic weaknesses such as selection bias or inadequate sample size. An additional problem is outcome definition. Low maternal nutriment levels are very different from clinical deficiency states and many of the important outcomes (preterm birth, perinatal mortality, fetal growth restriction) have other predictors to obscure the relationship between nutrition and adverse pregnancy outcomes. Despite the latter observations, nutriments whose supplementation may benefit deficiency states include zinc, selenium, chromium (diabetes), fluoride, magnesium, vitamin A (less than 5000 retinol equivalent [RE]), vitamin B_6, and vitamin C.

Vitamin toxicity

The clinician is occasionally confronted with a woman who is taking unorthodox amounts of vitamins or minerals. Much of the data on toxic risk are based on animal studies and anecdotal cases, especially those concerning the ingestion of more obscure vitamins and minerals. Results of animal studies should be interpreted with caution particularly given the lack of animal toxicity seen with thalidomide. Luckily, most water-soluble vitamins appear relatively safe for the mother and fetus; excess intake is readily excreted in the urine. Vitamin C taken in an amount greater than 6–8 g/day may cause loose stool. Vitamin B_6 intake greater than 500 mg/day is associated with a reversible peripheral neuropathy. Maternal or fetal toxicity has not been identified with the other water-soluble vitamins.

Toxicity is more of an issue with excess intake of fat-soluble vitamins. Vitamin A (retinol forms) is associated with a dose-dependent increase in fetal defects: hydrocephalus, microcephalus, and cardiac lesions. The risk of defects seems to be related to the retinol/retinyl ester forms of vitamin A. Carotenoid forms do not seem to have the same risks. The threshold intake where risk appears excessive has not been defined, but at doses lower than 10,000 RE of retinoid forms, the incidence of fetal abnormality is no greater than the baseline risk; with doses higher than 25,000 RE the risk of defects clearly exceeds the baseline risk. Huge doses (above 15 mg or 600,000 IU) of vitamin D have been associated with a variable degree of toxic symptoms (soft-tissue calcification). Excess vitamin E or vitamin K use has not been associated consistently with adverse outcome for the mother or fetus.

Toxicity associated with excess mineral intake is associated with primarily maternal symptoms. Iron intake at more than 200 mg/day is associated with gastrointestinal symptoms (heartburn, nausea, abdominal pain, constipation) in a dose-dependent fashion (placebo, 13%; 200 mg, 25%; 400 mg, 40%) [42]. Magnesium sulfate at more than 3 g/day is associated with catharsis and reduced iron absorption. Iodine excess is associated with goiter and hyperthyroidism. Selenium at more than 30 mg/day results in nausea, vomiting, fatigue, and nail changes. Molybdenum interferes with calcium absorption. Zinc intake at more than 45 mg/day has been associated with preterm delivery and reduced iron and copper absorption. Fluoride at doses higher than 2 mg/L (fluoridated water plus supplemental fluoride) is associated with dental fluorosis of the primary teeth in the fetus.

Lactation

Breastfeeding and breastmilk are unique gifts for the mother and newborn. Breastmilk has nutritional qualities far superior to artificial breastmilk formulas [62]. Artificial breastmilk formulas do not contain important enzymes and hormones to aid digestion, active or passive immunoglobulins, activated immune cells, or antibacterial compounds (lactoferrin). Breastmilk promotes growth of nonpathogenic bacterial flora in the infant's intestine (i.e., *Bifidobacterium* spp.). Formula contains inappropriate fatty acid and lactose concentrations for optimal brain growth, and inconsistent amounts of essential vitamins and other micronutriments.

The unique qualities of breastfeeding and breastmilk provide many benefits for the mother and infant. For the mother, the benefits include significant contraception and child spacing (lactational amenorrhea method), better mother–infant bonding, less cost for nutrition and equipment, less health care costs for the infant, less loss of work time and income to care for sick children, less postpartum retention of weight, and reduction in the risk of breast cancer. For the infant, the benefits include fewer deaths from infection, less morbidity from respiratory and gastrointestinal infections, appropriate growth patterns, less childhood obesity, less childhood cancer, better social interaction, higher intelligence, better oral–facial development, and protection from allergies.

The documented benefits of breastfeeding and breastmilk have prompted the World Health Organization, the US Surgeon General, and the American Academy of Pediatrics (AAP) [63] to recommend breastfeeding rather than artificial breastmilk feeding. The nutritional qualities of breastmilk are sufficient for infant growth until 6 months, after which gradual introduction of food is appropriate. The AAP recommends breastfeeding for at least 12 months. Until 100 years ago, the usual time for weaning was 2.5–4.0 years; this probably represents the biologic duration of breastfeeding.

As breastmilk is manufactured and secreted by the human breast, the nutritional quality and composition are remarkably constant regardless of the tremendous variation in maternal diet. The volume (700–1000 mL/day) of breastmilk produced for the infant determines the mother's nutritional needs during lactation. If the fully lactating woman has an average diet and takes one prenatal multivitamin daily (Table 2.6), her daily requirements for lactation are satisfied, except for magnesium and iodine. The deficiency in magnesium and iodine is not manifested by a variation in breastmilk concentration. The infant is not at risk for deficiency.

In the fully breastfed infant, the volume of breastmilk consumed determines the amount of energy, protein, vitamins, and minerals obtained by the infant. Therefore, a review of the factors that can affect breastmilk volume is appropriate. Less than 5% of women have anatomic limits for adequate volumes of breastmilk. These include congenital hypoplasia (small, tubular shape), cosmetic breast surgery (reduction or augmentation), severe nipple inversion, and periareolar breast surgery. Pain (nipple trauma, injections), stress, and maternal insecurity inhibit the release of oxytocin and contraction of the myoepithelial cells surrounding the breast acini (interference with the letdown reflex). Some medications (bromocriptine, ergotrate/methergine, combination birth control pills, or testosterone analogs) can reduce milk volume.

Analysis of levels of maternal energy intake and the volume of breastmilk reveals little risk for US women. Women who are below standards for BMI and who consume fewer than 1500 kcal/day preconceptually, during pregnancy, and during lactation (severely disadvantaged in developing countries) show little (less than 60 mL) difference in milk volume [63–66]. Nutritional supplementation studies in undernourished populations did not demonstrate an increase in milk volume. In developed countries, where the energy intake is at much higher levels, no reduction of milk volume is demonstrated. Short-term reduction in calorie intake (19–32%) in well-nourished lactating women did not reduce milk volume in those who restricted their intake to no less than 1500 kcal/day. In women who restricted their intake to less than 1500 kcal/day, the milk volume was reduced by 109 mL [64]. Gradual weight loss (2 kg/month) is associated with normal milk volumes. Regular postpartum exercise, which increases oxygen consumption by 25%, has no effect on breastmilk volume [64,65].

Dietary recommendations for pregnancy and lactation

In 1990 the Institute of Medicine, after an exhaustive review of the literature, published its recommendations, *Nutrition During Pregnancy* [11] and *Nutrition During Lactation* [65]. The recommendations support accurate measurement of BMI at the preconceptual (preferred) or initial visit (Table 2.4), subsequent measurement of weight at each prenatal and postpartum visit (Fig. 2.5), standardized assessment of maternal diet (Fig. 2.4), assessment of nutritional risk factors, patient education, and nutritional intervention.

One key component is different target levels of weight gain based on the mother's prepregnancy BMI. Table 2.4 describes the recommendations. Of equal importance, the amount and quality of the woman's diet should be assessed in a standardized fashion (Fig. 2.4). A good daily diet will contain seven 28 g (1 oz) servings of protein-rich foods (meat, poultry, fish, eggs, legumes, nuts), three 227 g (8 oz) servings of milk or an equivalent amount of other dairy products, six or more servings of grain products (each serving: 1 slice of bread, 1 oz of dry cereal, ½ cup of cooked pasta, hot cereal, or rice), and six or more servings of fruits and vegetables (each serving: ½ cup of cooked, 1 cup of raw, 6 oz juice). Pregnant women younger than 24 years should consume one extra serving of dairy products daily [11,66]. This diet, when taken with one tablet of a prenatal multivitamin daily, will supply 2500–2700 kcal energy per day and 1.3–1.5 g/kg ideal weight of protein per day as well as sufficient vitamins and minerals.

Once baseline information has been documented, the provider should counsel and educate the patient, continue accurate documentation of weight change, and intervene if necessary. Counseling and education involve setting a target goal (Table 2.4) of weight gain for prepregnancy BMI. Continued documentation of weight gain is simplified by the use of a chart (Fig. 2.5). Intervention (except for routine prenatal vitamins) is based on the presence of nutritional risk factors or abnormal weight gain patterns.

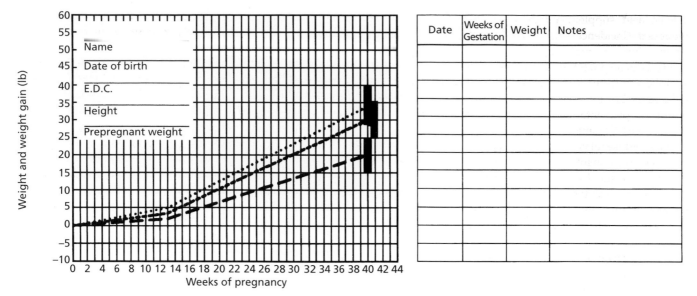

Fig. 2.5 Prenatal weight gain chart. Prepregnancy body mass index (BMI), 19.8 (·········); prepregnancy BMI 19.8–26.0 (normal body weight) (----------); prepregnancy BMI >26.0 (—————). (Reprinted with permission from *Nutrition during pregnancy and lactation*. Copyright 1992 by the National Academy of Sciences. Published by the National Academy Press, Washington, DC.)

Recently, the recommendations of the Institute of Medicine were evaluated using the Pregnancy Nutrition Surveillance System [67]. This analysis was limited to women who delivered liveborn, singleton infants between 37 and 41 weeks' gestation. According to women, infant, children (WIC) clinic data, less than 32% of subjects had missing data concerning BMI, weight gain, birth weight, or gestational age at delivery. The analysis included 220,170 women. Only 35% of non-Hispanic white women, 33.2% of non-Hispanic black women, and 36.4% of Hispanic-only women gained weight within the Institute's target range. Across the races, about 23% gained more than 4.5 kg (10 lb) above the Institute's recommendation. Overweight (38%) and obese (27.5%) women gained in excess of 4.5 kg (10 lb) above the recommendations; these are significant differences from the percent deviation seen in underweight (11%) and normal-weight women (20%). Among underweight women across all races, failure to gain at least the Institute's recommended weight was associated with adjusted odds ratios of 1.5–3.2 for delivery of a term infant weighing less than 2500 g. Excessive weight gain was associated with a significant decrease in the incidence of term small for gestational age infants. Weight gain in excess of 4.5 kg (10 lb) greater than the recommendations was associated with significant adjusted odds ratios (2.2–10.8) for a birth weight higher than 4500 g regardless of race. These data generally support the Institute's recommendations for weight gain based on prepregnancy BMI. The strong associations with adverse outcome, fetal growth restriction, and macrosomia, coupled with the frequency of excessive weight gain, predict the challenges of nutritional counseling in the late 20th century.

Conclusions

Maternal nutrition has an essential role in the health and well-being of the fetus and newborn. The single best evidence of adequate nutrition is appropriate weight gain for the woman's prepregnancy BMI: 11.3–13.6 kg (25–30 lb) for underweight and normal weight women, prepregnant BMI less than 26; and 6.8–9 kg (15–20 lb) for prepregnancy BMI over 26. Dynamic weight gain charts and food intake surveys are clinically practical as to allow intervention prior to term.

The average US woman who takes her prescribed prenatal vitamins consumes enough energy, protein, vitamins, and minerals (except for calcium) to prevent major adverse outcomes related to nutrition. Calcium deficiency is corrected easily by consuming an additional portion of dairy products each day. Unfortunately, many women gain much more than the recommended weight. Excessive nutrition can result in fetal macrosomia and postpartum weight retention. Postpartum weight retention has a key role in the obesity of adult women. As a result, obese women are at greater risk for future obstetric complications, adult-onset diabetes, hypertension, atherosclerotic vascular disease, and early death.

Despite numerous dietary and nutritional interventions, relatively few have been shown to be helpful in adequately controlled and powered trials. The beneficial inventions include the following.

1 Multiple micronutriments and protein/calorie supplements appear to be helpful in severely undernourished women who become pregnant (i.e., developing countries).

2 Folic acid supplementation of at least 0.4–0.8 mg/day reduces the incidence of neural tube defects in low-risk populations. Supplemental folic acid (4–5 mg/day) reduces the incidence of neural tube defects in high-risk populations.

3 Modest iron supplementation (30 mg/day elemental iron) reduces the incidence of anemia during pregnancy. The effect of iron supplementation on adverse pregnancy outcomes in the average US woman is less clear.

Massive doses of vitamin A are associated with birth defects, and excessive iron intake is associated with significant maternal gastrointestinal symptoms. Many other individual nutrients have great theoretical benefit; however, the data is mixed as to their benefit in low-risk patients from industrialized countries. These studies have major selection biases and are underpowered.

The publications of the Institute of Medicine, *Nutrition During Pregnancy* and *Nutrition During Lactation*, represent a unique resource and guide for the obstetric care provider. The assessment of maternal risk factors for nutritional risk factors, accurate measurement of weight and BMI, evaluation of current diet, establishment of target weight gain based on pre-pregnancy BMI, and ongoing assessment of weight gain during pregnancy are standards for preventative or therapeutic intervention.

Case presentation

A 24-year-old gravida 1, para 1 is seen at a family planning office visit 2 years after the birth of her healthy child. She wants to stop her birth control pills and become pregnant again. Her second cousin has recently delivered a child with spina bifida. She wishes to know what she can do to prevent the lesion in her fetus. The evaluation consists of a good dietary history, especially for folic acid intake, and ascertainment of any additional environmental, genetic, familial, or medical risk factors for developmental lesions including neural tube defects. If her other risk factors are absent, her risk remains slightly increased for a neural tube defect in her fetus. In counseling her about her slightly increased risk for neural tube defects, she is educated about folic acid-containing foods, advised to start prenatal vitamins with 1 mg/day folic acid immediately, and wait at least 3 months off hormonal contraception before attempting pregnancy. If she had a first- or second-degree relative with a neural tube defect, she should consume 4 mg/day folic acid in addition to prenatal vitamins.

References

1 Bergner L, Susser MW. Low birth weight and prenatal nutrition: an interpretative review. *Pediatrics* 1970;**46**:946–66.
2 Stein Z, Susser M, Saenger G, Marolla F. *Famine and Human Development: The Dutch Hunger Winter of 1944–1945*. New York: Oxford University Press, 1975.
3 Stein Z, Susser M. The Dutch famine, 1944–1945, and the reproductive process. I. Effects of six indices at birth. *Pediatr Res* 1975;**9**:70–6.
4 Stein Z, Susser M. The Dutch famine, 1944–1945, and the reproductive process. II. Interrelations of caloric rations and six indices at birth. *Pediatr Res* 1975;**9**:76–83.
5 Luke B. Nutritional influences on fetal growth. *Clin Obstet Gynecol* 1994;**37**:538–49.
6 Ananth CV, Vintzileos AM, Shen-Schwarz S, *et al.* Standards of birth weight in twin gestations stratified by placental chorionicity. *Obstet Gynecol* 1998;**91**:917–24.
7 Williams RL, Creasy RK, Cunningham GC, *et al.* Fetal growth and perinatal viability in California. *Obstet Gynecol* 1982;**59**:624–32.
8 Owen P, Donnet ML, Ogston SA, *et al.* Standards for ultrasound fetal growth velocity. *Br J Obstet Gynaecol* 1996;**103**:60–9.
9 Lubchenco LO. Assessment of gestational age and development of birth. *Pediatr Clin North Am* 1970;**17**:125–45.
10 Durnin JVGA. Energy requirements of pregnancy: an integration of the longitudinal data from the five-country study. *Lancet* 1987;**2**:1131–3.
11 Institute of Medicine. *Nutrition During Pregnancy*. Washington, DC: National Academy, 1990: 97, 102, 107, 152–9, 262–3, 273, 320–1.
12 Bakketeig LS, Hoffman HJ, Harley EE. The tendency to repeat gestational age and birth weight in successive births. *Am J Obstet Gynecol* 1979;**135**:1086–103.
13 Naeye RL. Weight gain and the outcome of pregnancy. *Am J Obstet Gynecol* 1979;**135**:3–9.
14 Taffel SM. Maternal weight gain and the outcome of pregnancy: United States. *Vital and Health Statistics*. Series 21, no. 44. DHHS publication no. (PHS) 86–1922. Hyattsville, MD: National Center for Health Statistics, Public Health Service, US Department of Health and Human Services, 1986: 25.
15 Kleiman JC. *Maternal weight gain during pregnancy: determinants and consequences*. NCHS working paper series no. 33. Hyattsville, MD: National Center for Health Statistics, Public Health Service, US Department of Health and Human Services, 1990.
16 Naeye RL, Blanc W, Paul C. Effects of maternal nutrition on the human fetus. *Pediatrics* 1973;**52**:494–503.
17 Mercer BM, Goldenberg RL, Das A, *et al.* The Preterm Prediction Study: a clinical risk assessment system. *Am J Obstet Gynecol* 1996;**174**:1885–93.
18 Papiernik E, Kaminski M. Multifactorial study of the risk of prematurity at 32 weeks of gestation. A study of the frequency of 30 predictive characteristics. *J Perinat Med* 1974;**2**:30–6.
19 Berkowitz GS. An epidemiologic study of preterm delivery. *Am J Epidemiol* 1981;**113**:81–92.
20 Picone TA, Allen NH, Olsen PN, Ferris ME. Pregnancy outcome in North American women. II. Effects of diet, cigarette smoking, stress, and weight gain on placentas, and on neonatal physical and behavioral characteristics. *Am J Clin Nutr* 1982;**36**:1214–44.
21 Cnattingius S, Bergstrom R, Lipworth L, Kramer M. Prepregnancy weight and the risk of adverse pregnancy outcomes. *N Engl J Med* 1998;**338**:147–52.
22 Goldenberg RL, Iams JD, Mercer BM, *et al.* The preterm prediction study: the value of new vs. standard risk factors in predicting early and all spontaneous preterm births. *Am J Public Health* 1998;**88**:233–8.

23 Parker JD. Postpartum weight change. *Clin Obstet Gynecol* 1994;**37**:528–37.

24 Greene GW, Smicikla-Wright H, School TO, Karp RJ. Postpartum weight change: how much of the weight gain in pregnancy will be lost after delivery? *Obstet Gynecol* 1988;**71**:701–7.

25 Campbell DM, MacGillivray I. Maternal physiological responses and birth weight in singleton and twin pregnancies by parity. *Eur J Obstet Gynecol Reprod Biol* 1977;**7**:17–24.

26 Brown JE, Schloesser P. Prepregnancy weight status, prenatal weight gain, birth weight, and perinatal mortality relationships in term, twin pregnancies. *FASEB J* 1998;**3**:A648.

27 Beaton GH, Milner J, Corey P, *et al.* Sources of variance in 24-hour dietary recall data: implications for nutrition study design and interpretation. *Am J Clin Nutr* 1979;**32**:2546–59.

28 Beaton GH, Milner J, McGuire V, *et al.* Source of variance in 24-hour dietary recall data: implications for nutrition study design and interpretation. Carbohydrate sources, vitamins and minerals. *Am J Clin Nutr* 1983;**37**:986–95.

29 Block G, Hartman AM. Issues in reproducibility and validity of dietary studies. *Am J Clin Nutr* 1989;**50**:1133–8.

30 Magkos F, Yannakoulia M. Methodology of dietary assessment in athletes: concepts and pitfalls. *Curr Opin Clin Nutr Metab Care* 2003;**6**:539–49.

31 Frank GC, Pelican S. Guidelines for selecting a dietary analysis system. *J Am Diet Assoc* 1986;**86**:72–5.

32 *Recommended Dietary Allowances*, 10th edn. Washington, DC: National Academy Press, 1989.

33 Henrik F, Gomo E, Nyazema N, *et al.* Effect of multmicronutrient supplementation on gestational length and birth size: a randomized, placebo-controlled, double-blind effectiveness trial in Zimbabwe. *Am J Clin Nutr* 2004;**80**:178–84.

34 Osrin D, Vaidya A, Shrestha Y, *et al.* Effects of antenatal multiple micronutrient supplementation on birthweight and gestational duration in Nepal: double-blind, randomised controlled trial. *Lancet* 2005;**365**:955–62.

35 Kramer MS. Tsocaloric balanced protein supplementation in pregnancy. *Cochrane Database Syst Rev* 2006;**2**: CD000133.

36 Kramer MS. High protein supplementation in pregnancy. *Cochrane Database Syst Rev* 2006;**2**.

37 Murphy JF, O'Riordan J, Newcombe RG, *et al.* Relation of haemoglobin levels in first and second trimesters to outcome of pregnancy. *Lancet* 1986;**1**:992–5.

38 Garn SM, Ridella SA, Petzold AS, Falkner F. Maternal hematologic level and pregnancy outcomes. *Semin Perinatol* 1981;**5**:155–62.

39 Chanarin I, Rothman D. Further observations on the relation between iron and folate status in pregnancy. *Br Med J* 1971;**2**:81–4.

40 Hallberg L, Bjorn-Rasmussen E, Ekenved G, *et al.* Absorption from iron tablets given with different types of meals. *Scand J Haematol* 1978;**21**:215–24.

41 Hallberg L, Brune M, Rossander L. Iron absorption in man: ascorbic acid and dose-dependent inhibition by phytate. *Am J Clin Nutr* 1989;**49**:140–4.

42 Hallberg L, Ryttinger L, Solvell L. Side effects of oral iron therapy: a double-blind study of different iron compounds in tablet form. *Acta Med Scand Suppl* 1967;**459**:3–10.

44 Hallberg L. Bioavailability of dietary iron in man. *Annu Rev Nutr* 1981;**1**:123–47.

46 Life Sciences Research Office, *Assessment of the iron nutritional status of the US population based on data collected in the Second National Health and Nutrition Examination Survey, 1976–1980.* Bethesda, MD: Federation of American Societies for Experimental Biology, 1984.

47 Mahomed K. Iron supplementation in pregnancy. *Cochrane Database Syst Rev* 2006;**2**.

48 Pitkin RM, Reynolds WA, Williams GA, Hargis GK. Calcium metabolism in normal pregnancy: a longitudinal study. *Am J Obstet Gynecol* 1979;**133**:781–90.

49 Grunewald C. Biochemical prediction of pre-eclampsia. *Acta Obstet Gynecol Scand Suppl* 1997;**164**:104–7.

50 Belizan JM, Villar J, Gonzales L, *et al.* Calcium supplementation to prevent hypertensive disorders of pregnancy. *N Engl J Med* 1991;**325**:1399.

51 Sanchez-Ramos L, Briones DK, Kaunitz AM, *et al.* Prevention of pregnancy-induced hypertension by calcium supplementation in angiotensin II-sensitive patients. *Obstet Gynecol* 1994;**84**:349–53.

52 Bucher HC, Guyatt GH, Cook RJ, *et al.* Effect of calcium supplementation on pregnancy-induced hypertension and preeclampsia: a meta-analysis of randomized control trials. *JAMA* 1996;**275**:1113–7.

53 Levine RJ, Hauth JC, Curet LB, *et al.* Trial of calcium to prevent preeclampsia. *N Engl J Med* 1997;**337**:69–76.

54 Duley L, Henderson-Smart D. Reduced salt intake compared to normal dietary salt, or high intake, in pregnancy. *Cochrane Database Syst Rev* 2006;**2**:CD001687.

55 Duley L, Henderson-Smart D, Meher S. Altered dietary salt for preventing pre-eclampsia, and its complications. *Cochrane Database Syst Rev* 2006;**2**:CD005548.

56 Spatling L, Spatling G. Magnesium supplementation in pregnancy. A double blind study. *Br J Obstet Gynaecol* 1988;**95**:120–5.

57 Mahomed K, Gulmezoglu AM. Vitamin D supplementation in pregnancy. *Cochrane Database Syst Rev* 2006;**2**:CD000228.

58 Rose NC, Mennuti MT. Periconceptional folate supplementation and neural tube defects. *Clin Obstet Gynecol* 1994;**37**:605–20.

59 Centers for Disease Control. Recommendations for the use of folic acid to reduce the number of cases of spina bifida and other neural tube defects. *Morbid Mortal Wkly Rep MMWR* 1992;**41**:1–7.

60 Czeizel AE, Dudas I. Prevention of the first occurrence of neural-tube defects by peri-conceptional vitamin supplementation. *N Engl J Med* 1992;**327**:1832–5.

61 Lumley J, Watson L, Watson M, Bower C. Periconceptional supplementation with folate and/or multivitamins for preventing neural tube defects. *Cochrane Database Syst Rev* 2006;**2**: CD001056.

62 Newton ER. Breastmilk: the gold standard. *Clin Obstet Gynecol* 2004;**47**:632–42.

63 American Academy of Pediatrics Work Group on Breastfeeding. Breastfeeding and the use of human milk. *Pediatrics* 1997;**100**:1035–9.

64 Strode MA, Dewey KG, Lonnerdal B. Effects of short-term caloric restriction on lactational performance of well-nourished women. *Acta Paediatr Scand* 1986;**75**:222–9.

65 Institute of Medicine. *Nutrition during lactation*. Washington, DC: National Academy, 1991;68–70.

66 Abrams B. Weight gain and energy intake during pregnancy. *Clin Obstet Gynecol* 1994;**37**:515–27.

67 Schieve LA, Cogswell ME, Scanlon KS. An empiric evaluation of the Institute of Medicine's pregnancy weight gain guidelines by race. *Obstet Gynecol* 1998;**91**:878–84.

3 Alcohol and substance abuse

William F. Rayburn

Substance use is most prevalent in reproductive age adults. Among women aged 15–44 years, almost 90% have used alcohol, approximately 44% have used marijuana, and at least 14% have used cocaine [1]. In 2002 and 2003, 4.3% of pregnant women used illicit drugs during the past month, 4.1% reported binge alcohol use, and 18.0% reported smoking cigarettes [2]. Pregnant women aged 15–25 years were more likely to use illicit drugs and smoke cigarettes during the past month than women aged 26–44 years [2]. Even though a woman may cease alcohol, illicit drug, or cigarette smoking during pregnancy, some women may not reduce or alter their patterns until pregnancy is actually diagnosed or well under way.

Care of alcohol or substance-using pregnant women is complex, difficult, and often demanding. Women's care providers must be aware of their unique psychological and social needs and the related legal and ethical ramifications surrounding pregnancy. This chapter discusses many issues related to pregnancies complicated by alcohol and other substance use. Screening for substance use, risks to the fetus, and comprehensive perinatal care are reviewed.

Screening for substance use

Identification of substance use before or during pregnancy most often depends on a history given voluntarily by the patient. Pregnant and postpartum women who use and abuse alcohol or other drugs are more stigmatized than nonpregnant women. They may therefore deny their drug habit and its potential harmful effects and not seek help. Young poor women can be especially fearful of the medical and social welfare system because of their naivety or desire to hide their pregnancy.

Questions about alcohol, illicit substances, and cigarette smoking should be routine at the initial prenatal visit. A history of past and present substance use should be obtained in a nonjudgmental manner and by questioning about the frequency and amount of specific substances [3]. If alcohol exposure was evident, the next step is to ask "Do you drink, smoke, or use street drugs?" Using the CAGE questionnaire, you may then ask the following: Have you ever felt that you should cut down on your drinking? Have people annoyed you by criticizing your drinking? Have you ever felt guilty about your drinking? Have you ever needed an "eye-opener" drink when you get up in the morning? [4].

Drug or metabolite testing with informed consent is recommended among those pregnant women with: (i) self-reporting of substance use; (ii) multiple medical, obstetric, and behavior characteristics (Table 3.1) suggesting substance use to facilitate referral to a comprehensive care program; or (iii) compliance requirements with treatment recommendations. Random testing of all gravidas raises several legal issues, however, including the right to privacy, lack of probable cause, and admissibility of test results [5].

Urine is the preferred source for drug testing, because it is easily available and in large quantities. Urine drug screening is usually performed using an immunoassay technique. Except for marijuana, most substances or their metabolites are measurable in urine for less than 72 hours and alcohol for less than 24 hours. Therefore, substances may not be identified unless urine specimens are tested frequently [6]. In the evaluations for cocaine and opiate exposure, hair analysis of the mother or newborn infant is also effective [7].

Effects on the fetus

Unlike prescription or nonprescription drugs, used medically, alcohol and substances of abuse may be intentionally or inadvertently taken at toxic doses. Consuming many drinks per occasion (i.e., binge drinking, ≥5 drinks) may be more harmful to the developing fetus than the same amount spread over several days, because of higher peak blood alcohol content [8].

Moreover, the impurity of most illicit drugs and the common practice of abusing multiple substances make it difficult to

Table 3.1 Examples of obstetric, behavior, and medical patterns in pregnant women suggestive of alcohol and substance use disorders.

Obstetric	Behavioral and Personal	Medical
Abruptio placentae	Alcohol—or drug-abusing partner	Anemia
Birth outside hospital	Bizarre or inappropriate behavior	Arrhythmias
Congenital anomalies	Child abuse or neglect	Bacterial endocarditis
Fetal alcohol spectrum disorder	Chronic unemployment	Cellulitis, abscesses, or phlebitis
Fetal distress	Difficulty concentrating	Cerebrovascular accident
Neonatal abstinence syndrome	Domestic violence	Drug overdose or withdrawal
No, sporadic, or late prenatal care	Family history of substance abuse	Hepatitis B and C
Preterm labor and delivery	Frequent emergency department visits	HIV seropositivity
Preterm rupture of the membranes	Incarceration	Lymphedema
Reduced fetal growth	Noncompliance with appointments	Myocardial ischemia or infarction
Spontaneous abortion	Poor historian	Pancreatitis
Stillbirth	Prostitution	Poor dental hygiene
Sudden infant death syndrome	Psychiatric history	Poor nutritional status
	Restless, agitation, demanding	Septicemia
	Slurred speech or staggering gait	Sexually transmitted diseases
		Tuberculosis

ascribe specific fetal effects and perinatal outcomes to a certain drug. Accurate evaluation of dosage and the exact period of exposure are rarely possible.

Table 3.2 lists effects in human fetuses from *in utero* exposure to certain substances [9]. This list was compiled using data from two or more reports in humans. Although this table serves as a guideline, counseling about absolute risk is unreasonable. The risk of structural anomalies is not increased in most cases of substance exposure, although the background risk of birth defects is 3% in the general pregnancy population [10]. Maternal alcohol and substance use place the fetus at risk for problems including low birthweight, small head circumference, prematurity, and a variety of developmental complications.

Fetal alcohol spectrum disorder, the term to encompass all levels of an outcome associated with prenatal alcohol exposure, affects approximately 1 in 100 births [11]. In the case of illicit drugs, evidence is neither sufficient nor consistent to identify with reasonable certainty which substance produced which effect and at what level. Furthermore, evidence to untangle the environmental factors (such as poverty and the corresponding poor nutrition and lack of access to prenatal care) from alcohol and substance abuse-related factors is limited, conflicting, or nonexistent.

The impact of prenatal alcohol and other substances on infant and child development presents other challenges. Although animal studies have shown that ethanol and drugs reduce the density of cortical neurons and change dendritic connections, the significance to human development is unclear [12]. Studies of behaviors in animals have shown long-term changes, and abnormal neurobehavioral findings in the newborn raise concerns about how those conditions may affect subsequent development.

Specific therapy for pregnancy

Psychologic and pharmacologic treatments are intertwined in managing pregnant patients with a chemical dependence. Support includes individual counseling, group therapy, exercise, lifestyle change training, and self-help groups such as Alcoholics Anonymous and Cocaine Anonymous. Relapse prevention methods, which utilize peer support and learning principles, are directed toward avoiding situations that elicit conditioned cravings for substances of abuse and toward developing better coping skills. Under supervision, mothers can become drug-free, learn effective parenting skills, and experience improved relationships with their children. This reunification model with her family also unburdens foster care systems by assuring the safety of the child(ren) in a therapeutic milieu.

Forms of behavioral therapy include self-management procedures, relaxation training, contingency contracting, and skills training. Contingency contracting involves rearranging that individual's environment so that positive consequences follow desired behavior, while either negative or neutral consequences follow undesired behaviors. These techniques require reinforcement from others, such as spouse or boyfriend, other family members, employers, or health care providers. Individuals admitting to a relapse of substance use or having positive urine drug screening are subject to negative consequences.

Psychiatric disorders among substance users are so common that it is difficult to ascertain whether it contributed to or resulted from the substance use. In many instances, abstinence from substance use results in an amelioration of those conditions. Specific pharmacotherapy may result in resolution

Table 3.2 Impact of *in utero* exposure of specific substances on the fetus and newborn infant and on obstetric complications*.

	Fetal/Neonatal Effects	Obstetric Complications
Alcohol	Microcephaly; growth deficiency; CNS dysfunction including mental retardation and behavioral abnormalities; craniofacial abnormalities (i.e., short palpebral fissures, hypoplastic philtrum, flattened maxilla); behavioral abnormalities	Spontaneous abortion
Cigarettes	No anomalies; reduced birthweight (200 g lighter)	Preterm birth Placenta previa Placental abruption Reduced risk of preeclampsia
Cannabis Marijuana THC Hashish	No anomalies; corresponding decrease in birthweight; subtle behavioral alterations	Reduction of 0.8 weeks in length of gestation
CNS sedatives Barbiturates Diazepam Flurazepam Meprobamate Methaqualone	No anomalies; depression of interactive behavior	
CNS stimulants Antiobesity drugs Amphetamines Cocaine Methylphenidate Phenmetrazine	Excess activity *in utero*; congenital anomalies (heart? biliary atresia?); depression of interactive behavior; urinary tract defects; symmetric growth restriction; placental abruption; cerebral infarction; brain lesions; fetal death; neonatal necrotizing enterocolitis	Spontaneous abortion
Hallucinogens LSD Ketamine Mescaline Dimethyltryptamine Phencyclidine (PCP)	No anomalies; chromosomal breakage (?) (LSD); dysmorphic face; behavioral problems	Spontaneous abortion
Narcotics Codeine Heroin Hydropmorphone Hydrocodone Meperidine Morphine Opium Pentazocine (and tripelennamine)	No anomalies; intrauterine withdrawal with increased fetal activity; depressed breathing movements; fetal growth restriction; perinatal mortality	Preterm delivery Preterm rupture of the membranes Meconium stained amniotic fluid
Inhalants Gasoline Glue Hairspray Paint	Similar to the fetal alcohol and fetal hydantoin syndromes (?); growth restriction; increased risk of leukemia in children; impaired heme synthesis	Preterm labor

CNS, central nervous system; LSD, lysergic acid diethylamide; THC, tetrahydrocannibalol (marijuana).
* ≥Two investigations in humans as reported in reference [9].

of both the psychiatric disorder and the substance use among women whose psychiatric disorder either antedated the substance use or coexisted with the addiction process [12,13].

We constantly look for signs of substance overdose and withdrawal. Unusual behavior, agitation, dilated or constricted pupils, elevated or decreased blood pressure, rapid or slow heart rate or respiratory rate, and altered reflexes are sought. These should not be confused with physiologic adaptive changes of pregnancy.

Select drug therapy with extensive counseling is an important modality. A prime example is methadone, which has been prescribed for years in treating opiate dependence during pregnancy. Opiate addiction leads to receptor system dysfunction and affects a patient's ability to remain abstinent. Methadone maintenance (usually 40–120 mg/day) reduces the risk of relapse, enhances retention in treatment and prenatal programs, and improves perinatal outcome [14,15]. We do permit breastfeeding during methadone maintenance therapy. Unfortunately, other forms of maintenance therapy for alcohol or other substance use (cocaine, methamphetamine) are not prescribed during pregnancy [13]. Benzodiazepines and phenobarbital are used to withdraw pregnant women who abuse alcohol and sedative-hypnotics. There is no conclusive evidence about effects of these drugs on withdrawal and long-term consequences during pregnancy.

Cocaine dependence remains a major public health problem because of the high relapse rates and poor treatment responses. Drug trials for cocaine addiction (tricyclic antidepressants, dopamine agonists, lithium, amino acids, and vitamins) have not been conducted during gestation and are not universally effective. Cocaine blocks the uptake of neurotransmitters, leading to their depletion. Further research is needed to determine whether dopamine agonists (bromocriptine, amantadine), used to replenish neurotransmitters from cocaine exposure, are effective and safe.

The obstetrician and other care givers can approach the pregnant woman who smokes in a stepwise manner. Patients who smoke should be advised to stop by providing clear, strong advice to quit with personalized messages about the benefits of quitting and the impact of continued smoking on the woman, fetus, and newborn [16]. Her willingness to attempt to quit smoking should be assessed within the next 30 days. Patients interested in quitting should be assisted by providing pregnancy-specific, self-help smoking cessation materials. Regular follow-up visits are encouraged to track the progress of the patient's attempt to quit smoking. Nicotine gum and patches should be considered for use during pregnancy only when nonpharmacologic treatments (e.g., counseling) have failed, and if the increased likelihood of smoking cessation, with its potential benefits, outweighs the unknown risk of nicotine replacement and potential concomitant smoking.

Comprehensive prenatal care

Care should be conducted by professionals with expertise and training in the area of substance use. The most common complaint by health care professionals is the feeling of ineffectiveness, because their patients are generally unmotivated, noncompliant, and difficult to retain in treatment [3,17]. Involving patients with treatment of their substance use is not a guarantee that they will seek prenatal care. Certain persons have either "kicked the habit" or feel that their habit is too infrequent for multidisciplinary care. Professionals willing to work with this population must tackle the many issues associated with substance use: poverty, lack of education and job training, poor parenting skills, domestic violence in the form of physical and sexual abuse, child abuse, family and other personal relations, communicable disease, child development, and such psychiatric disorders as depression, anxiety, post-traumatic stress disorder, and psychosis.

The most important aspect of this comprehensive preventive care is to encourage a woman to take an active role in reaching her ultimate goal: a drug-free environment for the fetus. Several reports exist about substance use treatment in multidisciplinary prenatal settings. These studies suggest that even minimal drug interventions (such as methadone maintenance) and counseling, combined with prenatal care, can lead to better pregnancy and infant outcomes [17,18]. Although comprehensive interventions such as this show promise for reducing substance use and harm to the fetus, few clinics in any community are solely dedicated to screening, assessing, and treating pregnant addicts.

Favorable outcomes relate directly to the time dedicated by the experienced multidisciplinary team [18,19]. Providers need to be sensitive to the feelings and cultural background of pregnant substance-using women and offer care in an environment that is supportive, nurturing, and nonjudgmental. As the patient becomes more involved, a strong and more positive relationship develops between patient and staff. The ability to be flexible and to provide an environment that is safe and fosters self-esteem and interpersonal growth is essential. Comfort levels of medical students toward pregnant women with substance use disorders can improve with experience at these clinics during their clerkship training [20].

Organization of primary/preventive care, laboratory, and behavioral services at our specialized prenatal clinic are shown in Table 3.3 [18]. This comprehensive program serves not only chemically dependent pregnant and postpartum women, but also their infants and children. It has long been our goal to promote not only cessation of alcohol, tobacco, and other substance use, but also to effect change in patients' lifestyles in a holistic sense. Substance use in pregnancy involves not only the woman, but entangles the family and whole community.

Each patient enrolled in our program receives prenatal care using a protocol established for chemically dependent women.

Table 3.3 Organization of laboratory, behavioral, and primary/prenatal care services in a comprehensive prenatal care program. Adapted from Bolnick J and Rayburn W. Substance use disorders in women: special considerations. *Obstet Gynecol Clin North Am* 2003;**30**:545–59 with permission.

Visit	Primary/Prenatal Care	Labs/Studies/Consents	Behavioral Counseling
New OB	Discuss proper nutrition and supplements Focus on any poor obstetric history (IUFD, repeated losses, anomalies, preterm deliveries, LBW) Smoke cessation, alcohol avoidance	Thorough drug use history (past and present) Thorough physical exam (signs of current/recent use) New OB labs, HIV (need consent); UDM; Urine C&S Place Tbc skin test and order hepatitis panel, LFTs Dating ultrasound	Assess patient's willingness/attempt to quit Encourage attendance at Milagro counseling sessions/methadone group Identify barriers to quitting and help identify solution Counsel patient regarding potential anomalies, fetal effects, and high risk problems (preterm labor, abruption, preeclampsia) that could occur with the particular drug being abused Discuss/treat comorbid disorders (depression, anxiety)
15–19 wk	Examine oral cavity; review oral hygiene Discuss elements of prenatal care; avoid frequent emergency visits Review STD labs	MSAFP (need consent) Check UDM Consider ultrasound to r/o anomalies	Motivational counseling for successes/failures Encourage continued attendance at counseling sessions/groups Educate and answer questions regarding effects of particular drug on her fetus at this stage
20–24 wk	Encourage compliance with appointments Fitness counseling; smoke cessation Discuss asthma and URIs		Observe for signs of withdrawal/overdose Inquire about job satisfaction Discuss any issues relating to prostitution or incarceration
25–28 wk	Examine skin (cellulitis, abscesses, phlebitis, acne, lymphedema, dermatitis) Discuss signs and symptoms of hepatitis, pancreatitis Explain about preterm labor/PPROM precautions	1 h glucola and Hct Check UDM Rh-immunoglobulin (if Rh neg)	Encourage continued attendance at counseling sessions/groups Educate regarding effects of particular drug on her fetus at this stage and on neonatal withdrawal symptoms and complications
29–30 wk	Use of safety belts; firearms Discuss about urinary tract infections Postpartum contraception counseling	Consent for any tubal ligation	Observe for signs of overdose/withdrawal Focus on any psychiatric history
31–32 wk	Discuss headaches Encourage childbirth classes Discuss safe sex	Begin daily fetal movement charting	Encourage attendance of counseling sessions Ask about current drug use Discuss domestic violence
33–34 wk	Review vaccination history (rubella, tetanus, travel immunizations, influenza, pneumococcal) Encourage childbirth classes Discuss asthma and upper airway problems	Repeat hepatitis panel, LFTs (if Hep C+) Repeat RPR and HIV Check UDM	Motivational counseling for successes/failures Observe for signs of overdose/withdrawal Discuss/make plans for ongoing counseling/drug treatment postpartum

Table 3.3 *Continued.*

Visit	Primary/Prenatal Care	Labs/Studies/Consents	Behavioral Counseling
35–36 wk	Discuss breastfeeding issues related to particular drug being abused Discuss breast conditioning and disorders	Consider ultrasound for fetal growth GC/chlamydia/GBS cultures	Inquire about support at home Educate about potential neonatal withdrawal symptoms and complications Discuss future employment
37 wk	Rediscuss labor precautions Confirm pediatrician/family physician Review plans for postpartum contraception	Check UDM	Motivational counseling for successes/failures Encourage continued attendance at counseling sessions/groups Ask about current drug use Review social work support (Los Pasos) and ongoing counseling/drug treatment
≥38 wk	Explain about postpartum "blues" and anatomic changes		Educate about analgesic options during labor Educate about potential neonatal withdrawal symptoms and complications
6 wk PP	Provide birth control counseling and prescriptions Review written information about general health care/annual exam	Pap; GC/C	Ask about current drug use Screen for depression Encourage continued attendance at counseling sessions/groups Discuss employment plans

C&S, culture and sensitivity; GBS, group B streptococcus; GC/C, gonorrhea/chlamydia; Hct, hematocrit; IUFD, intrauterine fetal death; LBW, low birth weight; LFT, liver function test; MSAFP, maternal serum alpha fetoprotein; OB, obstetric; Pap, Papanicolaou smear; PPROM, preterm premature rupture of the membranes; Rh, Rhesus; r/o, risk of/rule out; RPR, rapid plasma reagin test; STD, sexually transmitted disease; Tbc, tuberculosis; UDM, urine, drug and metabolites; URI, upper respiratory infection.

This protocol includes bi-monthly prenatal visits (until 32 weeks, then weekly), ultrasound to monitor fetal growth and to promote maternal bonding with the unborn baby, proper dating of the pregnancy, and 24-hour-a-day on-call staff. Patients are screened at least twice during pregnancy for hepatitis B and C, HIV, chlamydia, gonorrhea, and syphilis. Tuberculosis skin testing is undertaken at the initial visit. Routine counseling about healthy pregnancy includes nutrition counseling, childbirth classes, tours of the inpatient obstetrics and newborn facilities, analgesia/anesthesia classes (including regional, IV, and local anesthesia), and breastfeeding.

Hospital and postpartum care

Ideally, the same physicians or midwives providing prenatal care will see the patient in the hospital. The residents, fellows, and staff rotate at our clinic, and these doctors will be the caregivers during the labor process. Notification of anesthesia staff about any substance use is recommended. In this manner, continuity of care is maintained and patients feel more secure during the transition from pregnancy to care of the infant.

Many states require hospitals to report pregnant women suspected of heavy alcohol and other drug use to local public health authorities or the criminal justice system when the women present for delivery [17]. This reporting may cause women to be even more wary of acknowledging their problem and of seeking prenatal care and hospital delivery, particularly if they have other children who are in the custody of Child Protective Services (CPS) or who are living with relatives. In many states, protective services, foster care placements, and review boards base their decisions on whether to return a child to the mother on the length of time the child is away from the mother. These decisions serve as deterrents to women seeking effective long-term substance abuse treatment if childcare is unavailable.

Many chemically dependent women lose interest in the clinics once the baby has been delivered. If the neonate is healthy, the new mother may feel that her drug use is not that dangerous. It is the moral responsibility of the substance use program not to let these patients become lost to follow-up.

Once this happens, the patient is set up for failure and often reverts back to substance use.

Among nonpregnant women, substance use rates are lower for recent mothers than for women who are not recent mothers [2]. Health professionals need to continue monitoring women after delivery for signs and symptoms of substance use. These nonpunitive monitoring efforts are intended to identify behaviors in adults that can reduce attention to children and to spot developmental delays in children before beginning early intervention services.

Case presentation

VC is a 26-year-old G3P1021, seen for a postpartum examination after scant prenatal care. Six weeks ago, she delivered vaginally a 32w 2d fetus weighing 4 lbs 5 oz after preterm ruptured membranes and labor. The nonanomalous infant was discharged from the intensive care nursery 4 weeks later and is now being cared for by the grandmother. The patient declined to breastfeed.

She admits to using heroin and crack cocaine during the pregnancy but has not been using for 3 months. She was begun on 95 mg methadone late during her pregnancy and increased her dose after delivery. There is a history of poor family relationships, sexual and physical abuse, depression, housing and transportation difficulties, and limited prostitution. She was charged with drug possession once and with parole violations three times. Her prenatal laboratory tests were positive for hepatitis C, atypical squamous cells of undetermined significance (ASCUS) on Papanicolaou (Pap) test, and hematocrit 34% (microcytic hypochromic anemia).

Her pelvic examination revealed normal reparative changes. A Pap test and cultures were obtained. She is not currently sexually active, although the baby's father is on parole. Our plan was to arrange for an intrauterine device (IUD) placement following discussion about various methods of contraception. If an ASCUS result persists on cervical cytology, human papillomavirus (HPV) testing may be useful to detect high risk (16 or 18) serotypes and colposcopy would be performed.

The patient is currently living at a shelter. Our social work staff continue to assist on housing, employment, and legal issues. Counseling has already helped her in overcoming her drug abuse and in developing a more stable family relation to maintain social support and a closer relation with her infant. Precautions were given about hepatitis C transmission. She is aware that there is no good treatment for hepatitis C. Interferon is very expensive, has many side-effects, and is not 100% effective in eradicating the infection.

References

1 American College of Obstetricians and Gynecologists. Substance abuse in pregnancy. *ACOG Tech Bull* 1994;**195**:825–31.

2 National Survey on Drug Use and Health. *Substance use during pregnancy: 2002 and 2003 update*. DHHS Publication No. SMA 03-3836, NSDOH Series H-22. Rockville, MD: Office of Applied Studies, 2003.

3 Chasnoff I, Neuman K, Thornton C, Callaghan M. Screening for substance use in pregnancy: a practical approach for the primary care physician. *Am J Obstet Gynecol* 2001;**184**: 112–9.

4 Ewing JA. Detecting alcoholism: the CAGE questionnaire. *JAMA* 1984;**252**:1905–7.

5 Foley E. Drug screening and criminal prosecution of pregnant women. *J Obstet Gynecol Neonatal Nurs* 2002;**31**: 133–7.

6 Wolff K, Farrell M, Marsden J, *et al*. A review of biological indication of illicit drug use, practical considerations and clinical usefulness. *Addiction* 1999;**94**:1279–98.

7 Macgregor S, Keith L, Bachicha J, Chasnoff I. Cocaine abuse during pregnancy: correlation between prenatal care and perinatal outcome. *Obstet Gynecol* 1989;**74**:882–5.

8 Bailey B, Delaney-Black V, Covington C, *et al*. Prenatal exposure to binge drinking and cognitive and behavioral outcomes at age 7 years. *Am J Obstet Gynecol* 2004;**191**: 1037–43.

9 Reprotox® database, Reproductive Toxicology Center, Bethesda MD, 2005. Available at http://reprotox.org/

10 Cunningham F, Gant N, Leveno K, Gilstrap L, Hauth J, Wentsworth K. *Teratology, Drugs, and Medications: Williams Obstetrics*, 22nd edn. New York: McGraw-Hill, 2005: 1006.

11 Sampson PD, Streissguth AP, Bookstein FL. Incidence of fetal alcohol syndrome and prevalence of alcohol-related neurodevelopmental disorder. *Teratology* 1997;**56**:317–26.

12 Kranzler H, Amin H, Lowe V, Oncken C. Pharmacologic treatments for drug and alcohol dependence. *Psychiatr Clin North Am* 1999;**22**:212–39.

13 Rayburn WF, Bogenschutz MP. Pharmacotherapy for pregnant women with addictions. *Am J Obstet Gynecol* 2004;**191**:1885–97.

14 Archie C. Methadone in the management of narcotic addiction in pregnancy. *Curr Opin Obstet Gynecol* 1998;**10**:435–40.

15 Dashe J, Sheffield J, Jackson G, *et al*. Relationship between maternal methadone dosage and neonatal withdrawal. *Am J Obstet Gynecol* 2002;**100**:1244–9.

16 American College of Obstetricians and Gynecologists. *Smoking cessation during pregnancy*. Washington DC: ACOG Committee Opinion 316, Oct 2005.

17 *Outreach to and identification of women: practical approaches in the treatment of women who abuse alcohol and other drugs*. Rockville MD: US Dept Health and Human Services, Public Health Service, 1994: 124–6.

18 Bolnick J, Rayburn W. Substance use disorders in women: special considerations during pregnancy. *Obstet Gynecol Clin North Am* 2003;**30**:545–58.

19 Bauer C, Shankaran S, Bada HS, *et al*. The maternal lifestyle study: drug exposure during pregnancy and short-term maternal outcomes. *Am J Obstet Gynecol* 2002;**186**:487–95.

20 Ramirez W, Strickland L, Meng C, Beraun C, Rayburn W. Medical students' comfort levels toward pregnant women with substance use disorders. *Birth Defects Res* 2005;**73**:346.

4 Environmental agents and reproductive risk

Laura Goetzl

Obstetricians are frequently asked about the reproductive risks of specific environmental, work-related, or dietary exposures. While few exposures have been associated with a measurable increase in risk of congenital anomaly, fetal death, or growth impairment, ongoing research continues to identify new areas of concern. Research linking low levels of environmental exposures is hampered by the cost and difficulty of prospective cohort studies with accurate ascertainment of exposure to specific agents at various gestational periods. In this chapter, we discuss the principles concerning the evaluation of the developmental toxicity of occupational and environmental exposures in general, and review selected agents that have been associated with reproductive toxicity.

Background incidence of adverse outcome

Increased attributable risk of an individual environmental agent must be placed in the context of the background incidence of adverse pregnancy outcome in the general population. Approximately 30% of recognized pregnancies result in miscarriage and 3% result in children with major malformations, defined as a malformation requiring medical or surgical attention, or resulting in functional or cosmetic impairment. This high background risk introduces statistical problems in the identification of toxicity. If the increase in adverse outcome is relatively small, it is likely to go undetected unless the study sample size is quite large.

Biologic evidence of toxicity

Two types of evidence are generally employed when evaluating agents for evidence of reproductive toxicity: animal studies and epidemiologic studies in human populations.

Studies with experimental animals offer the advantage of studying varying levels of exposure (from minimal to substantial) at specific key developmental time periods. In addition, outcomes are standardized and typically include measures of fertility, fetal weight, viability, and presence and patterns of malformations. If low doses of a compound produce an increase in malformations, a role for the agent in disrupting embryo development is possible. Limitations of animal testing include species variations in toxicity (i.e., compounds may be toxic to human embryos but not to various animal embryos, and vice versa). Further, evaluation of functional attributes such as behavior or immunocompetence is not a part of standard testing schemes. Therefore, absence of toxicity in animal protocols provides only limited information on possible adverse effects on human development.

Human epidemiologic studies can be subdivided, in increasing order of scientific merit, into case reports, case–control studies, retrospective cohort studies, and well-designed prospective cohort studies. Often, case reports of malformations or pregnancy loss will emerge first, raising hypotheses that lead to further study. However, case reports alone are insufficient evidence to establish the presence or degree of risk. The evaluation of toxicity requires comprehensive assessment of both exposures and of outcomes. Accurate occupational and environmental exposures are difficult to measure in humans and it is even more difficult to pinpoint precise exposure at a specific gestational age. Outcome assessment can also be difficult because the identification of abnormalities in children is affected by the age of the child and the thoroughness with which abnormalities are sought. Relying on birth certificates or obstetrician reports, for example, will yield a lower rate of identification of abnormalities than will examination by a trained dysmorphologist using a standardized assessment protocol.

General principles

Principles of reproductive toxicity apply to environmental agents just as they do to pharmaceuticals and these principles are summarized here. These ideas were popularized by Wilson

Table 4.1 Reproductive toxicology sources.

Source	Web Address	Individual Practitioner Cost 2005
Reprotox	http://www.reprotox.org	$199.00/year
Teris	http://depts.washington.edu/terisweb/teris/ Individual Toxin Summary	$1000.00/year $3.50–15.00/report
Reprorisk	http://www.micromedex.com/products/reprorisk/	$500.00/year
OTIS	http://www.otispregnancy.org/ Limited number of fact sheets for download	Free
Toxnet	http://toxnet.nlm.nih.gov/	Free
DART	Developmental and Reproductive Toxicology Database http://toxnet.nlm.nih.gov/cgi-bin/sis/htmlgen?DARTETIC	Free

[1] in the 1950s based on his work with experimental animals, but they remain applicable decades later in a discussion of human risk.

1 A large proportion of adverse outcomes are unrelated to exposures. Only 5% of congenital malformations are estimated to be attributable to exposure to a chemical agent or pharmaceutical [2].

2 A specific agent may be nontoxic at low doses but toxic at higher doses. For example, X-ray exposures during pregnancy of ≥50 rad have been associated with microcephaly and mental retardation, but X-ray exposures in the range of most diagnostic procedures (<1 rad) are not associated with an increase in adverse pregnancy outcome.

3 Each fetus will respond differently to a given exposure based on their genetic susceptibility and other factors. For a given toxic exposure, responses can range from unaffected to significantly affected.

4 The timing of exposure during pregnancy will influence the response. Target tissues will have different sensitivities to toxicity at different times during gestation. Although the first trimester is the most typically sensitive time period for many congenital malformations (e.g., limb and heart defects), there are a number of examples of severe toxicity from exposures at other times in pregnancy. For example, agents that affect fetal growth and neurologic development, such as mercury and ethanol, will continue to be toxic throughout the second and third trimesters.

5 Toxicity must occur via a biologically plausible mechanism. Therefore, chemicals that cannot cross the placenta or agents such as microwaves that cannot penetrate into the uterus are unlikely causes of reproductive toxicity.

Specific agents

Research demonstrating adverse reproductive effects of various chemical and environmental agents is continuously evolving. In this section we present a snapshot of the current knowledge. Computerized databases are available and can provide access to regularly updated summaries of chemical exposures (Table 4.1).

Lead

Lead can cross the placenta readily [3,4]. In women with significant occupational lead exposure (pottery glazes, batteries), rates of stillbirth and miscarriage are increased [5] as well as rates of premature rupture of membranes and premature birth [6–8]. Over time, with the reduction in lead alkyl additives in gasoline and the use of lead-based paints, lead levels in women of reproductive age have declined. Surveillance from the 1980s suggested that 9% of white women and 20% of African-American women exceeded blood lead levels of 10 μg/dL [9]. More recently, overall percentages have declined to 0.5% [10].

While significant occupational exposures are rare in the USA, lower levels of perinatal lead exposure have been linked to adverse reproductive outcomes. Even mild elevations in maternal lead levels have been associated with an increased risk of miscarriage (5–9 μg/dL, odds ratio [OR] 2.8; 10–14 μg/dL, OR 5.4; ≥15 μg/dL, OR 12.2) [11]. Increased maternal bone lead levels, but not serum levels, have also been associated with a minor increased risk of pregnancy-induced hypertension [12]. Cord blood concentrations less than 30 μg/dL, and perhaps as low as 10 μg/dL [13,14], have been linked to measurable deficits in early cognitive development. Although the results are not consistent, elevated maternal lead levels during pregnancy have been associated with lower IQ scores at age 8 [15] and tests of attention and visuoconstruction at ages 15–17 [16]. Although isolated studies have linked maternal lead exposure to an increased fetal risk of neural tube defects [17] and total anomalous pulmonary venous return [18], these findings have not been consistent.

Sources of lead exposure include lead solders, pipes, storage batteries, construction materials (e.g., lead-based paints), dyes, and wood preservatives. A validated questionnaire for screening pregnant women is not available. Risk factors for maternal lead levels that exceed 10 µg/mL include occupational exposures and house remodeling; however, screening high-risk women still fails to identify approximately 30% of cases [19]. Women at risk of lead exposure should be evaluated prior to pregnancy. If the blood level is higher than 30 µg/dL, chelation therapy should be considered prior to conception. There is no agreement on how to manage women with lower levels of blood lead, although our preference at the time of writing would be to use chelation therapy to reduce blood lead concentrations to 10 µg/dL or less. Pregnancy itself may lead to a mobilization of bone stores of lead, with increased exposure [20–22]. Calcium treatment (1000–1200 mg/day) decreases bone mobilization during pregnancy and may provide modest reduction of maternal blood lead levels during pregnancy (–1 µg/dL) [21,23]. Current pregnancy is a relative contraindication to chelation therapy as ethylenediaminetetra-acetic acid (EDTA) may chelate other key minerals necessary for development and has been linked to malformations in animal models [24]. Chelation therapy during pregnancy should be individualized based on the maternal serum lead level and the gestational age.

Mercury

Methyl mercury, a byproduct of such industries as incineration of solid waste and fossil fuel combustion facilities, pollutes our oceans and waterways. Methyl mercury crosses the placenta freely and accumulates in fetal tissues at concentrations exceeding maternal levels [25,26]. At high levels, methyl mercury can result in fetal neurotoxicity with microcephaly, cerebral palsy, deafness, and blindness (Minimata Bay, Japan [27,28]), but is not reproducibly associated with congenital malformations. However, most exposure to mercury occurs at low levels from fish consumption (methyl mercury), dental amalgams (mercury vapor), or the vaccine preservative thimerosal (ethyl mercury). Thimerosal has been removed from most vaccines in the USA and is therefore an unlikely potential source of exposure.

Fish consumption remains a modifiable source of fetal and childhood mercury exposure. Several large cohort studies have addressed the effects of low levels of *in utero* mercury exposure from maternal fish consumption on neuropsychologic development. Studies from the Faroe Islands (>1000 mother–infant pairs) and New Zealand (237 pairs) [29,30] found subtle deficits in language, attention, intelligence, and memory in school-aged children. Another, more recent study from the Seychelles (779 mother–infant pairs) did not find an association between *in utero* mercury exposure and outcome at 9 years; however, the final power to detect these outcomes was only 50% [31]. In 2001, based on these findings and a 2000 report from the National Research Council (NRC) [32], the

Environmental Protection Agency (EPA) issued advice urging pregnant women to limit consumption of fish high in mercury (Table 4.2). A benchmark blood level of <5.8 µg/L was recommended by the NRC; exposure above this level was associated with a doubling in the risk of adverse neurologic outcomes. Among women of childbearing age in the USA between 1999 and 2002, between 4 and 8% exceeded this benchmark level [33]. More recent iterations of this advice balance concerns over mercury exposure with the known benefits of fish consumption (www.epa.gov/ost/fishadvice/factsheet.html). Moderate intake of relatively safer fish should not be discouraged, as increasing fish consumption has been linked with higher measures of infant cognition [34,35].

Mercury exposure from dental amalgams is usually a low level and is not easily modified. Both placement and removal of dental amalgams is associated with transient increased levels of mercury exposure and should be avoided during pregnancy [36,37]. Dental personnel may also be exposed to inorganic mercury in vapors released from dental amalgams. Although evidence of documented harm in dental personnel is limited, current studies lack the power to detect subtle neurodevelopmental deficits. Safe levels of mercury during

Table 4.2 Commercial fish and levels of mercury

High levels. Avoid in pregnancy
Swordfish
Shark
King mackerel
Tile fish

Moderate levels. Limit consumption to 6 oz/week
Canned albacore tuna
Fresh tuna
Orange roughy
Halibut
Grouper
Sea bass
Local fish if no specific information is available

Low levels. Limit consumption to 12 oz/week
Shrimp
Canned light tuna
Salmon
Pollack
Catfish
Haddock
Scallops
Tilapia

Web Links
http://epa.gov/waterscience/fish/states.htm
Provides state by state links on local fish advisories

http://www.cfsan.fda.gov/~frf/sea-mehg.html
Provides mercury levels in commercially bought fish

pregnancy have not been established although suggested guidelines are that environments have a mercury vapor concentration less than $0.01\,mg/m^3$ (one fifth of Occupational Safety and Health Administration [OSHA] limits of $0.05\,mg/m^3$).

Pesticides and herbicides

A diverse group of agents is used to control pests such as insects and unwanted plants. While most exposures are agricultural, significant household exposure can occur, especially in the inner city [38]. The majority of pesticides cross the placenta readily [38]. Methodologically, it is difficult to isolate a single agent in epidemiologic studies; exposure to pesticides has been estimated by maternal recall, proximity to agricultural pesticide use, or maternal pesticide levels. Several studies have linked occupational exposure to pesticides with an increased risk of miscarriage [39,40] and birth defects such as musculoskeletal [41,42] and limb reduction abnormalities [43]. No association or weak associations have been found between parental pesticide exposure and adverse pregnancy outcomes including low birthweight [44], preterm delivery, or early neurodevelopmental outcomes [45]. While several maternal recall case–control studies have linked household pesticide use with an increased risk of childhood cancer [46,47], no association was found when exposure was estimated by proximity to agricultural pesticide use [48]. Minimizing occupational pesticide exposure through the use of protective clothing, adequate ventilation, respiratory masks, and hand washing is recommended. Limiting everyday exposure by minimizing household pesticide use (especially aerosolized pesticides), washing fruits and vegetables or buying organic produce is of uncertain benefit, but is easily accomplished.

Polychlorinated biphenyls

Polychlorinated biphenyls (PCBs) are a heterogeneous group of more than 200 lipid-soluble chemicals that were used extensively in industry until 1979, particularly in the manufacture of electrical transformers. Low-level maternal exposure is largely related to meat, dairy, and fish consumption, particularly fish from contaminated areas such as the Great Lakes. PCBs cross the placenta easily (fetal to maternal serum ratios of 0.6 : 1.1) and also accumulate in human breastmilk (breastmilk to maternal ratios of 0.6 : 1.8) contributing to postnatal exposure [49]. The overall effect on birthweight appears to be modest (290 g difference between <10th and >90th percentile exposure) [50] in some studies and insignificant in others [51]. Studies of *in utero* exposure to low levels of PCBs and subsequent neurodevelopment have produced various results. Several studies have shown no relationship between maternal serum levels of PCBs and mental and motor development in infancy/early childhood [52] and at school age [53,54]. Other

studies have suggested minor deficits in attention, memory, and motor skills in vulnerable populations of children; deficits were not observed in children in more advantageous circumstances or in those who were breastfed [55,56]. Local fish advisories should be consulted to determine which fish should not be eaten during pregnancy (http://epa.gov/waterscience/fish/states.ht).

Organic solvents

Many women work in industries where they may be exposed to organic solvents including dry cleaning and manufacturing using solvent-based adhesives, paints, or lacquers. Common organic solvents include toluene, benzene, and xylene. Significant occupational exposure has been associated with small (160 g) reductions in birthweight and an increased risk of major malformations (relative risk [RR] 13.0; 95% confidence interval [CI] 1.8–99.5) [57]. The risk of any major malformation was 10% and the overwhelming majority of malformations occurred in women with symptomatic exposure. Maternal occupational exposure to solvents is also associated with increased rates of hyperactivity [58] and with subtle decreases in visual acuity and abnormalities in red/green color vision [59]. Purposeful maternal solvent abuse (sniffing) has been associated with a fetal syndrome similar to fetal alcohol syndrome in 12.5% of cases, as well as major malformations (16.1%) and neonatal hearing loss (10.7%) [60]. Occupational exposure to solvents should be identified and minimized; similarly women should avoid exposure to solvents at home, especially in poorly ventilated areas.

Video display terminals

Initial concerns regarding the reproductive risks of video display terminals (VDTs) centered on early reports linking occupational exposure with an increased risk of spontaneous pregnancy loss [61]. However, subsequent well-designed studies suggested no increased risk [62,63]. Therefore patients can be reassured that there are no known fetal risks associated with working at VDTs.

Case presentation

Your patient, a 38-year-old G1, presents at 8 weeks' gestation for her first prenatal visit. She reports that her husband is an avid fisherman and she is concerned about the risks of mercury and other toxins to her pregnancy from eating fish that he has caught. On the other hand, she does not want to mortally offend him by spurning his fish if the risks are low.

Adequately counseling this patient requires knowledge both of the amount of fish that your patient is consuming and local fish advisories. Local fish advisories are common (Fig. 4.1) and links to those in your area can be reached on the

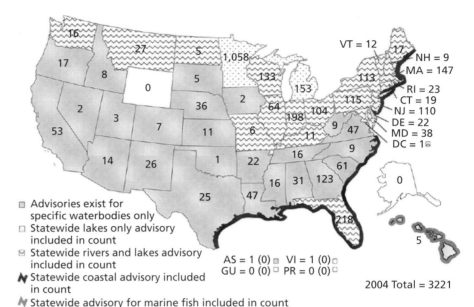

Fig. 4.1 Fish consumption advisories by state (2004 data, from Environmental Protection Agency [EPA]). Please note that states may have a different counting method for fish advisories from the national method, so advisory in the figure may be slightly different from those reported by individual states.

Legend:
- Advisories exist for specific waterbodies only
- Statewide lakes only advisory included in count
- Statewide rivers and lakes advisory included in count
- Statewide coastal advisory included in count
- Statewide advisory for marine fish included in count
- No advisories for chemical contaminants

AS = 1 (0) VI = 1 (0)
GU = 0 (0) PR = 0 (0)

2004 Total = 3221

Internet at http://epa.gov/waterscience/fish/states.htm. Possible fish contaminants triggering a local advisory include mercury, PCBs, chlordane, dioxins, and DDT. Patients should be advised not to consume any locally caught fish covered by a fish advisory during pregnancy. If no advisory is found, the patient may be counseled that she can eat up to 6 oz (one average meal) per week of fish her husband catches from local waters. However, she should not consume any other fish during that week. At the same time, the potential health benefits to her fetus of fish consumption during pregnancy should be reviewed. Ideally, fish consumption should continue during pregnancy, but should be limited to fish and shellfish with relatively low levels of contaminants, especially mercury. Locally caught fish may not be ideal for this purpose, especially in the Great Lakes area. Refrigerator magnets with the EPA Fish Advisories' website address and a message on the risks and benefits of fish consumption can be obtained free of charge by calling (800) 490-9198.

References

1 Wilson JG. Current status of teratology: general principles and mechanisms derived from animal studies. In: Wilson JG, Fraser FC, eds. *Handbook of Teratology*. New York: Plenum, 1977: 47–74.

2 Czeizel A, Rácz J. Evaluation of drug intake during pregnancy in the Hungarian case–control surveillance of congenital anomalies. *Teratology* 1990;**42**:505–12.

3 McClain RM, Becker BA. Teratogenicity, fetal toxicity, and placental transfer of lead nitrate in rats. *Toxicol Appl Pharmacol* 1975;**31**:72–82.

4 Barltrop D. Transfer of lead to the human feotus. In: Barltrop D, Burland WL, eds. *Mineral Metabolism in Pediatrics*. Oxford: Blackwell Science, 1969: 135–51.

5 Scanlon JW. Dangers to the human fetus from certain heavy metals in the environment. *Rev Environ Health* 1975;**2**:39–64.

6 Nogaki K. On action of lead on body of lead refinery workers: particularly conception, pregnancy and parturition in case of females and on vitality of their newborn. *Igaku Kenkyu* 1957;**27**:1314–38.

7 Fahim MS, Fahim Z, Hall DG. Effects of subtoxic lead levels on pregnant women in the state of Missouri. *Res Commun Chem Pathol Pharmacol* 1976;**13**:309–31.

8 Wilson AT. Effects of abnormal lead content of water supplies on maternity patients. *Scott Med J* 1966;**11**:73–82.

9 Crocetti AF, Mushak P, Schwartz J. Determination of numbers of lead-exposed women of childbearing age and pregnant women: an integrated summary of a report to the US Congress on childhood lead poisoning. *Environ Health Perspect* 1990;**89**:121–4.

10 Brody DJ, Pirkle JL, Kramer RA, *et al*. Blood lead levels in the US population. Phase I of the Third National Health and Nutrition Examination Survey (NHANES III). *JAMA* 1994;**272**:277–83.

11 Borja-Aburto VH, Hertz-Picciotto I, Lopez MR, *et al*. Blood lead levels measured prospectively and risk of spontaneous abortion. *Am J Epidemiol* 1999;**150**:590–7.

12 Rothenburg SJ, Kondrashov V, Manalo M, *et al*. Increases in hypertension and blood pressure during pregnancy with increased bone lead levels. *Am J Epidemiol* 2002;**156**;1079–87.

13 Bellinger D, Leviton A, Waternaux C, Needleman H, Rabinowitz M. Longitudinal analyses of prenatal and postnatal lead exposure and early cognitive development. *N Engl J Med* 1987;**316**:1037–43.

14 Dietrich KN, Krafft KM, Bornschein RL, *et al*. Low-level fetal lead exposure effect on neurobehavioral development in early infancy. *Pediatrics* 1987;**80**:721–30.

15 Wasserman GA, Liu X, Popovac D, *et al*. The Yugoslavia Prospective Lead Study: contributions of prenatal and postnatal lead exposure to early intelligence. *Neurotoxicol Teratol* 2000;**22**:811–8.

16 Ris MD, Dietrich KN, Succop PA, *et al*. Early exposure to lead and neurophyschological outcome in adolescence. *J Int Neuropsychol Soc* 2004;**10**; 261–70.

17 Bound JP, Harvey PW, Francis BJ, *et al*. Involvement of deprivation and environmental lead in neural tube defects: a matched case–control study. *Arch Dis Child* 1997;**76**:107–12.

18 Jackson LW, Correa-Villasenor A, Lees PS, *et al*. Parental lead exposures and total anomalous pulmonary venous return. *Birth Defects Res Part A Clin Mol Teratol* 2004;**70**:185–93.

19 Fletcher AM, Gelberg KH, Marshall EG. Reasons for testing and exposure sources among women of childbearing age with moderate blood lead levels. *J Community Health* 1999;**24**: 215–27.

20 Gulson BL, Mizon KJ, Korsch MR, *et al*. Mobilization of lead from human bone tissue during pregnancy and lactation: a summary of long term research. *Sci Total Environ* 2003;**303**:79–104.

21 Gulson BL, Mizon KJ, Palmer JM, *et al*. Blood lead changes during pregnancy and postpartum with calcium supplementation. *Environ Health Perspect* 2004;**112**:499–507.

22 Manton WI, Angle CR, Stanek KL, *et al*. Release of lead from bone in pregnancy and lactation. *Environ Res* 2003;**92**:139–51.

23 Hernandez-Avila M, Gonzalez-Cossio T, Hernandez-Avila JE, *et al*. Dietary calcium supplements to lower blood lead levels in lactating women: a randomized placebo-controlled trial. *Epidemiology* 2003;**14**:206–12.

24 Brownie CF, Brownie C, Noden D, Krook L, Haluska M, Aronson AL. Teratogenic effect of calcium edetate (CaEDTA) in rats and the protective effect of zinc. *Toxicol Appl Pharmacol* 1986;**82**:426–43.

25 Tsuchiya H, Mitani K, Kodama K, *et al*. Placental transfer of heavy metals in normal pregnant Japanese women. *Arch Environ Health* 1984;**39**:11.

26 Bjornberg KA, Vahter M, Berglund B, Niklasson B, Blennow M, Sandborgh-Englund G. Transport of methylmercury and inorganic mercury to the fetus and breast-fed infant. *Environ Health Perspect* 2005;**113**:1381–5.

27 Matsumoto H, Koya G, Takeucki T. Fetal Minimata disease: a neuropathological study of two cases of intrauterine intoxication by a methyl mercury compound. *J Neuropathol Exp Neurol* 1965;**24**:563–74.

28 Muramaki U. The effect of organic mercury on intrauterine life. *Acta Exp Biol Med Biol* 1972;**27**;301–36.

29 Grandjean P, Weihe P, White RF, *et al*. Cognitive deficit in 7-year old children with prenatal exposure to methylmercury. *Neurotoxicol Teratol* 1997;**19**:417–28.

30 Crump KS, Kjellstrom T, Shipp AM, Silvers A, Stewart A. Influence of prenatal mercury exposure upon scholastic and psychological test performance: benchmark analysis of a New Zealand cohort. *Risk Anal* 1998;**18**:701–13.

31 Myers GJ, Davidson PW, Cox C, *et al*. Prenatal methylmercury exposure from ocean fish consumption in the Seychelles child development study. *Lancet* 2003;**361**:1686–92.

32 National Research Council. *Toxicological effects of methylmercury.* Washington D.C.: National Academy Press, 2000.

33 Blood mercury levels in young children and childbearing-aged women, United States, 1999–2002. *MMWR Morb Mortal Wkly Rep* 2004;**53**:1018–20.

34 Oken E, Wright RO, Kleinman KP, *et al*. Maternal fish consumption, hair mercury, and infant cognition in an US cohort. *Environ Health Perspect* 2005;**113**:1376–80.

35 Daniels JL, Longnecker MP, Rowland AS, Golding J and the ALSPAC Study Team. Fish intake during pregnancy and early cognitive development of offspring. *Epidemiology* 2004;**15**:394–402.

36 Molim M, Bergman B, Marklund SI, Schutz A, Skerfving S. Mercury, selenium and glutathione peroxidase before and after amalgam removal in man. *Acta Odontol Scand* 1990;**48**:189–202.

37 Razagui IB, Haswell SJ. Mercury and selenium concentrations in maternal and neonatal scalp hair: relationship to amalgam-based dental treatment received during pregnancy. *Biol Trace Elem Res* 2001;**81**:1–19.

38 Whyatt RM, Barr DB, Camann DE, *et al*. Contemporary-use pesticides in personal air samples during pregnancy and blood samples at delivery among urban minority mothers and newborns. *Environ Health Perspect* 2003;**111**:749–56.

39 Arbuckle TE, Lin Z, Mery LS, Curtis KM. An exploratory analysis of the effect of pesticide exposure on the risk of spontaneous abortion in an Ontario farm population. *Environ Health Perspect* 2001;**109**:851–7.

40 Garry VF, Harkins M, Lybuvimov A, Erickson L, Long L. Reproductive outcomes in the women of the Red River Valley of the North. The spouses of pesticide applicators: pregnancy loss, age at menarche and exposures to pesticides. *J Toxicol Environ Health* 2002;**65**:769–86.

41 Hemminki K, Mutanen P, Luoma K, Saloniemi I. Congenital malformations by the parental occupation in Finland. *Int Arch Occup Environ Health* 1980;**46**:93–8.

42 Garry VF, Schreinemachers D, Harkins ME, Griffith J. Pesticide appliers, biocides and birth defects in rural Minnesota. *Environ Health Perspect* 1996;**104**:394–9.

43 Engel LS, O'Meara ES, Schwartz SM. Maternal occupation in agriculture and risk of adverse birth outcomes in Washington state, 1980–1991. *Am J Epidemiol* 2000;**26**:193–8.

44 Kristensen P, Ingens LM, Andersen A, Bye A, Sundheim L. Gestational age, birth weight, and perinatal death among births to Norwegian farmers, 1967–1991. *Am J Epidemiol* 1997;**146**:329–38.

45 Young JG, Eskenazi B, Gladstone EA, *et al*. Association between *in utero* organophosphate pesticide exposure and abnormal reflexes in neonates. *Neurotoxicol* 2005;**26**:199–209.

46 Daniels JL, Olshan AF, Savitz DA. Pesticides and childhood cancers. *Environ Health Perspect* 1997;**105**:1068–77.

47 Zahm SH, Ward MH. Pesticides and childhood cancer. *Environ Health Perspect* 1998;**106**:893–908.

48 Reynolds P, Von Behren J, Gunier RB, Goldberg DE, Harnly M, Hertz A. Agricultural pesticide use and childhood cancer in California. *Epidemiology* 2005;**16**:93–100.

49 DeKoning EP, Karmaus W. PCB exposure *in utero* and via breastmilk: a review. *J Expo Anal Environ Epidemiol* 2000;**10**:285–93.

50 Hertz-Picciotto I, Charles MJ, James RA, Keller JA, Willman E, Teplin S. *In utero* polychlorinated biphenyl exposure in relation to fetal and early childhood growth. *Epidemiology* 2005;**16**:648–56.

51 Longnecker MP, Klebanoff MA, Brock JW, Guo X. Maternal levels of polychlorinated biphenyls in relation to preterm and small for gestational age birth. *Epidemiology* 2005;**16**:641–7.

52 Daniels JL, Longnecker MP, Klebanoff MA, *et al*. Prenatal exposure to low level polychlorinated biphenyls in relation to mental and motor development at 8 months. *Am J Epidemiol* 2003;**157**:485–92.

53 Gray KA, Klebanoff MA, Brock JW, *et al*. *In utero* exposure to background levels of polychlorinated biphenyls and cognitive functioning among school age children. *Am J Epidemiol* 2005;**162**:17–26.

54 Gladen BC, Rogan WJ. Effects of perinatal polychlorinated biphenyls and dichlorodiphenyl dichloroethene on later development. *J Pediatr* 1991;**119**:58–63.

55 Vreugdenhil HJI, Lanting CI, Mulder PGH, Boersma ER, Weisglas-Kuperus N. Effects of prenatal PCB and dioxin background exposure on cognitive and motor abilities in Dutch children at school age. *J Pediatr* 2002;**140**:48–56.

56 Jacobsen JL, Jacobsen SW. Perinatal exposure to polychlorinated biphenyls and attention at school age. *J Pediatr* 2003;**143**:780–8.

57 Katthak S, K-Moghtader G, McMartin K, Barrera M, Kennedy D, Koren G. Pregnancy outcome following gestational exposure to organic solvents. *JAMA* 1999;**281**:1106–9.

58 Laslo-Baker D, Barrera M, Knittel-Keren D, *et al*. Child neurodevelopment outcome and maternal occupational exposure to solvents. *Arch Pediatr Adolesc Med* 2004;**158**:956–61.

59 Till C, Westall CA, Koren G, Nulman I, Rovet JF. Vision abnormalities in young children exposed prenatally to organic solvents. *Neurotoxicology* 2005;**26**:599–613.

60 Scheeres JJ, Chudley AE. Solvent abuse in pregnancy: a perinatal perspective. *J Obstet Gynaecol Can* 2002;**24**:22–6.

61 Gold EB, Tomich E. Occupational hazards to fertility and pregnancy outcome. *Occup Med (Lond)* 1994;**9**:435–69.

62 Blackwell R, Chang A. Video display terminals and pregnancy: a review. *Br J Obstet Gynaecol* 1988;**95**:446–53.

63 Rothenberg SJ, Manalo M, Jiang J, *et al*. Maternal blood lead level during pregnancy in South Central Los Angeles. *Arch Environ Health* 1999;**54**:151–7.

5 Medications in pregnancy and lactation

Catalin S. Buhimschi and Carl P. Weiner

Almost 100% of pregnant women are exposed to medications during pregnancy [1]. While thousands of pregnant and breastfeeding women ingest either a prescribed or over-the-counter (OTC) drug preparation daily, the study of medication use in pregnancy is one of the least developed areas of clinical pharmacology and drug research. Caregivers are encouraged to seek updated reference material such as *Drugs For Pregnant and Lactating Women* (Churchill Livingston, 2004) whose electronic version is updated yearly and refer to it frequently when making a prescribing decision.

Physiologic changes during pregnancy and drug clearance

The effect of any medication used during pregnancy reflects the dose and route of delivery, the plasma level achieved, its distribution, the availability and coupling of its effector mechanism, its clearance, and the physiologic adaptations of pregnancy that can alter these properties (Table 5.1) [2]. Plasma volume begins to rise in early gestation, and reaches almost 140% in the third trimester [3,4]. There are also increases in extracellular space and total body water which vary with body mass index (BMI) [5]. Thus, dilution may explain some of the effects of pregnancy on drug efficacy.

Cardiac output and renal glomerular filtration rates (GFRs) rise early in gestation [6]. There is also a change in the distribution of cardiac output; the percent delivered to the liver, crucial for drug disposal, and to skeletal muscle, decline during pregnancy [7]. These adaptations of normal pregnancy can increase the clearance of drugs excreted by the kidney, but decrease clearance that is predominantly hepatic. Gastric emptying and gastrointestinal transit slow, reducing the absorption of some drugs.

A large number of drugs are bound by albumin, which normally declines during pregnancy, increasing their availability. In the absence of binding to albumin, the clearance of a drug is increased and this may interfere with achieving a therapeutic drug level [8]. In addition to the decrease in albumin, pregnancy causes a partially compensated respiratory alkalosis, which also may affect the protein binding of some drugs.

Teratogens

Teratogens are agents that act during embryonic or fetal development to permanently alter growth, structure, or function. Currently recognized teratogens include viruses (e.g., rubella), environmental factors (e.g., hyperthermia, irradiation), chemicals (e.g., mercury, alcohol), and therapeutic drugs (e.g., thalidomide, isotretinoin).

Time of exposure

A teratogen acts during a critical period of embryonic (*embryopathy*) or fetal (*fetopathy*) development. The pre-implantation period is the 2 weeks between fertilization and implantation. Traditionally, this window is believed to be an "all or nothing" period because the injury of a large number of cells will inevitably cause an embryonic loss. However, if only a small number of cells are disrupted, a phenomenon called *compensation* can facilitate survival without malformation [9]. In contrast, a teratogenic agent can cause malformation during organogenesis (2–8 weeks postconception). Yet, the fetus (9 weeks postconception, 11 menstrual weeks through to delivery) can also be affected by alterations in structure and function of the organs which have initially developed normally during embryogenesis.

Factors involved in determining the nature of teratogens

Because most drugs reach the fetus via the maternal bloodstream, fetal exposure depends on the gestational age at the time of exposure, absorption of the drug, maternal serum levels, and/or maternal and placental clearance system. The

Table 5.1 Effects of pregnancy on organ systems and drug pharmacokinetics.

Organ		↑↓	Affects	Mechanism	PK/PD	Gestational age/timing of major effects
Cardiovascular system	Plasma volume	↑	Drug conc.		↑ Volume of distribution	Week 6–3rd trimester
	Albumin	↓	Drug protein binding	↓ Synthesis (partly)	↑ Unbound drug plasma conc.	NS†
Lung	Respiratory alkalosis		Drug protein binding		↑ Drug unbound plasma concentrations	NS
Heart	Cardiac output	↑				Gestation–10 wks & labor
Kidney	Glomerular filtration rate	↑	Creatinine/insulin clearance	↑ CO (partly)	↑ Drug clearance	6 wks–3rd trimester
	Diuresis	↑			↑ Drug clearance	96 h postpartum
GI tract	Gastric emptying/pH	↑		↓ Acid production	↓ Drug bioavailability	NS
	Intestinal transit time	↓				NS
Epithelial tissues	PXR	↔*	CYP, Pgp, MRP, BCRP	Estrogen-induced PXR transcription	↑ Drug metabolism, tissue efflux	NS

BCRP, breast cancer resistance protein; CYP, cytochrome-P450; MRP, multidrug resistance-associated protein; PD, pharmacodynamics; Pgp, P-glycoprotein; PK, pharmacokinetics; PXR, pregnane X receptor.

* Tissue-dependent.

† No specific time period, unknown, or not studied.

delivery of a teratogenic drug to the fetus requires placental passage. The placenta contains numerous transporters, some of which appear specifically dedicated to the removal of xenobiotic and toxic endogenous compounds [10]. Most substances with molecular mass below 500 daltons diffuse rapidly across the placental tissue, while agents of higher molecular weight have more variable transplacental passage rates. Ionization and high fat solubility (anesthetic gases) ensure rapid transplacental transfer of these drugs by simple diffusion. Steroid hormones directly influence the expression and function of some of these transporters. Investigating the relationship between hormones and drug efflux transporters may provide a deeper understanding of placental drug transfer and the consequent fetal drug exposure [11]. Of particular interest is the manipulation of transporter activity proteins to optimize the fetal therapeutic impact.

The increased circulating sex hormone levels characteristic of pregnancy have a profound impact on at least some drug metabolizing enzymes, drug bioavailability, and receptor coupling. Genetic variation is also a relevant determinant of drug clearance in both pregnant and nonpregnant women. The effect of pregnancy on the systems subject to genetic variation is likely to impact on dose and efficacy. Several drug groups whose metabolic pathways are known for genetic heterogeneity are widely used during pregnancy and changes in their clearances are reported [12–15]. Traditionally, maternal and fetal factors are considered responsible for drug teratogenicity. However, paternal exposure to certain drugs or environmental factors may also increase the risk of fetal teratogenicity. Induction of gene mutations early in the sperm development is one of the postulated mechanisms. Some of these effects are epigenetic in behavior, being transmitted to second and third generations [16].

FDA pregnancy safety category

Obstetric caregivers often rely on Food and Drug Administration (FDA) pregnancy safety categories (A, B, C, D, or X) (Table 5.2) before making a decision to initiate, continue, discontinue,

Table 5.2 Pregnancy drug categories from several countries.

Category	Pregnancy Category Definition
FDA Category (USA)	
A*	Adequate, well-controlled studies in pregnant women have not shown any risk to the fetus in the first 3 months of pregnancy, nor is there evidence of later risk *Very few medications have been tested to this level*
B†	There have been no adequate, well-controlled studies in women but studies using animals have not found any risk to the fetus, or animal studies have found risk that was not confirmed by adequate studies in pregnant women *Not many adequate studies have been performed in pregnant women, so the first situation (not enough information) usually applies if a medication is assigned to this category*
C†	There have been no adequate, well-controlled studies in women, but studies using animals have shown a harmful effect on the fetus, or there have not been any studies in either women or animals. Caution is advised, but the benefits of the medication may outweigh the potential risks
D‡	There is clear evidence of risk to the human fetus, but the benefits may outweigh the risk for pregnant women who have a serious condition that cannot be treated effectively with a safer drug
X‡	There is clear evidence that the medication causes abnormalities in the fetus. The risks outweigh any potential benefits for women who are (or may become) pregnant
FASS Category (Sweden)	
A*	Drugs taken by a large number of pregnant women with no proven increase in the frequency of malformations or other observed harmful effects on the fetus
B1*	Limited experience in pregnant women, no increase observed in the frequency of malformations or other observed harmful effects on the fetus Animal studies reassuring
B2*	Limited experience in pregnant women, no increase observed in the frequency of malformations or other harmful effects on the fetus Animal studies inadequate or lacking
B3†	Limited experience in pregnant women, no increase observed in the frequency of malformations or other harmful effects on the fetus Animal studies have shown evidence of an increased occurrence of fetal damage
C†	May cause pharmacologic adverse effects on the fetus or neonate
D‡	Suspected or proven to cause malformations or other irreversible damage
ADEC Category (Australia)	
A–D	Categories A,a B1,a B2,a B3,b C,b Dc similar to the FASS definitions
X‡	Limited experience in pregnant women, no increase observed in the frequency of malformations or other observed harmful effects on the fetus Animal studies reassuring

ADEC, Australian Drug Evaluation Committee (Australian categorization); FASS, Farmaceutiska Specialiteter i Sverige (Swedish categorization); FDA, Food and Drug Administration (US categorization).

* Drugs grouped as probably safe.

† Drugs grouped as potentially harmful.

‡ Drugs grouped as clearly harmful.

or replace a medication. However, only approximately 30 drugs or drug groups are known or strongly suspected to be teratogens (Table 5.3). Although major congenital abnormalities complicate 2–3% of all pregnancies, less than 10% of these (<0.2%) can be associated with a particular drug exposure.

The pregnancy risk categories are suboptimal: many are outdated, and are too superficial to account for the physiology and health care needs of pregnant and breastfeeding women. They are rarely revised as new information becomes available. Although there are commonalities among the classifications

Table 5.3 Drugs or drug groups known or strongly suspected to cause developmental defects, and their pregnancy safety categorization (see Table 5.1 for an explanation of the safety categories). After Weiner [17].

Drug	FASS	ADEC	FDA
Agents acting on renin–angiotensin system B (1st trimester), D (2nd and 3rd trimesters)	D	D	C
Antiepileptic drugs (valproic acid, carbamazepine, phenytoin)	D	D	D
Alkylating agents	D	D	D
Androgens	No code	D	X
Antimetabolites	D	D	D, X
Carbimazole	No code	C	D
Coumarin derivatives	D	D	X
Fluconazole (doses used in systemic mycoses)	B3	B3	C
Lithium	D	D	D
Misoprostol	D	X	X
Penicillamine	No code	D	D
Retinoids	D	X	X
Thalidomide	No code	No code	X

ADEC, Australian Drug Evaluation Committee (Australian categorization); FASS, Farmaceutiska Specialiteter i Sverige (Swedish categorization); FDA, Food and Drug Administration (US categorization).

used by industrialized countries, subjective interpretations of the same data can lead to disparate classifications. Two-thirds of all drugs sold in the USA are classified Category C, and less than 1% are Category A (i.e., shown to be safe during pregnancy). With the benefit of added experience, usually obtained after the drug has been marketed, we find that some Category X drugs are not absolutely contraindicated during pregnancy, and several Category C or D drugs are either clear human teratogens or have frequent and serious adverse fetal effects [17]. The result is often confusion among drug prescribers. So, what information is needed to assess the teratogenic risk of a given drug?

Evaluation of teratogenicity

Teratology is the study of the biologic mechanisms and causes of abnormal development as well as the study of appropriate preventative measures. While most organs develop during the first trimester, some, like the central nervous system (CNS), continue to develop throughout fetal life and even after birth. Many, if not most, potent human teratogens act during very specific developmental stages. For example, angiotensin-converting enzyme (ACE) inhibitors (e.g., enalapril) cross the placenta but have no adverse effects during the first trimester. However, later exposure is associated with cranial hypoplasia, irreversible renal failure, patent ductus arteriosus, or death. Thalidomide is another known human teratogen causing limb, face, and ears abnormalities after first trimester exposure. Similarly, nonsteroidal anti-inflammatory agents (NSAIDs; e.g., indomethacin, ibuprofen) may be associated with gastroschisis and other fetal sequelae are common

after 32 weeks (irreversible closure of the ductus or kidney failure).

The finding of a neonatal birth defect raises concern as to whether it was the consequence of prenatal exposure to a teratogen. Patients, drug prescribers, and policymakers often assume that the most serious short-term adverse effects of a drug are identified in premarketing studies, so recognition of unexpected harm after widespread use raises concern about "failures of the system" [18]. The unfortunate reality is that we learn about virtually all teratogenic effects only after a drug has already received marketing approval. Often, animal studies are seriously limited in their ability to predict human teratogenesis because of considerable variations in species-specific effects, even among mammalian species. Furthermore, teratogens are rarely detected in the human trials conducted before approval for marketing because most studies are too small and typically exclude women at reproductive ages, particularly if there is any suspicion a drug might be teratogenic generated by the preceding animal studies.

Two main approaches are used to identify teratogens: follow-up studies and case–control surveillance [18]. The former, often called "pregnancy registries," are developed to permit the efficient identification of drugs that are high-risk teratogens (or drugs that put a child at high risk for other common adverse pregnancy outcomes, such as developmental delay). For these purposes, a small number of patients will suffice. There is concern that pregnancy registries are often operated by drug manufacturers, and patients receiving multiple drugs may be recruited into multiple, uncoordinated registries.

Case–control surveillance studies developed as a system to identify serious illnesses caused by medications used in an ambulatory population [19]. By including information on infants with any of a wide range of specific birth defects and interviews with the mothers focusing on details of their antenatal exposure to all prescription and OTC medications (including herbal products), case–control surveillance studies can provide opportunities to examine large numbers of specific defects in relation to the wide range of medications taken by pregnant women.

Breastfeeding

Medication use by breastfeeding women may be beneficial, and even essential, for the health of mother and child. Although very few medications are contraindicated by breastfeeding, there are few data on the risk of most medications used in human pregnancy and lactation at the time they are initially marketed [20]. Many therapeutic and environmental substances can be transferred into the milk and for these the risk of breastfeeding may be exceeded by its great benefit to the infant, mother, or both [21]. Passive diffusion, lipid solubility, protein binding, and the degree of ionization are mechanisms governing the transfer of drugs across the basal membrane of the mammary gland alveoli.

Several studies have investigated drug concentrations in breastmilk [22]. The ideal information on breastfeeding exposure includes the weight-corrected percent of the maternal dose ingested by the unsupplemented 3-kg newborn and the resulting neonatal blood levels. Unfortunately, this information is reported for very few agents. More often, only a milk : maternal plasma (M : P) ratio or concentration is reported, which is often misleading as it ignores the quantity ingested and its oral bioavailability. Designing studies to quantify the amount of drug passed to the neonate and provide clinically reliable recommendations based on infant clearance, which is itself dependent on the ontogeny of elimination pathways and pharmacogenetics, are critically needed.

Research into environmentally related chemical contaminants in breastmilk remains an important field [23]. Diet is one major factor influencing breastmilk levels of organic pollutants (e.g., mercury in fish). Improved global breastmilk monitoring programs would allow for more consistent data on trends over time, the detection of xenobiotics in breastmilk, and the identification of disproportionately exposed populations.

Drugs with known human teratogenic effect

A list of medication drugs known to be human teratogens is provided in Table 5.3.

Agents acting on renin–angiotensin system ACE-I/A2R-antagonists; antihypertensives (enalapril, captopril, lisinopril)

Maternal considerations

There are no adequate reports or well-controlled studies in pregnant women because these agents are contraindicated. ACE inhibitors should not be used in pregnancy. In exceptional cases, they may be indicated for the control of severe hypertension when the patient is refractory to other medications [24]. Use of ACE inhibitors during the second and third trimesters of pregnancy is contraindicated because of their association with an increased risk of fetopathy. However, most recently it was also demonstrated that exposure to ACE inhibitors during the first trimester cannot be considered safe and should also be avoided [25]. Infants exposed to ACE inhibitors were at increased risk for malformations of the cardiovascular system and the central nervous system. Improved pregnancy outcome was noted in mothers treated prenatally with low doses of captopril, especially patients with insulin-dependent diabetes [26]. The lowest dose effective should be used when captopril is required during pregnancy [27]. In such situations, close monitoring of amniotic fluid and fetal well-being is recommended [28]. If oligohydramnios is detected, lisinopril should be discontinued unless life-saving for the mother.

Fetal considerations

There are no adequate reports or well-controlled studies in human fetuses. Lisinopril and enalapril cross the human placenta [29,30]. In humans, first trimester exposure appears reasonably safe. Later exposure to ACE inhibitors is associated with cranial hypoplasia, anuria, reversible or irreversible renal failure, death, oligohydramnios, prematurity, intrauterine growth restriction (IUGR), and patent ductus arteriosus [31]. The mechanism of renal dysfunction is likely related to fetal hypotension and prolonged decreased GFR. Antenatal surveillance should be initiated if there has been inadvertent exposure and the fetus is potentially viable. *Oligohydramnios* may not appear until after the fetus has irreversible injury. Neonates exposed *in utero* to ACE inhibitors should be observed closely for hypotension, oliguria, and hyperkalemia. If oliguria occurs despite adequate pressure and renal perfusion, exchange transfusion or peritoneal dialysis may be required [32].

Breastfeeding considerations

There are no adequate reports or well-controlled studies in nursing women. Trace amounts of enalapril are detected in breastmilk, although the kinetics remains to be elucidated [33]. Captopril is excreted in breastmilk at a very low concentration and is generally considered compatible with breastfeeding [34]. It is unknown whether lisinopril enters human breastmilk. Until further study, the infant should be monitored for possible adverse effects, the drug given at the lowest effective dose, and breastfeeding avoided at times of peak drug levels if breastfeeding continues.

Antiepileptic drugs (valproic acid, carbamazepine, phenytoin)

Maternal considerations

Valproate is the sodium salt of valproic acid. There are no adequate reports or well-controlled studies of valproate or carbamazepine in pregnant women. There is long clinical experience with valproate, which does not alter the efficacy of hormonal contraception [35]. Phenytoin is a first generation, enzyme-inducing anticonvulsant. Stable phenytoin serum levels are achieved in most pregnant women, although there is wide variability with equivalent doses [36]. Patients with unusually low levels may be either noncompliant or hypermetabolizers. Unusually high levels can result from hepatic disease, congenital enzyme deficiency, or other drugs that interfere with metabolism. Clearance of phenytoin is increased during pregnancy, with concentrations declining to half of prepregnancy if the dose is not adjusted. Dose adjustments should be based on clinical symptoms, and not solely on serum drug concentrations. Phenytoin may impair the effect of corticosteroids, Coumadin, digitoxin, doxycycline, estrogens, furosemide, oral contraceptives, quinidine, rifampin, theophylline, and vitamin D [37]. Drug interactions between enzyme-inducing anticonvulsants such as phenytoin and contraceptives are well documented. Either a higher dose of oral contraceptive or a second contraceptive method is recommended. Patients planning pregnancy should be counseled on the risks and the importance of periconceptual folate supplementation [38].

Fetal considerations

Valproic acid is a recognized human teratogen, increasing the relative risk by a factor of 4 [39]. The risk is compounded by a low serum folate. Valproic acid is rapidly and actively transported across the human placenta reaching a fetal:maternal ratio exceeding 2 [40]. For unknown reasons, valproic acid accumulates in the fetal plasma. A distinct facial appearance, coupled with a cluster of minor and major anomalies and CNS dysfunction characterize the fetal valproate syndrome [41,42]. The likelihood of an affected offspring is dose-dependent. Ten percent die in infancy, and 1 of 4 survivors have either developmental deficits or mental retardation. Affected fetuses may have an increased nuchal translucency measurement [43]. A maternal–fetal

medicine specialist should evaluate women taking valproic acid during pregnancy. Carbamazepine rapidly crosses the human placenta, and accumulates in fetal organs including the brain. Epidemiologic study suggests carbamazepine is a teratogen causing facial dysmorphism, spina bifida, distal phalange hypoplasia, and developmental delay [44]. Carbamazepine increased the rate of neural tube, cardiovascular, urinary tract, and cleft palate anomalies. Phenytoin is specifically associated with congenital heart defects, and cleft palate. There is evidence that a phenytoin-induced embryonic arrhythmia is one mechanism of teratogenicity. As for most psychotropic drugs, monotherapy and the lowest effective quantity given in divided doses to minimize the peaks can theoretically minimize the risks [45].

Breastfeeding considerations

Valproic acid enters human breastmilk, but the neonatal concentration is less than 10% that of maternal concentration [46]. Carbamazepine is excreted in human breastmilk. Although it is generally considered safe for breastfeeding women, neonatal sequelae reported include cholestatic hepatitis. The infant should be monitored for possible adverse effects, the drug given at the lowest effective dose, and breastfeeding avoided at times of peak drug levels. The transfer of phenytoin into human breastmilk appears relatively low and it is generally considered safe for breastfeeding [47].

Alkylating agents (cyclophosphamide)

Maternal considerations

Cyclophosphamide is an alkylating agent used to treat cancer of the ovary, breast, and blood and lymph systems. Transient sterility is common after cyclophosphamide, and there is a risk of secondary malignancy. There are no adequate reports or well-controlled studies in pregnant women. There are multiple case reports suggesting it can be used with a good pregnancy outcome [48–50].

Fetal considerations

Cyclophosphamide crosses the human placenta. Population studies have demonstrated neonatal hematologic suppression and secondary malignancies in the offspring are reported [51,52].

Breastfeeding considerations

Cyclophosphamide enters human breastmilk in high concentration and is generally considered not compatible with breastfeeding. Neonatal neutropenia has been reported [53,54].

Hormones: androgens (methyl-testosterone, medroxyprogesterone acetate)

Maternal considerations

Methyl-testosterone is used with modest results for the treatment of endometriosis in infertile women, palliation with advancing inoperable breast cancer, and also in combination with estrogen to enhance libido in women [55]. Numerous pregnant women are exposed to medroxyprogesterone because many pregnancies will not be recognized until after the first trimester [56]. Progestational agents (i.e., not native progesterone) such as medroxyprogesterone were long used during early pregnancy to prevent first trimester spontaneous abortion. The wisdom of this practice cannot be substantiated. While there are no adequate reports or well-controlled studies of medroxyprogesterone in pregnant women, epidemiologic studies are reassuring and there is not demonstrable increase in the prevalence of ectopic pregnancy.

Fetal considerations

There are no adequate reports or well-controlled studies in human fetuses. It is unknown whether methyl-testosterone crosses the human placenta, and animal studies (rodents, dog) reveal pseudohermaphroditism in female fetuses exposed to methyl-testosterone [57]. Animal studies show that *in utero* exposure of male fetuses to methyl-testosterone increases the risk of hypospadias [58,59], but not limb development and endochondral ossification [60]. While in humans there are insufficient data to quantify the risk for the female fetus, some synthetic progestins may cause mild virilization of the external genitalia [61,62]. Defects outside the external genitalia are not noted in either humans or rodents. First trimester exposure is an indication for a detailed anatomic ultrasound at 18–22 weeks' gestation.

Breastfeeding considerations

It is unknown whether methyl-testosterone enters human breastmilk. It is ineffective for suppressing lactation. Trace amounts of medroxyprogesterone are excreted into human breastmilk [63]. It does not appear to either suppress lactation or affect the nursing newborn [64]. It is typically given for contraception 3 days after delivery because progesterone withdrawal may be one stimulus for the initiation of lactogenesis.

Hormones: estrogens (diethylstilbestrol—DES)

Maternal considerations

Diethylstilbestrol was administered to approximately 3 million pregnant women in the USA and in the Netherlands between 1947 and 1975 [65]. There was an increased risk of mammary carcinomas in exposed women [66].

Fetal considerations

There are no adequate reports or well-controlled studies in human fetuses. Diethylstilbestrol exposed daughters frequently have developmental disorders of the cervix and corpus uteri (hypoplasia of the uterine cavity, uterine corpus, and cervix; T-shaped uterine cavity, constrictions of the uterine cavity, and bilateral hydrosalpinges) [67]. They have an increased risk of spontaneous abortion, ectopic pregnancy, and infertility, and possibly an increased risk of cervical incompetence. Spontaneous uterine rupture at term has also been described [68]. An increased risk of hypospadias in male fetuses exposed to diethylstilbestrol *in utero* was reported [69]. Rodent experiments reveal that diethylstilbestrol increases the incidence of genital tumors in not only second generation, but also third generation animals. However, recent studies report no increased risk of lower genital tract abnormalities in third generation women [70].

Breastfeeding considerations

Estrogens are contraindicated for lactation suppression. Diethylstilbestrol does not effectively suppress lactation [71].

Antimetabolites (methotrexate)

Maternal considerations

Methotrexate is an antimetabolite with multiple uses in reproductive-age women including the treatment of ectopic pregnancy, neoplastic disease, autoimmune disorders, and inflammatory conditions [72]. Methotrexate has been used to induce a medical abortion of an intrauterine pregnancy. It is more effective combined with misoprostol than alone [73]. As it is not 100% effective, women must be followed clinically until there is complete normalization of beta human chorionic gonadotropin (beta-hCG) titers from their serum [74,75].

Fetal considerations

There are no adequate reports or well-controlled studies in human fetuses. First trimester exposure results in an increased risk of internal and external malformations (craniofacial, axial skeletal, cardiopulmonary, and gastrointestinal abnormalities) and developmental delay, although most pregnancies exposed to low doses are successful [76,77]. Others report no association between later pregnancy exposure and congenital abnormalities [78].

Breastfeeding considerations

There are no adequate reports or well-controlled studies in nursing women. It is unknown whether methotrexate enters human breastmilk. Despite the lack of information, methotrexate is generally considered contraindicated in nursing mothers [79].

Antithyroid (methimazole-carbimazole)

Maternal considerations

The most common cause of maternal hyperthyroidism during pregnancy is Graves' disease. The mainstay of treatment is an antithyroid drug, either propylthiouracil (PTU) or methimazole [80,81]. Thyroid function tests should be obtained during gestation in women with hyperthyroidism and the dose of PTU or methimazole adjusted accordingly to keep 3,5,3'-triiodothyronine (T3) and thyroxine (T4) within the upper normal range for these women [82]. The lowest effective dose is recommended. Women previously treated with either a radioactive cocktail or thyroidectomy may still be producing thyroid-stimulating immunoglobulin even though they are themselves euthyroid. If the level is elevated, the fetus is at risk and should be referred to a fetal center for evaluation [83].

Fetal considerations

There are no adequate reports or well-controlled studies in human fetuses. Methimazole crosses the human placenta and is an alternative to PTU for the treatment of fetal hyperthyroidism secondary to thyroid-stimulating immunoglobulin [84]. The fetal response is often different to the maternal and some recommend it be tested directly. Methimazole can induce fetal goiter and even cretinism in a dose-dependent fashion. Recent studies of exposed children followed until 3–11 years reveal no deleterious effects on either thyroid function or physical and intellectual development with doses up to 20 mg/day. However, rare instances of aplasia cutis (manifest as scalp defects), esophageal atresia with tracheoesophageal fistula, and choanal atresia with absent/hypoplastic nipples (methimazole syndrome) are reported, suggesting methimazole may be a weak human teratogen. This reinforces the designation of PTU as the drug of choice [85,86].

Breastfeeding considerations

Methimazole is excreted in human breastmilk, but the kinetics remain to be clarified [87]. PTU is the drug of choice in this situation, because it does not cross membranes readily, and milk concentrations are therefore quite low [88]. Several recent studies observe no deleterious effects on neonatal thyroid function or on physical and intellectual development of breastfed infants whose mothers were treated with this medication [89].

Coumarin derivatives (warfarin)

Maternal considerations

Thromboembolic disease remains a major cause of maternal morbidity and mortality. There are no adequate reports or well-controlled studies of warfarin in pregnant women. It is most likely that a woman with a prior thromboembolic event unrelated to a permanent risk factor does not require prophylaxis during a subsequent pregnancy [90]. The risk of a bleeding complication during pregnancy approximates 18% with warfarin. An international normalized ratio (INR) of 3.0 is sufficient for either prophylaxis or treatment of venous thromboembolism, thus minimizing the risk of hemorrhage associated with higher INRs [91]. Women on warfarin planning pregnancy should switch to a heparinoid agent immediately after conception if possible. However, therapeutic heparin is not effective prophylaxis in women with a prosthetic heart valve [92]. In this instance, it is best to continue warfarin, although some recommend replacement with heparin at 6–12 weeks [93]. A daily dose >5 mg is associated with a greater risk of an adverse outcome. If the mother's condition requires anticoagulation with warfarin, it should be substituted with heparin at 36 weeks to decrease the risk to the fetus. Neuraxial anesthesia is contraindicated because of the risk of puncture-associated bleeding [94]. Warfarin treatment should be resumed postpartum.

Fetal considerations

Warfarin is a known teratogen. While there are no adequate reports or well-controlled studies in human fetuses, exposure at 6–10 weeks' gestation is associated with an embryopathy, and exposure subsequently with a fetopathy. The fetal warfarin syndrome includes nasal hypoplasia (failure of nasal septum development), microphthalmia, hypoplasia of the extremities, IUGR, heart disease, scoliosis, deafness, and mental retardation [95,96]. While the embryopathy appears secondary to a fetal vitamin K deficiency, the fetopathy results from microhemorrhages. The most common CNS malformations include agenesis of the corpus callosum, Dandy–Walker malformation, and optic atrophy. In a large series of women treated the duration of pregnancy for a prosthetic valve, the overall incidence of fetal warfarin syndrome was 5.6% [92]. The pregnancy loss rate was 32% and the stillbirth rate 10% of pregnancies achieving at least 20 weeks. School-age children exposed *in utero* have an increased frequency of mild neurologic dysfunction and an IQ <80 [97].

Breastfeeding considerations

Warfarin does not enter human breastmilk and is compatible with breastfeeding [98,99].

Fluconazole

Maternal considerations

There are no adequate reports or well-controlled studies of fluconazole in pregnant women. It has been used for the treatment of coccidioidomycosis during pregnancy and *Candida* sepsis postpartum [100].

Fetal considerations

There are no adequate reports or well-controlled studies in human fetuses. It is unknown whether fluconazole crosses the human placenta. A few children have been described with a similar and rare pattern of anomalies following fluconazole use. The features include brachycephaly, abnormal facies, abnormal calvarial development, cleft palate, femoral bowing, thin ribs and long bones, arthrogryposis, and congenital heart disease [101]. Each case was associated with chronic, parenteral use in the first trimester. Limited duration oral therapy is unlikely to pose a teratogenic risk. Fluconazole does not appear to increase the risks of IUGR or preterm delivery. It has been used for the treatment of congenital candidiasis [102].

Breastfeeding considerations

There are no adequate reports or well-controlled studies in nursing women. Fluconazole enters human breastmilk at concentrations similar to maternal plasma [103]. It is generally recommended that breastfeeding be avoided.

Lithium

Maternal considerations

Lithium is used for the treatment of psychiatric disorders. It is typically inadequate for the rapid control of acute mania [104]. The usefulness of lithium lies in the long-term prevention of recurrent mania and bipolar depression and in reducing risk of suicidal behavior. Pregnancy and especially the puerperium are times of high risk for recurrence of bipolar disease. Recommendations during pregnancy include discontinuing therapy for at least the first trimester, switching to an agent with a higher safety profile (e.g., tricyclics), using smaller doses of lithium, and avoiding sodium restriction or diuretics while under treatment [105]. The dose used should be titered to maintain a serum level at 0.5–1.2 mEq/L [106]. Toxicity develops at 1.5–2.0 mEq/L. Ideally, the drug should be tapered gradually over a month. Lithium levels should be monitored weekly after 35 weeks' gestation, and therapy either discontinued or decreased by one-quarter 2–3 days before delivery.

Fetal considerations

Lithium crosses the placenta and may be a weak human teratogen [107]. Several studies note an increased prevalence of Ebstein's anomaly, although this was not confirmed in a prospective, multicenter study. A targeted ultrasound performed by a fetal medicine expert is suggested [108]. Other neonatal complications often attributed to lithium include poor respiratory effort and cyanosis, rhythm disturbances, nephrogenic diabetes insipidus, thyroid dysfunction and goiter, hypoglycemia, hypotonia and lethargy, polyhydramnios, hyperbilirubinemia, and large-for-gestational-age infant [109]. As a result, the delivery of a mother taking lithium should be considered a high-risk delivery. The results of long-term follow-up studies are reassuring. Lithium is associated with cleft palate in mice [110,111].

Breastfeeding considerations

Lithium is excreted into human milk and can be measured in the nursing newborn [112]. There is no agreement whether nursing mothers should continue lithium while breastfeeding [113]. There is a lack of prospective studies confounded by polypharmacy. The neonatal clearance rate is slower than in the adult; thus, the level of circulating drug might be much higher than expected. If lithium use must be continued during breastfeeding, it should be measured in the neonatal blood if any adverse effects are noted.

Misoprostol

Maternal considerations

Misoprostol is a prostaglandin E analog. The only FDA-approved indication is the treatment and prevention of intestinal ulcer disease resulting from NSAID use. Although still not approved by the FDA for other indications, misoprostol is well studied and widely used for both cervical ripening and the induction of labor during either the second or third trimesters [114]. Combined with mifepristone, misoprostol is safe and effective for medical termination of early pregnancy [115]. Misoprostol is effective in ripening the cervix and inducing labor at term. The manufacturer of misoprostol issued in August 2000 a warning letter to US health care providers, cautioning against the use of misoprostol in pregnant women secondary to the lack of safety data for its use in obstetric practice. The American College of Obstetricans and Gynecologists (ACOG) took issue with that position, as there was a multitude of studies supporting its use. In 2002, the ACOG Committee Opinion on Obstetric Practice concluded the risk of uterine rupture during vaginal birth after cesarean (VBAC) is substantially increased by the use of misoprostol as well as other prostaglandin cervical ripening agents [116].

Fetal considerations

There are no adequate reports or well-controlled studies in human fetuses. Misoprostol is associated with a higher rate of uterine hyperstimulation, more variable decelerations, and likely as a result, a higher prevalence of meconium [117]. However, compared with oxytocin, there is no increase in the incidence of cesarean delivery for fetal distress or umbilical acidemia. Congenital defects after extremely high-dose exposures during unsuccessful medical abortions have been reported. Several reports in the literature associate the use of misoprostol during the first trimester with skull defects, cranial nerve palsies, facial malformations, and limb defects [118].

Breastfeeding considerations

Orally administered misoprostol is secreted in colostrum, but it is essentially undetectable by 5 hours [119].

Penicillamine

Maternal considerations

There are no adequate reports or well-controlled studies in pregnant women. Penicillamine is contraindicated during pregnancy except for the treatment of Wilson's disease and some cases of cystinuria [120].

Fetal considerations

There are no adequate reports or well-controlled studies in human fetuses. Penicillamine apparently crosses the human placenta, because congenital cutis laxa and associated defects are reported in neonates of treated women. Adverse effects include skeletal deformities, cleft palate, and embryotoxicity [121].

Breastfeeding considerations

There is no published experience in nursing women. It is unknown whether penicillamine enters human breastmilk.

Retinoids (isotretinoin)

Maternal considerations

Isotretinoin is contraindicated during pregnancy. Patients must be capable of complying with mandatory contraceptive measures. Only manufacturer-approved physicians may prescribe it [122].

Fetal considerations

Isotretinoin and its active metabolites crosses the human (and subhuman primate) placenta and is a known human tera-togen. Multiple organ systems are affected including CNS, cardiovascular, and endocrine organs [123]. Mental retardation without external malformation has also been reported. Similar malformations occur in rodents.

Breastfeeding considerations

There is no published experience in nursing women. It is unknown whether isotretinoin enters human breastmilk. Considering its effect on the fetus, breastfeeding is considered contraindicated.

Thalidomide

Maternal considerations

Thalidomide is a known human teratogen and contraindicated during pregnancy [124]. It is also excreted in semen and treated males should wear a condom during coitus [125]. Initially banned in the USA, its potential indications are growing, increasing the likelihood of an inadvertent pregnancy. There are no adequate reports or well-controlled studies of thalidomide in pregnant women.

Fetal considerations

There are no adequate reports or well-controlled studies in human fetuses. Thalidomide crosses the placenta and is a potent human teratogen causing limb abnormalities after first trimester exposure [126]. Even a single 50-mg dose can cause defects [127]. If pregnancy occurs, the drug should be discontinued and the patient referred to a fetal medicine expert for evaluation and counseling. Any suspected fetal exposure to thalidomide must be reported to the FDA [124].

Breastfeeding considerations

There is no published experience in nursing women. It is unknown whether thalidomide enters human breastmilk.

Drugs with minimal or not known human teratogenic effect

Steroids (betamethasone, dexamethasone)

Maternal considerations

Betamethasone and dexamethasone are used widely for the acceleration of fetal lung maturity [128,129]. Steroids may increase the risk of maternal infection in women with preterm premature rupture of the fetal membranes (PPROM), although most large studies reveal no increased risk [130].

They can transiently cause an abnormal glucose tolerance test [131], will worsen existing diabetes mellitus, and are associated with pulmonary edema when given with a tocolytic agent in the setting of an underlying infection [132]. Dexamethasone does not reduce the maternal perception of fetal movements and short-term variability [133]. It is not contraindicated in women with severe preeclampsia requiring preterm delivery. Women chronically treated must be monitored closely for hypertension or glucose intolerance, and treated with stress replacement doses postoperatively and postpartum. Dexamethasone is an effective antiemetic for nausea and vomiting after general anesthesia for pregnancy termination [134]. There are reports that intravenous dexamethasone helps modify the clinical course of the so-called HELLP syndrome both ante and postpartum [135]. However, most recent data contradict such findings [136].

Fetal considerations

Betamethasone and dexamethasone cross the human placenta and are two of the few drugs proven to improve perinatal outcome [137]. An increased risk of neonatal sepsis was suggested but not confirmed. Multiple courses of betamethasone are not recommended [138]. Adverse effects noted in animal and human studies are magnified by repeated courses of steroids [139]. They include a profound suppression of fetal breathing, movement, impaired myelination, IUGR, and microcephaly [140]. The fetal heart rate pattern may become transiently nonreactive. Intellectual and motor development and school achievement are not adversely influenced by steroid treatment. Epidemiologic studies report an association between oral clefting and exposure to corticosteroids during organogenesis [141]. IUGR, shortening of the head and mandible are also suggested as sequelae of chronic steroid use during pregnancy, although it is difficult to separate drug from disease impact. The Collaborative Perinatal Project followed women treated during the first trimester. While the number of exposures was limited, no increase in congenital malformations was detected. There was no increase in risk of anomalies when steroids were initiated after organogenesis. Complete fetal heart block has been treated with dexamethasone during pregnancy with positive results [142]. Some studies suggest that in contrast to betamethasone, dexamethasone does not alter biophysical parameters of the fetus (i.e., fetal breathing) when administered for the enhancement of lung maturation [143]. However, oligohydramnios is reportedly more common. When initiated by 6–7 weeks, dexamethasone can prevent or diminish virilization resulting from congenital adrenal hyperplasia [144,145].

Breastfeeding considerations

There are no adequate reports or well-controlled studies in breastfeeding women. Cortisone is present in human milk, but it is unclear whether maternal treatment with betamethasone or dexamethasone increases the concentration [146].

Benzodiazepines (diazepam)

Maternal considerations

There are no adequate reports or well-controlled studies of diazepam in pregnant women. Diazepam is a beneficial adjunct to intravenous fluids and vitamins for the treatment of first trimester hyperemesis. Diazepam was previously used for prophylaxis and treatment of eclamptic convulsions, but proved less effective than magnesium sulfate [147–149]. Diazepam is a useful antianxietal in women undergoing fetal therapy procedures such as cordocentesis.

Fetal considerations

There are no adequate reports or well-controlled studies in human fetuses. Diazepam rapidly crosses the human placenta [150]. Several studies suggest an increased risk of fetal malformation when diazepam is used during the first trimester. These have not been confirmed subsequently. Postnatal follow-up until age 4 years is likewise reassuring, revealing no adverse effects on neurodevelopment. Decreased fetal movement frequently accompanies intravenous administration. Prolonged CNS depression may occur in neonates, apparently because of their inability to metabolize diazepam. The shortest course and the lowest dose should be used when indicated during pregnancy. Some newborns exposed antenatally exhibit either the floppy infant syndrome, or marked neonatal withdrawal symptoms [151]. Symptoms vary with mild sedation, hypotonia, reluctance to suck, apneic spells, cyanosis, and impaired metabolic responses to cold stress. Such symptoms may persist for hours to months after birth.

Breastfeeding considerations

Diazepam and other benzodiazepines are excreted into human breastmilk [152]. The maximum neonatal exposure is estimated at 3% of the maternal dose. Problems may arise if the neonate is premature, or the maternal dose particularly high. Neonatal lethargy, sedation, and weight loss have been reported.

Antidepressants (fluoxetine, sertraline)

Maternal considerations

Depression is common during and after pregnancy, but typically goes unrecognized. Pregnancy is not a reason a priori to discontinue psychotropic drugs [153]. Fluoxetine is effective treatment for postpartum depression, and is as effective as a course of cognitive–behavioral counseling in the short term

[154]. There are no adequate reports or well-controlled studies of sertraline in pregnant women, although there is growing experience with its use for the treatment of postpartum depression [154]. In general, women taking selective serotonin reuptake inhibitors (SSRIs) during pregnancy for depression require an increased dose to maintain euthymia [155].

Fetal considerations

There are no adequate reports or well-controlled studies in human fetuses. Fluoxetine and sertraline cross the human placenta [156]. Maternal doses predict the umbilical cord concentration. Prospectively ascertained pregnancy outcomes after SSRIs, mainly fluoxetine and sertraline, reveal no teratogenic effect. Maternal use of high doses of fluoxetine throughout pregnancy may be associated with a risk for low birthweight [157]. Exposure throughout gestation does not adversely affect cognition, language development, or the temperament of preschool and early school-age children. *In utero* exposure to novel antipsychotics has not been associated with congenital malformations; however, the data are still limited [158]. Previous cohort study suggested a possible association between maternal use of the SSRI fluoxetine late in the third trimester of pregnancy and the risk of persistent pulmonary hypertension of the newborn (PPHN) in the infant. Small studies (only 14 infants) support an association between the maternal use of SSRIs in late pregnancy and PPHN in the offspring, and thus further study of this association is warranted [159].

Breastfeeding considerations

Maternal serum and peak breastmilk concentrations of fluoxetine and its active metabolite, norfluoxetine, predict nursing infant serum norfluoxetine concentrations. Breastfeeding is not contraindicated with either fluoxetine or sertraline [160]. If breastfed, the infant should be monitored for possible adverse effects, the drug given at the lowest effective dose, and breastfeeding avoided at times of peak drug levels. All psychotropic medications are transferred to breastmilk in varying amounts, and thus are passed on to the nursing infant. In theory, discarding breastmilk obtained at the time of peak drug concentration could allow the mother to reduce the infant's exposure to her medication; however, it is often impractical to do this [160].

Analgesics (aspirin, acetaminophen, ibuprofen, propoxyphene)

Maternal considerations

Aspirin is a potent drug with complex and still unclear mechanisms of action. Women ingesting large quantities of aspirin are at risk for myriad complications (gastrointestinal lesions, renal or hepatic dysfunction, asthma, hypoprothrombinemia, tachypnea, hyperthermia, lethargia) [161]. In a recent prospective case–control study, prenatal use of ibuprofen, naproxen, and possibly aspirin but not acetaminophen increased the risk of spontaneous abortion [162]. These findings need confirmation in studies designed specifically to examine the apparent association. The association was stronger if the initial use was around conception or if it lasted more than a week. Chronically high salicylate levels are associated with prolonged pregnancy, increased puerperal bleeding, decreased birthweight, and stillbirth. It is generally recommended that high doses of aspirin be avoided during the last trimester. Aspirin plus heparin remains the most efficacious treatment of antiphospholipid syndrome [163]. The evidence on the efficacy and safety of thromboprophylaxis with aspirin and heparin in women with a history of at least two spontaneous miscarriages or one later intrauterine fetal death without apparent causes other than inherited thrombophilias is too limited to recommend the use of anticoagulants in this setting [164]. However, one randomized trial sought to compare the efficacy of low-dose aspirin alone versus low-dose aspirin plus low molecular weight heparin in pregnant women with antiphospholipid syndrome and recurrent miscarriage as prophylaxis against pregnancy loss. A high success rate was achieved when low-dose aspirin was used for antiphospholipid syndrome in pregnancy. The addition of low molecular weight heparin did not significantly improve pregnancy outcome [165]. Controversy continues regarding the benefit of low-dose aspirin for the prevention of preeclampsia [166], although no complications of treatment have been documented and several meta-analyses suggest a modest reduction in preeclampsia and IUGR [167]. Acetaminophen is a component of a long list of analgesic medications. Chronic abuse and overdose are the most common problems. The damage appears secondary to free radical toxicity with consumption of glutathione during metabolism. *N*-acetylcysteine is the treatment of choice for an acute overdose [168]. Chronic abuse and overdose are the most common problems. Approximately 5% of women report prenatal use of either ibuprofen or naproxen near conception or during pregnancy. In a recent prospective case–control study, prenatal ibuprofen or naproxen use increased the risk of spontaneous abortion by 80%. Propoxyphene is a narcotic. There are no adequate reports or well-controlled studies in pregnant women.

Fetal considerations

Aspirin crosses the placenta [169]. Maternal aspirin ingestion has been linked to gastroschisis and small intestine atresia independent of fever or cold symptoms [170]. However, the overall risk of malformations was not increased following usage of aspirin [171]. Acetaminophen use during labor to treat the fever of chorioamnionitis is associated with improved fetal umbilical blood gases, presumably by reducing fetal oxygen demand as the maternal core temperature declines [172]. Although it was previously suggested that exposure to acetaminophen was associated with clubfoot and digital abnormalities, these reports are not sustained in large series. However, there appears to be a link between the drug and gastroschisis and small bowel atresia. Unlike aspirin, acetaminophen has no antiplatelet activity and does not pose a hemorrhagic risk to the fetus [173]. Ibuprofen also crosses the human placenta. Fetal levels are dependent on maternal, as NSAIDs are not metabolized by the fetal kidney. It is linked epidemiologically to both gastroschisis and persistent pulmonary hypertension in the neonate. Ibuprofen is as effective as indomethacin in closing the ductus, but does not affect renal function to the same extent [174]. No adverse effects were reported for propoxyphene.

Breastfeeding considerations

The use of aspirin in single doses should not pose any risk to the breastfeeding newborn [175]. In contrast, women on high doses of aspirin such as that for arthritis or rheumatic fever might best avoid breastfeeding, as the neonatal salicylate level may reach therapeutic levels. Acetaminophen is generally considered compatible with breastfeeding [176]. While low levels of ibuprofen and propoxyphene are excreted into human breastmilk, their use is generally considered compatible with breastfeeding.

Antihypertensives (methyldopa, hydralazine, labetalol, propranolol)

Maternal considerations

Hypertension predating pregnancy should be differentiated from preeclampsia. While treatment is indicated for women with a systolic blood pressure >170 mmHg and/or a diastolic blood pressure >109 mmHg, there is no consensus whether lesser degrees of hypertension require treatment during pregnancy. In women with mild to moderate chronic hypertension, antihypertensive therapy improves the maternal but apparently not the fetal outcome. Methyldopa is perhaps the best-studied antihypertensive agent during pregnancy [177]. It remains a first-line agent for the treatment of moderate to mild hypertension [178]. Methyldopa requires 48–72 h to exert its effect. Methyldopa is less effective than metoprolol, but as effective as nifedipine, labetalol and ketanserin, in decreasing both systolic and diastolic blood pressure in women with chronic hypertension [179]. Hydralazine and labetalol are the most widely used drug for the treatment of acute hypertension during pregnancy [180]. Propranolol is used extensively during pregnancy for the treatment of maternal hypertension, arrhythmia, and migraine headache, and is generally considered safe [181]. It is also used acutely to provide symptomatic relief of symptoms from thyrotoxicosis and pheochromocytoma [182,183]. The studies of propranolol as an oral hypotensive are small. It appears as effective as methyldopa, and is often coupled with other hypotensive agents such as hydralazine [184].

Fetal considerations

Most antihypertensive agents cross the placental barrier. Methyldopa is the only drug accepted for use during the first trimester of pregnancy [185]. Methyldopa does not significantly alter fetal cardiac activity or produce any fetal hemodynamic changes as measured by Doppler flow studies [186]. In contrast, methyldopa decreases placental vascular resistance in mild preeclampsia and in chronic hypertension. There are no adequate reports or well-controlled studies in human fetuses for hydralazine, but limited use during the first trimester reveals no evidence of teratogenicity. Intravenous labetalol can cause fetal bradycardia, hypoglycemia, bradycardia, hypotension, pericardial effusion, myocardial hypertrophy, and fetal death resulting from acute hypotension [187,188]. Overall, neonatal outcome is similar to that achieved with hydralazine [189]. Labetalol may be useful for the treatment of fetal thyrotoxicosis [190].

Breastfeeding considerations

Methyldopa, hydralazine, labetalol and propranolol enter human breastmilk [191]. Breastfed neonates delivered by women who are using antihypertensive medications are normotensive. The risk of hypoglycemia in breastfed neonates is increased by labetalol and may be blunted with glucose-fortified formula [192].

Antihistamines (diphenhydramine)

Maternal considerations

There are no adequate reports or well-controlled studies of antihistaminics during pregnancy. Diphenhydramine has a long history of use in obstetrics and is a useful adjunct for women who have allergic reactions to local anesthesia, laminaria, and serum albumin, or for the treatment of severe migraine headaches [193,194].

Fetal considerations

Although diphenhydramine crosses the human placenta, the kinetics remain to be elucidated. There is no evidence of increased fetal risk if administered during any stage of pregnancy. Diphenhydramine may cause neonatal depression if administered during labor [195].

Breastfeeding considerations

There is no published experience in nursing women. It is unknown whether diphenhydramine enters human breastmilk. Irritability is the most common adverse reaction reported in the newborns of women using antihistamines while breastfeeding [195].

Antibiotics (penicillin-G, tetracyclines, ciprofloxacin, metronidazole)

Maternal considerations

Penicillin and its derivatives, ampicillin, and cephalosporins are safe and commonly used during pregnancy [196–199]. Tetracycline is a broad-spectrum antibiotic. Tetracycline is generally avoided during pregnancy because of fetal considerations [200]. When penicillin is contraindicated, tetracycline-class agents (erythromycin) are alternatives for the treatment of gonorrhea and syphilis [201,202]. However, fluoroquinolone-resistant disease is being identified more frequently. A test for cure is essential. Despite this fluoroquinolone therapy (ciprofloxacin) is widely used as a treatment for gonorrhea because it is a relatively inexpensive, oral, and single-dose therapy [203]. Ciprofloxacin is also usually selected when penicillin-class agents have no effect on Gram-negative rods. Ciprofloxacin has the best safety profile of second-line drugs for drug-resistant tuberculosis [204]. It is the drug of choice for prophylaxis among asymptomatic pregnant women exposed to *Bacillus anthracis*, and treatment of Q fever during pregnancy [205,206]. Metronidazole is used widely during pregnancy and has multiple therapeutic benefits such as bacterial vaginosis (BV), trichomoniasis, inflammatory bowel disease, *Clostridium difficile* colitis, and anaerobic and protozoal infections [207,208]. Several large randomized trials seeking to determine whether successful treatment of BV reduced the prevalence of adverse outcomes ended in controversy [209–212]. Women who deliver preterm with symptomatic BV have a lower risk of preterm birth in a subsequent pregnancy if treated with clindamycin and erythromycin but not metronidazole [213]. Unfortunately, the treatment of women with asymptomatic BV and no prior preterm birth apparently does not alter their preterm delivery rate [214]. High-risk conditions that require treatment of BV with oral clindamycin and erthromycin include: women with prior preterm birth, BMI below $19.8 \, kg/m^2$ and women with evidence of endometritis before pregnancy. A "test of cure" should be obtained 1 month later [215].

Fetal considerations

Most penicillins cross the human placenta to some extent [216,217]. The extensive clinical experience is reassuring, as are the animal studies, which reveal no evidence of teratogenicity or IUGR despite the use of doses higher than those used clinically [218]. Tetracycline crosses the human placenta and may cause a yellow–gray–brown tooth discoloration in adults after fetal/childhood exposure [218,219].

However, treatment with doxycycline during pregnancy presents very little if any teratogenic risk to the fetus [220]. Ciprofloxacin crosses the human placenta [221], and can be found in amniotic fluid in low quantities. Short-duration treatment with ciprofloxacin appears free of adverse fetal responses. As a class, the new quinolones do not appear associated with an increased risk of malformation or musculoskeletal problems in humans [221]. There are no clinically significant musculoskeletal dysfunctions reported in children exposed to fluoroquinolones *in utero* [222,223]. However, longer follow-up and magnetic resonance imaging of the joints may be warranted to exclude subtle cartilage and bone damage. Similarly, metronidazole also crosses the human placenta but it does not pose a major teratogenic risk when used in the recommended dosage [224]. The safety of drug therapy for inflammatory bowel disease during pregnancy is an important clinical concern [225].

Breastfeeding considerations

Only trace amounts of penicillin-G enter human breastmilk [226]. It is generally considered compatible with breastfeeding. Tetracycline enters human breastmilk, although the kinetics remain to be elucidated [227]. Clinical experience suggests that maternal oral ingestion is compatible with breastfeeding. Ciprofloxacin enters human breastmilk, and oral doses of this drug are concentrated in breastmilk at levels higher than serum [228]. *Clostridium difficile* pseudomembranous colitis has been reported in a breastfed neonate whose mother was taking ciprofloxacin. Metronidazole is excreted into human breastmilk and is not associated with adverse effects in breastfed neonates [229].

Antivirals (acyclovir)

Maternal considerations

Treatment of genital herpes with acyclovir during pregnancy is not curative, but rather intended to reduce the duration of symptoms and viral shedding [230]. There is a long clinical experience free of adverse effects. Prophylactic acyclovir beginning at 36 weeks' gestation reduced the risks at delivery of clinical recurrence of genital herpes, caesarean section for recurrence, and herpes shedding at delivery [231]. Suppression therapy is both effective and cost-effective whether or not the primary infection occurred during the current pregnancy.

Fetal considerations

It is unknown whether acyclovir crosses the human placenta. Postmarketing surveillance has not revealed any increase in or pattern of malformations after exposure during the first trimester [232].

Breastfeeding considerations

Although acyclovir is passively secreted and achieves concentrations in breastmilk higher than maternal serum [233]. It is used to treat neonatal herpetic infection and is generally considered compatible with breastfeeding.

Case presentation

Dr. Howard was late for the office that day as a hypertensive patient had kept her in the hospital until early morning. It was a cold winter day. The waiting room was full of walk-ins and three new maternity patients. First in the examination room was a long-time patient now at 9 weeks' gestation. She has upper respiratory tract symptoms and received the influenza vaccine in October. Acetaminophen coupled with an antihistamine was prescribed. The next patient had a newly positive pregnancy test and was diagnosed with a seizure disorder several years back, although she has had no difficulties over the last 3 years. Recognizing the risk of an unnecessary prescription medication, and following consultation with the patient's neurologist, Dr. Howard recommended an ultrasound, discontinuation of her phenytoin, and a neurology follow-up in the following week. The next new patient was a 42-year-old in the 11th week of her fourth pregnancy with twins after in vitro fertilization. Three years ago, the patient was started by her general practitioner on a diuretic agent for mild hypertension. Her weight was 80 kg. Dr. Howard noticed that her blood pressure was now near normal (130/84 mmHg). Dr. Howard elected to discontinue the diuretic and made a note to test her for gestational diabetes a little earlier than usual, perhaps around 26 weeks.

Dr. Howard recalled that winter day vividly as she sat to complete her quarterly QA report. Strange, each of the pregnancies had suffered an unexpected complication. The first patient's child was doing well now after a gastroschisis repair with bowel resection for atretic loops of intestine. The second patient's child, who had a cleft palate and lip, required multiple surgical repairs. Her third patient was diagnosed with diabetes at 26 weeks, but despite the initiation of insulin therapy, delivered a 3.5-kg child at 31 weeks after she had been induced for what the high-risk specialist felt was superimposed preeclampsia.

References

1 Lacroix I, Damase-Michel C, Lapeyre-Mestre M, Montastruc JL. Prescription of drugs during pregnancy in France. *Lancet* 2000;**356**:1735–6.

2 Frederickson MC. Physiologic changes in pregnancy and their effect on drug distribution. *Semin Perinatol* 2001;**25**:120–3.

3 Plentl AA, Gray MJ. Total body water, sodium space and total exchangeable sodium in normal and toxemic pregnant women. *Am J Obstet Gynecol* 1959;**78**:472–8.

4 Verkeste CM, Slangen BF, Dubelaar ML, van Kreel BK, Peeters LL. Mechanism of volume adaptation in the awake early pregnant rat. *Am J Physiol* 1998;**274**:H1662–6.

5 Peterson VP. Body composition and fluid compartments in normal, obese and underweight human subjects. *Acta Med Scand* 1957;**108**:103–11.

6 Spaanderman ME, Meertens M, van Bussel M, Ekhart TH, Peeters LL. Cardiac output increases independently of basal metabolic rate in early human pregnancy. *Am J Physiol Heart Circ Physiol* 2000;**278**:H1585–8.

7 Robson SC, Mutch E, Boys RJ, Woodhouse KW. Apparent liver blood flow during pregnancy: a serial study using indocyanine green clearance. *Br J Obstet Gynaecol* 1990;**97**:720–4.

8 Wood M, Wood AJ. Changes in plasma drug binding and alpha 1-acid glycoprotein in mother and newborn infant. *Clin Pharmacol Ther* 1981;**29**:522–6.

9 Clayton-Smith J, Donnai D. Human malformations. In: Rimoin DL, Connor JM, Pyeritz RE, eds. *Emery and Rimoin's Principles and Practice of Medical Genetics*, 3rd edn. New York: Churchill Livingstone, 1996: 383.

10 Audus KL. Controlling drug delivery across the placenta. *Eur J Pharm Sci* 1999;**8**:161–5.

11 Young AM, Allen CE, Audis KL. Efflux transporters of the human placenta. *Adv Drug Deliv Rev* 2003;**55**:125–32.

12 Schatz M. The efficacy and safety of asthma medications during pregnancy. *Semin Perinatol* 2001;**25**:145–52.

13 Yerby M. The use of anticonvulsants during pregnancy. *Semin Perinatol* 2001;**25**:153–8.

14 Sibai BM. Antihypertensive drugs during pregnancy. *Semin Perinatol* 2001;**25**:159–64.

15 Newport DJ, Wilcox MM, Stowe ZN. Antidepressants during pregnancy and lactation: defining exposure and treatment issues. *Semin Perinatol* 2001;**25**:145–58.

16 Nelson BK, Moorman WJ, Schrader SM. Review of experimental male-mediated behavioral and neurochemical disorders. *Neurotoxicol Teratol* 1996;**18**:611–6.

17 Weiner CP. Introduction. In: Weiner CP, Buhimschi C, eds. *Drugs for Pregnant and Lactating Women*. Philadelphia: Churchill Livingston, 2004: xiii.

18 Mitchell AA. Systematic identification of drugs that cause birth defects: a new opportunity. *N Engl J Med* 2003;**349**:2556–9.

19 Slone D, Shapiro S, Miettinen O. Case–control surveillance of serious illnesses attributable to ambulatory drug use. In: Colombo F, Shapiro S, Slone D, Tognoni G, eds. *Epidemiological Evaluation of Drugs*. Amsterdam: Elsevier/North Holland Biomedical Press, 1977: 59–70.

20 Lagoy CT, Joshi N, Cragan JD, Rasmussen SA. Medication use during pregnancy and lactation: an urgent call for public health action. *J Womens Health (Larchmt)* 2005;**14**:104–9.

21 Berlin CM, Briggs GG. Drugs and chemicals in human milk. *Semin Fetal Neonatal Med* 2005;**10**:149–59.

22 McNamara PJ, Abbassi M. Neonatal exposure to drugs in breast milk. *Pharm Res* 2004;**21**:555–66.

23 Solomon GM, Weiss PM. Chemical contaminants in breast milk: time trends and regional variability. *Environ Health Perspect* 2002;**110**:A339–47.

24 Tomlinson AJ, Campbell J, Walker JJ, Morgan C. Malignant primary hypertension in pregnancy treated with lisinopril. *Ann Pharmacother* 2000;**34**:180–2.

25 Cooper WO, Hernandez-Diaz S, Arbogast PG, *et al.* Major congenital malformations after first-trimester exposure to ACE inhibitors. *N Engl J Med* 2006;**354**:2443–51.

26 Bar J, Chen R, Schoenfeld A, *et al.* Pregnancy outcome in patients with insulin dependent diabetes mellitus and diabetic nephropathy treated with ACE inhibitors before pregnancy. *J Pediatr Endocrinol Metab* 1999;**12**:659–65.

27 August P, Mueller FB, Sealey JE, Edersheim TG. Role of renin-angiotensin system in blood pressure regulation in pregnancy. *Lancet* 1995;**345**:896–7.

28 Easterling TR, Carr DB, Davis C, Diederichs C, Brateng DA, Schmucker B. Low-dose, short-acting, angiotensin-converting enzyme inhibitors as rescue therapy in pregnancy. *Obstet Gynecol* 2000;**96**:956–61.

29 Tabacova SA, Kimmel CA. Enalapril: pharmacokinetic/dynamic inferences for comparative developmental toxicity: a review. *Reprod Toxicol* 2001;**15**:467–78.

30 Miller RK, Jessee L, Barrish A, Gilbert J, Manson JM. Pharmacokinetic studies of enalaprilat in the *in vitro* perfused human placental lobule system. *Teratology* 1998;**58**:76–81.

31 Burrows RF, Burrows EA. Assessing the teratogenic potential of angiotensin-converting enzyme inhibitors in pregnancy. *Aust NZ J Obstet Gynaecol* 1998;**38**:306–11.

32 Filler G, Wong H, Condello AS, *et al.* Early dialysis in a neonate with intrauterine lisinopril exposure. *Arch Dis Child Fetal Neonatal Ed* 2003;**88**:F154–6.

33 Redman CW, Kelly JG, Cooper WD. The excretion of enalapril and enalaprilat in human breast milk. *Eur J Clin Pharmacol* 1990;**38**:99.

34 Devlin RG, Fleiss PM. Captopril in human blood and breast milk. *J Clin Pharmacol* 1981;**21**:110–3.

35 Crawford P. Interactions between antiepileptic drugs and hormonal contraception. *CNS Drugs* 2002;**16**: 263–72.

36 McAuley JW, Anderson GD. Treatment of epilepsy in women of reproductive age: pharmacokinetic considerations. *Clin Pharmacokinet* 2002;**41**:559–79.

37 Leppik IE, Rask CA. Pharmacokinetics of antiepileptic drugs during pregnancy. *Semin Neurol* 1988;**8**:240–6.

38 Crawford P. Interactions between antiepileptic drugs and hormonal contraception. *CNS Drugs* 2002;**16**: 263–72.

39 Azarbayjani F, Danielsson BR. Embryonic arrhythmia by inhibition of HERG channels: a common hypoxia-related teratogenic mechanism for antiepileptic drugs? *Epilepsia* 2002;**43**:457–68.

40 Nakamura H, Ushigome F, Koyabu N, *et al.* Proton gradient-dependent transport of valproic acid in human placental brush-border membrane vesicles. *Pharm Res* 2002;**19**:154–61.

41 Lindhout D, Omtzigt JG, Cornel MC. Spectrum of neural-tube defects in 34 infants prenatally exposed to antiepileptic drugs. *Neurology* 1992;**42**:111–8.

42 Kozma C. Valproic acid embryopathy: report of two siblings with further expansion of the phenotypic abnormalities and a review of the literature. *Am J Med Genet* 2001;**98**:168–75.

43 Witters I, Van Assche F, Fryns JP. Nuchal edema as the first sign of fetal valproate syndrome. *Prenat Diagn* 2002;**22**:834–5.

44 Matalon S, Schechtman S, Goldzweig G, Ornoy A. The teratogenic effect of carbamazepine: a meta-analysis of 1255 exposures. *Reprod Toxicol* 2002;**16**:9–17.

45 Iqbal MM, Sohhan T, Mahmud SZ. The effects of lithium, valproic acid, and carbamazepine during pregnancy and lactation. *J Toxicol Clin Toxicol* 2001;**39**:381–92.

46 Chaudron LH. When and how to use mood stabilizers during breastfeeding. *Prim Care Update Ob Gyns* 2000;**7**: 113–7.

47 Shimoyama R, Ohkubo T, Sugawara K, *et al.* Monitoring of phenytoin in human breast milk, maternal plasma and cord blood plasma by solid-phase extraction and liquid chromatography. *J Pharm Biomed Anal* 1998;**17**:863–9.

48 Kart Koseoglu H, Yucel AE, Kunefeci G, Ozdemir FN, Duran H. Cyclophosphamide therapy in a serious case of lupus nephritis during pregnancy. *Lupus* 2001;**10**:818–20.

49 Ozalp SS, Yalcin OT, Tanir HM. A hospital-based multicentric study results on gestational trophoblastic disease management status in a developing country. *Eur J Gynaecol Oncol* 2001;**22**:221–2.

50 Peters BG, Bray JJ, Masidonski P, Mahon SM. Issues surrounding adjuvant chemotherapy for breast cancer during pregnancy. *Oncol Nurs Forum* 2001;**28**:639–42.

51 Enns GM, Roeder E, Chan RT, Ali-Khan Catts Z, Cox VA, Golabi M. Apparent cyclophosphamide (cytoxan) embryopathy: a distinct phenotype? *Am J Med Genet* 1999;**86**:237–41.

52 Meirow D, Epstein M, Lewis H, Nugent D, Gosden RG. Administration of cyclophosphamide at different stages of follicular maturation in mice: effects on reproductive performance and fetal malformations. *Hum Reprod* 2001;**16**:632–7.

53 Ostensen M. Treatment with immunosuppressive and disease modifying drugs during pregnancy and lactation. *Am J Reprod Immunol* 1992;**28**:148–52.

54 Amato D, Niblett JS. Neutropenia from cyclophosphamide in breast milk. *Med J Aust* 1977;**1**:383–4.

55 Hammond MG, Hammond CB, Parker RT. Conservative treatment of endometriosis externa: the effects of methyltestosterone therapy. *Fertil Steril* 1978;**29**:651–4.

56 Borgatta L, Murthy A, Chuang C, Beardsley L, Burnhill MS. Pregnancies diagnosed during Depo-Provera use. *Contraception* 2002;**66**:169–72.

57 Shane BS, Dunn HO, Kenney RM, Hansel W, Visek WJ. Methyl testosterone-induced female pseudohermaphroditism in dogs. *Biol Reprod* 1969;**1**:41–8.

58 Grote K, Stahlschmidt B, Talsness CE, Gericke C, Appel KE, Chahoud I. Effects of organotin compounds on pubertal male rats. *Toxicology* 2004;**202**:145–58.

59 Tuffli GA. Testosterone and micropenis. *J Pediatr* 1974;**84**: 927.

60 Carbone JP, Figurska K, Buck S, Brent RL. Effect of gestational sex steroid exposure on limb development and endochondral ossification in the pregnant C57Bl/6J mouse. I. Medroxyprogesterone acetate. *Teratology* 1990;**42**:121–30.

61 Duck SC, Katayama KP. Danazol may cause female pseudohermaphroditism. *Fertil Steril* 1981;**35**:230–1.

62 Minh HN, Belaisch J, Smadja A. [Female pseudohermaphroditism.] *Presse Med* 1993;**22**:1735–40.

63 Baluchuci A, Ardsetani N, Ghazizadeh S. Effects of progestogen-only contraceptives on breast-feeding and infant growth. *Int J Gynaecol Obstet* 2001;**74**:203–5.

64 Ratchanon S, Taneepanichskul S. Depot medroxyprogesterone acetate and basal serum prolactin levels in lactating women. *Obstet Gynecol* 2000;**96**:926–8.

65 Treffers PE, Hanselaar AG, Helmerhorst TJ, Koster ME, van Leeuwen FE. Consequences of diethylstilbestrol during pregnancy: 50 years later still a significant problem. *Ned Tijdschr Geneeskd* 2001;**145**:675–80.

66 Mano MS, Kerr J, Kennedy J. Management of breast cancer in patients prenatally exposed to diethylstilbestrol: are we prepared? *Breast* 2005;**14**:408–10.

67 van Gils AP, Tham RT, Falke TH, Peters AA. Abnormalities of the uterus and cervix after diethylstilbestrol exposure: correlation of findings on MR and hysterosalpingography. *Am J Roentgenol* 1989;**153**:1235–8.

68 Porcu G, Courbiere B, Sakr R, Carcopino X, Gamerre M. Spontaneous rupture of a first-trimester gravid uterus in a woman exposed to diethylstilbestrol *in utero*: a case report. *J Reprod Med* 2003;**48**:744–6.

69 Klip H, Verloop J, van Gool JD, Koster ME, Burger CW, van Leeuwen FE, OMEGA Project Group. Hypospadias in sons of women exposed to diethylstilbestrol *in utero*: a cohort study. *Lancet* 2002;**359**:1102–7.

70 Carriers to pay NJ hospitals preset fees for services. *Med World News* 1978;**19**:37–8.

71 Brown DD. Inhibition of lactation with oestrogens. *Br Med J* 1969;**1**:51.

72 Kaya H, Babar Y, Ozmen S, *et al*. Intratubal methotrexate for prevention of persistent ectopic pregnancy after salpingotomy. *J Am Assoc Gynecol Laparosc* 2002;**9**:464–7.

73 Kulier R, Gulmezoglu AM, Hofmeyr GJ, Cheng LN, Campana A. Medical methods for first trimester abortion. *Cochrane Database Syst Rev* 2004;CD002855.

74 Gracia CR, Brown HA, Barnhart KT. Prophylactic methotrexate after linear salpingostomy: a decision analysis. *Fertil Steril* 2001;**76**:1191–5.

75 Dilbaz S, Caliskan E, Dilbaz B, Degirmenci O, Haberal A. Predictors of methotrexate treatment failure in ectopic pregnancy. *J Reprod Med* 2006;**51**:87–93.

76 Yedlinsky NT, Morgan FC, Whitecar PW. Anomalies associated with failed methotrexate and misoprostol termination. *Obstet Gynecol* 2005;**105**:1203–5.

77 Del Campo M, Kosaki K, Bennett FC, Jones KL. Developmental delay in fetal aminopterin/methotrexate syndrome. *Teratology* 1999;**60**:10–2.

78 Ostensen M. Related treatment with immunosuppressive and disease modifying drugs during pregnancy and lactation. *Am J Reprod Immunol* 1992;**28**:148–52.

79 Sorosky JI, Sood AK, Buekers TE. The use of chemotherapeutic agents during pregnancy. *Obstet Gynecol Clin North Am* 1997;**24**:591–9.

80 Koren G, Soldin O. Therapeutic drug monitoring of antithyroid drugs in pregnancy: the knowledge gaps. *Ther Drug Monit* 2006;**28**:12–3.

81 Azizi F. The safety and efficacy of antithyroid drugs. *Expert Opin Drug Saf* 2006;**5**:107–16.

82 Mestman JH. Diagnosis and management of maternal and fetal thyroid disorders. *Curr Opin Obstet Gynecol* 1999;**11**:167–75.

83 Nachum Z, Rakover Y, Weiner E, Shalev E. Graves' disease in pregnancy: prospective evaluation of a selective invasive treatment protocol. *Am J Obstet Gynecol* 2003;**189**:159–65.

84 Azizi F, Khamseh ME, Bahreynian M, Hedayati M. Thyroid function and intellectual development of children of mothers taking methimazole during pregnancy. *J Endocrinol Invest* 2002;**25**:586–9.

85 Nakamura S, Nishikawa T, Isaji M, *et al*. Aplasia cutis congenita and skull defects after exposure to methimazole *in utero*. *Intern Med* 2005;**44**:1202–3.

86 Karg E, Bereg E, Gaspar L, Katona M, Turi S. Aplasia cutis congenita after methimazole exposure in utero. *Pediatr Dermatol* 2004;**21**:491–4.

87 Johansen K, Andersen AN, Kampmann JP, Molholm Hansen JM, Mortensen HB. Excretion of methimazole in human milk. *Eur J Clin Pharmacol* 1982;**23**:339–41.

88 Cooper DS. Antithyroid drugs: to breast-feed or not to breast-feed. *Am J Obstet Gynecol* 1987;**157**:234–5.

89 Shepard TH, Brent RL, Friedman JM, *et al*. Update on new developments in the study of human teratogens. *Teratology* 2002;**65**:153–61.

90 Brill-Edwards P, Ginsberg JS, Gent M, *et al*. Recurrence of clot in this pregnancy study group. Safety of withholding heparin in pregnant women with a history of venous thromboembolism. *N Engl J Med* 2000;**343**:1439–44.

91 Vitale N, De Feo M, De Santo LS, Pollice A, Tedesco N, Cotrufo M. Dose-dependent fetal complications of warfarin in pregnant women with mechanical heart valves. *J Am Coll Cardiol* 1999;**33**:1637–41.

92 Suri V, Sawhney H, Vasishta K, Renuka T, Grover A. Pregnancy following cardiac valve replacement surgery. *Int J Gynaecol Obstet* 1999;**64**:239–46.

93 Vitale N, De Feo M, Cotrufo M. Anticoagulation for prosthetic heart valves during pregnancy: the importance of warfarin daily dose. *Eur J Cardiothorac Surg* 2002;**22**:656.

94 Hall JG, Pauli RM, Wilson KM. Maternal and fetal sequelae of anticoagulation during pregnancy. *Am J Med* 1980;**68**:122–40.

95 Tyagi A, Bhattacharya A. Central neuraxial blocks and anticoagulation: a review of current trends. *Eur J Anaesthesiol* 2002;**19**:317–29.

96 Zakzouk MS. The congenital warfarin syndrome. *J Laryngol Otol* 1986;**100**:215–9.

97 Wesseling J, Van Driel D, Smrkovsky M, *et al*. Neurological outcome in school-age children after *in utero* exposure to coumarins. *Early Hum Dev* 2001;**63**:83–95.

98 Dardick KR. Warfarin during lactation. *Conn Med* 1980;**44**:693.

99 Orme ML, Lewis PJ, de Swiet M, *et al*. May mothers given warfarin breast-feed their infants? *Br Med J* 1977;**1**:1564–5.

100 Busowski JD, Safdar A. Treatment for coccidioidomycosis in pregnancy? *Postgrad Med* 2001;**109**:76–7.

101 Aleck KA, Bartley DL. Multiple malformation syndrome following fluconazole use in pregnancy: report of an additional patient. *Am J Med Genet* 1997;**72**:253–6.

102 Sorensen HT, Nielsen GL, Olesen C, *et al*. Risk of malformations and other outcomes in children exposed to fluconazole *in utero*. *Br J Clin Pharmacol* 1999;**48**:234–8.

103 Force RW. Fluconazole concentrations in breast milk. *Pediatr Infect Dis J* 1995;**14**:235–6.

104 Carney SM, Goodwin GM. Lithium: a continuing story in the treatment of bipolar disorder. *Acta Psychiatr Scand Suppl* 2005;**426**:7–12.

105 Gelenberg AJ. Lithium efficacy and adverse effects. *J Clin Psychiatry* 1988;**49**(Suppl):8–11.

106 Teixeira NA, Lopes RC, Secoli SR. Developmental toxicity of lithium treatment at prophylactic levels. *Braz J Med Biol Res* 1995;**28**:230–9.

107 Giles JJ, Bannigan JG. Teratogenic and developmental effects of lithium. *Curr Pharm Des* 2006;**12**:1531–41.

108 van Gent EM, Verhoeven WM. Bipolar illness, lithium prophylaxis, and pregnancy. *Pharmacopsychiatry* 1992;**25**:187–91.

109 Pinelli JM, Symington AJ, Cunningham KA, Paes BA. Case report and review of the perinatal implications of maternal lithium use. *Am J Obstet Gynecol* 2002;**187**:245–9.

110 Wright TL, Hoffman LH, Davies J. Lithium teratogenicity. *Lancet* 1970;**2**:876.

111 Szabo KT. Teratogenic effect of lithium carbonate in the foetal mouse. *Nature* 1970;**225**:73–5.

112 Arnon J, Shechtman S, Ornoy A. The use of psychiatric drugs in pregnancy and lactation. *Isr J Psychiatry Relat Sci* 2000;**37**:205–22.

113 Schou M, Amdisen A. Lithium and pregnancy. 3. Lithium ingestion by children breast-fed by women on lithium treatment. *Br Med J* 1973;**2**:138.

114 Dodd JM, Crowther CA, Robinson JS. Oral misoprostol for induction of labour at term: randomised controlled trial. *Br Med J* 2006;**332**:509–13.

115 Zikopoulos KA, Papanikolaou EG, Kalantaridou SN, *et al*. Early pregnancy termination with vaginal misoprostol before and after 42 days gestation. *Hum Reprod* 2002;**17**:3079–83.

116 ACOG Committee Opinion. American College of Obstetricians and Gynecologists. Related ACOG Committee Opinion. Number 283, May 2003. New US Food and Drug Administration labeling on Cytotec (misoprostol) use and pregnancy. *Obstet Gynecol* 2003;**101**:1049–50.

117 Alfirevic Z, Weeks A. Oral misoprostol for induction of labour. *Cochrane Database Syst Rev* 2006;CD001338.

118 Yedlinsky NT, Morgan FC, Whitecar PW. Anomalies associated with failed methotrexate and misoprostol termination. *Obstet Gynecol* 2005;**105**:1203–5.

119 Vogel D, Burkhardt T, Rentsch K, *et al*. Misoprostol versus methylergometrine: pharmacokinetics in human milk. *Am J Obstet Gynecol* 2004;**191**:2168–73.

120 Furman B, Bashiri A, Wiznitzer A, Erez O, Holcberg G, Mazor M. Wilson's disease in pregnancy: five successful consecutive pregnancies of the same woman. *Eur J Obstet Gynecol Reprod Biol* 2001;**96**:232–4.

121 Pinter R, Hogge WA, McPherson E. Infant with severe penicillamine embryopathy born to a woman with Wilson disease. *Am J Med Genet A* 2004;**128**:294–8.

122 Brinker A, Kornegay C, Nourjah P. Trends in adherence to a revised risk management program designed to decrease or eliminate isotretinoin-exposed pregnancies: evaluation of the accutane SMART program. *Arch Dermatol* 2005;**141**:563–9.

123 Charakida A, Mouser PE, Chu AC. Safety and side effects of the acne drug, oral isotretinoin. *Expert Opin Drug Saf* 2004;**3**:119–29.

124 Uhl K, Kennedy DL, Kweder SL. Risk management strategies in the Physicians' Desk Reference product labels for pregnancy category X drugs. *Drug Saf* 2002;**25**:885–92.

125 Teo SK, Harden JL, Burke AB, *et al*. Thalidomide is distributed into human semen after oral dosing. *Drug Metab Dispos* 2001;**29**:1355–7.

126 Holmes LB. Teratogen-induced limb defects. *Am J Med Genet* 2002;**112**:297–303.

127 Gollop TR, Eigier A, Guidugli Neto J. Prenatal diagnosis of thalidomide syndrome. *Prenat Diagn* 1987;**7**:295–8.

128 Lieman JM, Brumfield CG, Carlo W, Ramsey PS. Preterm premature rupture of membranes: is there an optimal gestational age for delivery? *Obstet Gynecol* 2005;**105**:12–7.

129 Walfisch A, Hallak M, Mazor M. Multiple courses of antenatal steroids: risks and benefits. *Obstet Gynecol* 2001;**98**:491–7.

130 Egerman RS, Mercer BM, Doss JL, Sibai BM. A randomized, controlled trial of oral and intramuscular dexamethasone in the prevention of neonatal respiratory distress syndrome. *Am J Obstet Gynecol* 1998;**179**:1120–3.

131 Gurbuz A, Karateke A, Ozturk G, Kabaca C. Is 1-hour glucose screening test reliable after a short-term administration of antenatal betamethasone? *Am J Perinatol* 2004;**21**:415–20.

132 Elliott JP, O'Keeffe DF, Greenberg P, Freeman RK. Pulmonary edema associated with magnesium sulfate and betamethasone administration. *Am J Obstet Gynecol* 1979;**134**:717–9.

133 Mushkat Y, Ascher-Landsberg J, Keidar R, Carmon E, Pauzner D, David MP. The effect of betamethasone versus dexamethasone on fetal biophysical parameters. *Eur J Obstet Gynecol Reprod Biol* 2001;**97**:50–2.

134 Fujii Y, Uemura A. Dexamethasone for the prevention of nausea and vomiting after dilatation and curettage: a randomized controlled trial. *Obstet Gynecol* 2002;**99**:58–62.

135 Martin JN Jr, Thigpen BD, Rose CH, Cushman J, Moore A, May WL. Maternal benefit of high-dose intravenous corticosteroid therapy for HELLP syndrome. *Am J Obstet Gynecol* 2003;**189**:830–4.

136 Fonseca JE, Mendez F, Catano C, Arias F. Dexamethasone treatment does not improve the outcome of women with HELLP syndrome: a double-blind, placebo-controlled, randomized clinical trial. *Am J Obstet Gynecol* 2005;**193**:1591–8.

137 Effect of corticosteroids for fetal maturation on perinatal outcomes. *NIH Consensus Statement* 1994;**12**:1–24.

138 Spinillo A, Viazzo F, Colleoni R, *et al*. Two-year infant neurodevelopmental outcome after single or multiple antenatal courses of corticosteroids to prevent complications of prematurity. *Am J Obstet Gynecol* 2004;**191**:217–24.

139 Huang WL, Harper CG, Evans SF, Newnham JP, Dunlop SA. Repeated prenatal corticosteroid administration delays myelination of the corpus callosum in fetal sheep. *Int J Dev Neurosci* 2001;**19**:415–25.

140 Whitelaw A, Thoresen M. Antenatal steroids and the developing brain. *Arch Dis Child Fetal Neonatal Ed* 2000;**83**:F154–7.

141 Walker BE. Induction of cleft palate in rats with antiinflammatory drugs. *Teratology* 1971;**4**:39–42.

142 Costedoat-Chalumeau N, Georgin-Lavialle S, Amoura Z, Piette JC. Anti-SSA/Ro and anti-SSB/La antibody-mediated congenital heart block. *Lupus* 2005;**14**:660–4.

143 Mulder EJ, Derks JB, Visser GH. Antenatal corticosteroid therapy and fetal behaviour: a randomised study of the effects of betamethasone and dexamethasone. *Br J Obstet Gynaecol* 1997;**104**:1239–47.

144 Hughes I. Prenatal treatment of congenital adrenal hyperplasia: do we have enough evidence? *Treat Endocrinol* 2006;**5**:1–6.

145 Brook CG. Antenatal treatment of a mother bearing a fetus with congenital adrenal hyperplasia. *Arch Dis Child Fetal Neonatal Ed* 2000;**82**:F176–81.

146 Lockshin MD, Sammaritano LR. Corticosteroids during pregnancy. *Scand J Rheumatol Suppl* 1998;**107**:136–8.

147 Belfort MA, Anthony J, Saade GR. Prevention of eclampsia. *Semin Perinatol* 1999;**23**:65–78.

148 Duley L, Gulmezoglu AM. Magnesium sulphate versus lytic cocktail for eclampsia. *Cochrane Database Syst Rev* 2001;**1**: CD002960.

149 Duley L, Henderson-Smart D. Magnesium sulphate versus diazepam for eclampsia. *Cochrane Database Syst Rev* 2003;**4**: CD000127.

150 Kanto J, Erkkola R. The feto-maternal distribution of diazepam in early human pregnancy. *Ann Chir Gynaecol Fenn* 1974;**63**:489–91.

151 Gonzalez de Dios J, Moya-Benavent M, Carratala-Marco F. "Floppy infant" syndrome in twins secondary to the use of benzodiazepines during pregnancy. *Rev Neurol* 1999;**29**: 121–3.

152 McElhatton PR. The effects of benzodiazepine use during pregnancy and lactation. *Reprod Toxicol* 1994;**8**:461–75.

153 Cohen LS, Altshuler LL, Harlow BL, *et al.* Relapse of major depression during pregnancy in women who maintain or discontinue antidepressant treatment. *JAMA* 2006;**295**: 499–507.

154 Howard LM, Hoffbrand S, Henshaw C, Boath L, Bradley E. Antidepressant prevention of postnatal depression. *Cochrane Database Syst Rev* 2005;**2**:CD004363.

155 Heikkinen T, Ekblad U, Palo P, Laine K. Pharmacokinetics of fluoxetine and norfluoxetine in pregnancy and lactation. *Clin Pharmacol Ther* 2003;**73**:330–7.

156 Hendrick V, Stowe ZN, Altshuler LL, Hwang S, Lee E, Haynes D. Placental passage of antidepressant medications. *Am J Psychiatry* 2003;**160**:993–6.

157 Hendrick V, Smith LM, Suri R, Hwang S, Haynes D, Altshuler L. Birth outcomes after prenatal exposure to antidepressant medication. *Am J Obstet Gynecol* 2003;**188**:812–5.

158 Eberhard-Gran M, Eskild A, Opjordsmoen S. Treating mood disorders during pregnancy: safety considerations. *Drug Saf* 2005;**28**:695–706.

159 Chambers CD, Hernandez-Diaz S, Van Marter LJ, *et al.* Selective serotonin-reuptake inhibitors and risk of persistent pulmonary hypertension of the newborn. *N Engl J Med* 2006;**354**: 579–87.

160 Stowe ZN, Hostetter AL, Owens MJ, *et al.* The pharmacokinetics of sertraline excretion into human breast milk: determinants of infant serum concentrations. *J Clin Psychiatry* 2003;**64**:73–80.

161 Everson GW, Krenzelok EP. Chronic salicylism in a patient with juvenile rheumatoid arthritis. *Clin Pharm* 1986;**5**:334–41.

162 Li DK, Liu L, Odouli R. Exposure to non-steroidal anti-inflammatory drugs during pregnancy and risk of miscarriage: population based cohort study. *Br Med J* 2003;**327**:368.

163 Empson M, Lassere M, Craig JC, Scott JR. Recurrent pregnancy loss with antiphospholipid antibody: a systematic review of therapeutic trials. *Obstet Gynecol* 2002;**99**: 135–44.

164 Di Nisio M, Peters L, Middeldorp S. Anticoagulants for the treatment of recurrent pregnancy loss in women without antiphospholipid syndrome. *Cochrane Database Syst Rev* 2005;**2**: CD004734.

165 Farquharson RG, Quenby S, Greaves M. Antiphospholipid syndrome in pregnancy: a randomized, controlled trial of treatment. *Obstet Gynecol* 2002;**100**:408–13.

166 Caritis S, Sibai B, Hauth J, *et al.* Low-dose aspirin to prevent preeclampsia in women at high risk. National Institute of Child Health and Human Development Network of Maternal-Fetal Medicine Units. *N Engl J Med* 1998;**338**:701–5.

167 Vainio M, Kujansuu E, Iso-Mustajarvi M, Maenpaa J. Low dose acetylsalicylic acid in prevention of pregnancy-induced hypertension and intrauterine growth retardation in women with bilateral uterine artery notches. *Br J Obstet Gynaecol* 2002;**109**:161–7.

168 Acetylcysteine (Acetadote) for acetaminophen overdosage. *Med Lett Drugs Ther* 2005;**47**:70–1.

169 Anderson DF, Phernetton TM, Rankin JH. The placental transfer of acetylsalicylic acid in near-term ewes. *Am J Obstet Gynecol* 1980;**136**:814–8.

170 Martinez-Frias ML, Rodriguez-Pinilla E, Prieto L. Prenatal exposure to salicylates and gastroschisis: a case–control study. *Teratology* 1997;**56**:241–3.

171 Kozer E, Nikfar S, Costei A, Boskovic R, Nulman I, Koren G. Aspirin consumption during the first trimester of pregnancy and congenital anomalies: a meta-analysis. *Am J Obstet Gynecol* 2002;**187**:1623–30.

172 Kirshon B, Moise KJ Jr, Wasserstrum N. Effect of acetaminophen on fetal acid–base balance in chorioamnionitis. *J Reprod Med* 1989;**34**:955–9.

173 Collins E. Maternal and fetal effects of acetaminophen and salicylates in pregnancy. *Obstet Gynecol* 1981;**58**:57S–62S.

174 Thomas RL, Parker GC, Van Overmeire B, Aranda JV. A meta-analysis of ibuprofen versus indomethacin for closure of patent ductus arteriosus. *Eur J Pediatr* 2005;**164**:135–40.

175 Bleyer WA, Breckenridge RT. Studies on the detection of adverse drug reactions in the newborn. II. The effects of prenatal aspirin on newborn hemostasis. *JAMA* 1970;**213**:2049–53.

176 Spigset O, Hagg S. Analgesics and breast-feeding: safety considerations. *Paediatr Drugs* 2000;**2**:223–38.

177 Borghi C, Esposti DD, Cassani A, Immordino V, Bovicelli L, Ambrosioni E. The treatment of hypertension in pregnancy. *J Hypertens Suppl* 2002;**20**:S52–6.

178 Kirsten R, Nelson K, Kirsten D, Heintz B. Clinical pharmacokinetics of vasodilators. Part II. *Clin Pharmacokinet* 1998;**35**:9–36.

179 Livingstone I, Craswell PW, Bevan EB, Smith MT, Eadie MJ. Propranolol in pregnancy three year prospective study. *Clin Exp Hypertens B* 1983;**2**:341–50.

180 Scardo JA, Vermillion ST, Newman RB, Chauhan SP, Hogg BB. A randomized, double-blind, hemodynamic evaluation of

nifedipine and labetalol in preeclamptic hypertensive emergencies. *Am J Obstet Gynecol* 1999;**181**:862–6.

181 Aube M. Migraine in pregnancy. *Neurology* 1999;**53**:S26–8.

182 Caswell HT, Marks AD, Channick BJ. Propranolol for the preoperative preparation of patients with thyrotoxicosis. *Surg Gynecol Obstet* 1978;**146**:908–10.

183 Sukenik S, Biale Y, Ben-Aderet N, Khodadadi J, Levi D, Stern J. Successful control of pheochromocytoma in pregnancy. *Eur J Obstet Gynecol Reprod Biol* 1979;**9**:249–51.

184 Bott-Kanner G, Schweitzer A, Reisner SH, Joel-Cohen SJ, Rosenfeld JB. Propranolol and hydralazine in the management of essential hypertension in pregnancy. *Br J Obstet Gynaecol* 1980;**87**:110–4.

185 Elhassan EM, Mirghani OA, Habour AB, Adam I. Methyldopa versus no drug treatment in the management of mild pre-eclampsia. *East Afr Med J* 2002;**79**:172–5.

186 Gunenc O, Cicek N, Gorkemli H, Celik C, Acar A, Akyurek C. The effect of methyldopa treatment on uterine, umbilical and fetal middle cerebral artery blood flows in preeclamptic patients. *Arch Gynecol Obstet* 2002;**266**:141–4.

187 Olsen KS, Beier-Holgersen R. Fetal death following labetalol administration in pre-eclampsia. *Acta Obstet Gynecol Scand* 1992;**71**:145–7.

188 Crooks BN, Deshpande SA, Hall C, Platt MP, Milligan DW. Adverse neonatal effects of maternal labetalol treatment. *Arch Dis Child Fetal Neonatal Ed* 1998;**79**:F150–1.

189 Hjertberg R, Faxelius G, Belfrage P. Comparison of outcome of labetalol or hydralazine therapy during hypertension in pregnancy in very low birth weight infants. *Acta Obstet Gynecol Scand* 1993;**72**:611–5.

190 Bowman ML, Bergmann M, Smith JF. Intrapartum labetalol for the treatment of maternal and fetal thyrotoxicosis. *Thyroid* 1998;**8**:795–6.

191 Beardmore KS, Morris JM, Gallery ED. Excretion of antihypertensive medication into human breast milk: a systematic review. *Hypertens Pregnancy* 2002;**21**:85–95.

192 Munshi UK, Deorari AK, Paul VK, Singh M. Effects of maternal labetalol on the newborn infant. *Indian Pediatr* 1992;**29**:1507–12.

193 Chanda M, Mackenzie P, Day JH. Hypersensitivity reactions following laminaria placement. *Contraception* 2000;**62**: 105–6.

194 Stafford CT, Lobel SA, Fruge BC, Moffitt JE, Hoff RG, Fadel HE. Anaphylaxis to human serum albumin. *Ann Allergy* 1988;**61**:85–8.

195 Miller AA. Diphenhydramine toxicity in a newborn: a case report. *J Perinatol* 2000;**20**:390–1.

196 Watson-Jones D, Gumodoka B, Weiss H, *et al.* Syphilis in pregnancy in Tanzania. II. The effectiveness of antenatal syphilis screening and single-dose benzathine penicillin treatment for the prevention of adverse pregnancy outcomes. *J Infect Dis* 2002;**186**:948–57.

197 Michelow IC, Wendel GD Jr, Norgard MV, *et al.* Central nervous system infection in congenital syphilis. *N Engl J Med* 2002;**346**:1792–8.

198 Ballard RC, Berman SM, Fenton KA. Azithromycin versus penicillin for early syphilis. *N Engl J Med* 2006;**354**:203–5.

199 Boyer KM, Gotoff SP. Prevention of early-onset neonatal group B streptococcal disease with selective intrapartum chemoprophylaxis. *N Engl J Med* 1986;**314**:1665–9.

200 Stauffer UG. Tooth changes caused by tetracycline in the fetus, infant and child. *Schweiz Med Wochenschr* 1967;**97**:291–3.

201 ElTabbakh GH, Elejalde BR, Broekhuizen FF. Primary syphilis and nonimmune fetal hydrops in a penicillin-allergic woman: a case report. *J Reprod Med* 1994;**39**:412–4.

202 Smith JR, Taylor-Robinson D. Infection due to *Chlamydia trachomatis* in pregnancy and the newborn. *Baillieres Clin Obstet Gynaecol* 1993;**7**:237–55.

203 Centers for Disease Control and Prevention (CDC). Increases in fluoroquinolone-resistant *Neisseria gonorrhoeae*: Hawaii and California, 2001. *MMWR Morb Mortal Wkly Rep* 2002;**51**: 1041–4.

204 Bothamley G. Drug treatment for tuberculosis during pregnancy: safety considerations. *Drug Saf* 2001;**24**:553–65.

205 Centers for Disease Control and Prevention (CDC). Updated recommendations for antimicrobial prophylaxis among asymptomatic pregnant women after exposure to *Bacillus anthracis*. *MMWR Morb Mortal Wkly Rep* 2001;**50**:960.

206 Ludlam H, Wreghitt TG, Thornton S, *et al.* Q fever in pregnancy. *J Infect* 1997;**34**:75–8.

207 Connell W, Miller A. Treating inflammatory bowel disease during pregnancy: risks and safety of drug therapy. *Drug Saf* 1999;**21**:311–23.

208 Gulmezoglu AM. Interventions for trichomoniasis in pregnancy. *Cochrane Database Syst Rev* 2002;**3**:CD000220.

209 Klebanoff MA, Hauth JC, MacPherson CA, *et al.* National Institute for Child Health and Development Maternal Fetal Medicine Units Network. Time course of the regression of asymptomatic bacterial vaginosis in pregnancy with and without treatment. *Am J Obstet Gynecol* 2004;**190**:363–70.

210 Klebanoff MA, Hillier SL, Nugent RP, MacPherson CA, Hauth JC, Carey JC. National Institute of Child Health and Human Development Maternal-Fetal Medicine Units Network. Is bacterial vaginosis a stronger risk factor for preterm birth when it is diagnosed earlier in gestation? *Am J Obstet Gynecol* 2005;**192**:470–7.

211 Okun N, Gronau KA, Hannah ME. Antibiotics for bacterial vaginosis or *Trichomonas vaginalis* in pregnancy: a systematic review. *Obstet Gynecol* 2005;**105**:857–68.

212 Hauth JC, Goldenberg RL, Andrews WW, DuBard MB, Copper RL. Reduced incidence of preterm delivery with metronidazole and erythromycin in women with bacterial vaginosis. *N Engl J Med* 1995;**333**:1732–6.

213 Goldenberg RL, Klebanoff M, Carey JC, Macpherson C. Metronidazole treatment of women with a positive fetal fibronectin test result. *Am J Obstet Gynecol* 2001;**185**:485–6.

214 Carey JC, Klebanoff MA, Hauth JC, *et al.* Metronidazole to prevent preterm delivery in pregnant women with asymptomatic bacterial vaginosis. National Institute of Child Health and Human Development Network of Maternal-Fetal Medicine Units. *N Engl J Med* 2000;**342**:534–40.

215 McGregor JA, French JI. Bacterial vaginosis in pregnancy. *Obstet Gynecol Surv* 2000;**55**(5 Suppl 1):S1–19.

216 Pacifici GM. Placental transfer of antibiotics administered to the mother: a review. *Int J Clin Pharmacol Ther* 2006;**44**:57–63.

217 Elek E, Ivan E, Arr M. Passage of penicillins from mother to foetus in humans. *Int J Clin Pharmacol* 1972;**6**:223–8.

218 Dashe JS, Gilstrap LC 3rd. Antibiotic use in pregnancy. *Obstet Gynecol Clin North Am* 1997;**24**:617–29.

219 Klastersky-Genot MT. Effects of tetracycline, administered during pregnancy, on the deciduous teeth: a double blind controlled study. *Acta Stomatol Belg* 1970;**67**:107–24.

220 Czeizel AE, Rockenbauer M. Teratogenic study of doxycycline. *Obstet Gynecol* 1997;**89**:524–8.

221 Polachek H, Holcberg G, Sapir G, *et al*. Transfer of ciprofloxacin, ofloxacin and levofloxacin across the perfused human placenta *in vitro*. *Eur J Obstet Gynecol Reprod Biol* 2005;**122**:61–5.

222 Berkovitch M, Pastuszak A, Gazarian M, Lewis M, Koren G. Safety of the new quinolones in pregnancy. *Obstet Gynecol* 1994;**84**:535–8.

223 Peled Y, Friedman S, Hod M, Merlob P. Ofloxacin during the second trimester of pregnancy. *DICP* 1991;**25**:1181–2.

224 Heisterberg L. Placental transfer of metronidazole in the first trimester of pregnancy. *J Perinat Med* 1984;**12**:43–5.

225 Moskovitz DN, Bodian C, Chapman ML, Marion JF, Rubin PH, Scherl E. The effect on the fetus of medications used to treat pregnant inflammatory bowel-disease patients. *Am J Gastroenterol* 2004;**99**:656–61.

226 Nau H. Clinical pharmacokinetics in pregnancy and perinatology. II. Penicillins. *Dev Pharmacol Ther* 1987;**10**:174–98.

227 Hendeles L, Trask PA. Tetracycline and lactation. *J Am Dent Assoc* 1983;**107**:12, 14.

228 Giamarellou H, Kolokythas E, Petrikkos G, Gazis J, Aravantinos D, Sfikakis P. Pharmacokinetics of three newer quinolones in pregnant and lactating women. *Am J Med* 1989;**87**:49S–51S.

229 Passmore CM, McElnay JC, Rainey EA, D'Arcy PF. Metronidazole excretion in human milk and its effect on the suckling neonate. *Br J Clin Pharmacol* 1988;**26**:45–51.

230 Scott LL, Hollier LM, McIntire D, Sanchez PJ, Jackson GL, Wendel GD Jr. Acyclovir suppression to prevent recurrent genital herpes at delivery. *Infect Dis Obstet Gynecol* 2002;**10**:71–7.

231 Little SE, Caughey AB. Acyclovir prophylaxis for pregnant women with a known history of herpes simplex virus: a cost-effectiveness analysis. *Am J Obstet Gynecol* 2005;**193**:1274–9.

232 Laerum OD. Toxicology of acyclovir. *Scand J Infect Dis Suppl* 1985;**47**:40–3.

233 Sheffield JS, Fish DN, Hollier LM, Cadematori S, Nobles BJ, Wendel GD Jr. Acyclovir concentrations in human breast milk after valaciclovir administration. *Am J Obstet Gynecol* 2002;**186**:100–2.

Genetics

6 Genetic screening for mendelian disorders

Deborah A. Driscoll

Genetic screening to identify couples at risk for having off-spring with inherited conditions such as Tay–Sachs disease, sickle cell disease, and cystic fibrosis has been integrated into obstetric practice. The number of genetic conditions for which carrier screening and genetic testing is available has increased as a result of the Human Genome Project and advances in technology. Further, the demand for genetic screening and testing has increased. The decision to offer population-based genetic screening is complex. Factors to consider include disease prevalence and carrier frequency; nature and severity of the disorder; options for treatment; intervention and prevention; availability of a sensitive and specific screening and diagnostic test; positive predictive value of the test; and cost [1]. Care must be taken to avoid the potential for psychologic harm to the patient and the misuse of genetic information and possible discrimination. Successful implementation of genetic screening programs requires adequate educational materials for providers and patients and genetic counseling services. This chapter reviews mendelian inheritance, indications for genetic screening, and the current carrier screening guidelines for common genetic disorders.

Family history

Genetic screening begins with an accurate family history, which should be a routine part of a patient's complete evaluation. It is useful to summarize this information in a pedigree to demonstrate the family relationships and which relatives are affected. The family history should include three generations; the sex and state of health should be noted. Stillbirths and miscarriage should be recorded. A history of the more common genetic diseases, chromosomal abnormalities, and congenital malformations such as cardiac defects, cleft lip and palate, and neural tube defects should be routinely sought. The history should also include cognitive and behavioral disorders such as mental retardation, autism, developmental delay, and psychiatric disorders. Cancer and age at diagnosis should be

noted. Genetic diagnoses should be confirmed by review of the medical records whenever possible. Pedigree analysis is important in determining the type of inheritance of a given mendelian disorder, and is important in providing accurate risk estimate.

Mendelian inheritance

Mendelian inheritance refers to genetic disorders that arise as a result of transmission of a mutation in a single gene. Most single-gene disorders are uncommon, usually occurring in 1 in 10,000–50,000 births. Over 11,000 single gene disorders or traits have been described and can be found in the Online Mendelian Inheritance in Man (www3.ncbi.nlm.nih.gov/omim/) [2]. Obstetricians should be familiar with the inheritance patterns and some of the common disorders for which carrier screening is available.

There are three basic patterns of mendelian inheritance:
1 autosomal dominant;
2 autosomal recessive; and
3 X-linked.

Genes occur in pairs; one copy is present on each one of a pair of chromosomes. If the effects of an abnormal gene are evident when the gene is present in a single dose, then the gene is said to be dominant. A carrier of an autosomal dominant disorder has a 50% chance of transmitting the disorder to his or her off-spring. In general, pedigree analysis shows the disease in every generation with some exceptions. In some families, the disorder may not be expressed in every individual who inherits the gene. This is referred to as incomplete or reduced penetrance. Affected relatives may have a variable phenotype as a result of differences in expression. Modifying genes and/or the environment can influence the phenotype and hence it may be difficult to predict the outcome accurately. Autosomal dominant disorders may also arise as a result of a sporadic mutation. If this occurs then a couple does not have a 50% risk of having a subsequent affected child unless germline mosaicism exists. Germline mosaicism refers to the existence of a population of cells with the mutation in the testes or ovary.

For autosomal recessive disorder to be expressed, both copies of the gene must be abnormal. Carriers of autosomal recessive disorders are detected either through carrier screening, or after the birth of an affected child or relative. Pedigree analysis typically shows only siblings to be affected. In general, carriers are healthy although at the cellular level they may demonstrate reduced enzyme levels; this is not sufficient to cause disease. For example, Tay–Sachs carriers have a reduced level of hexosaminidase A. When both parents are carriers there is a 25% chance of having an affected child in each pregnancy. There is a two-thirds likelihood that their offspring is a carrier.

X-linked diseases such as Duchenne muscular dystrophy or hemophilia primarily affect males because they have a single X chromosome. In contrast, female carriers are less likely to be affected because of the presence of two X chromosomes. A female carrier may show manifestations of the disease because of unfavorable lyonization or inactivation of the X chromosome with the normal copy of the gene. A female who carries a gene causing an X-linked recessive condition has a 50% chance of transmitting the gene in each pregnancy; 50% of the male fetuses will be affected and 50% of the females will be carriers. X-linked disorders can also occur as a result of a *de novo* mutation. The mother of a child with an X-linked condition is not necessarily a carrier. Similar to autosomal dominant disorders, germline mosaicism must also be considered. A male with an X-linked disorder will pass the abnormal gene on his X chromosome to all of his daughters who will be carriers; his sons receive his Y chromosome and hence will be unaffected. X-linked dominant disorders such as incontinentia pigmenti are rare and affect females; they tend to be lethal in males.

It is now recognized that some genetic conditions do not follow simple mendelian inheritance. Some genes contain a region of trinucleotide repeats (i.e., $(CCG)_n$) that are unstable and may expand during transmission from parent to offspring. When the number of repeats reaches a critical level, the gene becomes methylated and is no longer expressed (e.g., Fragile X syndrome). Testing is available to determine if an individual with a positive family history of mental retardation carries a premutation, which may expand to a full mutation in their offspring [3]. Trinucleotide repeats are also implicated in several neurologic disorders such as Huntington disease and myotonic dystrophy [4].

Carrier screening

Carrier screening refers to the identification of an individual who is heterozygous or has a mutation in one of two copies of the gene. The screening test may identify an individual with two mutations who is so mildly affected it has escaped medical attention. Ideally, carrier screening should be offered to patients and their partners prior to conception to provide them with an accurate assessment of their risk of having an affected child and a full range of reproductive options. Most screening takes place during pregnancy and should be performed as early as possible to allow couples an opportunity to have prenatal diagnostic testing. When both parents are carriers, genetic counseling is recommended and they are informed of the availability of prenatal diagnostic testing, pre-implantation genetic diagnosis, donor gametes (eggs or sperm), and adoption to avoid the risk for having an affected child. It is helpful to explore their attitudes towards prenatal testing and termination of pregnancy. In addition, they may consider contacting their relatives at risk and inform them of the availability of carrier screening.

In the USA, preconception or prenatal genetic screening tests are available for many inherited conditions. The decision to offer testing is based on family history, or ethnic or racial heritage associated with an increased risk for a specific condition. Information about specific genetic disorders and testing can be found at www.genetests.org. Screening should be voluntary and informed consent is desirable. Patients should be provided with information about the disorder, the prevalence, severity, and treatment options. Test information including detection rates and the limitations should be reviewed with the patient. When the detection rate is less than 100%, it is important for the patient to understand that a negative screening test reduces the likelihood that an individual is a carrier and at risk for having an affected offspring but does not eliminate the possibility. For some patients, genetic counseling may assist with the decision-making process. Patients should also be assured that their test results are confidential.

Guidelines for carrier screening for the hemoglobinopathies [5], cystic fibrosis [6], and genetic diseases more commonly found among individuals of Eastern European Jewish heritage [7] have been developed by the American College of Obstetricians and Gynecologists (ACOG). These disorders are briefly described below and in Table 6.1. DNA-based tests to assess an individual's carrier status for other inherited conditions such as spinal muscular atrophy or Huntington disease are available but in general are only offered if an individual is at an increased risk to be a carrier based on family history.

When a family history suggests that a patient or her partner may be at increased risk to be a carrier or to have a child with an inherited condition, the first step is to determine if the gene for that disorder has been identified. If the gene is known, the optimal strategy is to test the affected relative. Many disorders are caused by mutations unique to a family, and DNA sequencing is required to identify the disease-causing mutation. Once a mutation is confirmed in the affected individual, testing relatives at risk to be carriers is possible. In some cases, DNA

Table 6.1 Mendelian disorders frequent among individuals of Eastern European Jewish ancestry.

Disorder	Carrier Rate	Clinical Features
Tay–Sachs disease	1 in 30	Hypotonia, developmental delay, loss of developmental milestones, mental retardation beginning at 5–6 months; loss of sight at 12–18 months, usually fatal by age 6
Canavan disease	1 in 40	Hypotonia, developmental delay, seizures, blindness, large head, gastrointestinal reflux
Familial dysautonomia	1 in 32	Abnormal suck, feeding difficulties, episodic vomiting, abnormal sweating, pain and temperature instability, labile blood pressure, absent tearing, scoliosis
Cystic fibrosis	1 in 24	Chronic pulmonary infections, malabsorption, failure to thrive, pancreatitis, male infertility because of congenital absence of the vas deferens
Fanconi anemia type C	1 in 89	Limb, cardiac, and genitourinary anomalies; microcephaly, mental retardation, developmental delay; anemia, pancytopenia, and increased risk for leukemia
Niemann–Pick type A	1 in 90	Jaundice and ascites caused by liver disease; pulmonary disease; developmental delay and psychomotor retardation, progressive decline in cognitive ability and speech, dysphagia, seizures, hypotonia, abnormal gait
Bloom syndrome	1 in 100	Prenatal and postnatal growth deficiency; predisposition to malignancies; facial telangiectasias, abnormal skin pigmentation, learning difficulties, mental retardation
Mucolipidosis IV	1 in 127	Growth and severe psychomotor retardation; corneal clouding, progressive retinal degeneration, strabismus
Gaucher disease	1 in 15	Chronic fatigue, anemia, easy bruising, nosebleeds, bleeding gums, menorrhagia, hepatosplenomegaly, osteoporosis, bone and joint pain

Note: carrier rates apply to individuals of Eastern European Jewish ancestry; clinical features may vary in presentation, severity, and age of onset.

sequencing can be used as a carrier screening test but it is expensive and less reliable than testing the affected person. Testing for disorders that are the result of one or more common mutations can be utilized for carrier testing provided that the diagnosis in the affected relative is correct. For example, a carrier test has been developed for spinal muscular atrophy, a common autosomal recessive disorder caused by a deletion in exon 7 of the *SMN* gene [8]. This is a highly accurate carrier test because the vast majority of cases are caused by this deletion. Confirmatory testing of the affected individual is still recommended whenever possible. Many laboratories will accept postmortem tissue samples and paraffin blocks if the affected individual is deceased.

Carrier screening tests may be helpful when a particular diagnosis is suspected based on ultrasound findings in the pregnancy. The antenatal evaluation of a fetus with a congenital malformation typically includes a thorough ultrasound examination and fetal echocardiogram to look for associated anomalies, as well as a fetal karyotype. Single-gene disorders are often considered in the differential diagnosis but until recently were not amenable to prenatal testing. Now that the molecular basis of many of these disorders has been elucidated, either carrier screening of the parents or diagnostic testing of the pregnancy is possible when a particular diagnosis is suspected. For example, carrier screening for Fanconi anemia type C may be considered as part of the evaluation of a fetus with absent radius [9], particularly if the couple are of Eastern European Jewish ancestry, because the carrier frequency is 1 in 90 in this population and a single mutation accounts for 99% of the disease-causing mutations. Testing the parents to determine their carrier status can help establish or exclude a diagnosis in the fetus with an anomaly.

Carrier testing may be carried out on request because of heightened anxiety and concern. It is not uncommon for patients to request a test based on a personal experience, recent newspaper article, or television show. In these instances, it is important for them to understand their individual risk of being a carrier and having an affected child, as well as the risks, benefits, and limitations of testing. Pre- and post-test counseling is very important. For most rare disorders this is not a very cost-conscious approach but with the availability of high-throughput molecular technology testing is becoming more affordable. Although it has become feasible to perform these tests, our ability to predict outcome and future risks associated with carrier status is sometimes limited. In many cases, longitudinal studies of carriers will be needed to better define the risks and benefits of testing.

Hemoglobinopathies

The hemoglobinopathies include structural hemoglobin variants and the thalassemias. Sickle cell disease, a severe form of anemia, is an autosomal recessive disorder common among individuals of African origin but also found in Mediterranean,

Arab, southern Iranian, and Asian Indian populations. Approximately 1 in 12 African-Americans are carriers or have sickle cell trait (Hb AS). The underlying abnormality is a single nucleotide substitution (GAG to GTG) in the sixth codon of the beta-globin gene. This mutation leads to the substitution of the amino acid valine for glutamic acid. Sickle cell disorders also include other structural variants of beta-hemoglobin. Screening is best accomplished by complete blood count (CBC) with red blood cell (RBC) indices and a hemoglobin electrophoresis.

The thalassemias are a heterogeneous group of hereditary anemias brought about by reduced synthesis of globin chains. Alpha-thalassemia results from the deletion of two to four copies of the alpha-globin gene. The disorder is most common among individuals of South-East Asian descent. If one or two of the genes are deleted, the individual will have alpha-thalassemia minor, which is usually asymptomatic. Deletion of three genes results in hemoglobin H disease, which is a more severe anemia, and a fetus with deletions of all four alpha-chain genes can only make an unstable hemoglobin (Bart hemoglobin) that causes lethal hydrops fetalis and is associated with preeclampsia. Alpha-thalassemia is also common among individuals of African descent but typically does not result in hydrops.

The beta-thalassemias are caused by mutations in the beta-globin gene that result in defective or absent beta-chain synthesis. Beta-thalassemia is more common in Mediterranean countries, the Middle East, South-East Asia, and parts of India and Pakistan. The heterozygous carrier (beta-thalassemia minor) is not usually associated with clinical disability, except in periods of stress. Individuals who are homozygous (beta-thalassemia major or Cooley anemia) have severe anemia, failure to thrive, hepatosplenomegaly, growth retardation, and bony changes secondary to marrow hypertrophy. The mean corpuscular volume (MCV) is performed as an initial screening test for patients at risk. Individuals with low MCV ($<80\,\mu L^3$) should undergo hemoglobin electrophoresis; beta-thalassemia carriers have an elevated HbA_2 ($>3.5\%$). Diagnosis of alpha-thalassemia trait is by exclusion of iron deficiency and molecular detection of alpha-globin gene deletions.

Cystic fibrosis

In 2001, ACOG and the American College of Medical Genetics (ACMG) recommended that carrier screening for cystic fibrosis, an autosomal recessive disorder that primarily affects the pulmonary and gastrointestinal system, be offered to non-Hispanic Caucasian patients planning a pregnancy or currently pregnant [6]. Cystic fibrosis screening is available to any patient; however, the prevalence and carrier rates are lower in other populations and the detection rates are also reduced, resulting in a less effective screening test. ACMG recommends that a panel of 23 pan-ethnic mutations be used

for screening the general population [10]. For individuals with a family history of cystic fibrosis, screening with an expanded panel of mutations or complete analysis of the *CFTR* gene by sequencing may be indicated, if the mutation has not been previously identified in the affected relative. Patients with a reproductive partner with cystic fibrosis or congenital absence of the vas deferens may benefit from this approach to screening. Genetic counseling in these situations is usually beneficial. Cystic fibrosis carrier screening may also identify individuals with two mutations who have not been previously diagnosed as having cystic fibrosis. These individuals may have a milder form of the disease and should be referred to a specialist for further evaluation.

Jewish genetic diseases

There are a number of autosomal recessive conditions that are more common in individuals of Eastern European Jewish (Ashkenazi) descent. Several of these conditions are lethal or associated with significant morbidity. Tay–Sachs was the first disorder amenable to carrier screening based on the measurement of serum or leukocyte hexosaminidase A levels [11]. Today, similar detection rates can be achieved with mutation testing [12]. With the identification of the genes and disease-causing mutations for other disorders, carrier screening became feasible. ACOG recommended that in addition to Tay–Sachs, carrier testing for Canavan disease [13], familial dysautonomia, and cystic fibrosis be offered when one or both parents are of Eastern European Jewish descent [7]. These disorders share similar prevalence and carrier rates (Table 6.1). The sensitivity of these tests is also very high (95% or higher) and thus, a negative result indicates that the risk of having a child with the disorder is very low. However, it is important to recognize that, with the exception of Tay–Sachs and cystic fibrosis, the prevalence and the nature of the gene mutations in the non-Jewish population is unknown and hence carrier screening of a non-Jewish individual is of limited value. Table 6.1 lists the disorders for which carrier testing is available and provides a brief list of the clinical features. Many of these disorders are less frequent and therefore the decision to pursue screening is left to the patient.

Prenatal diagnosis

Invasive prenatal diagnostic testing is available for patients identified through carrier screening to be at increased risk for having an affected offspring (see Chapter 49). Molecular testing for the specific gene mutations can be performed on cells obtained through chorionic villus sampling (CVS) at 10–12 weeks' gestation or amniocentesis after 15 weeks' gestation. It is critical that the laboratory performs maternal cell contamination studies to ensure the accuracy of the test results.

Newborn screening

Carriers of mendelian disorders may also be identified through state newborn screening programs. Newborn screening was designed to identify newborns with inherited metabolic disorders who would benefit from early detection and treatment. However, advances in genetics and technology have led to expanded screening programs which include testing for hemoglobinopathies, endocrine disorders, hearing loss, and infectious diseases. Newborn screening for most mendelian disorders is performed by collecting capillary blood from a heel puncture onto a filter paper. Specimens are then sent to a reference laboratory where they are assayed for the specified diseases. Confirmatory testing is necessary because of the high false positive rate on the initial screen. In addition to the appropriate referral of the infant for treatment, genetic counseling of the couple is recommended to review the recurrence risk and reproductive options.

Case presentation

A 26-year-old healthy primigravida presents for prenatal care at 8 weeks' gestation. There is no family history of congenital malformations, genetic disorders, mental retardation, neurologic or psychiatric conditions. The patient's ancestors are Eastern European Jewish. Her partner is Caucasian and his ancestors are Northern European. She denies any medication use and has been taking multivitamins.

Based on the patient's Eastern European Jewish ancestry, the obstetrician discusses the availability of carrier screening tests to determine if she is a carrier of Tay–Sachs disease, Canavan disease, familial dysautonomia, and cystic fibrosis. The patient is provided with a pamphlet containing information about the disorders, the prevalence and carrier rate, risk of an affected child, test sensitivity, limitations, and possible outcomes. If the test is negative then her risk of being a carrier is markedly reduced and it is highly improbable that she will have a child with one of these disorders. If the test indicates that she is a carrier then her partner should be counseled and offered screening. The obstetrician informs the patient that the decision to proceed with carrier screening is hers and testing is voluntary.

The patient is informed of the following risks to be a carrier: about 1 in 30 for Tay–Sachs and familial dysautonomia, 1 in 24 for cystic fibrosis, and 1 in 40 for Canavan disease. The screening tests, performed on a sample of blood from the patient, analyze her DNA for the common mutations that cause each of these disorders. The detection rates are greater than 95%. Because the patient is pregnant, serum hexosaminidase A levels are unreliable; in lieu of DNA testing, leukocyte testing can be performed and has a high detection rate (98%). The patient enquires if there are other disorders she should be worried about. Her obstetrician informs her that carrier testing is available for a number of other inherited conditions that are common among individuals of Eastern European Jewish ancestry (Table 6.1). With the exception of Gaucher disease, which can be mild and is treatable, the other disorders occur less frequently and the chance that she is a carrier is approximately 1 in 90 or higher.

The patient asks if her partner should be tested. The obstetrician informs the patient that most of these disorders are less common among non-Jewish individuals and the detection rate is unknown. Therefore, carrier screening is not recommended for her partner unless the test indicates that she is a carrier. Cystic fibrosis is an exception; the carrier rate among Caucasians of Northern European ancestry is similar and the test detection rates are high. She may ask her partner to have cystic fibrosis carrier screening so that if they are both carriers she would learn early in the pregnancy and have the option of CVS if she desires prenatal diagnostic testing.

The patient elects to have the carrier screening performed for Tay–Sachs, Canavan, familial dysautonomia, and cystic fibrosis. Her obstetrician calls to inform her that the test results indicate that she is not a carrier of one of the common mutations that cause Tay–Sachs, Canavan, or familial dysautonomia and therefore she is unlikely to have an affected child. However, she is a carrier of ΔF508, the most common cystic fibrosis mutation found in approximately 70% of cystic fibrosis patients. The obstetrician recommends screening for cystic fibrosis in her partner and offers genetic counseling to obtain additional information. The partner agrees and the screening test demonstrates that he does not have any of the 23 common mutations that cause cystic fibrosis. Therefore, based on the partner's ethnicity and the test sensitivity, his risk of being a carrier has been reduced to approximately 1 in 208 and the risk that this couple will have an affected child is 1 in 832 ($1 \times 1/208 \times 1/4$). Prenatal testing is not recommended. The obstetrician informs the patient that she inherited the mutation from one of her parents so her siblings may also be carriers, and recommends she share this information with them.

References

1 Holtzman NA. *Newborn screening for genetic-metabolic diseases: progress, principles and recommendations.* Department of Health, Education, and Welfare. Publication no. (HSA) 78–5207, 1977.

2 *Mendelian Inheritance in Man, OMIM*^{TM}. Center for Medical Genetics, Johns Hopkins University (Baltimore, MD) and National Center for Biotechnology Information, National Library of Medicine (Bethesda, MD), 1998. World Wide WebURL: http://www.ncbi.nlm.nih.gov/omim/.

3 Sherman S, Pletcher BA, Driscoll DA. Fragile X syndrome: diagnostic and carrier testing. *Genet Med* 2005;**7**: 584–7.

4 Wenstrom KD. Fragile X and other trinucleotide repeat diseases. *Obstet Gynecol Clin North Am* 2002;**29**:367–88.

5 American College of Obstetricians and Gynecologists (ACOG) Practice Bulletin. Clinical Management Guidelines for Obstetrician Gynecologists Number 64, July 2005. Hemoglobinopathies in Pregnancy. *Obstet Gynecol* 2005;**106**:203–10.

6 ACOG, ACMG. *Preconception and Prenatal Carrier Screening for Cystic Fibrosis*. Washington DC: American College of Obstetricians and Gynecologists, 2001.

7 ACOG Committee on Genetics. Prenatal and preconceptional carrier screening for genetic diseases in individuals of Eastern European Jewish descent. *Obstet Gynecol* 2004;**104**:425–8.

8 Ogino S, Wilson RB. Genetic testing and risk assessment for spinal muscular atrophy (SMA). *Hum Genet* 2002;**111**:477–500.

9 Merrill A, Rosenblum-Vos L, Driscoll DA, Daley K, Treat K. Prenatal diagnosis of Fanconi anemia (Group C) subsequent to abnormal sonographic findings. *Prenat Diagn* 2005;**25**:20–2.

10 Watson MS, Cutting GR, Desnick RJ, *et al*. Cystic fibrosis population carrier screening: 2004 revision of American College of Medical Genetics mutation panel. *Genet Med* 2004;**6**:387–91.

11 ACOG Committee on Genetics. Number 318. Screening for Tay–Sachs disease. *Obstet Gynecol* 2005;**106**:893–4.

12 Eng CM, Desnick RJ. Experiences in molecular-based screening for Ashkenzi Jewish genetic disease. *Adv Genet* 2001;**44**:275–96.

13 American College of Obstetricians and Gynecologists. *Screening for Canavan disease*. ACOG Committee Opinion 212. Washington, DC: ACOG, 1998.

7 Screening for neural tube defects

Nancy C. Chescheir

Neural tube defects are among the most common significant congenital anomalies. The first fetal anomaly diagnosed by ultrasound was anencephaly [1]. Enormous public health and medical attention has been focused on the prenatal identification of pregnancies with this complication for several decades. Despite many years of attention to this problem, however, there is ongoing research to refine the diagnostic process.

Neural tube defects are a group of central nervous system disorders that result from the failure of normal primary neurulation, an embryologic process that is normally completed in the human by about day 26–28 postconception. Failure of normal closure of the anterior neuropore results in anencephaly. If the posterior neuropore fails to close, the resulting defect is known as spina bifida. The most significant form of spina bifida includes a failure of closure of the overlying dermis and also epidermis and is known as an open spina bifida (OSB) or spina bifida aperta. The prenatal diagnosis of OSB is the primary focus of this chapter. With OSB, the defect can be flat, with no overlying sac, in which case it is known as a rachischisis defect. When the sac contains only dural elements, the defect is a meningocele. When it also includes neural elements, it is a meningomyelocele. Anencephaly and spina bifida comprise the majority of neural tube defects. In addition, this spectrum of defects includes encephalocele, in which there is a defect in the skull (most commonly in the occipital area), with displacement of the meninges and usually brain tissue into the encephalocele, and iniencephaly, a rare disorder in which there is a skull defect with exposed brain in combination with a cervical neural tube defect with fusion to the cranium.

Among the neural tube defects, OSB is of the greatest public health interest, as this disorder is compatible with a near normal lifespan and varying degrees of impairment (both physical and cognitive). In addition, there is growing interest in whether its complications can be ameliorated with prenatal intervention. Thus, the pressure for early and accurate diagnosis is growing, in order to allow women reproductive options including pregnancy termination, selection of health care providers and hospitals in order to maximize neonatal well-being, and potential inclusion in the ongoing National Institute of Child Health and Human Development (NICHD) sponsored Management of Myelomeningocele Study (MOMS) of prenatal surgery for OSB. Increasingly, efforts are being made to more accurately predict the likely outcome for the child with a particular lesion to facilitate informed decision making by the parent(s).

Serum screening

In 1985, the American College of Obstetricians and Gynecologists (ACOG) [2] produced an alert from the Professional Liability Committee which recommended that all women be offered maternal serum alpha-fetoprotein (MSAFP) screening to increase the prenatal detection of open neural tube defects. This ushered in a new era in prenatal care in which specific maternal tests were offered in a large-scale fashion to detect fetal structural defects.

MSAFP is offered between 15 and 22 weeks of pregnancy [3]. AFP is a protein, produced originally in the yolk sac and then primarily in the fetal liver. The concentration in the fetal serum is approximately 40,000–50,000 times that in the maternal serum. The fetus excretes AFP in urine. It enters the maternal serum most likely by transport across the placenta and membranes. By performing population studies of the level of MSAFP in normal singleton, well-dated pregnancies, it was possible to develop a standard curve of how much AFP is normal in the maternal serum at different gestational ages. In situations in which there is an elevated production of AFP (such as in multiple gestations), increased excretion of AFP in the amniotic cavity (fetal nephrotic syndrome) or loss of fetal skin integrity such that the fetal intravascular AFP can "leak" into the amniotic fluid at higher levels (open neural tube defects, ventral wall defects, fetal dermatologic disorders), then the MSAFP levels are likely to be higher than normal. Fetal to maternal hemorrhage, such as in cases with early placental dysfunction, can also increase the MSAFP. This is likely the source of the association of elevated MSAFP levels with increased rates of growth restriction, preterm birth, and maternal preeclampsia.

As with any screening program, a decision has to be made about the balance of the sensitivity and specificity of the test. Historically, MSAFP levels ≥2.50 multiples of the median (MOM) had been associated with a detection rate of 88% of patients with anencephaly and 79% of those with spina bifida, for testing performed at 16–18 weeks' gestation. Typically, the cut-off value for prenatal screening is set so that the detection rate will be approximately 80%, and 5% of the population will be considered to have an abnormal test. Increasing the detection rate significantly results in many more women being identified falsely and put through the anxiety-provoking and expensive process of the evaluation of an abnormal MSAFP.

However, in the 20 plus years since MSAFP screening was recommended by ACOG for the general population, significant changes in the use of ultrasound and better understanding of the factors that place a woman at increased risk of bearing a child with spina bifida (and thus a candidate for diagnostic testing and not screening) have changed the utility of MSAFP screening. This screening is commonly performed in conjunction with measurement of other analytes to provide Down syndrome risk assessment. Bundling of the MSAFP with other screens may alter the uptake rate for the test overall, and thus the population of people screened. For instance, there may be a shift towards older women choosing to use the screening for Down syndrome because of increased concern in this population for aneuploidy. Another factor that has changed some of the dynamics of MSAFP screening is the earlier use of ultrasound, which has significant utility in the detection of anencephaly and OSB as well as providing improved dating criteria. As prenatal screening for Down syndrome with nuchal translucency and first trimester analytes is carried out more commonly, it is likely that fewer women will then also choose to undergo second trimester screening with MSAFP. However, that remains to be determined.

Despite the results of the RADIUS study [4], which showed no improvement in fetal perinatal morbidity or mortality by routine versus selected ultrasound in low-risk pregnant women, approximately 67% of pregnant women in the USA in 2000 received at least one basic ultrasound as learned from birth certificate data [5].

Dashe et al. [6] hypothesized that routine ultrasound might compare favorably with MSAFP screening in the primary identification of neural tube defects. In order to describe how these two common tests function, they performed a retrospective comparison of how neural tube defects were identified in their population of predominantly indigent women. Approximately half of their patients underwent MSAFP screening. Seventy-five percent who were eligible and were offered it, accepted. Approximately one-third of their patients began prenatal care after the window in which MSAFP can be performed. Sixty-six babies with neural tube defects were identified, 65 of them prenatally. Thirty-two were anencephalic, 27 had spina bifida, and there were five with either encephalocele or iniencephaly. Table 7.1 highlights that the MSAFP screening was abnormal in 65% overall—79% of those with anencephaly, but only 47% with OSB. The one OSB that was not identified prenatally was found to have hydrocephalus at 34 weeks, but the sacral spina bifida was not seen. As can be seen, inaccurate dating criteria significantly worsens the sensitivity of MSAFP screening, which is a gestational age-dependent test.

The mean MSAFP in those women with a fetus with anencephaly was 4.89 MOM; for those with OSB it was 2.22 MOM (below the 2.50 MOM cut-off). This is an important characteristic of MSAFP screening. Those lesions that have a larger surface area tend to have higher MSAFP than those with small surface areas.

The 53% of these women who did not have MSAFP screening were identified predominantly on the basis of their routine or standard ultrasound. This detected 100% of the anencephalic fetuses, all of the fetuses with iniencephaly or encephalocele, and 92% of the OSB.

Similarly, Norem et al. [7] reviewed the path to diagnosis of 189 patients with fetal neural tube defects. In this population, there were 67 with OSB, 104 anencephalics, and 18 with encephalocele. MSAFP screening was accepted by 79%. Routine sonography was offered to all patients between 15 and 20 weeks. Most of the Kaiser centers in this study offered standard ultrasound prior to MSAFP screening. There were 67 identified patients with OSB and, of these, 27 had no serum

Table 7.1 Likelihood of alpha-fetoprotein (AFP) elevation and likelihood of abnormality on routine ultrasound. (After Dashe et al. [6].)

	Overall	Anencephaly	Spina Bifida	Other
Serum AFP elevated	20/31 (65%)	11/14 (79%)	7/15 (47%)	2/2 (100)
Dated by US	13/15 (87%)	6/6/ (100%)	5/7 (71)	2/2 (100)
Dated by LMP, age confirmed by US	6/7 (86)	4/4	2/3 (67)	
Dated by LMP, no US confirmation	1/9 (11)	1/4 (25)	0/5	
Abnormality on standard ultrasound	35/36	20/20	12/13	3/3

LMP, last menstrual period; US, ultrasound.

screening. Among the 40 who had MSAFP screening, only 62% had an abnormally elevated result. Fifty-four of the 67 had routine sonography either alone or prior to MSAFP screening, and 93% of the cases were identified at the time of the routine ultrasound. The remainder were identified after referral because of an elevated MSAFP, or because of a known high-risk factor.

In conclusion, MSAFP screening under "real world" conditions in which routine sonography is offered to women appears to contribute little to the screening efficiency. In these two studies, routine ultrasound performed in the same window as AFP screening detected approximately 92% of patients with OSB. In settings in which routine sonography is not offered, MSAFP screening can be expected to identify approximately 50% of patients with a fetus with OSB, in part because of a higher rate of inaccurate dating of the pregnancies without the benefit of routine sonography.

Routine second trimester sonography

Both the American Institute of Ultrasound in Medicine [8] and ACOG [9] include an examination of the fetal spine and cranium in the required content of a routine second trimester fetal scan. The cranial abnormalities in the second trimester related to OSB include hydrocephalus with enlargement of the lateral ventricles, confluence of the lateral ventricles and the third ventricle, obliteration of the cisterna magna with cerebellar distortion from herniation of the cerebellum through the foramen magnum (Arnold–Chiari II malformation), and frontal notching. On ultrasound, these are commonly known as the "banana sign" and the "lemon sign" respectively. These findings are typically easier to detect than the actual spinal defect. To detect the spinal defect it is necessary to obtain serial "bread loaf" type views of all spinal levels from the cervical to the sacral levels both in coronal section through the ventral echo center and the midline of the spinal laminae, as well as cross-sectional views of each spinal level. Sacral lesions are less likely to be associated with the cranial abnormalities and are easier to miss than the higher lesions. Importantly, they are also associated with fewer sequelae for the neonate.

Limitations of second trimester ultrasound as a population screening tool include:

1 Late onset of prenatal care such that women miss this window.
2 In some centers, it is cost prohibitive.
3 Maternal acoustic characteristics.
4 Sonographer/sonologist skill and experience.
5 Resolution of the equipment used.

However, as shown in the data by Dashe *et al.* [6] and Norem *et al.* [7], it is reasonable to expect that routine second trimester sonography will detect 100% of cases of anencephaly and approximately 90% of cases of OSB.

Diagnostic ultrasound

Population screening methodologies such as maternal serum screening studies and routine second trimester sonography are not appropriate for women at increased risk of bearing a child with neural tube defects. In these women, diagnostic studies should be considered.

Table 7.2 lists those factors that should prompt referral to diagnostic studies for spina bifida. In essence, this is a list of identifiable factors that significantly increase the risk of neural tube defects.

Confirmation of the presence of an OSB relies on the same ultrasound findings as described above. However, diagnostic studies should also include identification of the lesion level and whether there are associated abnormalities. The anatomic lesion level is defined as the upper level of the spine that shows disruption of the skin overlying the defect. Landmarks such as identification of the 12th rib allow the sonographer reasonable accuracy in pinpointing the highest affected level. It has been demonstrated that ultrasound is accurate to within one vertebral level of the anatomic level [10].

In uncertain cases, when the diagnosis of spina bifida is unconfirmed by ultrasound but suspected, amniocentesis can be offered. Analyzing the level of amniotic fluid AFP and acetylcholinesterase measured against standards for gestational age can offer more certain diagnoses. The question of whether to offer karyotype analysis to all presumed isolated cases of neural tube defects is an important one. Sepulveda *et al.* [11] obtained karyotype analysis in 95% of 152 consecutive fetuses with a neural tube defect. Seven percent of these resulted in the diagnosis of a chromosomal abnormality. All chromosomally abnormal fetuses had sonographic evidence of abnormalities in addition to those anticipated with the neural tube defect itself. The seven patients with OSB who had abnormalities included three with trisomy 13 and four with trisomy 18. Other studies in the past have also shown an 8–10% rate of chromosome abnormalities amongst patients with spina bifida [12,13]. These studies did not uniformly evaluate for the presence or absence of additional structural abnormalities at the time of karyotype evaluation, although 12/31 aneuploid fetuses were

Table 7.2 Risk factors for fetal neural tube defects.

Previous infant with a neural tube defect
First-degree relative with a neural tube defect
Maternal serum AFP level greater than the laboratory cut-off with confirmed dates
Suspicious screening ultrasound
Maternal pre-existing diabetes
Maternal periconceptional use of valproic acid or Depakote
Maternal obesity

AFP, alpha-fetoprotein.

described as having no additional findings. Because these additional studies were published in the mid-1990s, it is unclear whether the lack of additional findings was related to improved sonographic technique or to a biologic finding that aneuploidy can occur in the setting of an otherwise normal fetus with a neural tube defect. Clinical judgment is recommended, therefore, in determining whether to obtain a karyotype. If amniocentesis is going to be performed to measure amniotic fluid AFP and acetylcholinesterase it would seem appropriate to obtain a karyotype. In the absence of additional structural abnormalities or other risk factors for aneuploidy such as advanced maternal age, karyotype analysis can be considered if it would affect the patient's decisions about future pregnancy management.

Predicting functional outcome prenatally

Natural history studies correlating prenatal findings with postnatal outcomes are very difficult to perform. Part of this relates to pregnancy termination in identified fetuses. Although there are wide regional variations, in the USA as many as 20–30% of fetuses with spina bifida are electively terminated [14]. In addition, there is a very wide spectrum of outcomes with spina bifida. Attempting to predict cognitive function, motor abilities, lifespan, and quality-of-life has to be undertaken with some trepidation. Nonetheless, several authors have studied prenatal findings and correlated them with postnatal outcomes in order to provide some guidance in this area.

In a study performed on 30 prenatally diagnosed fetuses with myelomeningocele [10] in Brazil where pregnancy termination is illegal, some interesting findings were noted. Seven of 30 infants (26.9%) were considered to have a good prognosis without detectable intellectual or motor impairment. Two of these seven infants had lesion levels at or above L4. One patient in this group had clubbed feet. The presence or absence of clubbed feet did not correlate with long-term outcome. However, fetuses with lesions at or below L3 without clubbed feet appeared to have a better prognosis than any other group. The degree of fetal ventriculomegaly considerably influences the postnatal intellectual performance regardless of the motor status. There were four patients in the overall study without ventriculomegaly and three of them had normal intellectual outcomes. Among all infants with prenatal ventricular enlargement, 82% had abnormal outcomes. There was, however, no cut-off for the measurements of the ventricular enlargement below which normal intellectual development could be assured.

There was a 13% overall mortality rate predominantly related to complications of surgery or hind brain herniation. In the 23 of 27 overall with a poor prognosis (premature death, intellectual or motor impairment) the site of the lesion was the most significant isolated outcome predictor. Lesions at L3 and

above fell into the poor prognosis category 79% of the time, with a positive predictive value of 88.2% and negative predictive value of 55.6%. Eighty-two percent of fetuses with ventriculomegaly (87% overall) fell in the poor prognosis group. Importantly, that means that 18% of fetuses with ventriculomegaly fell into the good prognosis group. This suggests that some of the intellectual impairment may be related to shunt complications which by the time of the neurologic evaluation at 23 months, had occurred in approximately 28% of the intellectually normal and 38% of the intellectually impaired infants. This group was unable to predict bowel or bladder function postnatally as the young age of the children precluded this analysis.

In a study performed at the University of Alabama, Biggio *et al.* [15] followed a cohort of patients with isolated spina bifida. They excluded from their series those patients who underwent *in utero* therapy and a significant number of women who had elected to terminate their pregnancies, leaving 33 ongoing pregnancies. Ventriculomegaly was present on the initial ultrasound in 65% of pregnancies that were terminated and in 55% of the continuing pregnancies. This was not different between groups. An additional 33% of those in the continuing group who did not have ventriculomegaly at the initial study developed it later on in pregnancy, usually around 28 ± 6 weeks. Those fetuses with ventriculomegaly at the first study tended to have larger ventricles at birth than those without (29 ± 10 mm vs. 15 ± 4 mm). Overall, 12% of their continuing fetuses did not develop ventriculomegaly prenatally. In general, the higher the spinal lesion the more likely was it for the fetus to develop large ventricles. Clubbed feet was present in 6% of the continuing pregnancies at the initial study but developed in 18% more as the pregnancy progressed. This group did not have neonatal follow-up.

In summary then, it seems clear that the lower the lesion level, the better the prognosis. In addition, the absence of ventriculomegaly at the initial diagnosis suggests a smaller ventricular size at birth than in those with ventriculomegaly at the time of the initial diagnosis. However, none of these findings accurately predict with a high degree of certainty what the outcome will be for the individual fetus being evaluated. Substantial work is to be done in this area as this is the critical question for families who have to consider their options and for patient selection if maternal-fetal surgery for spina bifida proves to be efficacious.

Conclusions

Fetuses with spina bifida are diagnosed commonly such that it is now unusual for a woman who is receiving prenatal care in the USA to receive the unexpected diagnosis in the delivery room. It is likely that as an increasing number of women undergo first trimester ultrasound in the setting of nuchal translucency screening, there will be an increased identification of fetuses with neural tube defects diagnosed in the first trimester. In a study by Weisz [16], 42% of fetuses with OSB were identified at the time of a first trimester ultrasound. MSAFP screening uptake rates are likely to change as first trimester screening increases in popularity. Policy decisions regarding performing a routine ultrasound will certainly have an impact on the detection rate of spina bifida. Once spina bifida is diagnosed, it is critical that a complete diagnostic evaluation be performed so that the family can be advised of the condition of their fetus. Rapid referral to a diagnostic center following prenatal detection of either a risk factor or the presence of spina bifida is critical. If this results in a decision to continue the pregnancy, accurate counseling with pediatric neurologists and neurosurgeons as well as coordination of care with local spina bifida clinics can be established early on.

Case presentation

A 26-year-old nulliparous woman presents for a second trimester prenatal visit at 15 weeks' gestation (based on first trimester sonogram) desiring information on the most cost-effective method to rule out spina bifida in her child. She and her husband are healthy and have no family history of birth defects. However, her friend has a child with spina bifida and she is concerned about the possibility of this for her baby. Her doctor explains that maternal serum screening with alphafetoprotein (MSAFP) with ultrasound confirmation of a firm last menstrual period (LMP) has approximately 80% sensitivity for spina bifida detection. Without confirmation of the dates, MSAFP screening has a substantially lower sensitivity. The doctor also explains that ultrasound in the first trimester is insensitive for screening for most structural abnormalities, but ultrasound at 18–20 weeks will detect as many as 95% of cases of spina bifida.

She decides to undergo maternal serum screening with MSAFP at that visit and the results came back at 1.3 MOM (within the range of normal). She then is referred for a sonogram at 18 weeks to evaluate for fetal anomalies, especially fetal spina bifida because not all are detected with maternal serum screening. The level II sonogram reveals an appropriate for gestational age male infant with no evidence of structural defects, including spina bifida. The physician performing the sonogram reviews with her that not all anomalies are detectable with sonography, and although 95% of cases are detected with ultrasound, small lesions may not be detectable until after delivery.

References

1 Campbell S, Johnstone FD, Holt EM, May P. Anencephaly: early ultrasonic diagnosis and active management. *Lancet* 1972;**2**:1226.

2 American College of Obstetricians and Gynecologists. *Professional liability implications of AFP tests*. DPL Alert. Washington, DC: ACOG, 1985.

3 Wald NJ. *MS-AFP: issues in the prenatal screen and diagnosis in NTDs*. Washington DC: US Government Printing Office, 1980: 280.

4 Ewigman BG, Crane JP, Frigoletto FD, LeFevre ML, Bain RP, McNellis D, for the RADIUS Study Group. Effect of prenatal ultrasound screening on perinatal outcome. *N Engl J Med* 1992;**329**;821–7.

5 Martin JA, Hamilton BE, Ventura SJ, Menacker F, Park MM. Births: final data for 2000. *Natl Vital Stat Rep* 2002;**50**:1–101.

6 Dashe JS, Twickler DM, Santos-Ramos R, McIntire DD, Ramus RR. Alpha-fetoprotein detection of neural tube defects and the impact of standard ultrasound. *Am J Obstet Gynecol* epub, June 2006.

7 Norem CT, Schoen EJ, Walton DL, *et al*. Routine ultrasonography compared with maternal serum alpha-fetoprotein for neural tube defect screening. *Obstet Gynecol* 2005;**106**:747–52.

8 AIUM. Practice Guideline for the performance of an antepartum obstetrical examination. June 4, 2003.

9 American College of Obstetricians and Gynecologists (ACOG). Ultrasonography in pregnancy. *ACOG Practice Bulletin*. December 2004;58.

10 Fabio C, Peralta A, Bunduki V, *et al*. Association between prenatal sonographic findings and postnatal outcomes and 30 cases of isolated spina bifida aperta. *Prenat Diagn* 2003;**23**:311–4.

11 Sepulveda W, Corral E, Ayala C, Bes C, Gutierrez J, Vasquez P. Chromosomal abnormalities in fetuses with open neural tube defects: prenatal identification with ultrasound. *Ultrasound Obstet Gynecol* 2004;**23**:352–6.

12 Kennedy D, Chitayat D, Winsor EJT, Silver M, Toi TT. Ultrasound, chromosome and autopsy or postnatal findings in 212 cases of prenatally diagnosed neural tube defects. *Am J Med Genet* 1998;**77**:317–21.

13 Hume RF, Drugan A, Reichler A, *et al*. Aneuploidy among prenatally detected neural tube defects. *Am J Med Genet* 1996;**61**:171–3.

14 Cragan JD, Roberts HE, Edmonds LD, *et al*. Surveillance for anencephaly and spina bifida and the impact of prenatal diagnosis, United States, 1985–1994. *MMWR CDC Surveill Summ* 1995;**44**:1–13.

15 Biggio JR, Wenstrom KD, Owen J. Fetal open spina bifida: a natural history of disease progression in utero. *Prenat Diagn* 2004;**24**:287–9.

16 Weisz B. Early detection of fetal structural abnormalities. *Reprod Biomed Online* 2005;**10**;541–53.

8 First and second trimester screening for fetal aneuploidy

Fergal D. Malone

Prenatal screening for Down syndrome and other aneuploidies, such as trisomy 18, has advanced significantly since its advent in the 1980s. Antenatal screening for Down syndrome began by selecting women over the age of 35 as candidates for amniocentesis. Maternal serum screening for Down syndrome in the second trimester started in the mid-1980s, with low levels of the analyte alpha-fetoprotein (AFP) associated with an increased risk of fetal Down syndrome. The panel of screening tests available has expanded considerably, and now includes first trimester serum and sonographic screening, second trimester serum and sonographic screening, and combinations of screening tests across both trimesters.

First trimester sonographic screening

The single most powerful discriminator of Down syndrome from euploid fetuses is first trimester sonographic measurement of the nuchal translucency space, generally performed between 10.5 weeks' gestation and the end of the 13th week [1]. Fetal nuchal translucency (NT) refers to the normal subcutaneous fluid-filled space between the back of the neck and the overlying skin (Fig. 8.1). The larger the NT measurement, the higher the association with Down syndrome, other chromosomal abnormalities, and adverse pregnancy outcome.

Because the average NT measurement is only 0.5–1.5 mm in thickness, it is absolutely essential that the sonographic technique is meticulous, follows an agreed protocol, and is performed only by those with adequate training and experience. An error of only a fraction of a millimeter can have a significant impact on the Down syndrome risk quoted to an individual patient. Critical components of good NT sonographic technique are demonstrated in Fig. 8.1, and include imaging the fetus in the mid-sagittal plane, adequate magnification to focus only on the fetal head and upper thorax, discrimination between the nuchal skin and amniotic membrane, and caliper placement on the inner borders of the echolucent space. NT sonography is a more powerful discriminator of Down syndrome fetuses from euploid fetuses at 11 weeks', rather than 13 weeks', gestation, and therefore this form of screening should be performed as close to 11 weeks as possible [1].

Several large prospective population screening studies have now been completed in the USA and in Europe, and each have confirmed that NT sonography, when performed by trained and experienced sonographers, is a powerful screening tool for fetal aneuploidy [1–4]. At a 5% false positive rate, NT sonography (combined with maternal age) detects 70% of cases of Down syndrome at 11 weeks, but decreases to 64% at 13 weeks' gestation [1].

Other sonographic tools that are available for first trimester screening for fetal aneuploidy include nasal bone sonography, ductus venosus Doppler waveform analysis, and tricuspid regurgitation. Fetuses with Down syndrome appear to have relatively short nasal bones, leading to the suggestion that failure to visualize the nasal bones at the time of first trimester NT sonography may be an additional useful tool for Down syndrome detection. While initial studies of high-risk patient populations demonstrated that in expert hands absence of the fetal nasal bone in the first trimester may detect as many as 67% of cases of Down syndrome, a subsequent large population screening trial failed to demonstrate a role for this form of sonography [5,6]. It is likely therefore that first trimester nasal bone sonography will not have a role for general population screening for Down syndrome, but may be a second-line tool in select expert centers for evaluating pregnancies already found to be at increased risk.

A normal first trimester ductus venosus Doppler waveform is triphasic in appearance, with constant forward flow (Fig. 8.2). Absence of forward flow, or retrograde flow, during the atrial contraction phase has been shown in some smaller studies to be a marker for fetal aneuploidy [7]. However, the reproducibility of this measurement has been questioned and, like nasal bone sonography, it is likely that this form of first trimester sonography will remain a second-line screening tool at select expert centers [8]. Finally, more recent research has suggested that the presence of significant tricuspid regurgitation

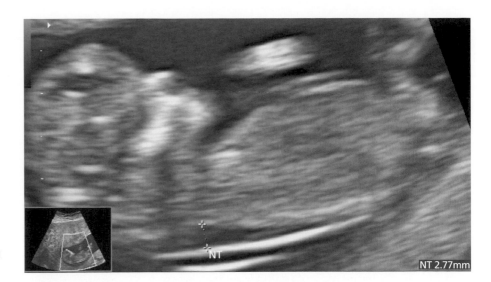

Fig. 8.1 First trimester ultrasound examination demonstrating measurement of the fetal nuchal translucency (NT) space.

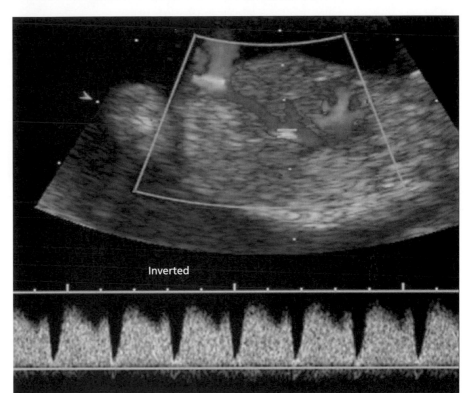

Fig. 8.2 Ductus venosus flow velocity waveform in a normal 13-week fetus. The Doppler gate is placed in the ductus venosus between the umbilical venous sinus and the inferior vena cava. Note that there is triphasic pulsatile flow with constant forward flow. The troughs of flow during the atrial contraction also demonstrate forward flow. (Reprinted from Malone *et al.* [16] with permission.)

at the time of NT sonography is also a useful marker for fetal Down syndrome [9]. However, further population screening studies are still needed to validate the role of first trimester tricuspid regurgitation for this indication. When considering newer forms of ultrasound evaluation for fetal Down syndrome, a balance needs to be struck between exciting new modalities and robust sonographic techniques that can be easily implemented at a general population level. Just because a new technique may perform well in select expert hands when evaluating high-risk patients does not imply that it will be a useful addition to general population screening.

Combined first trimester serum and sonographic screening

In Down syndrome pregnancies, first trimester serum levels of pregnancy-associated plasma protein A (PAPP-A) are decreased compared with euploid pregnancies, and human chorionic gonadotropin (hCG) levels are increased. Because these two serum markers are relatively independent of each other, and of both maternal age and NT measurements, improvements in Down syndrome risk assessment can be achieved by a combination serum and sonographic screening approach. Several large population studies have now confirmed that this combined first trimester screen is significantly better than screening for Down syndrome based on NT sonography alone [1,3]. At a 5% false positive rate, such combined first trimester screening detects 87% of cases of Down syndrome at 11 weeks, decreasing to 82% at 13 weeks' gestation (compared with 70% and 64% detection rates, respectively, for NT alone) [1]. Looked at differently, to achieve an 85% Down syndrome detection rate at 11 weeks' gestation, screening using NT sonography alone would yield a false positive rate of 20%, while combined first trimester screening would have a false positive rate of only 3.8% [1].

It is now clear that first trimester screening for fetal Down syndrome should be provided using the combination of NT sonography with appropriate serum markers. The only exception to this may be the presence of a multiple gestation where it can be very difficult to interpret the relative contributions of different placentas to maternal serum marker levels. In this latter situation it is reasonable to provide a Down syndrome risk assessment based on NT sonography alone.

Another practical problem for the implementation of first trimester combined screening in the USA is limited access to assays for the free beta subunit of hCG (fβhCG). Both total hCG and fβhCG are very effective discriminators of Down syndrome and euploid pregnancies, but when evaluated as univariate markers fβhCG is more powerful (15% versus 28% detection rates, respectively, for a 5% false positive rate at 11 weeks) [3]. However, in actual clinical practice fβhCG is never used on its own to screen for fetal Down syndrome, but instead will always be used in combination with other serum markers, such as PAPP-A and NT sonography. When the combination of first trimester NT, PAPP-A, and fβhCG is compared with the combination of NT, PAPP-A, and total hCG, their performance is actually very similar, with Down syndrome detection rates of 83% and 80%, respectively, for a 5% false positive rate [3]. Therefore, for clinicians in practice, if fβhCG is not available at their local laboratory it would still be possible to achieve almost as effective Down syndrome screening using the more widely available total hCG.

First trimester cystic hygroma

It has now become clear that there is a subgroup of fetuses with enlarged NT measurements that are at sufficiently high risk for aneuploidy and other adverse outcomes that delaying invasive diagnostic testing until serum markers are available is not necessary. The finding of an increased NT space, extending along the entire length of the fetus, and in which septations are clearly visible, is referred to as septated cystic hygroma, and is an easily identifiable feature during first trimester sonography (Fig. 8.3). Septated cystic hygroma will be encountered in approximately 1 in every 300 first trimester sono-

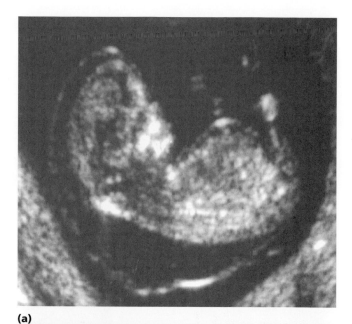

(a)

(b)

Fig. 8.3 (a) Septated cystic hygroma at 12 weeks' gestation: mid-sagittal view demonstrating increased nuchal translucency space extending along the entire length of the fetus. (Reprinted with permission from Malone *et al.* [10].) (b) Septated cystic hygroma at 12 weeks' gestation: transverse view through the fetal neck demonstrating septations.

graphic evaluations [10]. Once this diagnosis is made, patients should be counseled regarding a 50% incidence of fetal aneuploidy, with the most common abnormalities being Down syndrome, followed by Turner syndrome and trisomy 18 [10]. Less than 20% of such pregnancies will result in a healthy liveborn infant at term. Once this finding has been made, there is no need to delay until first trimester serum marker assays are completed, or until computerized Down syndrome risk assessments are calculated. Immediate invasive diagnosis using chorionic villus sampling (CVS) should be offered.

Second trimester sonographic screening

The mainstay for antenatal screening for Down syndrome for over 20 years has been second trimester sonographic evaluation of fetal anatomy, also frequently referred to as the genetic sonogram. Two general approaches have been used in the second trimester: sonographic detection of major structural fetal malformations, and sonographic detection of minor markers for Down syndrome.

The detection of certain major structural malformations that are known to be associated with aneuploidy should prompt an immediate consideration of genetic amniocentesis. The major structural malformations that are associated with Down syndrome include cardiac malformations (AV canal defect, ventricular septal defect, tetralogy of Fallot), duodenal atresia, cystic hygroma, and hydrops fetalis. The major malformations associated with trisomy 18 include cardiac malformations (AV canal defect, ventricular septal defect, double outlet right ventricle), meningomyelocele, omphalocele, esophageal atresia, rocker bottom feet, cleft lip or palate, cystic hygroma, and hydrops fetalis. While the genetic sonogram can be performed at any time during the second and third trimesters, the optimal time is likely to be at 17–18 weeks' gestation, which is late enough to maximize fetal anatomic evaluation, yet early enough to allow for amniocentesis results to be obtained. When a major structural malformation is found, such as an AV canal defect or a double-bubble suggestive of duodenal atresia, the risk of Down syndrome in that pregnancy can be increased by approximately 20- to 30-fold [11]. For almost all patients, such an increase in their background risk for aneuploidy will be sufficiently high to justify immediate genetic amniocentesis.

Second trimester sonography can also detect a range of minor markers for aneuploidy. The latter are not considered structural abnormalities of the fetus per se but, when noted, may be associated with an increased probability that the fetus is aneuploid. The minor markers that have been commonly linked to Down syndrome include nuchal fold thickening, nasal bone hypoplasia, mild ventriculomegaly, short femur or humerus, echogenic bowel, renal pyelectasis, echogenic intracardiac focus, clinodactyly, sandal gap toe, and widened iliac angle [12]. The minor markers that are associated with trisomy 18 include nuchal fold thickening, mild ventriculomegaly, short femur or humerus, echogenic bowel, enlarged cisterna magna, choroid plexus cysts, micrognathia, single umbilical artery, clenched hands, and fetal growth restriction. It should be noted that almost all data supporting the role of second trimester sonography for minor markers for aneuploidy are derived from high-risk populations, such as patients of advanced maternal age or with abnormal maternal

Table 8.1 Likelihood ratios for Down syndrome when an isolated minor sonographic marker is detected. The patient's a priori risk is multiplied by the appropriate positive likelihood ratio to yield an individualized post-test risk for fetal Down syndrome. (After Nyberg *et al.* [12].)

Minor Marker	Likelihood Ratio	95% Confidence Interval
Nuchal fold >5 mm	11	6–22
Echogenic bowel	6.7	3–17
Short humerus	5.1	2–17
Short femur	1.5	0.8–3
Echogenic intracardiac focus	1.8	1–3
Pyelectasis	1.5	0.6–4
Any two minor markers	10	6.6–14
Any three or more minor markers	115	58–229
No markers	0.4	0.3–0.5

serum screening results. It is still unclear what the relative contribution of screening for such minor markers will be in lower risk patients from the general population.

To objectively counsel patients following the prenatal diagnosis of a minor sonographic marker, likelihood ratios can be used to create a more precise risk assessment for the patient that their fetus might be affected with Down syndrome. Their use in clinical practice is simply to multiply the relevant likelihood ratio by the a priori risk. Table 8.1 summarizes the likelihood ratios that can be used to modify a patient's risk for Down syndrome, depending on which minor marker is detected. If no markers are present, the patient's a priori risk can be multiplied by 0.4, effectively reducing their chances of carrying a fetus with Down syndrome by 60% [12]. The likelihood ratio values listed for each marker assume that the marker is an isolated finding. By contrast, when more than one minor marker is noted in the same fetus different likelihood ratios must be used, with the risk for Down syndrome being increased by a factor of 10 when two minor markers are detected and by a factor of 115 when three or more minor markers are found [12]. It should also be noted that the 95% CI values for each marker's likelihood ratios are rather wide. These values should therefore be used only as a general guide for counseling patients, and care should be exercised to avoid implying too much precision in the final risk estimates. Accuracy of risk estimates, however, can be maximized by using the best available a priori risk value for a particular patient, such as the results of maternal serum marker screening or first trimester combined screening, rather than maternal age, when available.

Second trimester serum screening

Maternal serum levels of AFP and unconjugated estriol (uE3) are both approximately 25% lower in pregnancies complicated by Down syndrome compared with euploid pregnancies [13]. By contrast, levels of hCG and inhibin-A are approximately twice as high in pregnancies complicated by Down syndrome [13]. Maternal serum levels of AFP, uE3, and hCG all tend to be decreased in pregnancies complicated by trisomy 18. The combination of AFP, uE3, and hCG, commonly known as the triple screen, can detect 69% of cases of Down syndrome, for a 5% false positive rate [1]. When inhibin-A is added to this test, commonly known as the quad screen, the Down syndrome detection rate increases to 81%, for a 5% false positive rate [1,3]. Performance of serum screening tests can be maximized by accurate ascertainment of gestational age and, wherever possible, sonographic dating should be used instead of menstrual dating. It is optimal to provide serum screening between 15 and 16 weeks' gestation, thereby allowing the results to be available at the time of second trimester sonographic evaluation. Subsequently, if the genetic sonogram reveals any minor markers, the Down syndrome risk quoted from serum screening should be used with the appropriate likelihood ratio (as summarized in Table 8.1) to determine the final Down syndrome risk.

Combined first and second trimester screening

It is now clear that both first and second trimester approaches to screening for Down syndrome are highly effective, with first trimester combined screening being superior to second trimester serum quad screening only when performed as early as 11 weeks' gestation [1]. However, rather than restricting patients to one or another screening option, it is now possible to improve screening performance even further by combining screening tests across both trimesters. There are currently three approaches to this: integrated screening, sequential screening, and contingent screening.

Integrated screening

Integrated screening is a two-step screening protocol, with results not being released until all screening steps are completed. Sonographic measurement of NT, together with serum assay for PAPP-A, are obtained between 10 and 13 weeks' gestation, followed by a second serum assay for AFP, hCG, uE3 and inhibin-A obtained between 15 and 16 weeks' gestation. A single risk assessment is then calculated at 16 weeks' gestation. This "fully integrated" test has a Down syndrome detection rate of 95%, for a 5% false positive rate [1,3]. A variant of this approach, referred to as the "serum integrated" test, involves blood tests only, including PAPP-A in the first trimester, followed by AFP, hCG, uE3, and inhibin-A in the second trimester. This latter test, which does not require an NT ultrasound assessment, has a Down syndrome detection rate

of 86%, for a 5% false positive rate [1,3]. For some patients who are anxious to receive rapid screening results, or for those who might wish to avail of a first trimester CVS, it is possible that such integrated screening tests might not be acceptable, as a delay inevitably exists between the time of first trimester screening measurements and release of results in the second trimester. However, for patients who may not be interested in, or have access to, first trimester CVS, the efficiency of being provided with a single Down syndrome risk assessment result, which maximizes detection and minimizes false positives, may make such integrated screening tests appear attractive.

Sequential screening

In contrast to integrated screening, stepwise sequential screening refers to multiple different Down syndrome screening tests being performed, with risk estimates being provided to patients upon completion of each step. A key concept in performing stepwise screening is to ensure that each subsequent screening test that is performed should use the Down syndrome risk from the preceding test as the new a priori risk for later screening, or should include all previous marker results in risk calculation. If sequential screening tests are performed independently for Down syndrome without any modification being made for earlier screening results, the positive predictive value of the later tests will inevitably deteriorate, and it is likely that the overall false positive rate will increase [14]. A potential advantage of stepwise screening over integrated screening is that it allows patients in the first trimester to avail themselves of an immediate CVS, should their risk estimate justify this test, without having to wait until 16–18 weeks when the integrated screening results are provided. Patients could therefore achieve the benefit of early diagnosis associated with first trimester screening, as well as the higher detection rate for Down syndrome associated with integration of both first and second trimester screening tests.

Contingent screening

Finally, one of the major disadvantages of providing all possible first and second trimester screening tests for patients is the cost involved and the patient anxiety inherent with prolongation of the screening process over several months. A possible solution to this is to utilize contingent screening. With the contingent approach, patients have first trimester screening with NT, PAPP-A, and fβhCG, and only those patients with extremely high-risk results (e.g., greater than 1 in 30) are offered CVS. Patients with extremely low-risk results that are unlikely to be significantly changed by additional later tests (e.g., less than 1 in 1500) are reassured and are not offered additional Down syndrome screening tests. Finally, borderline risk patients (e.g., with risks between 1 in 30 and 1 in 1500) return at 15 weeks for quad serum markers and these are combined with the earlier first trimester markers to provide a final Down syndrome risk. The advantage of this approach is that it may focus the benefits of CVS with the highest risk patients, while significantly reducing the number of second trimester screening tests performed. Theoretical models have suggested that contingent screening may have performance similar to integrated screening (approximately 90–95% detection, at a 4–5% false positive rate), but with only 20% of patients needing to return in the second trimester for further screening [15]. While this appears to be an exciting approach that may be quite cost effective, it still requires validation by actual population trials before it can be endorsed for clinical application.

Case presentation

A 35-year-old white woman, G1P0, with no significant family history, presents at 11 weeks' gestation requesting reassurance regarding the possibility of fetal Down syndrome. After appropriate pretest counseling, in which the various screening tests and the relative advantages and disadvantages of screening versus invasive diagnostic tests are discussed, the patient agrees to proceed with combined first trimester screening. NT sonography is performed by a sonographer experienced in this technique, and the fetal crown rump length (CRL) is measured at 45 mm, while the NT space is measured at 1.6 mm. A maternal blood sample is obtained and sent to a prenatal screening laboratory for assay of PAPP-A and fβhCG, together with the sonographer's credentialing ID number (to facilitate an NT quality assurance scheme) and the fetal CRL and NT data. Four days later, the local physician's office receives a laboratory report confirming that the patient's a priori age-related risk for Down syndrome is 1 in 270, and that this has been reduced to 1 in 1500 by combined first trimester screening. The patient is informed of this result, feels reassured, and declines CVS.

Subsequently, the patient has a detailed sonographic fetal anatomic survey performed at 18 weeks' gestation at her physician's office. No major malformations are found, but the fetus is noted to have a single echogenic intracardiac focus in the left ventricle, but no other minor markers are seen. The patient is informed of this finding and its possible association with Down syndrome. The physician knows that this marker has a likelihood ratio of 1.8 for Down syndrome and calculates that the final risk of Down syndrome in this patient's case is 1 in 830 ([1/1500] × 1.8). The patient is again reassured and declines genetic amniocentesis. Approximately 5 months later, she delivers a healthy female infant at term.

References

1 Malone FD, Canick JA, Ball RH, *et al*. A comparison of first trimester screening, second trimester screening, and the combination of both for evaluation of risk for Down syndrome. *N Engl J Med* 2005;**353**:2001–11.

2 Snijders RL, Noble P, Sebire N, Souka A, Nicolaides KH. UK multicenter project on assessment of risk of trisomy 21 by maternal age and fetal nuchal-translucency thickness at 10–14 weeks of gestation. *Lancet* 1998;**351**:343–6.

3 Wald NJ, Rodeck C, Hackshaw AK, Walters J, Chitty L, Mackinson AM. First and second trimester antenatal screening for Down's syndrome: the results of the Serum, Urine and Ultrasound Screening Study (SURUSS). *Health Technol Assess* 2003;**7**:1–77.

4 Wapner R, Thom E, Simpson JL, *et al*. First-trimester screening for trisomies 21 and 18. *N Engl J Med* 2003;**349**:1405–13.

5 Cicero S, Rembouskos G, Vandecruys H, Hogg M, Nicolaides KH. Likelihood ratio for trisomy 21 in fetuses with absent nasal bone at the 11–14-week scan. *Ultrasound Obstet Gynecol* 2004;**23**:218–23.

6 Malone FD, Ball RH, Nyberg DA, *et al*. First trimester nasal bone evaluation for aneuploidy in the general population: results from the FASTER Trial. *Obstet Gynecol* 2004;**104**:1222–8.

7 Matias A, Gomes C, Flack N, Montenegro N, Nicolaides KH. Screening for chromosomal abnormalities at 10–14 weeks: the role of ductus venosus blood flow. *Ultrasound Obstet Gynecol* 1998;**12**:380–4.

8 Hecher K. Assessment of ductus venosus flow during the first and early second trimesters: what can we expect? *Ultrasound Obstet Gynecol* 2001;**17**:285–7.

9 Faiola S, Tsoi E, Huggon IC, Allan LD, Nicolaides KH. Likelihood ratio for trisomy 21 in fetuses with tricuspid regurgitation at the 11 to 13+6 week scan. *Ultrasound Obstet Gynecol* 2005;**26**:22–7.

10 Malone FD, Ball RH, Nyberg DA, *et al*. First trimester septated cystic hygroma: prevalence, natural history, and pediatric outcome. *Obstet Gynecol* 2005;**106**:288–94.

11 Nyberg DA, Luthy DA, Resta RG, Nyberg BC, Williams MA. Age-adjusted ultrasound risk assessment for fetal Down's syndrome during the second trimester: description of the method and analysis of 142 cases. *Ultrasound Obstet Gynecol* 1998;**12**:8–14.

12 Nyberg DA, Souter VL, El-Bastawissi A, Young S, Luthhardt F, Luthy DA. Isolated sonographic markers for detection of fetal Down syndrome in the second trimester of pregnancy. *J Ultrasound Med* 2001;**20**:1053–63.

13 Wald NJ, Kennard A, Hackshaw A, McGuire A. Antenatal screening for Down's syndrome. *J Med Screening* 1994;**4**:181–246.

14 Platt LD, Greene N, Johnson A, *et al*. Sequential pathways of testing after first-trimester screening for trisomy 21. *Obstet Gynecol* 2004;**104**:661–6.

15 Wright D, Bradbury I, Benn P, Cuckle H, Ritchie K. Contingent screening for Down syndrome is an efficient alternative to non-disclosure sequential screening. *Prenat Diagn* 2004;**24**:762–6.

16 Malone FD, D'Alton MD, for the Society for Maternal Fetal Medicine. First trimester sonographic screening for Down Syndrome. *Obstet Gynecol* 2003;**102**:1006–79.

Monitoring: Biochemical and Biophysical

9 Fetal endocrinology

Nebojsa Radunovic and Charles J. Lockwood

The fetal endocrine system differs from that which follows birth because of its interdependence on maternal and placental compartments. Our understanding of fetal endocrinology was originally based on animal models as well as from information derived from abortus' specimens, anencephalic fetuses, and from neonatal umbilical cord blood samples obtained after preterm or term delivery. More recently, direct assessment of the fetal hormonal milieu has become possible through the use of cordocentesis. This chapter reviews the ontogeny of the fetal endocrine system and clinical conditions that arise from its dysfunction.

Hypothalamus and pituitary

Ontogeny

The human fetal forebrain (prosencephalon) is identifiable by the third week of gestation. At the same point in development, a primitive endodermal invagination from the foregut (Rathke pouch) becomes visible anterior to the roof of the oral cavity. During the fourth and fifth weeks post-conception, the forebrain differentiates into the telencephalon and diencephalon, and the hypothalamus becomes visible as swelling on the inner surface of the diencephalic neural canal. Simultaneously, an outpouching of neural ectoderm from the diencephalon in the floor of the developing third ventricle fuses with the Rathke pouch. While the Rathke pouch forms the anterior and intermediate lobe of the pituitary (adenohypophysis), this neuroectodermal diverticulum gives rise to the posterior lobe of the pituitary (neurohypophysis).

The hypothalamus is largely developed by 7 weeks post-conception. By the 10th week post-conception, cells are arranged longitudinally into lateral, core, and midline hypothalamic zones [1] and norepinephrine, dopamine, and serotonin as well as several of hypothalamic hormones, including gonadotropin-releasing hormone (GnRH), thyrotropin-releasing hormone (TRH), and somatostatin can be detected [2,3]. Condensations of lateral and midline hypothalamic cells form the hypothalamic nuclei and interconnecting fiber tracts and cells display immunostaining for all the hypothalamic neuropeptides including growth hormone releasing hormone (GHRH), corticotropin-releasing hormone (CRH), GnRH, TRH, and somatostatin can be identified by the 13–16th weeks post-conception [4].

Immunocytochemical and electron microscopic assessment of the pituitary's adenohypophysis indicates that by 12 weeks cellular differentiation is virtually complete with four out of the five major cell types present: somatotrophs (growth hormone [GH] secreting cells), thyrotrophs (thyroid-stimulating hormone [TSH] secreting cells), corticotrophs (adrenocorticotropic hormone [ACTH] secreting cells), and gonadotrophs (luteinizing hormone [LH] and follicle-stimulating hormone [FSH] secreting cells). The exception to this pattern of pituitary hormone expression are the lactotrophs (prolactin [PRL] secreting cells) that can be identified by immunostaining only at mid-pregnancy [5]. However, it is not until the end of the seventh month that cells of the adenohypophysis terminally differentiate into the distinct cell types found in the adult gland.

Capillaries develop within the proliferating anterior pituitary mesenchymal tissue around the Rathke pouch and within the primordial hypothalamus by 8 weeks post-conception. Vascular cast studies suggest that the hypothalamic-pituitary portal system is intact by 12 weeks' gestation. However, local diffusion may allow communication between the phypothalamus and pituitary before that time. Maturation of the pituitary portal vascular system continues until 30–35 weeks.

Hypothalamic hormones

The hypothalamic hormones (Table 9.1) can be divided into those produced in the hypothalamus and released into the portal circulation (releasing hormones) and those

Table 9.1 Hypothalamic hormones.

Releasing hormones
Gonadotropin-releasing hormone (GnRH)
Growth hormone-releasing hormone (GHRH)
Somatostatin
Thyrotropin-releasing hormone (TRH)
Corticotropin-releasing hormone (CRH)

Neurohypophyseal hormones
Arginine vasotocin (AVT)
Antidiuretic hormone (ADH)
Oxytocin (OT)

synthesized in neuron cell bodies within the hypothalamus and transported via axons to the neurohypophysis where they are stored or released into the systemic circulation (neurohypophyseal hormones).

Releasing hormones

Most of the anterior pituitary hormones are controlled by stimulatory hormones, but GH and PRL are also regulated by inhibitory factors. The releasing hormones of the hypothalamus are secreted episodically, not continuously, and in some cases display a circadian rhythm.

Gonadotropin-releasing hormone. While GnRH is the major physiologic secretagogue of gonadotropins in adults, it has a lesser role in fetuses given the high levels of human chorionic gonadotropin (hCG). During early embryologic development, GnRH neurons originate in the nasal region near the developing olfactory bulbs and then migrate to the hypothalamus. Kallmann syndrome, which is associated with both anosmia (loss of sense of smell) and hypogonadic hypogonadism (deficits in GnRH expression), has been used to support a developmental origin of GnRH cells in the olfactory placode [6]. By 16 weeks post-conception, GnRH-containing neurons terminate in portal vessels.

The hypothalamic content of GnRH has been reported to rise during the first half of gestation and depend on fetal gender [7]. Maximum GnRH content was observed in females at 22–25 weeks' gestation and in males at 34–38 weeks' gestation [8]. *In vitro* studies indicate that the human fetal pituitary releases LH and FSH in response to GnRH by 14–15 weeks' gestation. The magnitude of the LH response to GnRH *in vitro* is greater in female fetal pituitaries. Exposure to estradiol by the second trimester enhances the sensitivity of human fetal pituitaries to GnRH, potentially explaining this gender difference.

Growth hormone-releasing hormone. Neurons immunostaining for GHRH are present by 18 weeks within the hypothalamic median eminence, with an increase in staining later in gesta-

tion [9]. Hypothalamic GHRH binds to specific receptors on pituitary somatotropes to increase intracellular cyclic adenosine monophosphate (cAMP) and selectively stimulate transcription of GH mRNA and GH secretory pulses.

Somatostatin. This potent suppressor of pituitary GH secretion is detectable in the fetal hypothalamus by 11 weeks, and hypothalamic content increases by 22 weeks post-conception [3]. At this age, the somatotropes respond to both GHRH and somatostatin. Somatostatin suppresses basal GH secretion without altering GH mRNA levels and it appears to be the primary regulator of GH pulses in response to physiologic stimuli. Because somatostatin crosses the human placenta, administration of somatostatin to the mother can suppress fetal pituitary GH release and reduce GH concentration in umbilical cord blood [3].

Thyrotropin-releasing hormone. TRH is detectable in the human fetal brain extracts by 5 weeks, the hypothalamus by 8 weeks, and the circulation by 20 weeks' gestation [3]. Thereafter, concentrations do not change with gestation. Extrahypothalamic sources of TRH such as brain, spinal cord, pancreas, placenta and stomach, and reduced fetal clearance may account for the elevated TRH levels found in fetuses. In humans, TRH crosses the placenta, and administration of TRH to the mother results in a rise in fetal cord plasma TSH from at least 25 weeks' gestation [10].

Corticotropin-releasing hormone. In postnatal life, CRH secretion into the hypophyseal–portal circulation promotes the release of pituitary ACTH, which, in turn, stimulates the release of cortisol by the adrenal glands. Hypothalamic CRH and pituitary ACTH release are, in turn, inhibited by cortisol. CRH mRNA and/or protein has also been localized to the placenta and immunoreactive CRH is released by and/or localized to amniocytes, cytotrophoblasts, and decidual cells. In contrast to the negative regulation of hypothalamic CRH secretion by cortisol, corticosteroids stimulate expression of CRH by cultured villous cytotrophoblasts, amnion, chorion, and decidual cells [11].

The ontologic development and functioning of the fetal hypothalamic-pituitary-adrenal (HPA) axis is greatly affected by placental sources of these hormones. We found that fetal serum CRH concentrations did not correlate with gestational age or fetal ACTH levels but did with maternal (i.e., placental-derived) values [12]. In turn, placental CRH levels most closely correlated with fetal cortisol values. While fetal CRH concentrations were significantly higher than neonatal and nonpregnant adult values, they were significantly lower than maternal values. Economides *et al.* [13] also noted an absence of correlation between fetal CRH and fetal ACTH. These findings strongly suggest the fetal HPA axis is largely controlled by placental CRH production.

Neurohypophyseal hormones

The hypothalamo-neurohypophysial system secretes three nonapeptides during the fetal period: arginine vasotocin (AVT), antidiuretic hormone (ADH, also known as arginine vasopressin), and oxytocin (OT). Each nonapeptide consists of a 6-amino acid ring connected by a disulfide bridge and a 3-amino acid carboxyl terminal side-chain. AVT is phylogenetically the ancestral peptide, with structural and functional similarities to both ADH and oxytocin. Between 12 and 19 weeks the ratio of AVT to ADH decreases, by term the pituitary content of AVT is low and synthesis ceases in postnatal life [14]. The ADH and OT peptides are synthesized in large cell bodies of hypothalamic magnocellular neurons in the supraoptic nuclei and the lateral and superior parts of the paraventricular nuclei, respectively. These hormones are transported to the posterior pituitary for storage and release with long axonal tracks which extend from the hypothalamus to nerve terminals in the posterior pituitary and median eminence (hypothalamo-hypophyseal tract). Both ADH and OT are rapidly cleared from the circulation, with a half-life of 3–6 minutes. Clearance occurs in the kidney and, to a lesser extent, in the liver. Additionally, vasopressinases and oxytocinases produced by the cytotrophoblasts of the human placenta are found in cord blood, maternal plasma and amniotic fluid, and increase across gestation [15]. There is little evidence to suggest that either ADH or OT crosses the human placenta during gestation. At term, the umbilical arterial ADH concentration is significantly higher than the level in umbilical venous blood confirming the fetal source of this hormone.

Antidiuretic hormone. ADH is an important vasoactive hormone because it maintains cardiovascular homeostasis under stressful conditions. At higher doses, ADH elevates venous pressure and paradoxically decreases blood volume. Fetal hypoxia, hemorrhage, and hyperosmolality stimulate the release of ADH, and ADH levels in amniotic fluid increase in patients with Rhesus isoimmunization [16]. High concentrations of ADH have been found in the umbilical cord blood of growth-restricted fetuses, and following fetal bradycardia or passage of meconium, consistent with its role in mediating stress. Maternal indometacin therapy decreases fetal urinary flow rates as a result of stimulation of circulating ADH levels and enhancement of peripheral ADH effects in the fetus [17]. ADH also regulates lung liquid secretion by decreasing the secretion rate in fetuses and increasing lung liquid reabsorption in neonates.

Oxytocin

Immunoreactive OT is detected in the fetal hypothalamus by 16 weeks' gestation, about 3 weeks after ADH. The initially high ratio of ADH to OT decreases with gestation, reaching unity in the neonatal period. Levels of these two hormones increase significantly after 20 weeks' gestation. From 20–26 weeks, there is a threefold increase in OT content, by 32 weeks reaching levels two to five times greater than at 14–17 weeks. This increase in OT content with gestational age is caused by a relative increase in OT synthesis [18]. Labor is associated with further increases in fetal OT production.

Anterior pituitary hormones

The anterior pituitary gland has five distinct cell types which produce seven different hormones (Table 9.2). Gonadotropes secrete LH and FSH while thyrotropes secrete TSH. All three hormones are heterodimeric polypeptides consisting of a common α-glycoprotein subunit (αGSU) and a distinct β subunit (FSHβ, LHβ and TSHβ). Somatotropes secrete GH, which regulates growth and metabolism. Lactotropes synthesize PRL that controls milk production. Corticotrope-melanotropes constitute the major cell type in the intermediate lobe and secrete both melanocyte-stimulating hormone-β (MSH-β) and ACTH. Both products are generated by proteolysis of the product of the pro-opiomelanocortin (POMC) gene.

Gonadotropins

Both LH and FSH are synthesized by human pituitary tissue incubated *in vitro* as early as 5 weeks and detectable in the fetal circulation by 12 weeks' gestation. Gonadotropin deficiency (hypogonadotropic hypogonadism) can be isolated but deficiency occurs more frequently in association with the deficiency of other pituitary-hypothalamic hormones. As noted, Kallmann syndrome is characterized by hypogonadotropic hypogonadism and anosmia (or hyposmia). Absence or abnormalities of the olfactory bulbs have been described in this condition. Failure of GnRH neurons to migrate from the olfactory placode to the hypothalamus during embryonic development appears to account for hypogonadotropic hypogonadism in these patients. Some patients with Kallmann syndrome have

Table 9.2 Anterior pituitary hormones.

Gonadotropins
Luteinizing hormone (LH)
Follicle-stimulating hormone (FSH)

Pro-opiomelanocortin (POMC) derivatives
Adrenocorticotrophic hormone (ACTH)
β-endorphin
α-melanocyte-stimulating hormone (α-MSH)
Corticotropin-like intermediate lobe peptide (CLIP)
β-lipotropin (β-LPH)

Growth hormone (GH)

Prolactin (PRL)

Thyroid-stimulating hormone (TSH)

defects on the short arm of the X chromosome and it has been suggested that this results in defective production of a key adhesion molecule that is needed for proper migration of GnRH neurons. Aside from anosmia, patients generally show physical manifestations similar to those with other forms of congenital hypogonadotropic hypogonadism. An isolated mutation of the β-subunit of FSH has been described. This rare condition represents a form of isolated hypogonadotropic hypogonadism, with selective impairment of FSH (in contrast to Kallmann syndrome).

Sexual dimorphism defines the prenatal patterns of fetal gonadotropin synthesis and secretion. Pituitary LH and FSH content peaks at 25–29 weeks' gestation in female fetuses and at term in males [19]. Elevated circulating levels of gonadotropins have been found in newborns and infants with gonadal failure, confirming the presence of an intact hypothalamic-pituitary-gonadal axis *in utero*. For example, in the syndrome of gonadal dysgenesis (Turner syndrome), levels of FSH and, to a lesser extent, LH are elevated above the normal range during infancy. Similarly, elevation of basal and stimulated gonadotropin levels has been described in male infants with anorchia, rudimentary testes, and other forms of primary testicular failure. The levels of FSH are lower than those seen in females with gonadal dysgenesis.

Females with congenital GnRH or gonadotropin deficiency as well as ovarian agenesis/dysgenesis have normal external genitalia because female sexual differentiation is the "default" pathway and does not appear to require GnRH, LH-FSH, or ovarian hormones. Conversely, males with congenital GnRH or gonadotropin deficiency (whether isolated as in Kallmann syndrome or associated with other pituitary hormone deficiencies) tend to have ambiguous genitalia including microphallus and undescended testes. The partial development of the male genitalia in these cases results from hCG stimulation of testicular testosterone production. However, in cases of gonadal agenesis/dysgenesis in males, female external genitalia will be present.

Male infants with certain forms of androgen resistance may have elevation of LH. Inactivating mutations of the LH receptor gene represent a recently recognized form of gonadal failure and may lead to inadequate virilization of male fetuses and to later failure of normal pubertal development in females. Infants with Down syndrome have also been found to have elevated gonadotropin (primarily FSH) levels, which is consistent with the diagnosis of primary hypogonadism.

Adrenocorticotropic hormone and β-endorphin

ACTH is synthesized by corticotrophes located predominantly in the anterior pituitary lobe. It is derived from the processing of a larger precursor molecule called pro-opiomelanocortin (POMC). Immunoreactive POMC, ACTH, and related peptides can be detected in the human pituitary by 8 weeks post-conception. Pituitary corticotrophes respond to

CRH by 10 weeks' gestation and this response does not appear to significantly change across gestation.

In postnatal life, the primary secretogogues controlling ACTH release are CRH and ADH, peptides that are produced in same region of hypothalamus. Conversely, glucocorticoids act on the hypothalamus to inhibit the release of CRH and act on the pituitary to inhibit synthesis and secretion of ACTH. However, in prenatal life, fetal ACTH levels rise across gestation commensurate with the increase in fetal cortisol. Paradoxically, serum CRH values do not fall across gestation, or correlate with fetal ACTH or cortisol, suggesting a decoupling of fetal HPA axis feedback inhibition resulting from cortisol-induced placental CRH production [12].

ACTH has long-term stimulatory effects on the expression of adrenal steroidogenic enzymes, the density of LDL receptors, and the rate of *de novo* adrenal cholesterol synthesis. Moreover, ACTH enhances adrenal hypertrophy and hyperplasia possibly by stimulating paracrine factor(s) such as insulin-like growth factor-II (IGF-II) which, in turn, induce adrenal cell division. Conversely, in the absence of ACTH, as in anencephaly, the fetal adrenal is reduced in size even at 15 weeks' gestation but its development can be induced by administration of ACTH. Thus, ACTH provides tropic and trophic stimulation to the fetal adrenal beginning in the second trimester.

The involution of the adrenal cortex following parturition reflects the normal reduction in plasma ACTH levels that occurs once the influence of placental CRH is removed. A histologic appearance similar to that of the fetal zone has been described in older children with untreated congenital adrenal hyperplasia (CAH) and in adults administered large amounts of ACTH.

The generation of ACTH from POMC also results in the production of β-endorphin. As expected, secretion of both ACTH and β-endorphin by the anterior pituitary appears to be subject to similar, perhaps identical, control mechanisms. Indeed, conditions that elevate or depress plasma ACTH concentrations exert the same effects on β-endorphin levels. Other peptides generated by POMC metabolism include α-melanocyte-stimulating hormone (α-MSH), corticotropin-like intermediate lobe peptide (CLIP), and β-lipotropin (β-LPH).

We observed that the fetal β-endorphin values were lower than those observed in neonates and found no correlation with gestational age [20]. We also noted a marked increase in the concentration of β-endorphin after multiple needle insertions at the time of cordocentesis [21]. These studies suggest that, *in utero*, the fetus responds to stress by increasing the β-endorphin secretion.

Growth hormone

Human pituitary organ cultures secrete GH by 5 weeks post-conception and immunoreactive GH is first detected in the human fetal pituitary by 8 weeks post-conception. The absolute number of GH-secreting cells increases progressively through pregnancy; however, it is unclear whether hypothalamic GHRH exerts trophic effect on the development and differentiation of pituitary somatotropes. For example, primordial cells obtained from the Rathke pouch can spontaneously differentiate in culture without hypothalamic influences.

Studies of fetal plasma GH concentrations from abortuses and neonatal cord blood at term suggest that concentrations peak at 20 weeks then decline rapidly toward term. Premature newborns have higher GH levels in umbilical cord blood than do term newborns. Gender differences in GH secretion were noted in samples obtained by fetoscopy, with male fetuses having higher concentrations than females. Cord blood GH concentrations appear to be higher in growth-restricted and "distressed" infants.

In postnatal life, GH secretion is regulated in a complex manner by an interaction between hypothalamic GHRH and somatostatin, both of which are secreted in a variable manner into the portal circulation as well as systemic IGF-I. It is now recognized that feedback within the somatotropic axis is mediated at both the hypothalamic and pituitary levels by GH. GHRH binds to specific receptors on somatotropes, increases intracellular cAMP, and selectively stimulates transcription of GH mRNA as well as GH secretory pulses while somatostatin suppresses basal GH secretion without altering GH mRNA levels acting as the primary regulator of GH pulses in response to physiologic stimuli. IGF-I, the peripheral target hormone of GH, participates in negative feedback regulation by inhibiting both GH gene transcription and GH secretion.

The fall in plasma GH concentration in the latter half of gestation may be caused by an increase in somatostatin release or a simultaneous decrease in GHRH release.

In anencephalic fetuses, pituitary GH content and plasma levels are low yet somatic growth is normal, suggesting that GH does not have a major role in regulating fetal growth. In addition, this finding is consistent with the concept that, in the term fetus, the hypothalamic influence on GH release is primarily stimulatory.

Prolactin

Lactotrophs are the primary PRL-secreting cells. They can be detected in fetal hypophysis at 12 weeks, and their number slightly increases toward mid-gestation. Simultaneously, PRL levels increase after 20 weeks in fetal blood obtained from abortuses and after preterm delivery. In studies where fetal blood has been collected from 14 to 37 weeks by cardiac puncture or cordocentesis, PRL levels increase linearly with gestation, but do not correlate with maternal blood levels. Following birth, PRL levels decline by more than 60% in the first week.

In postnatal life, PRL is controlled in a complex manner by hypothalamic releasing hormones, neurotransmitters, and steroid hormones. The dominant influence is tonic inhibition by dopamine directly secreted into the portal circulation by neurons arising in the medial-basal hypothalamus. Similarly, α-MSH, which stimulates tuberoinfundibular dopamine release, also inhibits PRL. On the other hand, TRH acts as a PRL-releasing factor and estrogen stimulates lactotroph proliferation and PRL synthesis.

At mid-gestation, fetal PRL secretion is not tonically inhibited because the dopaminergic control is not operative until the late third trimester. Similarly, human fetal lactotrophes do not respond to TRH stimulation until after 20 weeks. Thus, by term, reduced dopamine and increased TRH sensitivity and estrogen levels drive PRL production. This explains why high levels of PRL are present in the fetal circulation near term. Conversely, declining TRH and estrogen levels following delivery account for the observed fall in PRL levels in postnatal life. Observations in humans and animals suggest a role for PRL in the regulation of fluid and electrolyte balance. Indirect evidence suggests that PRL may influence fetal lung maturation by facilitating surfactant synthesis.

Thyroid-stimulating hormone

TSH can be detected in the human fetal pituitary by 12 weeks post-conception and in fetal circulation by 13 weeks. Thereafter, fetal TSH levels progressively increase during gestation, reaching concentrations that are well above adult ranges. Radunovic *et al.* [22] employed cordocentesis to study thyroid function in fetuses from 12 weeks' gestation to term, and demonstrated that fetal plasma TSH concentrations increased with gestation. Fetal TSH levels were higher than adult values.

In postnatal life, pituitary TSH secretion is stimulated by TRH and inhibited by TSH itself as well as somatostatin, dopamine, and iodothyronines. In the fetal period, however, this regulation does not appear to be operative. Therefore the persistent rise in TSH towards term may result from a progressive increase in pituitary sensitivity to TRH. Alternatively, several extrahypothalamic sources of TRH have been demonstrated, such as placental transfer of maternal TRH, placental synthesis of TRH analogs, and TRH synthesis by peripheral fetal tissues which may drive fetal TSH production.

Adrenal gland

The adrenal gland comprises two distinct endocrine organs. The cortex originates from the coelomic mesoderm in close association with the primordial genital ridge around the 4th week post-conception. The medulla arises from the primitive ganglia of the coeliac plexus of the autonomic nervous system, which is, in turn, derived from the neural crest. During intrauterine development, the adrenal gland is much larger in relation to total body size than it is in adults.

After 12 weeks' gestation, the morphology of the adrenal cortex remains relatively constant. The human fetal adrenal cortex consists of two primary anatomic zones: the outer definitive (adult) zone, and an inner fetal zone. The outer definitive (adult) zone of the human fetal adrenal cortex is the main site of mineralocorticoid synthesis, comprising only 15–20% of the fetal adrenal cortex. This zone is relatively quiescent until the third trimester of pregnancy, when it expresses CYP11A1 (P450 side-chain cleavage enzyme), the enzyme that catalyzes initial steroidogenesis and CYP11B2 (aldosterone synthase). Thus, it secretes primarily aldosterone and is analogous to the adult zona glomerulosa. Subsequently, an adjacent middle zone develops, the zona fasciculate, which expresses CYP11A1 and CYP11B1 (P450c11-beta, 11-beta-hydroxylase) enzymes that catalyze cortisol synthesis. This region is believed to be the site of *de novo* cortisol production after 28 weeks' gestation.

The normally hypertrophied fetal inner zone (fetal cortex) is the principal site of dehydroepiandrosterone sulfate (DHEAS) production, and involutes rapidly after birth. By 20 weeks, the fetal zone clearly dominates and is composed of large eosinophilic cells that exhibit ultrastructural characteristics typical of steroid-secreting cells. The inner androgen-secreting cortical layer of the adult adrenal gland, the zona reticularis, does not form until the third year of life.

Rapid growth of the human fetal adrenal cortex begins at approximately 10 weeks' gestation and continues to term, entirely as a result of enlargement of the fetal zone.

By 20 weeks, the gland becomes as large as the fetal kidney. Between 20 and 30 weeks, the size and weight of the fetal adrenal gland doubles, achieving a relative size 10- to 20-fold that of the adult adrenal. A further doubling in fetal adrenal weight occurs after 30 weeks' gestation such that by term the gland weighs approximately 3–4 g.

The medulla is essentially absent from the fetal adrenal throughout most of gestation except for small islands of chromaffin cells scattered through the body of the cortex. After the involution of the fetal zone during the first postnatal week the chromaffin cells coalesce around the central vein and begin to form a rudimentary medulla.

After mid-gestation, ACTH is the principal trophic factor for the adrenal cortex and its presence is obligatory. ACTH also induces the enzyme 3-β-hydroxysteroid dehydrogenase/Δ4-5-isomerase in the fetal zone to promote DHEAS synthesis which is also under the control of placental estrogen and placental-derived CRH. We analyzed a large number of paired maternal and fetal samples across pregnancy and observed that cortisol concentrations in the fetal and maternal blood both increased with increasing gestational age and correlated with each other [12]. Fetal cortisol levels were significantly lower than maternal, neonatal, and nonpregnant adult values [12].

Congenital adrenal hyperplasia (CAH) is a collection of autosomal recessive disorders characterized by a deficiency in

Table 9.3 Enzymes required for cortisol synthesis.

21-hydroxylase (21-OH) (CYP21A2, P450c21)
11-β-hydroxylase (CYP 11B1, P450c11)
17-hydroxylase (CYP 17, P450c17)
3-β-hydroxysteroid dehydrogenase
Cholesterol side-chain cleavage enzyme (CYP11A1, P450scc)

one or more of the five enzymes required for cortisol biosynthesis (Table 9.3). The most common abnormality (1 in 5000 to 1 in 15,000 births) is caused by a deficiency of the enzyme 21-hydroxylase (21-OH) (CYP21A2 deficiency). There are two major clinical presentations of 21-OH deficiency. The classic form results from a homozygous absence of 21-OH and presents with overt salt wasting and virilization of female infants. The far more common, nonclassical form results from a partial deficiency of enzymatic activity and presents with menstrual disturbances and hirsuitism in females after puberty. A third rare abnormality is associated with low but detectable activity (<2%) sufficient to prevent salt wasting but sufficient to cause virilization. Unfortunately, genotype does not always correlate with phenotype.

Since discovery and mapping of the allelic variants in the 1980s, direct DNA analysis of the CYP21A2 gene has become the routine approach. As with most autosomal recessive disorders, the majority of at-risk couples become known only after having an affected child. Nevertheless, in some families the mutations are not known, requiring sequencing of the whole gene or linkage studies. When sequencing is not practicable and linkage studies are not informative, biochemical analysis of the amniotic fluid for 17-hydroxyprogesterone may still be necessary. In addition, the sonographic detection of an abnormally enlarged clitoris in a female fetus should alert the physician to rule out CAH.

Because the differentiation of the external genitalia begins at approximately 6–7 weeks' gestation, diagnosis by amniocentesis and even chorionic villus sampling comes too late to prevent masculinization. Thus, for patients at risk of having an affected fetus, pharmacologic therapy with dexamethasone must be initiated prior to sex assignment. This implies that therapy needs to be administered to all patients at risk despite the fact that the chance of having an affected female fetus among carrier parents is only 1 in 8 (i.e., 1 in 4 to be affected × 1 in 2 to be a female). Therapy can be discontinued in 7/8 at-risk pregnancies as soon as the diagnosis of CAH is ruled out or a male fetus is identified.

Thyroid

The thyroid gland is derived from a medial outpouching in the floor of the primitive pharynx which gives rise to the thyroid follicular cells. In contrast, bilateral evaginations of the fourth pharyngeal pouch give rise to parafollicular or calcitonin-secreting cells. Organogenesis and migration of the thyroid bud caudally into the neck is complete by 10 weeks post-conception. Only after completion of migration do thyroid follicular cells differentiate and express thyroid-specific genes such as thyroglobulin (TG), TSH receptor, and thyroperoxidase (TPO). However, future follicular cells acquire the capacity to form TG as early as the 29th day post-conception whereas the capacity to concentrate iodide and synthesize thyroxine (T4) is delayed until about the 11th week. Thus, radioactive iodine inadvertently given to the mother at this point and beyond would be accumulated by the fetal thyroid.

By the 17th week, serum T4 concentrations begin to increase accompanied by progressive increases in fetal serum TSH concentrations. Because the capacity of the pituitary to synthesize and secrete TSH is not apparent until the 11th week, early growth and development of the thyroid do not seem to be TSH-dependent. Subsequently, rapid changes in pituitary and thyroid function take place in response to TSH.

The major thyroid hormone-binding protein in plasma, TG, is detectable in serum by the 10th gestational week and increases in concentration progressively to term. This increase accounts, in part, for the progressive increase in total serum T4 concentration during the second and third trimesters. However, increased secretion of T4 must also have a role because the concentration of unbound, or free, T4 also rises. This increase in free T4 secretion likely reflects the progressive rise in TSH release from the fetal pituitary after 18 weeks as well as an increased TSH receptor expression in the thyroid after 18 weeks' gestation, coincident with pituitary–hypothalamic maturation.

In contrast, 3,5,3'-triiodothyronine (T3) levels in the fetal blood rise after 28 weeks. Prior to this time 3,3',5'-triiodothyronine or reverse T3 (rT3) production is high, peaking in the second trimester and then declining toward term [22]. The rT3 molecule is formed when the iodine atom is removed from the inner ring of T4.

The placenta is freely permeable to TRH, TSH receptor stimulating IgG, and drugs used to treat thyroid disease, such as propylthiouracil (PTU), methimazole, iodine, and β-adrenergic receptor antagonists. We have observed a significant correlation between maternal total T3 and fetal total T4 and T3 levels, suggesting human placental transfer of T3 from mother to fetus even under physiologic conditions [22]. However, this correlation may simply reflect the parallel increase in maternal and fetal hormone concentrations during gestation.

Evidence that transfer of maternal T4 and T3 into the fetal circulation has a crucial physiological role in embryonic and fetal neurodevelopment comes from the work of Haddow *et al.* [23]. They observed that 62 children of women with high early second trimester serum TSH concentrations scored 4 points lower on the Wechsler Intelligence IQ Scale than those of the children of the 124 matched control women, and that 15% of the former children had scores of 85 or less compared with 5% of matched control children.

Conversely, there is evidence that normal maternal thyroid function can protect against adverse neurodevelopment in fetuses with anatomic or enzymatic thyroid defects. Vulsma *et al.* [24] evaluated T4 transfer from mother to fetus in 25 neonates with an autosomal recessive disorder resulting in the complete inability to iodinate thyroid proteins. They noted that among affected neonates, umbilical cord T4 levels ranged from 35 to 70 nmol/L, confirming that in infants with severe congenital hypothyroidism, substantial amounts of protective T4 are transferred from mother to fetus during late gestation.

We have shown that useful information about fetal thyroid function in the second half of pregnancy can be obtained from a single cordocentesis [22]. Such information may be useful in the prenatal diagnosis of hypothyroidism and hyperthyroidism, as well as in monitoring intrauterine therapy.

Fetal hypothyroidism

The combination of both maternal and fetal hypothyroidism can have severe fetal and neonatal consequences. Transient fetal hypothyroidism can result from maternal dietary iodine deficiency, as well as transfer of blocking antibodies or antithyroid drugs in mothers with Hashimoto disease and medically treated Graves disease, respectively. Paradoxically, inadequately treated maternal hyperthyroidism may suppress the fetal pituitary-thyroid axis. Iodine deficiency, blocking antibodies, and high-dose PTU therapy can lead to fetal goiter potentially obstructing the fetal esophagus or trachea. This can lead to polyhydramnios and preterm delivery. If the goiter is of sufficient size it can cause extension of the fetal neck leading to dystocia or birth injury. High-output cardiac failure with cardiomegaly and pleural effusion can occasionally result from arteriovenous shunting through the goiter [25]. Other manifestations of fetal hypothyroidism in which there is either inadequate levels of protective maternal T3 and T4 or their delivery is blocked by antibodies or drugs include delayed epiphyseal ossification, bradycardia, and growth lag.

Permanent fetal hypothyroidism can result from thyroid dysgenesis (anatomic defect) or mutations in the genes controlling crucial T4 synthetic enzymes. *In utero* manifestations are either absent or mild given the protective effects of transplacental transfer of maternal T3 and T4. However, without prompt postnatal treatment, growth delay and severe mental retardation will ensue in children (cretinism). Even with immediate diagnosis and treatment at birth, long-term follow-up of children with congenital hypothyroidism suggests they may be at risk for mild neurodevelopmental delays.

The diagnosis of fetal hypothyroidism begins with eliciting a history of maternal hypothyroidism. In patients with Hashimoto thyroiditis, blocking immunoglobulin levels can be measured, and if present the fetus will be at risk. Alternatively, mothers with iodine deficiency or those with Graves disease receiving high-dose PTU are at risk for fetal hypothyroidism. Biweekly fetal heart rate assessments should be obtained to detect bradycardia while monthly ultrasound examinations should be employed to screen for goiter, polyhydramnios, growth lag, and, after 32 weeks' gestation, delayed appearance of epiphyseal ossification centers.

In utero treatment includes intra-amniotic administration of T4 in dose ranges of 150–500 μg given weekly [26,27]. With such therapy fetal goiters have been shown to regress, and fetal and newborn TSH levels have normalized.

Fetal hyperthyroidism

Fetal thyrotoxic (hyperactive) goiter most commonly results from transplacental passage of TSH receptor binding (stimulating) antibodies (TSAb or TSI) in patients with Graves disease or, less commonly, Hashimoto thyroiditis. Approximately 5% (1.5–12%) of fetuses whose mothers have Graves disease develop fetal or neonatal thyrotoxicosis. This may even occur despite the fact that the mother is currently euthyrotic status post-thyroid ablation with replacement therapy. Fetal hyperthyroidism can be a cause of fetal morbidity and mortality because of hyperactive goiter, although these tend to be smaller than hypoactive goiters. Fetal hyperthyroidism may also cause growth restriction, tachycardia, premature ossification of the epiphyses, hydrops associated with high output cardiac failure, and craniosynostosis. Premature delivery occurs in up to 90% of cases with fetal hyperthyroidism, with a perinatal mortality of 12–50%.

Diagnosis again begins with a maternal history of thyroid disease. As with fetal hypothyroidism associated with maternal thyroid disease, such patients require evaluation of maternal thyroid function tests and immunoglobulin status. The fetal heart rate should be assessed biweekly to detect tachycardia. Ultrasound should be performed every 4 weeks to detect development of goiter, hydrops, fetal growth restriction, and, after 24 weeks, premature epiphyseal ossification. Occasionally, the investigation of fetal hyperthyroidism begins after incidental detection of a fetal goiter. This should prompt maternal history, thyroid antibody measurements, and, if necessary, cordocentesis to measure fetal thyroid hormones.

After confirming the diagnosis of fetal hyperthyroidism, treatment should be initiated with PTU [28]. The initial maternal dosage is 100 mg orally three times a day, which is decreased to 50 mg orally three times a day. Alternatively, maternal methimazole can be used [29]. For mothers who are status post-thyroid, ablative surgery or ^{131}I treatment and on T4 replacement therapy, PTU should be well tolerated.

Gonads

Gonadal development and steroidogenesis in the fetal testes is under the control of gonadotropins: placental hCG during early gestation and fetal pituitary LH and FSH in the second half of gestation. In the male fetus, the interstitial cells of the testis begin synthesizing testosterone from low-density lipoprotein cholesterol at approximately 8 weeks. The production rate is maximal at 17–21 weeks but declines thereafter. This pattern coincides closely with the differentiation of the male urogenital tract. In anencephalic male fetuses the testicular size is reduced but the steroid-producing capacity is normal. Estradiol synthesis in the fetal testes is negligible.

In the female fetus, ovarian formation of estradiol from testosterone is detectable at 10 weeks, suggesting the presence of aromatase activity at this early age.

Circulating levels of testosterone in the male fetus parallel the rise and fall of testicular testosterone production, whereas levels in the female fetus remain relatively low and constant throughout gestation. Estradiol concentrations in the circulation of male and female fetuses are low throughout gestation. The fetal ovary is relatively quiescent during early pregnancy, and anencephalic female fetuses have normal ovarian development until the third trimester.

Testosterone has two primary functions during the fetal period: first, to ensure the normal development of the male gonads, and second, to serve as the feedback-active agent in the regulation of pituitary LH secretion. FSH mediates the later stages of testicular maturation including seminiferous tubule development and spermatogenesis. The release of FSH from the fetal pituitary is also regulated by the feedback action of inhibin, which is produced by the fetal testes and ovary. Testes contain higher levels of inhibin than the ovary, accounting for the lower plasma concentration of FSH in the male than in the female fetus.

Inhibin is synthesized and secreted by testicular Sertoli cells and by ovarian granulosa cells and it inhibits the release of FSH but not LH from the pituitary. Inhibin is also synthesized by the placenta. Biologically active inhibin is present in the fetus, and administration of it suppresses serum FSH.

Pancreatic hormones and growth factors

The pancreas develops both dorsal and ventral foregut diverticula which fuse during embryogenesis to form both the exocrine and endocrine pancreas. By 10 weeks' gestation, insulin and other neuropeptides are present in clusters of immature endocrine cells and in the circulation. By 16 weeks' gestation these clusters become vascularized and during the second half of pregnancy developing islets become innervated and differentiated to contain a single pancreatic hormone type. Cordocentesis from 17 to 38 weeks indicate that fetal plasma insulin levels and the fetal insulin : glucose ratio increased exponentially across gestation and fetal β-cells display physiologic responses to changes in glucose levels *in utero* [30]. This fetal β-cell response to glucose and amino acids matures with increasing gestational age. By term, fetal β-cells respond readily to changes in the glucose and amino acid levels and are affected by circulating catecholamine levels and stress.

Fetal pancreatic α-cells are the first cell type to be identified clearly in the pancreas, mainly in the periphery. The α-cells appear before β-cells, with δ-cells detectable only later in gestation. Fetal α-cells respond rapidly to changes in the level of amino acids and catecholamines with glucagon to respond to inadequate maternal nutrition. The fetal pancreas also expresses IGF-I and II and IGF binding protein 3 during late gestation. IGF-I and II increase with gestation after 33 weeks, and levels correlate with placental lactogen. Impaired fetal nutrition and fetal corticosteroid treatment suppress IGF-I and II gene expression. Autonomic innervation is achieved by late gestation and involved in regulating islet cell responses to stressful stimuli.

Case presentation 1

A 24-year-old, G2P1001, patient presents for prenatal care. Her past medical, surgical, and gynecologic histories are unremarkable. Her first pregnancy was remarkable for the delivery of a virilized female who developed salt-wasting in the immediate neonatal period and was diagnosed with the classic form of 21-hydroxylase deficiency. Rapid DNA analysis based on allele-specific polymerase chain reaction (PCR) using mutation site-specific primers detected one of the eight most common mutations in the CYP21A2 gene. Both parents were noted to be heterozygotes for the mutation. An ultrasound was performed which confirmed a viable intrauterine pregnancy with a crown rump length consistent with 6 weeks' gestation. After informed consent was obtained, the patient was begun on dexamethasone at a dose of 0.25 mg four times a day. At 11 weeks, a chorionic villus sampling and the resultant genetic analysis identified a female carrier of the CYP21A2 mutation. Dexamethasone was weaned and the rest of the pregnancy was uneventful resulting in a term delivery.

It is currently recommended to start adrenal suppressive therapy as soon as a positive pregnancy test is obtained (<7 weeks' gestation) as cases of masculinization have been reported when treatment was initiated at 9 weeks' gestation. Treatment consists of the aforementioned dose of dexamethasone because it readily crosses the placenta. Therapy can be discontinued in seven out of eight at-risk pregnancies as soon as the diagnosis of CAH is ruled out. If the fetus is an affected female, the therapy is continued throughout gestation. When treatment is continued beyond the first trimester, serial maternal estriol levels should be obtained to confirm that complete fetal adrenal gland suppression has been achieved. Stress-dose corticosteroids should be given to the patient during labor and then tapered gradually postpartum. However, if the fetus is a male, the therapy can be discontinued at the time of diagnosis. Although this therapy is widely accepted, it is still considered experimental. A recently published commentary written in *JAMA* advocates Institutional Review Board approval be obtained on all patients offered this treatment as long-term follow-up has not been documented on individuals who received *in utero* steroid treatment for CAH [31].

Case presentation 2

A 33-year-old, G1 P0, patient at 30 weeks' gestation presents for consultation because of a possible fetal goiter detected in her physician's office ultrasound examination. Her past medical history is remarkable for Graves disease diagnosed in the first trimester and managed initially with 300 mg/day PTU. She remained poorly controlled on this regimen with hyper-reflexia, tachycardia, and blood pressures of 160/80 mmHg. The dosage of PTU was increased to 450 mg/day and she was begun on 50 mg/day atenolol which was subsequently raised to 100 mg/day. On evaluation, the maternal pulse is 90 beats/min, and she remains hyper-reflexive. The uterine fundus is 29 cm and fetal heart rate is 140 beats/min. On ultrasound, the fetus is noted to be in a vertex presentation, with normal amniotic fluid volume, an estimated fetal weight at the 25th percentile and both distal femoral epiphyses are evident. The fetal goiter measures 3 × 2 cm and blood flow is clearly evident on color Doppler examination. A cordocentesis is performed which demonstrates a fetal T4 value of 1.40 ng/dL (>3 standard deviations), and an undetectable TSH. The patient was managed by increasing her PTU dosage to 900 mg/day. This results in resolution of the fetal goiter, and a reduction in the maternal pulse to 80 beats/min off atenolol.

This case illustrates the difficult diagnostic dilemma posed by maternal Graves disease when patients have high levels of TSH receptor binding antibodies, and are receiving both high-dose PTU therapy and β-adrenergic receptor blocking agents. In such cases, the PTU and high maternal T4 and T3 levels may result in hypoactive fetal goiter and hypothyroidism, while the thyroid stimulating antibodies may stimulate fetal hyperthyroidism and cause thyroid hypertrophy and hyperplasia with a hyperfunctioning goiter. However, treatment with β-blockers may result in a normal fetal heart rate or actual bradycardia despite fetal thyrotoxicosis. The use of color Doppler may distinguish between the relatively hypovascular hypoactive goiter of fetal hypothyroidism from the highly vascular hyperactive goiter of fetal hyperthyroidism. The former in the setting of bradycardia and delayed epiphyseal ossification would suggest fetal hypothyoidism. The latter in the setting of tachycardia and premature epiphyseal ossification would suggest fetal hyperthyroidism. In either case, because the low fetal heart rate could be because of the β-blocker therapy, cordocentesis can be used to directly assess fetal T4.

References

1 Koutcherov Y, Mai JK, Ashwell KW, Paxinos G. Organization of human hypothalamus in fetal development. *J Comp Neurol* 2002;**446**:301–24.

2 Gilmore DP, Wilson CA. Indoleamine and catecholamine concentrations in the mid-term human fetal brain. *Brain Res Bull* 1983;**10**:395–8.

3 Aubert ML, Grumbach MM, Kaplan SL. The ontogenesis of human fetal hormones. IV. Somatostatin, luteinizing hormone releasing factor, and thyrotropin releasing factor in hypothalamus and cerebral cortex of human fetuses 10–22 weeks of age. *J Clin Endocrinol Metab* 1977;**44**:1130–41.

4 Mastorakos G, Ilias I. Maternal and fetal hypothalamic-pituitary-adrenal axes during pregnancy and postpartum. *Ann N Y Acad Sci* 2003;**997**:136–49.

5 Asa SL, Kovacs K, Horvath E, *et al*. Human fetal adenohypophysis: electron microscopic and ultrastructural immunocytochemical analysis. *Neuroendocrinology* 1988;**48**:423–31.

6 Quinton R, Hasan W, Grant W, *et al*. Gonadotropin-releasing hormone immunoreactivity in the nasal epithelia of adults with Kallmann's syndrome and isolated hypogonadotropic hypogonadism and in the early midtrimester human fetus. *J Clin Endocrinol Metab* 1997;**82**:309–14.

7 Paulin C, Dubois MP, Barry J, Dubois PM. Immunofluorescence study of LH-RH producing cells in the human fetal hypothalamus. *Cell Tissue Res* 1977;**182**:341–5.

8 Siler-Khodr TM, Khodr GS. Studies in human fetal endocrinology. I. Luteinizing hormone-releasing factor content of the hypothalamus. *Am J Obstet Gynecol* 1978;**130**:795–800.

9 Bresson JL, Clavequin MC, Fellmann D, Bugnon C. Ontogeny of the neuroglandular system revealed with HPGRF 44 antibodies in human hypothalamus. *Neuroendocrinology* 1984;**39**:68–73.

10 Thorpe-Beeston JG, Nicolaides KH. Fetal thyroid function. *Fetal Diagn Ther* 1993;**8**:60–72.

11 Fadalti M, Pezzani I, Cobellis L, *et al*. Placental corticotropin-releasing factor: an update. *Ann N Y Acad Sci* 2000;**900**:89–94.

12 Lockwood CJ, Radunovic N, Nastic D, Petkovic S, Aigner S, Berkowitz GS. Corticotropin-releasing hormone and related pituitary-adrenal axis hormones in fetal and maternal blood during the second half of pregnancy. *J Perinat Med* 1996;**24**:243–51.

13 Economides D, Linton E, Nicolaides K, Rodeck CH, Lowry PJ, Chard T. Relationship between maternal and fetal corticotrophin-releasing hormone-41 and ACTH levels in human mid-trimester pregnancy. *J Endocrinol* 1987;**114**:497–501.

14 Skowsky WR, Fisher DA. Fetal neurohypophyseal arginine vasopressin and arginine vasotocin in man and sheep. *Pediatr Res* 1977;**11**:627–30.

15 Fisher DA. Maternal–fetal neurohypophyseal system. *Clin Perinatol* 1983;**10**:695–707.

16 Weiner CP, Smith F, Robillard JE. Arginine vasopressin and acute, intravascular volume expansion in the human fetus. *Fetal Ther* 1989;**4**:69–72.

17 Walker MP, Moore TR, Brace RA. Indomethacin and arginine vasopressin interaction in the fetal kidney: a mechanism of oliguria. *Am J Obstet Gynecol* 1994;**171**:1234–41.

18 Khan-Dawood FS, Dawood MY. Oxytocin content of human fetal pituitary glands. *Am J Obstet Gynecol* 1984;**148**:420–3.

19 Asa SL, Kovacs K, Singer W. Human fetal adenohypophysis: morphologic and functional analysis in vitro. *Neuroendocrinology* 1991;**53**:562–72.

20 Radunovic N, Lockwood CJ, Alvarez M, Nastic D, Berkowitz RL. Beta-endorphin concentrations in fetal blood during the second half of pregnancy. *Am J Obstet Gynecol* 1992;**167**:740–4.

21 Radunovic N, Lockwood CJ, Ghidini A, Alvarez M, Berkowitz RL. Is fetal blood sampling associated with increased beta-endorphin release into the fetal circulation? *Am J Perinatol* 1993;**10**:112–4.

22 Radunovic N, Dumez Y, Nastic D, Mandelbrot L, Dommergues M. Thyroid function in fetus and mother during the second half of normal pregnancy. *Biol Neonate* 1991;**59**:139–48.

23 Haddow JE, Palomaki GE, Allan WC, *et al*. Maternal thyroid deficiency during pregnancy and subsequent neuropsychological development of the child. *N Engl J Med* 1999;**341**:549–55.

24 Vulsma T, Gons MH, de Vijlder JJ. Maternal–fetal transfer of thyroxine in congenital hypothyroidism due to a total organification defect or thyroid agenesis. *N Engl J Med* 1989;**321**:13–6.

25 Morine M, Takeda T, Minekawa R, *et al*. Antenatal diagnosis and treatment of a case of fetal goitrous hypothyroidism associated with high-output cardiac failure. *Ultrasound Obstet Gynecol* 2002;**19**:506–9.

26 Johnson RL, Finberg HJ, Perelman AH, Clewell WH. Fetal goitrous hypothyroidism: a new diagnostic and therapeutic approach. *Fetal Ther* 1989;**4**:141–5.

27 Agrawal P, Ogilvy-Stuart A, Lees C. Intrauterine diagnosis and management of congenital goitrous hypothyroidism. *Ultrasound Obstet Gynecol* 2002;**19**:501–5.

28 Porreco RP, Bloch CA. Fetal blood sampling in the management of intrauterine thyrotoxicosis. *Obstet Gynecol* 1990;**76**:509–12.

29 Wenstrom KD, Weiner CP, Williamson RA, Grant SS. Prenatal diagnosis of fetal hyperthyroidism using funipuncture. *Obstet Gynecol* 1990;**76**:513–7.

30 Economides DL, Proudler A, Nicolaides KH. Plasma insulin in appropriate- and small-for-gestational-age fetuses. *Am J Obstet Gynecol* 1989;**160**:1091–4.

31 Seckl JR, Miller WL. How safe is long-term prenatal glucocorticoid treatment? *JAMA* 1997;**277**:1077–9.

10 Fetal lung maturity

Steven G. Gabbe, Sarah H. Poggi, and Alessandro Ghidini

The lecithin:sphingomyelin (L:S) ratio for assessment of fetal pulmonary maturity was first introduced by Gluck *et al.* [1] in 1971 and over 30 years later this test is still the gold standard to which others are compared. However, there is increasing experience with a second generation of methods for evaluating fetal pulmonary maturation. These newer tests appear to be more specific than the L:S ratio and have advantages of being fast, yet accurate. Like the determination of L:S ratio, such tests are performed on amniotic fluid.

Indications for assessment of fetal pulmonary maturity

There are many clinical scenarios that may suggest the need to assess for fetal lung maturity. Examples would be preterm labor, as tocolysis is generally contraindicated in the presence of mature fetal lungs or iatrogenic preterm delivery, such as that indicated for a stable placenta previa. Even at more than 37 weeks, in the presence of unsure dates or obstetric complications affecting lung maturity such as diabetes, the American College of Obstetricians and Gynecologists has recommended that fetal pulmonary maturity should be confirmed before elective delivery at less than 39 weeks' gestation [2].

Techniques for obtaining amniotic fluid

Amniocentesis. Amniocentesis performed under ultrasonographic guidance in experienced hands is associated with low rates of failure or of bloody fluid collection, and a lower than 1% risk of complications, such as emergent delivery [3].

Vaginal pool collection. The assessment of fetal pulmonary maturity can be obtained from vaginal pool specimens in the presence of premature rupture of membranes. Blood, meconium, and mucus can alter the results. In the absence of these contaminants, vaginally free-flowing collected fluid can be evaluated for determination of L:S ratio, surfactant:albumin ratio (SAR), phosphatidylglcerol (PG), and lamellar body counts (LBC) yielding results similar to those observed with samples obtained with amniocentesis.

Specific tests for lung maturity

Lecithin:sphingomyelin ratio

The concentrations of these two substances are approximately equal until mid-third trimester of gestation, when the concentration of pulmonary lecithin increases significantly while the nonpulmonary sphingomyelin concentration remains unchanged. Thin-layer chromatography after centrifugation to remove the cellular component and organic solvent extraction is used on chilled amniotic fluid specimens.

An L:S ratio of 2.0 or greater predicts absence of respiratory distress syndrome (RDS) in 98% of neonates. With a ratio of 1.5–1.9, approximately 50% of infants will develop RDS. Below 1.5, the risk of subsequent RDS increases to 73% [4]. Maternal serum has a L:S ratio ranging from 1.3 to 1.9; thus, blood-tinged samples could falsely lower a mature result. The presence of meconium can interfere with test interpretation increasing the L:S ratio by 0.1–0.5, thus leading to an increase in falsely mature results.

Phosphatidylglycerol

Phosphatidylglycerol is a minor constituent of surfactant that becomes evident in amniotic fluid several weeks after the rise in lecithin [5]. Its presence indicates a more advanced state of fetal lung development and function, as PG enhances the spread of phospholipids on the alveoli. The original PG testing was performed by thin-layer chromatography and required time and expertise. More recently, enzymatic assay or slide agglutinations have been used successfully to determine the presence of PG.

The results are typically reported qualitatively as positive or negative, where positive represents an exceedingly low risk of RDS. PG determination is not generally affected by blood, meconium, or vaginal secretion.

Lung profile (combined approach)

Gluck has emphasized that complete assessment of fetal lung maturity requires determination of the L:S ratio, the percentage of acetone precipitable lecithin, and the presence of the acidic phospholipids phosphatidylinositol (PI) and phosphatidylglycerol (PG) [6]. Recognizing the presence of PG may be useful for timing the elective delivery of fetuses of diabetic patients. The lung profile will also reduce the number of false-immature predictions, as some infants with L:S ratios below 2.0 do show PG. This observation has been made in so-called stressed pregnancies complicated by severe hypertension, prolonged premature rupture of membranes, or diabetes with vascular involvement.

TDx test (surfactant:albumin ratio) (SAR)

The TDx test requires 1 mL amniotic fluid and can be run in less than 1 hour. The SAR is determined, with amniotic fluid albumin used as an internal reference. The fluorescence polarization assay uses polarized light to evaluate the competitive binding of a probe to both albumin and surfactant in amniotic fluid.

Recently, a SAR of 55 mg/g (using the TDx-FlxFLM II method) has been proposed as a better threshold to indicate maturity [7]. Approximately 50% of infants with an immature TDx result will develop RDS.

A disadvantage of the TDx-FLM method is the large quantification scale. However, while values greater than 55 are regarded as mature, values of 35–55 are considered "borderline." As for L:S ratio, red blood cell phospholipids may falsely lower the TDx-FLM result, but a mature test can reliably predict pulmonary maturity.

Lamellar body counts

Lamellar bodies, the storage form of surfactant, are released into the amniotic fluid by fetal type II pneumocytes. Because they are the same size as platelets, the amniotic fluid concentration of lamellar bodies may be determined using a commercial cell counter. The test requires less than 1 mL amniotic fluid and takes only 15 minutes to perform. Although initial studies employed centrifugation, it is now agreed that the sample should be processed without spinning as centrifugation reduces the number of lamellar bodies.

Values of 40,000–50,000/μL generally indicate pulmonary maturity, while a count below 15,000/μL suggests a significant risk for RDS [8]. The test compares favorably with L:S and PG with a negative predictive value of a mature cut-off of

97.7% vs 96.8% and 94.7%, respectively [9]. A meta-analysis calculated receiver-operating characteristic curves based upon data from six studies and showed the LBC performed slightly better than the L:S ratio in predicting RDS [10].

Meconium has a marginal impact on lamellar bodies counts, increasing the count by 5000/μL. Bloody fluid can initially slightly increase the count because the platelets are counted as lamellar bodies. Afterwards, the procoagulant activity of amniotic fluid produces an entrapment of both platelets and lamellar bodies, causing a decrease of LBC.

Foam stability index

The foam stability index (FSI) is derived from the shake test, an assay of surfactant function that evaluates the ability of pulmonary surfactant to generate stable foam in the presence of ethanol. The commercially prepared test kit contains wells with a predispensed volume of ethanol. Adding amniotic fluid to each test well produces final ethanol concentrations ranging from 44% to 50%. After shaking the amniotic fluid–ethanol mixture, one reads the FSI as the highest well in which a rim of stable foam persists. RDS has been reported unlikely with an FSI of 47 or higher; however, a negative test often occurs in the presence of a mature lung. The FSI cannot be derived from an amniotic fluid specimen contaminated by blood or meconium [11].

Multiple tests or cascade?

Faced with different assays for fetal lung maturity, some laboratories perform multiple tests simultaneously, leaving the clinician with the possibility of results both indicative and not of pulmonary maturity from the same amniotic fluid specimen. In general, any "mature" test result is indicative of fetal pulmonic maturity given the high predictive value of any single test (5% or less of false mature rates). Conversely, the use of a "cascade" approach has been proposed to minimize the risk of delivery of an infant with immature lungs, while avoiding unnecessary delay in delivery and costs. According to this approach, a rapid and inexpensive test is performed first, with follow-up tests performed only in the face of immaturity of the initial test (e.g., LBC or TDx-FLM as the initial test and L:S ratio as the final test).

Clinical conditions affecting risk of RDS and predictive value of pulmonary maturity tests

Several circumstances can affect the risk of RDS and modify the predictive value of pulmonary maturity tests. In African-Americans, lung maturity is achieved at lower gestational ages and at lower L:S ratios (1.2 or greater) than in white people. In addition, female gender is associated with acceleration of lung maturation. Intrauterine growth restriction and preeclampsia are associated with an acceleration of fetal lung maturity.

In contrast, maternal diabetes and Rhesus (Rh) isoimmunization are associated with a delay in fetal lung maturation. Some authors have recommended the use of higher thresholds of L:S ratio (e.g., a cut-off ratio of 3) to establish pulmonic maturity in these conditions [12]. Presence of a LBC of 50,000/μL has similarly been recommended to indicate mature fetal lungs in diabetic women. Presence of PG is commonly considered as gold standard for documentation of fetal lung maturity with diabetes or Rh-isoimmunization.

In twin gestations it is commonly recommended that the sac of the male twin or the larger twin be sampled at amniocentesis. The reasoning is that if the sampled twin has mature pulmonic results, the other-twin is even more likely to be mature.

Less need for testing?

Recent changes in clinical practice have, in many cases, reduced the need for determining fetal lung maturity. More obstetricians are scheduling ultrasound examinations early in pregnancy, thereby establishing gestational age more accurately. The result is that elective deliveries at term can be scheduled without determining fetal lung maturation. Similarly, in pregnancies complicated by diabetes mellitus, excellent maternal glucose control through self-monitoring of blood glucose levels and carefully planned insulin regimens, combined with intensive antepartum fetal surveillance, has reduced the fear of unexpected intrauterine death late in the third trimester. More patients with insulin-dependent diabetes mellitus are being allowed to enter spontaneous labor at term or are induced at 39 weeks or above, making amniocentesis to establish fetal lung maturity unnecessary.

However, the recent trend away from vaginal birth after cesarean back to elective repeat cesarean delivery will probably tend to increase the demand for amniocentesis to facilitate delivery scheduling, particularly if dates are uncertain or delivery is desired prior to 39 weeks. These effects remain to be seen.

Case presentation

A 32-year-old white, G3P2002, patient has a known complete previa in the setting of poorly controlled gestational diabetes and is carrying a male fetus. She is 35–37 weeks, with the uncertainty a result of her late entry to prenatal care and the possibility of an large for gestational age (LGA) baby because of her diabetes. An amniocentesis for lung maturity is recommended to aid with delivery planning. Curiously, although there is no

transplacental passage of the needle, the amniotic fluid is noted to be slightly blood tinged.

The lamellar count comes back within the hour at 42,000. Because of concern that this is not over the threshold value of 50,000 recommended for diabetic mothers and because results may be falsely increased, at least initially, by blood contamination, the decision is made to wait for L:S and PG results before delivery (a cascade approach).

Later that day, the L:S ratio is noted to be 1.9 and the PG is negative. Although the L:S may be falsely lowered by the presence of blood, it would be hard to imagine the ratio would be above 3.0, the value required in a diabetic patient. PG should not be affected by blood at all and the presence of PG (or its equivalent such as LBC >50,000 or L:S >3.0) must be achieved to indicated delivery on the basis of pulmonary maturity in a diabetic. The decision is made to defer delivery and continue antepartum testing. Assuming no bleeding from the previa or fetal issues that would prompt delivery regardless of fetal lung maturity status, the amniocentesis will be repeated in 1 week.

References

1 Gluck L, Kulovich MV, Boerer RC Jr, *et al.* Diagnosis of the respiratory distress syndrome by amniocentesis. *Am J Obstet Gynecol* 1971;**109**:440.

2 American College of Obstetricians and Gynecologists (ACOG). Assessment of fetal lung maturity. ACOG Educational Bulletin no. 230. Washington, DC: ACOG, November 1996.

3 Stark CM, Smith RS, Lagrandeur RM, Batton DG, Lorenz RP. Need for urgent delivery after third-trimester amniocentesis. *Obstet Gynecol* 2000;**95**:48–50.

4 Harper MA, Lorenz WB. Immature lecithin/sphingomyelin ratios and respirator course. *Am J Obstet Gynecol* 1993;**168**:495.

5 Towers CV, Garite TJ. Evaluation of the new Amniostat-FLM test for the detection of phosphatidylglycerol in contaminated fluids. *Am J Obstet Gynecol* 1989;**160**:298.

6 Kulovich MV, Hallman MB, Gluck L. The lung profile. I. Normal pregnancy. *Am J Obstet Gynecol* 1979;**135**:57.

7 Kesselman EJ, Figueroa R, Garry D, Maulik D. The usefulness of the TDx/TDxFLx fetal lung maturity II assay in the initial evaluation of fetal lung maturity. *Am J Obstet Gynecol* 2003;**188**:1220–2.

8 Neerhof MG, Dohnal JC, Ashwood ER, Lee IS, Anceschi MM. Lamellar body counts: a consensus on protocol. *Obstet Gynecol* 2001;**97**:318–20.

9 Ghidini A, Poggi SH, Spong CY, Goodwin KM, Vink J, Pezzullo JC. Role of lamellar body count for the prediction of neonatal respiratory distress syndrome in non-diabetic pregnant women. *Arch Gynecol Obstet* 2005;**271**:325–8.

10 Wijnberger LD, Huisjes AJ, Voorbij HA, Franx A, Bruinse HW, Moll BV. The accuracy of lamellar body count and lecithin/ sphingomyelin ratio in the prediction of neonatal respiratory distress syndrome: a meta-analysis. *Br J Obstet Gynaecol* 2001;**108**:585–8.

11 Lipshitz J, Whybrew W, Anderson G. Comparison of the Lumadex-foam stability test, lectithin : sphingomyelin ratio, and simple shake test for fetal lung maturity. *Obstet Gynecol* 1984;**63**:349.

12 Ghidini A, Spong CY, Goodwin K, Pezzullo JC. Optimal thresholds of lecithin/sphingomyelin ratio and lamellar body count for the prediction of the presence of phosphatidylglycerol in diabetic women. *J Matern Fetal Neonatal Med* 2002;**12**:95–8.

11 Antepartum fetal monitoring

Brian L. Shaffer and Julian T. Parer

The goal of antenatal surveillance is to prevent fetal injury and death. Antenatal testing should improve long-term neurologic outcome through optimal timing of delivery while avoiding unnecessary intervention, such as cesarean delivery or preterm delivery. The US National Center for Health Statistics (NCHS) defines intrauterine fetal death (IUFD) as death prior to birth, 20 or more weeks in gestation, without neonatal breathing, pulsation of the umbilical cord, a heartbeat, and without voluntary movements. However, gasping, fleeting movements, transient cardiac contractions, and respiratory efforts are not considered signs of life [1].

In 2002, the incidence of IUFD was 6.4/1000 live births plus fetal deaths [2], short of the national health objective of 4.1/1000 [3]. Half of the fetal deaths occur in fetuses of 20–27 weeks' gestation (3.3/1000), and the remaining in those 28 or more weeks (3.2/1000). The fetal mortality rate has declined considerably since 1950 and late fetal mortality (≥28 weeks) has decreased 23% from 1990 [4].

To assist in reaching the Healthy People 2010 goal of an IUFD incidence of 4.1/1000 [3], the etiology of IUFD must be clarified. Several approaches based on the timing of the event, gestational age, and specifying the abnormal "compartment" (i.e., maternal, fetal, and placental) have been proposed [5]. The most common etiologies in those less than 27 weeks include infection, abruption, and lethal congenital anomalies. In comparison, the most frequent causes of stillbirth at more than 28 weeks are growth restriction and abruption. However, unexplained deaths account for 27–60% of cases of IUFD after 20 weeks [5,6]. Because of this large proportion of "unexplained" IUFDs, there has been a focus on associated risk factors for stillbirth. Maternal race, age, socioeconomic status, medical illnesses, and biologic markers, such as abnormal serum markers, have been associated with increased risks of IUFD [5]. However, up to 50% of those with IUFD have no known risk factors [7].

Those mothers who are at increased risk for IUFD are often referred for antenatal testing. Despite performing antepartum surveillance for several decades, unequivocal evidence does not clearly illustrate when, how frequently, or at what gestational age to perform testing. The standard should be determined by the performance of the specific test—in this case the sensitivity and specificity, compared with the rate of stillbirth and the week-specific mortality rate.

There are several antepartum testing modalities from which to choose, including fetal movement or "kick counts," the non-stress test (NST), the amniotic fluid index (AFI) combined with the NST (modified biophysical profile), the contraction stress test (CST), the biophysical profile (BPP), and use of Doppler velocimetry. Our aim is to present a reasonable guide of who to test, when to begin, how frequently, and which test to choose.

Fetal movement or "kick counts"

Decreased fetal movement may precede fetal death by several days [8]. Because up to 50% of those with IUFD have no risk factors and thus undergo no formal antepartum surveillance, some have recommended kick counts for all patients [8,9]. Several studies of intervention after decreased movements have been associated with decreasing the IUFD rate [9]. Defining what constitutes "decreased movement" varies, and regardless of the method, once decreased fetal movement has been diagnosed, a back-up test is employed. One evaluation of maternal perception of kick counts used 10 movements in 2 hours. The authors found a decreased stillbirth rate from 8.7/1000–2.1/1000 after implementing formal fetal movement counts [9]. However, Grant et al. [10] found no difference in mortality in those who presented after decreased fetal movement. The authors reported that women with decreased movement presented earlier with stillborns, whereas those in routine care were diagnosed at the next visit. The authors asserted that fetal death was predictable but not preventable and large amounts of provider and maternal time were necessary to prevent a single IUFD [10]. In contrast, Froen [11], in a meta-analysis, highlights the shortcomings of that study and asserts that vigilance toward maternal perception of fetal movements significantly reduces avoidable stillbirth rates while costing only an additional antenatal visit in 2.1% of pregnancies. With few patients returning for unscheduled visits, this low "false alarm" rate seems acceptable as fetal movement monitoring may improve the IUFD rate, especially in low-risk pregnancies.

The NST is a recording of fetal heart rate and uterine activity and is performed with the patient in the semi-Fowler position with left lateral tilt. The fetal heart rate transducer and tocodynamometer are placed on the maternal abdomen. A "reactive" or normal test is one in which there is a normal fetal heart rate tracing (FHT) baseline (110–160 beats per minute [beats/min]), with moderate variability (6–25 beats/min), and two accelerations (FHT peaks 15 beats/min above the baseline for ≥15 seconds). A reactive or "normal" NST is associated with survival for 7 days in 99% of cases [12]. The duration of an NST is normally 20 minutes, but an additional 20 minutes may be added if needed.

The variability and baseline of the FHT is governed by a functioning cortex, brainstem, and cardiac conduction system. However, a reactive NST does not reflect an entirely normal central nervous system, as a fetus affected by holoprosencephaly may still have a reactive NST [13].

The value of the NST relies on several assumptions, which can be made after a few characteristics are observed. In the presence of a normal baseline rate, variability, and accelerations, the fetus is presumed to be nonacidemic and nonasphyxiated. The acceleration is a response to fetal movement. Adequate accelerations have been associated with sonographically detected fetal movement in 99% of cases [14]. Several factors have been identified as modulators of accelerations, including sympathetic discharge, fetal circadian rhythm, gestational age, and maternal medication exposure or illicit drug use. Maternal smoking has been associated with decreased FHT reactivity [15,16]. Similarly, assumptions can be made about the fetal status when accelerations are absent during an NST. Fetal sleep cycles usually last 20–40 minutes but may be longer. Fetal movement and accelerations are less likely to occur during sleep. Also, non-REM sleep is associated with reduced FHT variability [17]. Thus, extending the NST duration to 40 minutes allows for variation in sleep–wake cycle. Lack of accelerations, however, may indicate a fetal state of hypoxemia or acidemia, central nervous system (CNS) depression, or congenital anomalies.

Variable decelerations during an NST are not infrequent and may occur in up to 50% of those undergoing testing. If variable decelerations are nonrepetitive, lasting less than 30 seconds, and occur in the setting of an otherwise reactive NST, there is no need for intervention [18]. However, three or more variable decelerations in 20 minutes have been associated with increased cesarean rates for nonreassuring FHT [19,20]. Decelerations lasting more than 60 seconds have been associated with IUFD and cesarean for nonreassuring FHT [21–23].

Table 11.1 False negative and false positive rates for antenatal testing modalities.

Test	False Negative*	False Positive[†] (%)
Nonstress test	1.9–5 [32–36]	50% [33]
Modified biophysical profile	0–0.8 [26,27,40,41]	60% [27]
Contraction stress test	0.4 [33,47,48]	40% [50]
Biophysical profile	0.6 [45]	40% [45]

* Risk of fetal mortality (per 1000 live births) <1 week after a negative test result.
[†] Fetal survival >1 week after a positive test result.

A nonreactive NST over a 40-minute testing period may indicate fetal compromise, but the gestational age must be considered because in one study 50% of healthy fetuses between 24 and 28 weeks had a nonreactive NST [24]. At 28–32 weeks, only 15% of normal fetuses were not reactive [25].

Vibroacoustic stimulation (VAS) can be used without compromising the detection of the impaired fetus while shortening the time to produce a reactive test [26–29]. Often, VAS is used after a period of nonreactive FHT. The provider gives a 1-second stimulation and may repeat after 60 seconds if no fetal acceleration occurs. A third stimulation may be administered for up to 3 seconds in duration if no acceleration occurs after previous attempts. Using VAS may not actually decrease the duration of testing, producing prolonged accelerations, in approximately one-third of cases [30]. Despite common assumptions, manual stimulation and maternal administration of a glucose-containing drink do not improve the reactivity of the NST [31].

The nonreactive NST has a false positive rate (fetal survival >1 week after a nonreactive NST) of up to 50%, requiring back-up testing (e.g., CST/BPP). Poor fetal outcome (e.g., perinatal death, low 5-minute Apgar score, late decelerations during labor) occurs only in 20% of cases with a nonreactive NST. In the largest series of patients (n=5861) undergoing antepartum surveillance with the NST, the false negative (fetal death <1 week after a reactive NST) rate was 3.1/1000, while others have found similar results (1.9–5/1000) (Table 11.1) [32–36]. However, the use of the NST is "widely integrated into clinical practice" [37] and despite no definitive evidence of a beneficial effect on fetal mortality it will probably continue to be utilized liberally in modern obstetric practice [38].

Modified BPP (NST/AFI)

The risk of short-term hypoxemia is addressed with the NST. Measuring the AFI is a surrogate for fetal renal perfusion and reflects long-term placental function via the amniotic fluid status. The AFI acts as a measure of redistribution of fetal blood flow as hypoxemia can lead to decreased renal perfusion, urine output, and oligohydramnios [26,39]. The modified BPP has a lower false negative rate than the NST alone, 0–0.8/1000, but the false positive rate (i.e., a normal fetus despite a positive test result) remains 60% [26,27,40,41]. When utilizing the modified BPP, a back-up test must be performed for any of the following: nonreactive NST, significant variable or late decelerations, or AFI <5.

Intervention based on surveillance with the modified BPP may not be without consequence as its use in one study was associated with a higher rate of cesarean (relative risk [RR] 2.09; 95% confidence interval [CI], 1.69–2.57). Further, intervention in those with a false positive test led to iatrogenic premature delivery in 1.5% of women tested [27]. However, it appears that the modified BPP is similar in its incidence of adverse outcomes following a negative result (risk of fetal mortality after a negative test result) compared with the contraction stimulation test (CST) with a risk of IUFD of approximately 1 in 1000 in both tests. The modified BPP is probably currently the primary means for antenatal surveillance [41,42].

Biophysical profile

The BPP consists of an NST with ultrasound observation of the fetus for up to 30 minutes, and reflects potential acute and chronic fetal hypoxia. The BPP has five separate variables: the NST, fetal breathing, movement, tone, and the AFI (Table 11.2). The AFI is the chronic marker while the other four components reflect acute asphyxia. Each component scores either 0 or 2 points. Each component score is tallied and a composite score is given, yet not all measures are equal. Indeed, low AFI is independently associated with increased level of acidemia [43]. The BPP can be employed for primary antepartum surveillance, follow-up of nonreactive NST, or for further information after positive or suspicious CST.

The management is the BPP as follows (Table 11.3).

Eight and 10 out of 10 are normal and repeat testing should be performed as typically scheduled. However, if points were lost for oligohydramnios, this confers fetal jeopardy and delivery should be considered if the gestational age permits. Alternatively, more frequent surveillance, including assessment of fetal growth, should be carried out.

A score of 6/10 is equivocal and should be repeated within 12–24 hours if less than 34 weeks. However, it the fetus is 34 or more weeks, delivery should be considered. If oligohydramnios is present, delivery should be considered, as the test is likely a true positive if the fetus loses points for nonreactive NST or breathing movements. In contrast, the test is more likely a false positive if the fetus has normal fluid and loses points for nonreactive NST and another parameter [44].

A score of 4/10 requires immediate evaluation and intervention and may warrant delivery unless the fetus is very premature (i.e., <28 weeks). If delivery is not carried out, repeat assessments are needed every 12–24 hours.

A score of 2/10 requires delivery if the score persists after extending testing for 120 minutes [45].

Table 11.2 Scoring for biophysical profile. Modified from [45,65].

Variable	Normal (Score = 2 for 1–5)	Abnormal (Score = 0 for 1–5)
1 Fetal breathing movement (FBM)	≥1 episode of FBMs of ≥30 seconds in duration	<30 seconds of sustained FBMs
2 Fetal movement	≥3 discrete body/limb movements (simultaneous limb and trunk movements are counted as a single movement)	≤2 movements
3 Fetal tone	≥1 episode of active extension with rapid return to flexion of fetal limb(s)	Either slow extension with return to partial flexion or movement of limb in full trunk, or hand extension, or absent fetal movement
4 Reactive FHT	≥2 accelerations of ≥15 beats/min, peak amplitude lasting ≥15 seconds from the baseline in 20 minutes	<2 accelerations or accelerations <15 beats/min peak amplitude or accelerations <15 seconds duration in 20 minutes
5 Amniotic fluid index	>5.0 cm	≤5.0 cm
For twins, deepest vertical pocket in each sac	≥2.0 cm	<2.0 cm

FHT, fetal heart rate tracing.

Table 11.3 Biophysical profile scoring and management.

Score	Risk of Asphyxia	Management	Perinatal Mortality*
10/10	Nearly zero	Follow as clinical course dictates	<1/1000
8/10 (AFI nl)			
8/10 (Oligo)	Chronic asphyxia likely	If normal urinary tract, no ROM—delivery after corticosteroids	20–30
6/10 (AFI nl)	Asphyxia not excluded	Repeat testing. If persistent 6/10, deliver at >37 weeks; if	50
6/10 (Oligo)	Chronic asphyxia likely	immature repeat within 24 h—if less than 6/10 delivery	>50
4/10	Acute likely, if oligo, risk of acute and chronic increases	Delivery, continuous FHT	115 >115 if oligo
2/10	Acute with chronic asphyxia likely	Delivery, typically via cesarean	220
0/10	Nearly certain	Deliver immediately	550

AFI, amniotic fluid index; FHT, fetal heart rate tracing; ROM, rupture of membranes; oligo, oligohydramnios.

* Risk of fetal mortality (per 1000 live births) within 1 week without any fetal intervention [65].

Contraction stress test

The CST is a measure of fetal response to stress. The uterus contracts and the spiral arteries are occluded, decreasing flow to the intervillous space and resulting in decreased oxygenation of the fetus. In the suboptimally oxygenated fetus, the baseline O_2 deficit will be worsened and late decelerations on the FHT will be apparent. The advantage of the CST is that subtle hypoxia prior to acidosis is more easily detected when compared with the BPP/NST, and the CST is helpful in predicting tolerance of labor.

The CST is performed with the patient in the semi-Fowler position. An adequate test is assessment of the FHT and uterine contractions with three contractions in 10 minutes, each lasting at least 40 seconds in duration. Oxytocin can be employed for uterine contractions (0.5 mU/min, increased every 20 minutes to a maximum of 10 mU/min) or manual stimulation of the maternal nipple may be used. This is done by rubbing one nipple through the clothing for 2 minutes or until a contraction begins. If no contractions are observed after 2 minutes, a second stimulation is performed after 5 minutes. An alternative technique is to apply warm packs to the breasts for a maximum of 2 minutes followed by a 5-minute interval prior to restimulation.

Nipple stimulation was approximately 50% faster than intravenous oxytocin in one evaluation of the time to an adequate CST [46]. Contraindications to the CST include preterm labor, preterm premature rupture of the membranes (PPROM), abnormal vaginal bleeding, and contraindications for vaginal delivery (e.g., placenta previa, prior classic cesarean, extensive uterine surgery).

The CST test result is "negative" if there are no late decelerations or significant variable decelerations in the setting of a normal baseline fetal heart rate. After three adequate contractions occur in 10 minutes, a negative and reactive CST has a false negative rate of 0.4–1/1000 and more than 99% survival over a week [47–49]. A CST is deemed positive if more than 50% of uterine contractions have associated late decelerations. A positive CST is associated with a 50% rate of poor perinatal outcome including perinatal death, increased cesarean for nonreassuring fetal status, and low 5-minute Apgar score.

While a positive CST is associated with adverse outcomes, the fetus may tolerate labor and therefore a trial of labor induction is recommended, unless there is an obstetric contraindication to vaginal delivery [50]. A reactive, positive CST is one with normal FHT variability and baseline but late decelerations after more than 50% of contractions. This generally calls for delivery, or close follow-up surveillance at a very early gestational age. A test deemed equivocal or suspicious is one in which there are 50% or fewer late decelerations, variable decelerations (i.e., possibly indicating IUGR, oligohydramnios), or an abnormal FHR baseline. These can be managed by delivery or more frequent testing, depending on gestational age.

If there are five or more uterine contractions in 10 minutes or contractions lasting more than 90 seconds in the setting of fetal heart rate decelerations then the CST is equivocal—hyperstimulation. Finally, a tracing is considered unsatisfactory if there are fewer than three contractions or the FHT is of poor quality (see Table 11.4 for management of CST results).

Doppler velocimetry

Doppler velocimetry is used as an adjunct to other testing modalities and is particularly useful in the growth restricted

Table 11.4 Follow-up for contraction stress test (CST).

CST result	Follow-up
Reactive–negative	Repeat, 7 days
Nonreactive–negative	Repeat, 24 hours Evaluation for nonreactivity Fetus <28 weeks, normal variability, repeat in 7 days
Reactive–equivocal	Repeat, 24 hours
Nonreactive–equivocal	Repeat, 24 hours
Reactive–positive	Gestational age >37 weeks, trial of induction Preterm: further evaluation
Nonreactive–positive	Term: delivery via cesarean Preterm: further testing

fetus [51]. It is not generally used as a primary means of surveillance, nor for screening in a low-risk population. The fetal umbilical artery (UA) is used to assess the hemodynamic components of placental vascular impedance. In some fetuses with IUGR, there is increased systolic : diastolic (S : D ratio above 3) blood flow velocity in the umbilical artery signifying increased umbilical vascular impedance. In severe IUGR, with high placental impedance, there may be absent or reversed flow [52–54]. Fetal mortality is increased with reversed or absent end-diastolic flow [55] and asphyxia in small for gestational age fetuses is associated with absent end-diastolic flow in the umbilical artery [56]. The use of Doppler velocimetry in high-risk pregnancies was associated with decreases in induction of labor, antepartum admission, and may result in decreased perinatal mortality (adjusted odds ratio [OR] 0.71; 95% CI, 0.50–1.01) [57].

Increased S : D ratios in those with a "high-risk" pregnancy were more likely to have "abnormal" perinatal outcome than those with values of less than 3.0 (2.3–2.9). The S : D ratio was a better predictor of poor outcome than suboptimal fetal growth [58]. The best predictor of poor long-term outcomes may be in those with IUGR and associated with umbilical cord S : D ratio abnormalities [59].

Poorer neurodevelopmental outcome in children aged 5–12 years was associated with reversed end-diastolic flow compared with normal and absent flow [59]. Other adverse outcomes have been associated with absent and reversed end-diastolic flow in the umbilical artery: mortality (28–45%), neonatal intensive care unit (NICU) admission (84–98%), and cesarean section (73%) for fetal distress [55,60]. Abnormal Doppler indices alone should not dictate intervention, but rather indicate the level of antenatal surveillance needed. For instance, a growth restricted fetus less than 32 weeks' gestation, with absent end-diastolic flow in the umbilical artery, continuous FHT and a reassuring BPP, may allow for maternal and fetal evaluation, corticosteroid administration, and preparation for delivery. In the setting of IUGR, absent end-diastolic flow should trigger continuous fetal surveillance with prolongation of the pregnancy dictated only by a reassuring BPP score, NST, and early gestational age.

In normal fetuses, the impedance of the vessels in the brain is relatively higher than in the UA and S : D ratios average above 5. In the fetus with IUGR and especially in those with asymmetrical IUGR, the impedance decreases further to increase perfusion and presumably oxygen delivery. Measurements of the middle cerebral artery (MCA) in fetuses with IUGR may reveal decreased S : D ratios. This increase in the umbilical artery S : D ratio, and decrease in the MCA S : D ratio, can be used as an index of the fetal compensatory mechanisms, and indicates a more severe response to IUGR [61–63].

Doppler interrogation of the MCA using the peak systolic velocity (PSV) is a tool for predicting fetal anemia in at-risk pregnancies. In contrast to the management of IUGR, measurement of the PSV has good sensitivity for moderate or severe anemia in the fetus affected by Rh alloimmunization [64].

Specific indications and onset of testing

The appropriate initiation and frequency of testing is determined by the indication for the test as well as gestational age. Typically, testing is begun at 32 weeks and is performed on a weekly to twice weekly basis. However, maternal or fetal situations may dictate daily testing (e.g., unstable hypertension, poorly controlled diabetes) [43]. The specifics of many recommendations are often based on sparse evidence while others are opinion-based and quite controversial. Table 11.5 shows the antenatal testing guidelines for the University of California San Francisco.

Case presentation

A 36-year-old white gravida 1, para 0 had chronic hypertension. She began prenatal care at 8 weeks and was maintained on labetalol, 400 mg twice daily. Baseline urine analysis revealed 465 mg protein and a serum creatinine of 1.3 mg/dL. At 15 weeks an amniocentesis was performed for advanced maternal age, revealing a chromosomally normal male fetus.

Serial sonograms were performed for fetal growth, beginning at 26 weeks. At 28 weeks, antenatal testing was initiated with twice weekly modified BPP. The initial NST result was nonreactive despite acoustic stimulation after 20 minutes. The AFI was 11.0.

Although the NST result may have been nonreactive as a result of the prematurity of the fetus, other etiologic factors were explored. She was questioned about her eating and drug

Table 11.5 Fetal surveillance: diagnostic conditions and frequency. The basic formal testing scheme is NST/AFI (modified BPP).

Indicator	GA of initiation	Frequency
1 Post dates	41 weeks (earlier if EDD unsure)	Twice weekly
2 Hypertensive diseases:		
(a) Preeclampsia (including r/o preeclampsia)	At Dx	Twice weekly (or more frequently depending on severity)
Chronic hypertension	32 weeks	Weekly
(b) Chronic hypertension with IUGR	See IUGR	See IUGR
3 Diabetes mellitus		
(a) GDM		
(i) On diet and exercise (A1)—good control (FBG < 95 mg/dL, PPBG < 140 mg/dL)	Kick counts only	
(ii) On insulin or oral agent (A2)—good or poor control	32 weeks	Twice weekly
(b) Pregestational (Type I, Type II)		
(i) W/out complications—good control	32 weeks	Twice weekly
(ii) W/out complications—poor control	28 weeks	Twice weekly
(iii) W/complications (e.g., poor growth, vascular disease)	28 weeks or when complications arise	Twice weekly
4 Advanced maternal age ≥40 years	32 weeks	Weekly
5 Severe maternal conditions (e.g., cardiac, pulmonary, severe asthma, sickle cell)	32 weeks	Weekly or more frequently
6 Active drug/ETOH abuse or methadone use	32 weeks	Weekly
7 SLE or antiphospholipid syndrome	32 weeks (earlier if microvascular disease)	Weekly or more frequently
8 Thyroid disease		
(a) Uncontrolled	32 weeks	Twice weekly
(b) Maternal Graves disease w/TSI > 130%	36 weeks	Weekly
9 Cholestasis	At Dx (begin before bile acid results)	Twice weekly
10 Herpes gestationis	At Dx	Weekly
11 HIV (on combination Rx)	32 weeks	Weekly
12 Seizure disorder (poorly controlled)	28 weeks	Weekly
13 IVF	36 weeks / 40 weeks	Weekly / Twice weekly
14 History abruption previous pregnancy	2 weeks prior to GA of previous abruption	Weekly
15 Increased MSAFP, increased MSHCG, or low PAPP-A (<1st percentile)	32 weeks	Weekly
16 Oligohydramnios	At Dx	As indicated
17 Polyhydramnios	At Dx	Weekly
18 IUGR (<10th percentile) or R/O IUGR (sono pending)	At Dx	Twice weekly

Table 11.5 *Continued.*

Indicator	GA of Initiation	Frequency	
19 Twins:			
(a) di/di w/normal growth and normal AFV	32 weeks	Weekly	
	36 weeks	Twice weekly	
(b) mono/di w/normal growth and concordant/normal AFV	28 weeks	Weekly	
	32 weeks	Twice weekly	
(c) di/di w/IUGR and/or discordant growth (>20%) and/or abnormal AFV	at Dx	Twice weekly	NST/Deepest pocket in each sac
(d) mono/di w/IUGR and/or discordant growth (>20%) and/or discordant AFV	at Dx	Twice weekly	
(e) mono/mono	at GA of intervention	Daily	
20 Triplets	same as mono/di twins	same as mono/di twins	
21 Hx previous IUFD	32 weeks or if previous demise <32 weeks, then begin 2 weeks prior to date of previous demise	Weekly	
22 Fetuses with certain abnormalities (e.g., CDH, gastroschisis, persistent echogenic bowel, increased NT (>3.5 mm))	32 weeks	Weekly	
23 Fetal arrhythmia (i.e., SVT, PACs, etc.)	At Dx	Weekly (BPP if unable to obtain FHR strip)	
24 Fetal heart block	At Dx (≥28 weeks)	Weekly BPP	
25 Fetal anemias (e.g., Rh alloimmunization, parvovirus, NAIT)	≥28 weeks or at onset of disease	Weekly or more frequently	

AFV, amniotic fluid volume; BPP, biophysical profile; CDH, congenital diaphragmatic hernia; di, dichorionic/diamnionic; Dx, diagnosis; EDD, estimated date of delivery; ETOH, alcohol; FBG, fasting blood glucose; FHR, fetal heart rate; GA, gestational age; GDM, gestational diabetes mellitus; Hx, history; IUGR, intrauterine growth restriction; IVF, *in vitro* fertilization; mono di, monochorionic diamniotic; MSAFP, maternal serum alpha-fetoprotein; MSHCG, maternal serum human chorionic gonadotropin; NAIT, neonatal alloimmune thrombocytopenia; NT, nuchal translucency; PAC, premature atrial contractions; PAPP-A, pregnancy-associated plasma protein A; PPBG, postprandial blood glucose; R/O, rule out; Rh, Rhesus; Rx, therapy; SLE, systemic lupus erythematosus; SVT, supraventricular tachycardia; TSI, thyroid stimulating immunoglobulin.

habits; she had a normal breakfast prior to the test and denied any illicit drug use. A BPP was performed to follow-up the nonreactive NST, with a score of 8/10 (loss of 2 points for NST result). With a reassuring BPP, the nonreactive tracing was attributed to the fetal prematurity.

At 29 weeks, there was a reactive NST result and an AFI of 9.7. However, blood pressure was 167/105 mmHg and the fundal height was 26 cm. She was hospitalized, and biometry revealed that the fetus was 820 g (<5%), and a presumptive diagnosis of IUGR was made. Umbilical artery Doppler velocimetry was performed which revealed an increased S:D ratio of 5.3–6.0, with end-diastolic flow. In addition, the MCA S:D ratio measured 3.0–3.8. During her hospitalization, she experienced a severe exacerbation of hypertension, the labetalol was increased and a second agent, nifedipine, was begun. On admission, the complete blood cell count (CBC), liver function test (LFT), and urine protein values were normal. An NST on the day of admission was reactive; the AFI was 5.0. Owing to the severity of the hypertension and abnormal cord Doppler indicies, twice daily NST testing was initiated and a course of

betamethasone was given for acceleration of fetal pulmonary maturity.

A plan for twice weekly AFI monitoring and weekly Doppler velocimetry was devised. Three days later, the NST result was nonreactive and the AFI was 4.0. A BPP was performed, with an equivocal score of 6/10 (loss of 2 points for nonreactive NST and oligohydramnios). Repeat testing was scheduled for the next morning (12 hours later). On hospital day 5, she complained of mid-epigastric pain. Laboratory tests revealed a hematocrit of 42%, platelet count of $102,000 \times 10^9$/L, and serum aspartate transaminase and alanine transaminase levels of 960 U/L and 1020 U/L, respectively.

The repeat BPP score was 4/10 with the additional loss of fetal breathing. Preparations for induction of labor were made because of the deteriorating fetal and maternal conditions, and a male infant weighing 875 g was delivered vaginally. Apgar scores were 5 at 1 minute and 8 at 5 minutes. Umbilical artery (CUA) and vein (CUV) blood gas values were obtained: CUA pH 7.27, P_{CO_2} 48 mmHg, P_{O_2} 33 mmHg, base excess –4.4 and CUV pH 7.30, P_{CO_2} 42 mmHg, P_{O_2} 39 mmHg, base excess –3.4.

The newborn required intubation for 48 hours, was weaned from all oxygen support by day 12 of life, and discharged on day 46 of life. The mother was treated with magnesium sulfate for 48 hours postpartum, her abnormal laboratory values were normal by day 5 postpartum, and she was discharged.

References

1 Procedures for coding cause of fetal death under ICD-10 2005. http://www.cdc.gov/nchs/about/major/fetaldth/abfetal.htm

2 Martin JA, Kochanek KD, Strobino DM, Guyer B, MacDorman MF. Annual Summary of Vital Statistics—2003. *Pediatrics* 2005;**115**:619–34.

3 US Department of Health and Human Services. *Healthy People 2010*, 2nd edn. *Understanding and Improving Health and Objectives for Improving Health*. 2 vols. Part 16: *Maternal, Infant, and Child Health*. Washington DC: US Government Printing Office, Nov 2000.

4 Barfield W, Martin JA, Hoyert DL. Racial/ethnic trends in fetal mortality: United States, 1990–2000. *MMWR Morb Mortal Weekly Rep* 2004;**53**:529–32.

5 Fretts RC. Etiology and prevention of stillbirth. *Am J Obstet Gynecol* 2005;**193**:1923–35.

6 Huang DY, Usher RH, Kramer MS, *et al*. Determinants of unexplained antepartum fetal deaths. *Obstet Gynecol* 2000;**95**:215–21.

7 Incerpi MH, Miller DA, Samadi R, Settlage RH, Goodwin TM. Stillbirth evaluation: what tests are needed? *Am J Obstet Gynecol* 1998;**178**:1121–5.

8 Pearson JF, Weaver JB. Fetal activity and fetal wellbeing: an evaluation. *Br Med J* 1976;**1**:1305–7.

9 Moore TR, Piacquadio K. A prospective evaluation of fetal movement screening to reduce the incidence of antepartum fetal death. *Am J Obstet Gynecol* 1989;**160**:1075–80.

10 Grant A, Elbourne D, Valentin L, Alexander S. Routine formal fetal movement counting and risk of antepartum late death in normally formed singletons. *Lancet* 1989;**8659**:345–9.

11 Froen JF. A kick from within: fetal movement counting and the canceled progress in antenatal care. *J Perinat Med* 2004;**32**: 13–24.

12 Schifrin BS. The rationale for antepartum fetal heart rate monitoring. *J Reprod Med* 1979;**23**:213–21.

13 Cardosi RJ, Heffron JA, Spellacy WN. Reactive nonstress test despite severe congenital brain damage. What does the test measure? *J Reprod Med* 1997;**42**:251–2.

14 Rabinowitz R, Persitz E, Sadovsky E. The relation between fetal heart rate accelerations and fetal movements. *Obstet Gynecol* 1983;**61**:16–8.

15 Graca LM, Cardoso CG, Clode N, Calhaz-Jorge C. Acute effects of maternal cigarette smoking on fetal heart rate and fetal body movements felt by the mother. *J Perinat Med* 1991;**19**:385–90.

16 Oncken C, Kranzler H, O'Malley P, Gendreau P, Campbell WA. The effect of cigarette smoking on fetal heart rate characteristics. *Obstet Gynecol* 2002;**99**:751–5.

17 Nijhuis JG, Prechtl HF, Martin CB Jr, Bots RS. Are there behavioural states in the human fetus? *Early Hum Dev* 1982;**6**:177–95.

18 Meis PJ, Ureda JR, Swain M, Kelly RT, Penry M, Sharp P. Variable decelerations during nonstress tests are not a sign of fetal compromise. *Am J Obstet Gynecol* 1986;**154**:586–90.

19 Anyaegbunam A, Brustman L, Divon M, Langer O. The significance of antepartum variable decelerations. *Am J Obstet Gynecol* 1986;**155**:707–10.

20 O'Leary JA, Andrinopoulos GC, Giordano PC. Variable decelerations and the nonstress test: an indication of cord compromise. *Am J Obstet Gynecol* 1980;**137**:704–6.

21 Druzin ML, Gratacos J, Keegan KA, Paul RH. Antepartum fetal heart rate testing. VII. The significance of fetal bradycardia. *Am J Obstet Gynecol* 1981;**139**:194–8.

22 Bourgeois FJ, Thiagarajah S, Harbert GM Jr. The significance of fetal heart rate decelerations during nonstress testing. *Am J Obstet Gynecol* 1984;**150**:213–6.

23 Pazos R, Vuolo K, Aladjem S, Lueck J, Anderson C. Association of spontaneous fetal heart rate decelerations during antepartum nonstress testing and intrauterine growth retardation. *Am J Obstet Gynecol* 1982;**144**:574–7.

24 Bishop EH. Fetal acceleration test. *Am J Obstet Gynecol* 1981;**141**:905–9.

25 Druzin ML, Fox A, Kogut E, Carlson C. The relationship of the nonstress test to gestational age. *Am J Obstet Gynecol* 1985;**153**:386–9.

26 Clark SL, Sabey P, Jolley K. Nonstress testing with acoustic stimulation and amniotic fluid volume assessment: 5973 tests without unexpected fetal death. *Am J Obstet Gynecol* 1989;**160**:694–7.

27 Miller DA, Rabello YA, Paul RH. The modified biophysical profile: antepartum testing in the 1990s. *Am J Obstet Gynecol* 1996;**174**:812–7.

28 Smith CV, Phelan JP, Platt LD, Broussard P, Paul RH. Fetal acoustic stimulation testing. II. A randomized clinical comparison with the nonstress test. *Am J Obstet Gynecol* 1986;**155**:131–4.

29 Zimmer EZ, Divon MY. Fetal vibroacoustic stimulation. *Obstet Gynecol* 1993;**81**:451–7.

30 Newnham JP, Burns SE, Roberman BD. Effect of vibratory acoustic stimulation on the duration of fetal heart rate monitoring tests. *Am J Perinatol* 1990;**7**:232–4.

31 Tan KH, Sabapathy A. Maternal glucose administration for facilitating tests of fetal wellbeing. *Cochrane Database Syst Rev* 2001;**4**:CD003397.

32 Boehm FH, Salyer S, Shah DM, Vaughn WK. Improved outcome of twice weekly nonstress testing. *Obstet Gynecol* 1986;**67**:566–8.

33 Freeman RK, Anderson G, Dorchester W. A prospective multi-institutional study of antepartum fetal heart rate monitoring. I. Risk of perinatal mortality and morbidity according to antepartum fetal heart rate results. *Am J Obstet Gynecol* 1982;**143**:771–7.

34 Druzin ML, Gratacos J, Paul RH. Antepartum fetal heart rate testing. VI. Predictive reliability of "normal" tests in the prevention of antepartum deaths. *Am J Obstet Gynecol* 1980;**137**:745–7.

35 Devoe LD. The non stress test. In: Eden RD, Boehm FH, eds. *Assessment and Care of the Fetus: Physiological, Clinical, and Medicolegal Principles*. Norwalk, CT: Appleton & Lange, 1990.

36 Phelan JP, Lewis PE Jr. Fetal heart rate decelerations during a nonstress test. *Obstet Gynecol* 1981;**57**:228–32.

37 American College of Obstetricians and Gynecologists Practice Bulletin. *Antepartum fetal surveillance*. ACOG Educational Bulletin 238. Washington, DC: American College of Obstetricians and Gynecologists, 1999.

38 Pattison N, McCowan L. Cardiotocography for antepartum fetal assessment. *Cochrane Database Syst Rev* 1999;**1**:CD001068.

39 Seeds AE. Current concepts of amniotic fluid dynamics. *Am J Obstet Gynecol* 1980;**138**:575–86.

40 Vintzileos AM, Knuppel RA. Multiple parameter biophysical testing in the prediction of fetal acid–base status. *Clin Perinatol* 1994;**21**:823–48.

41 Nageotte MP, Towers CV, Asrat T, Freeman RK, Dorchester W. The value of a negative antepartum test: CST and modified BPP. *Obstet Gynecol* 1994;**84**:231–4.

42 Nageotte MP, Towers CV, Asrat T, Freeman RK, Dorchester W. The value of a negative antepartum test: CST and modified BPP. *Obstet Gynecol* 1994;**84**:231–4.

43 Devoe LD, Gardner P, Dear C, Castillo RA. The diagnostic values of concurrent nonstress testing, amniotic fluid measurement, and Doppler velocimetry in screening a general high-risk population. *Am J Obstet Gynecol* 1990;**163**:1040–7.

44 Hanley ML, Vintzileos AM. Biophysical testing in premature rupture of the membranes. *Semin Perinatol* 1996;**20**:418–25.

45 Manning FA, Morrison I, Lange IR, Harman CR, Chamberlain PF. Fetal assessment based on fetal biophysical profile scoring: experience in 12,620 referred high-risk pregnancies. I. Perinatal mortality by frequency and etiology. *Am J Obstet Gynecol* 1985;**151**:343–50.

46 Huddleston JF, Sutliff G, Robinson D. Contraction stress test by intermittent nipple stimulation. *Obstet Gynecol* 1984;**63**:669–73.

47 Evertson LR, Gauthier RJ, Collea JV. Fetal demise following negative contraction stress tests. *Obstet Gynecol* 1978;**51**:671–3.

48 Lagrew DC. The contraction stress test. *Clin Obstet Gynecol* 1995;**38**:11–25.

49 Schrifrin BS. The rationale for antepartum fetal heart rate monitoring. *J Reprod Med* 1979;**23**:213–21.

50 Thacker SB, Berkelman RL. Assessing the diagnostic accuracy and efficacy of selected antepartum fetal surveillance techniques. *Obstet Gynecol Surv* 1986;**41**:121–41.

51 Haley J, Tuffnell DJ, Johnson N. Randomised controlled trial of cardiotography versus umbilical artery Doppler in the management of small for gestational age fetuses. *Br J Obstet Gynaecol* 1997;**104**:431–5.

52 Erskine RL, Ritchie JW. Umbilical artery blood flow characteristics in normal and growth-retarded fetuses. *Br J Obstet Gynaecol* 1985;**92**:605–10.

53 Gudmundsson S, Marsal K. Umbilical and uteroplacental blood flow velocity waveforms in pregnancies with fetal growth retardation. *Eur J Obstet Gynecol Reprod Biol* 1988;**27**:187–96.

54 Reuwer PJ, Bruinse HW, Stoutenbeek P, Haspels AA. Doppler assessment of the fetoplacental circulation in normal and growth-retarded fetuses. *Eur J Obstet Gynecol Reprod Biol* 1984;**18**:199–205.

55 Karsdorp VH, van Vugt JM, van Geijn HP, *et al*. Clinical significance of absent or reversed end diastolic velocity waveforms in umbilical artery. *Lancet* 1994;**344**:1664–8.

56 Nicolaides KH, Bilardo CM, Soothill PW, Campbell S. Absence of end diastolic frequencies in umbilical artery: a sign of fetal hypoxia and acidosis. *Br Med J* 1988;**297**:1026–7.

57 Neilson JP, Alfirevic Z. Doppler ultrasound for fetal assessment in high risk pregnancies. *Cochrane Database Syst Rev* 1996;**4**:CD000073.

58 Maulik D, Yarlagadda P, Youngblood JP, Ciston P. The diagnostic efficacy of the umbilical arterial systolic/diastolic ratio as a screening tool: a prospective blinded study. *Am J Obstet Gynecol* 1990;**162**:1518–23.

59 Schreuder AM, McDonnell M, Gaffney G, Johnson A, Hope PL. Outcome at school age following antenatal detection of absent or reversed end diastolic flow velocity in the umbilical artery. *Arch Dis Child Fetal Neonatal Ed*. 2002;**86**:108–14.

60 Maulik D, ed. *Doppler Ultrasound in Obstetrics and Gynecology*. New York: Springer-Verlag, 1997.

61 Strigini FA, De Luca G, Lencioni G, Scida P, Giusti G, Genazzani AR. Middle cerebral artery velocimetry: different clinical relevance depending on umbilical velocimetry. *Obstet Gynecol* 1997;**90**:953–7.

62 Fong KW, Ohlsson A, Hannah ME, *et al*. Prediction of perinatal outcome in fetuses suspected to have intrauterine growth restriction: Doppler US study of fetal cerebral, renal, and umbilical arteries. *Radiology* 1999;**213**:681–9.

63 Bahado-Singh RO, Kovanci E, Jeffres A, *et al*. The Doppler cerebroplacental ratio and perinatal outcome in intrauterine growth restriction. *Am J Obstet Gynecol* 1999;**180**:750–6.

64 Mari G, Deter RL, Carpenter RL, *et al*. Noninvasive diagnosis by Doppler ultrasonography of fetal anemia due to maternal red-cell alloimmunization. Collaborative Group for Doppler Assessment of the Blood Velocity in Anemic Fetuses. *N Engl J Med* 2000;**342**:9–14.

65 Manning FA. Fetal biophysical profile. *Obstet Gynecol Clin* 1999;**26**:557–78.

12 Interpreting intrapartum fetal heart tracings

Michael Nageotte

Over the past 30 years, electronic fetal heart rate monitoring (EFM) has become an accepted means of assessing fetal status during labor. More than 85% of live births in the USA are so monitored despite a frequent lack of agreement on strip interpretation and management decisions [1]. This has resulted in an increased rate of cesarean delivery in patients monitored with EFM accompanied by a lack of clear evidence of efficacy. EFM is unquestionably a labor-saving device for nurses and is unlikely to be displaced from what is an accepted standard obstetric practice. Further, monitoring of the fetal heart rate (FHR) is a highly reliable modality in identifying the well-oxgenated fetus. This is because the brain controls the heart rate and changes in both cerebral blood flow and blood oxygenation in turn affect the FHR. Certain patterns in the heart rate of the fetus can be used to determine oxygen status with excellent concordance between normal fetal oxygenation and the presence of normal baseline FHR accompanied by FHR accelerations. While the concordance between normal oxygenation and the presence of FHR accelerations provides clinical reassurance, the absence of accelerations does not necessarily predict abnormality in fetal oxygenation. In fact, the correlation between abnormalities of the FHR (e.g., late or variable decelerations, elevated baseline) and adverse neonatal outcomes is at best tenuous [2]. That is to say, the positive predictive value of a nonreassuring FHR pattern to predict adverse outcome is very poor. Consequently, EFM should be understood and employed cautiously and used only as a diagnostic tool in the management of a woman's labor. It is only with the correct interpretation of the information provided from such a modality that appropriate management decisions can be made.

Interpretation guidelines for EFM

In order to understand the FHR and communicate interpretation accurately among health care providers there needs to be an appreciation of certain aspects of the FHR. These include baseline rate, variability, accelerations, and decelerations. The overall pattern appearance, changes over time, and response to certain clinical interventions must also be considered. In 1997, the National Institute of Child Health and Human Development Research Planning Workshop convened and proposed specific definitions for these various aspects of the FHR [3]. These definitions have been recently recommended for use in FHR monitoring by the American College of Obstetricians and Gynecologists [4].

Evaluation frequency

Assessment of FHR should occur frequently during active labor. For women with complicated pregnancies, such evaluations using auscultation should be every 15 min in the first stage of labor and every 5 min in the second stage [5]. The recommended evaluation frequency for laboring women without complications is auscultation every 30 min in the first stage of labor and every 15 min in the second stage. Similarly, when using EFM the frequency of tracing review would apply. Unfortunately, at times there is lack of concordance in the FHR strip interpretation among physicians and nurses. While there is generally excellent agreement when a strip is reassuring, for those FHR patterns that are not reassuring there is poor agreement regarding interpretation and management. Such interpretation is further challenged by clinically important confounders including gestational age, parity, maternal vital signs, medications, and progress in labor.

FHR pattern definitions

1 *Baseline* The baseline FHR is the mean rate rounded in increments of 5 beats/min over a minimum of 10 min. Bradycardia is when the baseline is less than 110 beats/min and tachycardia is when the baseline is greater than 160 beats/min.

2 *Variability* Irregular fluctuations in the baseline FHR of two

or more cycles per minute describe variability. FHR variability is either absent, minimal (amplitude range ≤5 beats/min), moderate (amplitude range >5–25 beats/min), or marked (amplitude range >25 beats/min). Of note, the sinusoidal heart rate has a smooth sine wave-like pattern of regular amplitude and frequency. The sinusoidal pattern is excluded from the FHR variability definition.

3 *Accelerations* An abrupt increase from baseline FHR to peak within 30 seconds of at least 15 beats/min lasting at least 15 seconds is termed an acceleration. Gestational age has a role in this definition, with fetuses less than 32 weeks having accelerations defined as increases at least 10 beats/min above baseline lasting at least 10 seconds.

4 *Decelerations*

(a) *Late deceleration:* a gradual and visually apparent decrease of baseline FHR lasting at least 30 seconds with return to baseline associated with a uterine contraction. Late decelerations are delayed in onset with the nadir of deceleration occurring after the contraction peak. Early deceleration is defined as a gradual and visually apparent decrease and return to baseline of the FHR associated with a contraction.

(b) *Early deceleration:* a gradual and visually apparent decrease and return to baseline of the FHR associated with contraction. An early deceleration has its nadir occur with the peak of the uterine contraction and mirrors the onset, peak, and ending of the contraction.

(c) *Variable deceleration:* a sudden, rapid decrease of the FHR to its nadir in less than 30 seconds. The decrease must be at least 15 beats/min lasting at least 15 seconds with return to baseline in less than 2 min.

(d) *Prolonged deceleration:* a decrease in the FHR of at least 15 beats/min lasting for longer than 2 min but less than 10 min before return to baseline.

Reassuring FHR

The most reliable marker of adequate fetal oxygenation and normal acid–base status is the presence of FHR accelerations. An additional marker of reassurance is the presence of normal FHR variability. Caution must be employed in the interpretation of EFM when variability is present when accompanied by concerning characteristics of the FHR such as persistent decelerations [6].

Nonreassuring FHR

The absence of accelerations in the FHR particularly when accompanied by persistent decelerations may be a concerning finding in the EFM. The presence of recurrent late, variable, or prolonged decelerations with absent FHR variability are nonreassuring patterns and require close attention by the health care providers. Possible causes of such decelerations and their remedies should be considered. Treatment options include cervical examination to determine dilation and assess for umbilical cord prolapse. Repositioning the patient to the left or right lateral recumbent position is recommended. Discontinuation or diminishing of Pitocin or other uterine stimulants and consideration of treatment with a tocolytic agent are additionally recommended. Employing one or more of these treatments will often result in rapid improvement of the concerning FHR.

Further assessment of such FHR patterns should include ancillary tests of the fetus status. The most commonly used modalities are scalp stimulation or vibroacoustic stimulation of the fetus with observation for the occurrence of an immediate acceleration of the FHR. Specifically, if there is an acceleration of the FHR accompanying either direct digital scalp or vibroacoustic stimulation, fetal acidosis is excluded (pH ≥7.21) at that point in time [7]. This allows for the continuation of labor in a patient with nonreassuring FHR changes. In the absence of accelerations of the FHR with such stimulation, there is the possibility of an abnormal fetal scalp pH. Traditionally, obtaining a sample of fetal blood from the scalp has been utilized as a means to determine the fetal pH. However, this technique is currently rarely employed and for most practitioners is not even available. Further, there is poor sensitivity and specificity of a scalp pH less than 7.21 predicting umbilical artery acidosis (pH <7.0) or adverse neonatal neurologic outcome. Consequently, direct assessment of fetal blood pH levels no longer occurs in most centers.

Fetal resuscitation

Management of nonreassuring FHR patterns is often limited to immediate delivery, commonly by cesarean section. However, use of various ancillary techniques should be considered and frequently result in improved FHR tracing. The association of maternal hypotension and concerning changes in the FHR is commonly seen. Correction of such hypotension with maternal position change or ephedrine infusion (following epidural) is encouraged. Perhaps the most common technique is the administration of oxygen to the laboring patient along with rapid intravenous infusion of fluids. Not surprisingly, such interventions have not been shown to be efficacious but nonetheless are widely employed. What has been shown to have efficacy is the use of various forms of tocolytic therapy [8]. These most commonly include beta agonists such as terbutaline and ritodrine although other agents such as magnesium sulfate or calcium-channel blockers can be considered. However, while improvement of the FHR commonly occurs following such therapy, there is no evidence to suggest overall improvement in newborn or neonatal outcome. Additionally, use of amnioinfusion in patients experiencing recurrent variable decelerations of the FHR has been

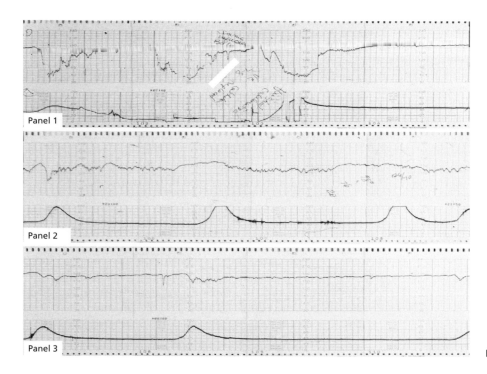

Fig. 12.1 Fetal heart rate (FHR) measurements.

shown to reduce the frequency and severity of variable decelerations as well as the need for cesarean delivery for fetal intolerance to labor [9]. This is a simple technique which is readily available in most labor and delivery units.

Case presentation

The patient is a 32-year-old, G3 P2002, at 39 weeks' gestation in active labor. Cervical examination reveals 5 cm dilation with vertex well applied to the cervix. Artificial rupture of the membranes is performed with return of clear amniotic fluid. Within minutes, the FHR changes from a normal pattern without deceleration to one of persistent variable decelerations (Fig. 12.1, panel 1). Through the previously placed intrauterine pressure catheter, amnioinfusion of normal saline was begun at 10 mL/min for 1 hour. The subsequent FHR revealed marked change in the FHR to a persistently reassuring pattern (panels 2, 3). The patient subsequently had a vaginal delivery of a health newborn with Apgars of 8 and 9 at 1 and 5 min, respectively.

This case demonstrates the potential value of amnioinfusion in patients experiencing recurrent variable decelerations. Although the exact mechanism of action is unknown, it is thought that the infused fluid relieves compression of the umbilical cord which is the etiology of the FHR decelerations.

References

1 Martin JA, Hamilton BE, Venture SJ, Menacker F, Park MM, Sutton PD. Births: final data for 2002. *Natl Vital Stat Rep* 2003;**52**:1–113.

2 Nelson KB, Dambrosia JM, Ting TY, Grether JK. Uncertain value of electronic fetal monitoring in predicting cerebral palsy. *N Engl J Med* 1996;**324**:613–8.

3 NICHD Research Planning Workshop. Electronic fetal heart rate monitoring: research guidelines for interpretation. *Am J Obstet Gynecol* 1997;**177**:1385–90.

4 Intrapartum fetal heart rate monitoring. ACOG Practice Bulletin No 62, American College of Obstetricians and Gynecologists. *Obstet Gynecol* 2005;**105**:1161–9.

5 Vitzileos AM, Nochimson DJ, Antsakis A, Vavarigos I, Guzman EF, Knuppel RA. Comparison of intrapartum electronic fetal heart rate monitoring versus intermittently auscultation in detecting fetal academia at birth. *Am J Obstet Gynecol* 1995;**173**:1021–4.

6 Samueloff A, Langer O, Berkus M, Field N, Xenakis E, Ridgway L. Is fetal heart rate variability a good predictor of fetal outcome? *Acta Obstet Gynecol Scand* 1994;**73**:39–44.

7 Skupzki DW, Rosenberg CR, Egllinton GS. Intrapartum fetal stimulation tests: a meta-analysis. *Obstet Gynecol* 2001;**99**:129–34.

8 Kulier R, Hofmeyr GJ. Tocolytics for suspected intrapartum fetal distress. *Cochrane Database Sys Rev* 1998;**1**:CD00035.

9 Hofmeyr GJ. Amnioinfusion for umbilical cord compression in labor. *Cochrane Database Syst Rev* 1998;**1**:CD00013.

Maternal Disease

13 Sickle cell disease

Scott Roberts

Sickle cell disease is composed of a group of genetic disorders involving abnormal hemoglobin. Each hemoglobin is made up of two alpha-globin (141 amino acids) and two beta-globin chains (146 amino acids). These chains conform in a way that allows solubility, oxygen affinity and transport, and stable biconcavity in the red blood cell. Solubility and reversible oxygen binding are the key properties deranged in hemoglobinopathies. Sickle hemoglobin (S) results from the substitution of glutamic acid by valine in the beta-globin chain at position 6; and hemoglobin C from substitution of the same amino acid, but by lysine. The beta-globin genes are expressed codominantly so that homozygous SS or the compound heterozygote SC must be expressed for clinical morbidity to be significant. In contrast, the abnormal beta-thalassemia variant of beta-globin causes the production of normal hemoglobin A to be absent or reduced.

The most prevalent disorder is sickle cell anemia resulting from the homozygous SS genotype. One of every 12 African-Americans is a carrier for the hemoglobin S gene and hence ($1/12 \times 1/12 \times 1/4 = 1/576$) approximately 1 in 600 African-American newborns have sickle cell anemia [1]. The overall rate of sickle cell disorders at birth for African-Americans is 1 in 300 [2]. The prevalence of the hemoglobin C allele is approximately 1 in 40 and the abnormal gene for beta-thalassemia approximately 1 in 40 to 1 in 50 in this population. These disorders are associated with increased maternal and perinatal morbidity and mortality.

Red blood cells with hemoglobin S undergo sickling under conditions of decreased oxygen tension. This results in hemolysis, increased viscosity, and vaso-occlusion (VOC), and leads to further decreased oxygenation. This VOC leads to local infarction in all major organ systems, and all surviving adults with sickle cell anemia have undergone autosplenectomy after multiple episodes of VOC and infarction. The bone pain, so typical of sickle cell crises, represents VOC in the bone marrow. Other chronic and acute changes from sickling include bony abnormalities such as osteonecrosis of the femoral and humeral heads; renal medullary damage; hepatomegaly; ven-tricular hypertrophy; pulmonary infarctions; pulmonary hypertension; cerebrovascular accidents; leg ulcers; and a propensity to infection and sepsis [3–5].

Because of hemolysis of defective red blood cells, most patients with sickle cell anemia have hemoglobin values of approximately 7–8 g/dL. Iron therapy will not correctly treat their anemia and may worsen their condition. Folic acid requirements, however, are considerable as there is an intense hematopoiesis occurring to compensate for the markedly shortened red blood cell lifespan. Patients with SC disease are usually less anemic, with hemoglobin levels near 10 g/dL, and painful crises occur less frequently. Manifestations of S/beta-thalassemia disease are quite variable, but can present similarly to severe SS disease. In either SC disease or S/beta-thalassemia, iron studies should be performed and iron supplemented if indicated.

Pregnancy is a serious burden to women with sickle hemoglobinopathies, especially those with hemoglobin SS disease. Pregnancy usually results in an increased frequency of sickle cell crises. Infections and pulmonary complications are common. Maternal mortality has decreased dramatically over the years because of improvements in medical care, but remains high [6,7]. In addition, more than one-third of pregnancies in women with sickle syndromes end in abortion, stillbirth, or neonatal death (Table 13.1).

Hemoglobin SC disease

In nonpregnant women, morbidity and mortality from sickle cell/hemoglobin C disease are much lower than that seen with SS homozygous disease. Fewer than half of the women with SC disease have ever been symptomatic prior to pregnancy. However, during pregnancy and the puerperium, attacks of severe bone pain and episodes of pulmonary infarction and embolization become more common [8]. A particularly worrisome complication is acute chest syndrome seen in both SS and SC disease related to embolization of necrotic fat and

Table 13.1 Pregnancy outcomes in patients with S/S anemia. Data from 309 pregnancies in eight reports [6,8,16,19–23].

	Range	Mean
Spontaneous abortion (%)	7–16	12.2
Stillbirth (%)	1–8	4.1
Neonatal death (%)	0–9	2.0
Low birthweight (%)	7–33	21.3
Perinatal mortality	10.5–121.1/1000	57.4/1000

Table 13.2 Pregnancy outcomes reported since 1956 for women with sickle cell anemia and hemoglobin SC disease [6,7,22–28].

	Sickle Cell Disease (SS)	Hemoglobin SC Disease
Women	1213	351
Pregnancies	2214	798
Maternal deaths (per 100,000)	~2500	~2300
Perinatal mortality (per 1000)	~175	~75

cellular bone marrow, and VOC sickling, with resultant respiratory insufficiency. This syndrome is characterized by a noninfectious pulmonary infiltrate with fever, leading to hypoxemia and acidosis, and, infrequently, death. Acute chest syndrome is the leading cause of death among patients with sickle cell disease [9].

Maternal death is as common with SC disease as it is with homozygous SS disease (2300–2500 in 100,000). Perinatal mortality is higher in SC disease (75 in 1000) than in the general population, but not as high as with SS disease (175 in 1000) (Table 13.2).

Hemoglobin S/beta-thalassemia disease

This heterozygous condition usually is much milder than either SS or SC disease. Variable amounts of hemoglobin A are produced depending on the variant of the beta-thal allele inherited. Hemoglobin F is made in abundance with extramedullary hematopoiesis to make up for abnormally low hemoglobin A. In its most usual form, a level of A2 above 3.5% on hemoglobin electrophoresis is diagnostic. In the most severe form of S/beta-thalassemia disease, no hemoglobin F is made and the resulting phenotypic expression is of severe SS disease.

Either of the above sickle cell variants can have symptoms as bad or worse than any particular SS patient. Particularly unnerving and dangerous is the previously asymptomatic SC or S/beta-thalassemia patient who presents with acute chest syndrome in pregnancy.

Management during pregnancy

Close observation of these patients is mandatory during pregnancy. They are at increased risk for infection, which in turn can aggravate sickling crises. With the increased red cell mass typically required during pregnancy, folate supplementation is important. Any strain that impairs erythropoiesis or increases red blood cell destruction aggravates the anemia. Clinical presentations that cause anemia and pain may be overlooked (e.g., placental abruption, ectopic pregnancy, appendicitis, and pyelonephritis). The diagnosis of sickle cell crisis should be reserved until other possible causes are ruled out.

Covert bacteriuria and acute pyelonephritis are increased in these patients. Frequent (monthly or every trimester) screening urine cultures should be employed to discover asymptomatic bacteriuria and treat before it becomes symptomatic. Acute pyelonephritis can result in the release of endotoxin which lyses sickle cells and suppresses hematopoiesis resulting in severe anemia and sickle crises. Pneumonia is common, caused by *Streptococcus pneumoniae*, and the polyvalent pneumococcal vaccine is recommended. Annual inactivated influenza vaccine should be administered. Hepatitis B vaccination is recommended. For patients who have undergone autosplenectomy, vaccination against *Hemophilus influenza* type B is recommended.

Crises are hallmarked by intense pain, usually from involved bone marrow. As many as 40% of sickle cell patients have acute chest syndrome [9]. Episodes can develop acutely and do so more often late in pregnancy. Intravenous hydration along with opioid analgesics should be given. Oxygen by nasal cannula will decrease the sickling at the capillary level and improve symptoms. Any focus of infection should be discovered and treated as it may be responsible for the crisis. The risk of low birthweight, fetal growth restriction, preterm delivery, and preeclampsia are increased. Cardiac dysfunction is prevalent in sickle cell disease. After years of pulmonary infarction, restrictive airway disease can lead to ventricular hypertrophy and pulmonary hypertension [10]. There is increased preload and decreased afterload with a normal ejection fraction. This condition is augmented by the increasing volume of pregnancy. Chronic hypertension can aggravate the pre-existing cardiac dysfunction. Severe preeclampsia, sepsis, or secondary pulmonary hypertension can lead to heart failure. A multidisciplinary approach should be used involving obstetricians, hematologists, and anesthesiologists [11].

Prophylactic red blood cell transfusions

Some institutions utilize prophylactic red blood cell transfusions. Managed correctly, sickle crises can be held to a minimum. Hematocrit and hemoglobin electrophoresis are monitored monthly and transfusion effected to keep the hematocrit between 25 and 30% and the A : S ratio at 60 : 40. Prophylactic transfusions will not modify an existing sickle crisis. However, exchange transfusion in the face of crisis, acute chest syndrome, stroke, and infection can be valuable. Transfusion is not without its complications. Transfusion-related lung injury occurs in approximately 1 in 5000 units of blood products transfused [12]. Delayed hemolytic transfusion reactions are reported in as many as 10% of patients [13]. The rate of viral infection from transfusion is exceedingly low with modern pretransfusion blood screening techniques. The highest rate is from hepatitis B at 1 in 100,000 and that from hepatitis C and HIV at approximately 1 in 2,000,000 [14]. The rate of alloimmunization has been reported at 3% per unit in the sickle disease population [15]. Because of the concern for the aforementioned and the usual need for repeated transfusions in this population, all blood should be typed and crossed and leukocyte reduced. There is no reported benefit in maternal or perinatal mortality from the use of prophylactic transfusions [16]. Much of the decrease in perinatal and maternal morbidity and mortality is ascribed to improved perinatal care in the sickle disease population. Managing without prophylactic transfusions, however, can involve multiple long and painful hospitalizations [8,16].

Fetal assessment

Pregnancies in women with sickle cell disease are at increased risk for spontaneous abortion, preterm labor, fetal growth restriction, and stillbirth [17]. Frequent assessment for the detection of fetal growth restriction, oligohydramnios, and assurance of fetal activity is important. Formal antepartum surveillance may be used to augment fetal assessment (e.g., biophysical profile, umbilical artery Doppler in the presence of fetal growth restriction). Published data concerning antepartum surveillance in pregnancies complicated by sickle cell disease are limited.

Labor and delivery

Management should take into account the degree of underlying cardiac dysfunction. Preparatory consultation with an anesthesiologist is helpful. Route of delivery otherwise should be based solely on obstetric indications. Epidural anesthesia is ideal and will keep the patient comfortable during a long labor process. If a difficult vaginal or cesarean delivery is foreseen, and the patient's hematocrit is less than 20%, packed red blood cells should be administered. Blood should be typed and crossed and readily available. Fluid administration should be conservative to avoid circulatory overload and pulmonary edema.

Genetic evaluation

Prenatal genetic evaluation is possible for the sickle hemoglobinopathies. Maternal and paternal electrophoresis will elucidate the potential genotypes. When there is reasonable suspicion and probability, amniocentesis or chorionic villous sampling should be offered and polymerase chain reaction (PCR) utilized to detect abnormal fetal genotypes. Most couples with foreknowledge of an SS fetus will opt to carry the pregnancy forward [18], but some will not.

Case presentation

The patient is a 28-year-old, G1P0, Nigerian woman with SS disease. She was first seen at 15–16 weeks with painful sickle crisis involving her extremities and pleuritic chest pain. She was found to have a hematocrit of 28.5% and had been previously transfused during the pregnancy prior to obstetric presentation, with electrophoresis revealing S 60% and A 40%. She was alloimmunized with anti-c and anti-E antibodies, titers too low to report. Ultrasound showed diamnionic/dichorionic twins. Baseline renal function showed 24 hour urine protein of 122 mg and urine culture was negative. Chest X-ray revealed left retrocardiac opacity which was stable in appearance from a previous chest X-ray 1 year prior and probably represented old pulmonary infarction. Cardiomegaly and a small calcified spleen were noted on computed tomography (CT) scan from 1 year prior. Influenza vaccination was given. Pneumococcal vaccine had been given previously. Significant pathology (e.g., appendicitis, acute chest syndrome) were ruled out. Her crisis was managed with intravenous hydration, opioid analgesics, and oxygen by nasal cannula. She remained hospitalized for the next 2 weeks and was discharged on 4 mg/day folate.

She was seen in the clinic thereafter every 2 weeks. At 20, 26, and 30 weeks ultrasound evaluation revealed size = dates with 4, 8, and 14% discordance, respectively, between twins. The father of the babies was unavailable for zygosity testing concerning maternal antibodies, and fortunately anti-c and anti-E titers were never significantly elevated. From 18 weeks onward the patient was transfused approximately every month to achieve a hematocrit >25% with hemoglobin S <40%. She presented to the hospital three more times during gestation for painful VOC, one of which was complicated by an hemoglobin S fraction of 78% with a hematocrit of 23.6%. However, because of subsequent and continued adequate hematocrit and hemoglobin A versus S fractions and absence of objective morbidity, exchange transfusion was not performed.

Her last admission occurred at 32–33 weeks. At this time she had mildly elevated blood pressures and a hematocrit of

22.7%. With limited IV access, the patient had a peripherally inserted central catheter (PICC) line placed and received transfusion to a hematocrit of 30%. Her 24-hour urine protein was 3.8 g. She was managed with ward rest and maternal fetal surveillance. At 33–34 weeks her hypertension exacerbated and the decision to deliver for severe preeclampsia was made. A low transverse cesarean was performed and seizure prophylaxis was instituted until 24 hours postpartum. She recovered unremarkably, without further crises or transfusions, during the puerperal period. Both babies did well in the special care nursery and went home within 2 weeks.

We note the lack of apparent benefit in this patient with prophylactic transfusions on significantly decreasing the number of painful crises she endured. We believe that this patient's management was complicated by opioid tolerance and/or dependence. She was never pain free beginning with her first admission at 15–16 weeks, and was managed as an outpatient with oral hydromorphone between admissions. Difficulties were also encountered in achieving IV access in this patient who had received multiple transfusions in her lifetime. Although premature and complicated by preeclampsia, both maternal and perinatal outcome were good.

We believe this case highlights some of the significant and not atypical problems with SS disease in pregnancy. It should be emphasized that some of the worst morbidity occurs in SC and S/beta-thalassemia disease, and that evaluation and management should be similar to that of the SS patient.

References

1 Angastiniotic M, Modell B. Global epidemiology of hemoglobin disorders. *Ann N Y Acad Sci* 1998;**850**:251–69.

2 Motulsky AG. Frequency of sickling disorders in US Blacks. *N Engl J Med* 1973;**288**:31–3.

3 Driscoll MC, Hurlet A, Styles L, *et al*. Stroke risk in siblings with sickle cell anemia. *Blood* 2003;**101**:2401–4.

4 Gladwin MT, Sachdev V, Jison ML, *et al*. Pulmonary hypertension as a risk factor for death in patients with sickle cell disease. *N Engl J Med* 2004;**350**:886–95.

5 Weatherall DJ, Provan AB. Red cell I: Inherited anaemias. *Lancet* 2000;**355**:1169–75.

6 Powars DR, Sandhu M, Niland-Weiss J, *et al*. Pregnancy in sickle cell disease. *Obstet Gynecol* 1986;**67**:217–28.

7 Poddar D, Maude GH, Plant MJ, Scorer H, Serjeant GR. Pregnancy in Jamaican women with homozygous sickle cell disease: fetal and maternal outcome. *Br J Obstet Gynaecol* 1986;**93**:927–32.

8 Cunningham FG, Pritchard JA, Mason R. Pregnancy and sickle hemoglobinopathy: results with and without prophylactic transfusions. *Obstet Gynecol* 1983;**62**:419–24.

9 Vichinsky EP, Neumayr LD, Earles AN, *et al*. Causes and outcomes of the acute chest syndrome in sickle cell disease. *N Engl J Med* 2000;**342**:1855–65.

10 Powars D, Weidman JA, Odom-Maryon T, Niland JC, Johnson C. Sickle cell chronic lung disease: prior morbidity and the risk of pulmonary failure. *Medicine (Baltimore)* 1988;**67**:66–76.

11 Rees DC, Olujohungbe AD, Parker NE, Stephens AD, Telfer P, Wright J. Guidelines for the management of the acute painful crisis in sickle cell disease. British Committee for standards in Haematology General Haematology Task Force by the Sickle Cell Working Party. *Br J Haematol* 2003;**120**:744–52.

12 Silliman CC, Boshkov LK, Mehdizadehkashi Z, *et al*. Transfusion-related acute lung injury: epidemiology and a prospective analysis of etiologic factors. *Blood* 2003;**101**:454–62.

13 Garratty G. Severe reactions associated with transfusion of patients with sickle cell disease. *Transfusion* 1997;**37**:357–61.

14 Jackson BR, Busch MP, Stramer SL, AuBuchon JP. The cost-effectiveness of NAT for HIV, HCV, and HBV in whole-blood donations. *Transfusion* 2003;**43**:721–9.

15 Cox JV, Steane E, Cunningham G, Frenkel EP. Risk of alloimmunization and delayed hemolytic transfusion reactions in patients with sickle cell disease. *Arch Intern Med* 1988;**148**:2485–9.

16 Koshy M, Burd L, Wallace D, Moawad A, Baron J. Prophylactic red-cell transfusions in pregnant patients with sickle cell disease: a randomized cooperative study. *N Engl J Med* 1988;**319**:1447–52.

17 Serjeant GR, Loy LL, Crowther M, Hambleton IR, Thame M. Outcome of pregnancy in homozygous sickle cell disease. *Obstet Gynecol* 2004;**103**:1278–85.

18 Alter BP. Prenatal diagnosis of hematologic diseases: 1986 update. *Acta Haematol* 1987;**78**:137–41.

19 Morrison JC, Wiser WL. The effect of maternal partial exchange transfusion on the infants of patients with sickle cell anemia. *J Pediatr* 1976;**89**:286–9.

20 Morrison JC, Schneider JM, Whybrew WD, Bucovaz ET, Menzel DM. Prophylactic transfusions in pregnant patients with sickle cell hemoglobinopathies: benefit versus risk. *Obstet Gynecol* 1980;**56**:274–80.

21 Miller JM Jr, Horger EO 3rd, Key TC, Walker EM Jr. Management of sickle cell hemoglobinopathies in pregnant patients. *Am J Obstet Gynecol* 1981;**141**:237–41.

22 Smith JA, Espeland M, Bellevue R, Bonds D, Brown AK, Koshy M. Pregnancy in sickle cell disease: experience of the cooperative study of sickle cell disease. *Obstet Gynecol* 1996;**87**:199–204.

23 Charache S, Scott J, Niebyl J, Bonds D. Management of sickle cell disease in pregnant patients. *Obstet Gynecol* 1980;**55**:407–10.

24 el-Shafei AM, Dhaliwal JK, Sandhu AK. Pregnancy in sickle cell disease in Bahrain. *Br J Obstet Gynaecol* 1992;**99**:101–4.

25 Howard RJ, Tuck SM, Pearson TC. Pregnancy in sickle cell disease in the UK: results of a multi-centre survey of the effect of prophylactic blood transfusion on maternal and fetal outcome. *Br J Obstet Gynaecol* 1995;**102**:947–51.

26 Milner PF, Jones BR, Dobler J. Outcome of pregnancy in sickle cell anemia and sickle cell-hemoglobin C disease. *Am J Obstet Gynecol* 1980;**138**:239–45.

27 Seoud MA, Cantwell C, Nobles G, Levy DL. Outcome of pregnancies complicated by sickle cell and sickle-C hemoglobinopathies. *Am J Perinatol* 1994;**11**:187–91.

28 Sun PM, Wilburn W, Raynor BD, Jamieson D. Sickle cell disease in pregnancy: twenty years of experience at Grady Memorial Hospital, Atlanta, Georgia. *Am J Obstet Gynecol* 2001;**184**:1127–30.

14 Thrombocytopenia

Robert M. Silver and Erin A.S. Clark

The antepartum diagnosis of maternal thrombocytopenia has become more common because platelet counts are now routinely obtained as part of prenatal screening. Although thrombocytopenia is classically defined as a platelet count of less than 150,000/μL, there is a physiologic drop in platelet count during pregnancy of 10–30% secondary to hemodilution and increased consumption. The most common causes of maternal thrombocytopenia include gestational thrombocytopenia, preeclampsia/HELLP (hemolysis, elevated liver enzymes, and low platelet count) syndrome, and autoimmune thrombocytopenia. These conditions have implications for both mother and fetus. Thus, it is important to consider both maternal and fetal thrombocytopenia.

Maternal thrombocytopenia

Gestational thrombocytopenia (GTP), also termed incidental thrombocytopenia of pregnancy, describes a mild (usually more than 70,000/μL platelet count), common (up to 5%), asymptomatic thrombocytopenia that occurs during pregnancy [1,2]. This accounts for more than 70% of thrombocytopenias in pregnant women [2,3]. The cause of thrombocytopenia in these women is unclear, but may be an acceleration of the physiologic pattern of increased platelet destruction [1]. Women with this diagnosis are healthy, not at risk for fetal thrombocytopenia or bleeding complications, and have no history of autoimmune thrombocytopenia. Platelet counts return to normal after delivery. It can be difficult to distinguish GTP from autoimmune thrombocytopenia. If thrombocytopenia is found late in pregnancy and counts are more than 70,000/μL, GTP is the most likely diagnosis. However, other causes of thrombocytopenia, including preeclampsia, should be excluded. Women with GTP do not require additional testing or specialized care.

Autoimmune thrombocytopenia, also termed *idiopathic thrombocytopenic purpura* (ITP), is a syndrome characterized by immunologically mediated thrombocytopenia. The disorder is caused primarily by autoantibodies to platelet membrane glycoproteins, leading to increased platelet destruction. In adults, ITP is typically a chronic disorder. It can be difficult to distinguish from other causes of thrombocytopenia and is a diagnosis of exclusion. The most common signs and symptoms include petechiae, ecchymoses, easy bruising, epistaxis, gingival bleeding, and menorrhagia. Serious spontaneous bleeding complications are rare, even in severely thrombocytic individuals with platelet counts of less than 10,000/μL [4]. When thrombocytopenia is profound and detected early in pregnancy, suspicion is high that the diagnosis is ITP. It often coexists with pregnancy because the disease usually presents in the second to third decade of life and has a female preponderance of 3 : 1 [5].

Few diagnostic tests are useful in the evaluation of ITP. A complete blood count (CBC) and peripheral blood smear are helpful to exclude other causes of thrombocytopenia (e.g., pancytopenia, leukemias). The peripheral smear may show an increased proportion of slightly enlarged platelets. Bone marrow biopsy is sometimes helpful to clarify the diagnosis as increased numbers of immature megakaryocytes may be seen and inadequate platelet production may be excluded. Although antiplatelet antibodies are present in most individuals with ITP, they are very nonspecific, and testing is not recommended for the routine evaluation of maternal thrombocytopenia [6].

The focus of maternal therapy is to avoid bleeding complications associated with severe thrombocytopenia. Because labor and delivery pose a substantial risk for bleeding, most authorities recommend more aggressive medical therapy for women in the late second or third trimesters. Current recommendations about maternal therapy for ITP are derived largely from expert opinion. Pregnant women who are asymptomatic and who have platelet counts of over 50,000/μL do not require treatment. In the first and second trimesters, asymptomatic women with platelet counts of 30,000–50,000/μL also do not require treatment. Treatment is considered appropriate for women with:

1 Platelet counts of less than 10,000/μL at any gestational age;

2 Platelet counts of 10,000–30,000/μL during the second or third trimesters; or

3 Platelet counts of 10,000–30,000/μL with bleeding at any gestational age.

It is controversial as to whether women with counts between 30,000 and 50,000/μL should be treated during the third trimester.

Glucocorticoids are standard first-line treatment in both pregnant and nonpregnant adults. Prednisone is initiated at a dosage of 1–2 mg/kg/day and is typically continued for 2–3 weeks. If platelet counts reach acceptable levels, the drug is tapered by 10–20% per week until the lowest dosage required to maintain the platelet count at an acceptable level is achieved. Some increase in platelet count occurs in approximately 70% of patients, and complete remission has been reported in up to 25% of cases [7]. A response to glucocorticoids is usually apparent in 3–7 days and will reach a maximum in 2–3 weeks [5]. The benefits of steroids appear to outweigh the risks in women requiring treatment for ITP.

Intravenous immunoglobulin (IVIG) is an appropriate initial treatment for pregnant women with:

1 Platelet counts of less than 10,000/μL in the third trimester; and

2 Platelet counts of 10,000–30,000/μL who are bleeding.

IVIG is also used in cases refractory to treatment with glucocorticoids. The optimal dose for treatment is uncertain. IVIG 400 mg/kg/day given for 2–5 consecutive days is the most widely used regimen, although similar results have been obtained using higher doses for a shorter duration. This dose of IVIG will substantially increase the platelet count in 75% of patients and will restore normal platelet counts in 50% of patients [6,8]. However, in 70% of cases, the platelet count will return to pretreatment levels within 1 month after treatment [6,8]. Mild side-effects of IVIG are common, but serious side-effects are rare. The most substantial drawback of IVIG therapy may be expense. It should therefore be used in cases of severe thrombocytopenia, hemorrhage, or nonresponse to steroids.

Intravenous anti-D immunoglobulin has been used to successfully treat ITP in Rhesus (Rh) positive individuals, although experience is limited [9–11]. There is a theoretical risk of causing fetal anemia by administering high doses to pregnant women with Rh positive fetuses. Acute hemolysis and disseminated intravascular coagulation (DIC) may be rare but potentially severe complications of anti-D administration [12]. In general, anti-D antibodies appear to be safe for both mother and fetus [11]. The use of anti-D is attractive because it is less expensive and has a shorter infusion time than IVIG.

Splenectomy was the first therapy recognized to be effective for ITP and induces complete remission in approximately 80% of patients. The postsplenectomy platelet counts increase rapidly and are often normal within 1–2 weeks. The procedure is usually avoided during pregnancy but can be safely accomplished, although preferably in the second trimester. Splenectomy during pregnancy is reserved for women with platelet counts of less than 10,000/μL who are bleeding and who fail to respond to steroids and IVIG [6]. The procedure is not recommended for asymptomatic women with platelet counts of more than 10,000/μL.

Platelet transfusions should be used only as a temporary measure to prepare a patient for splenectomy or surgery, or for life-threatening hemorrhage. However, the usual elevation in platelet counts of approximately 10,000/μL per unit of platelet concentrate transfused is not achieved in patients with ITP because antiplatelet antibodies also bind to donor platelets. Thus, 6–10 units of platelet concentrate should be transfused. The ITP practice guideline panel recommends platelet transfusions before delivery in women with platelet counts of less than 10,000/μL undergoing planned cesarean delivery or with mucous membrane bleeding and anticipated vaginal delivery [6].

Mothers with ITP require little specialized care beyond attention to platelet count. These patients should be instructed to avoid salicylates, nonsteroidal anti-inflammatory agents, and trauma. Regardless of route of delivery, platelets, fresh frozen plasma (FFP), and IVIG should be readily available.

Other causes

Other causes of thrombocytopenia during pregnancy include preeclampsia/HELLP syndrome, systemic lupus erythematosus, antiphospholipid syndrome, human immunodeficiency virus infection, DIC, drug-induced thrombocytopenia, thrombotic thrombocytopenic purpura, hemolytic uremic syndrome, and pseudo-thrombocytopenia as a result of laboratory artefact. These disorders can be excluded with an appropriate history, physical examination, assessment of blood pressure, human immunodeficiency virus (HIV) serology, and laboratory studies (e.g., liver function tests).

Fetal thrombocytopenia

Autoimmune thrombocytopenia

Fetal thrombocytopenia and, rarely, bleeding complications may occur with ITP because maternal immunoglobulin-G (IgG) antiplatelet antibodies are actively transported across the placenta. Avoidance of fetal hemorrhagic complications is the central issue in the obstetric management of these women. Occasionally, minor clinical bleeding such as purpura, ecchymoses, hematuria, or melena is observed. Rarely, fetal thrombocytopenia can lead to intracranial hemorrhage (ICH) which can result in severe neurologic impairment or even death. It is important to emphasize that the risk of serious fetal bleeding with maternal ITP is very low [3].

Strategies intended to minimize or avoid fetal bleeding complications include corticosteroids, IVIG, and splenectomy. Currently, no maternal treatment has been found to be consistently effective in the prevention of fetal/neonatal thrombocytopenia or to improve fetal outcome [13–16]. The risk of neonatal bleeding is inversely proportional to the platelet count and bleeding complications are rare with platelet counts over 50,000/µL [3,15]. Attempts have been made to determine which fetuses are severely thrombocytopenic and at higher risk for ICH. Unfortunately, no maternal factor has been identified that can predict fetal thrombocytopenia in all cases and current evidence does not support the routine use of fetal scalp sampling and cordocentesis in women with ITP [17,18].

Route of delivery was once considered critical to neonatal outcome in women with ITP. Passage through the birth canal was proposed as the reason for bleeding in thrombocytopenic fetuses and this together with anecdotal reports and case series led to recommendations for delivery by cesarean section [19]. However, vaginal delivery has never been proven to cause ICH and several studies have shown no association between route of delivery and neonatal bleeding complications [3,15,20]. At this time, it seems prudent to deliver by cesarean section for the usual obstetric indications without determination of the fetal platelet count in most women. However, the matter remains controversial.

In all cases of possible fetal thrombocytopenia, whether secondary to ITP or alloimmune thrombocytopenia, a neonatologist or other clinician familiar with the condition should be present to care for potential bleeding complications and the anticipated decrease in neonatal platelet count during the first several days after birth. The use of scalp electrodes, forceps, and vacuum extractors should be avoided in these patients. Although there is a theoretical risk of neonatal thrombocytopenia, women with ITP should not be discouraged from breastfeeding [21].

Alloimmune thrombocytopenia

Fetal and neonatal alloimmune thrombocytopenia (NAIT) is a serious and potentially life-threatening disorder that affects 1 in 1000–2000 live infants [22–25]. The condition is analogous to Rh isoimmunization, except that maternal IgG alloantibodies are directed against fetal platelet antigens. Several polymorphic, di-allelic platelet antigen systems are responsible for this condition. Uniform nomenclature has been adopted describing these antigen systems as human platelet antigens (e.g., HPA-1, HPA-2), with alleles designated as "a" or "b." The most frequent cause of severe NAIT in white people is the HPA-1a antigen. Although approximately 1 in 42 pregnancies are incompatible for HPA-1a, NAIT develops in only a small fraction of these cases. This may be because the disorder is sub-

clinical in some cases, and it may also be because, in addition to antigen exposure, an immunologic susceptibility (possibly related to HLA type) is necessary.

In contrast to Rh isoimmunization, NAIT can occur during a first pregnancy without prior exposure to the offending antigen. It is usually diagnosed after birth when an infant is found to have thrombocytopenia, petechiae, or ecchymoses. Affected infants are often severely thrombocytopenic, and 10–20% have ICH [26,27]. Fetal ICH can occur *in utero* and a significant number of cases can be diagnosed by antenatal ultrasound. The recurrence risk is substantial and has been estimated to be up to 100% in cases of HPA-1a incompatibility, depending upon paternal zygosity for HPA-1a [23,28]. Thrombocytopenia tends to worsen as pregnancy progresses in untreated fetuses.

The goal of the obstetric management of pregnancies at risk of NAIT is to prevent ICH and its associated complications. In contrast to ITP, the dramatically higher frequency of ICH associated with NAIT justifies more aggressive interventions. Also, therapy must be initiated antenatally because of the risk of *in utero* ICH. Possible NAIT should be suspected in cases of otherwise unexplained fetal or neonatal thrombocytopenia, ICH, or porencephaly. In most cases, the diagnosis of NAIT can be determined by testing the parents; testing fetal or neonatal blood is confirmatory and occasionally helpful. Appropriate assays include serologic confirmation of maternal antiplatelet antibodies that are specific for paternal or fetal/neonatal platelets. In addition, individuals should undergo platelet typing with paternal zygosity testing. This can be determined serologically or with DNA-based tests. It is unnecessary to repeat testing in a family with a previously confirmed case of NAIT. Antibody titers are poorly predictive of risk to the current pregnancy and need not be obtained once the diagnosis is made. If the father is heterozygous for the offending antigen, fetal HPA typing can be accomplished with chorionic villi or amniocytes. Fetal genotyping avoids additional expensive and risky interventions in approximately 50% of such cases.

If the fetus is determined to be at risk, cordocentesis should be considered to determine the fetal platelet count. This strategy avoids treatment of fetuses that have normal platelet counts and provides feedback about treatment response in cases of thrombocytopenia. The risk of hemorrhagic complications with cordocentesis is increased in pregnancies affected by NAIT [29]. The overall perinatal loss rate for cordocentesis has been reported to be 2.7% [30] and is likely higher in the setting of severe fetal thrombocytopenia. Even with prophylactic transfusion of maternal platelets at the time of cordocentesis, the percentage of bleeding complications may be unchanged [31]. The risk of bleeding at the site of cordocentesis has prompted some clinicians to empirically treat pregnancies at risk for NAIT without determining the fetal platelet count. This strategy is usually reserved for cases of HPA-1a sensitization with a known antigen-positive fetus.

Disadvantages include the potential for unnecessary and expensive treatment and the inability to assess treatment efficacy or to institute salvage therapy in cases of treatment failure. The benefits of cordocentesis may outweigh the risks in most cases, but the matter remains controversial. The number of cordocenteses should be minimized, especially in early gestation when the consequence of hemorrhage is greatest.

The optimal timing of the initial cordocentesis also is uncertain. ICH can occur early in gestation, but such cases are rare [32,33]. Active transport of IgG is limited until the late second and third trimesters. It is therefore likely that in most instances fetal blood sampling and treatment can be delayed until viability. It seems prudent to individualize management of these cases depending on the antigen involved and the severity of NAIT during previously affected pregnancies.

Proposed therapies to increase fetal platelet counts and prevent ICH include maternal treatment with steroids and IVIG, fetal treatment with IVIG, and fetal platelet transfusions. No therapy is effective in all cases. Low-dose maternal steroids do not appear to improve fetal platelet counts. The efficacy of high-dose steroids is uncertain. IVIG administered directly to the fetus has had inconsistent results. Platelet transfusions are effective but the short half-life of transfused platelets requires weekly procedures. The potential risks involved with multiple transfusions as well as the potential for increased sensitization limits the attractiveness of this treatment. Platelet transfusions are likely best reserved for severe cases refractory to other therapies. Administration of IVIG to the mother appears to be the most consistently effective antenatal therapy for NAIT. Weekly infusions of 1 g/kg maternal weight of IVIG will often stabilize or increase the fetal platelet count [27,34,35]. ICH is extremely rare in pregnancies treated with IVIG [27].

Most authorities recommend cesarean delivery for fetuses with platelet counts less than 50,000/μL. As discussed in the section on ITP, vaginal delivery has never been shown to cause ICH and cesarean delivery has never been shown to prevent it. Nonetheless, the substantial rate of ICH probably justifies cesarean delivery in pregnancies with severe NAIT.

A typical strategy is to assess fetal platelet count between 20 and 26 weeks' gestation in fetuses at risk. The procedure can usually be safely delayed until viability. Thrombocytopenic fetuses are treated with maternally administered IVIG and the fetal platelet count is reassessed in 4–6 weeks. High-dose steroids (nonflourinated corticosteroids; e.g., prednisone) are added if there is no response to IVIG. The fetal platelet count is again determined at term to guide the route of delivery. This strategy limits the number of cordocenteses to three or fewer per pregnancy.

There are no current data to support population-wide screening for HPA incompatibility. Studies are ongoing to address the efficacy and cost-effectiveness of such programs. Screening relatives of affected women also remains of unproven benefit.

Case presentation 1

A healthy 34-year-old G3P2002, at 36 weeks' gestation, presents for evaluation of regular contractions. The cervix is 3 cm dilated and 50% effaced. Routine CBC is notable for a platelet count of 94,000/μL. Her blood pressure is 116/72 mmHg. She denies headache, vision changes, abdominal pain, or bleeding of any type. Prenatal HIV serology is negative, and hematocrit, liver enzymes, and a creatinine are normal. A platelet antibody test is positive. The clinician is concerned about possible ITP and wonders about the need for treatment.

When a clinician evaluates a mother with thrombocytopenia, a careful history should be obtained with emphasis on discovering a history of underlying bleeding diathesis, medication use, and medical conditions associated with thrombocytopenia. A physical examination should be performed to look for petechiae or ecchymoses. A peripheral smear should be considered to evaluate platelet morphology and to exclude platelet clumping. Although antiplatelet antibodies are present in most individuals with ITP, tests for these antibodies are nonspecific, poorly standardized, and subject to a large degree of interlaboratory variation. Antiplatelet antibody tests cannot distinguish between GTP and ITP and are not recommended for the routine evaluation of maternal thrombocytopenia.

In this case, there is no evidence of preeclampsia or other medical conditions associated with thrombocytopenia. Gestational thrombocytopenia is the most likely diagnosis and no additional testing or treatment is warranted.

Case presentation 2

A 26-year-old G2P1001 presents for prenatal care at 8 weeks' gestation. Her prior pregnancy was uncomplicated resulting in vaginal birth of a healthy infant at 39 weeks' gestation. However, her infant had petechiae and neonatal platelet count was determined to be 22,000/μL. There was no evidence of sepsis, preeclampsia, or other explanation for the thrombocytopenia. The platelet count increased after platelet transfusion and the child has had no medical problems or persistent thrombocytopenia. The couple asks whether the current fetus is at risk for thrombocytopenia and if anything can be done to prevent it.

The clinician should consider a diagnosis of NAIT in any case of current or prior unexplained fetal or neonatal thrombocytopenia. Both parents should be tested for platelet antigen type, zygosity, and the mother should be tested for specific antiplatelet antibodies against paternal platelet antigens. Testing is best accomplished in a specialized laboratory with expertise in NAIT; testing for generic antiplatelet antibodies in the mother is not clinically useful.

In this case, the mother is HPA-1b homozygous and the father is HPA-1a/HPA-1b heterozygous. The mother has specific antibodies against HPA-1a. The couple should be advised that there is a 50% chance that the fetus carries the HPA-1a gene and is at risk for NAIT. Amniocentesis for fetal platelet antigen genotyping should be offered. If the fetus is HPA-1b, no further evaluation is required. If the fetus is HPA-1a, consideration should be given to evaluation of the fetal platelet count and treatment with IVIG. The couple should be referred for consultation with a maternal–fetal medicine specialist to discuss the risks and benefits of specific management options. Trial of labor should only be allowed in cases wherein fetal platelet count is documented to be more than 50,000/μL and delivery should occur in a setting with neonatal expertise in NAIT.

References

1 Burrows RF, Kelton JG. Incidentally detected thrombocytopenia in healthy mothers and their infants. *N Engl J Med* 1988;**319**:142–5.

2 Burrows RF, Kelton JG. Thrombocytopenia at delivery: a prospective survey of 6715 deliveries. *Am J Obstet Gynecol* 1990a;**162**:731–4.

3 Burrows RF, Kelton JG. Fetal thrombocytopenia and its relation to maternal thrombocytopenia. *N Engl J Med* 1993;**329**:1463–6.

4 Lacey JV, Penner JA. Management of idiopathic thrombocytopenic purpura in the adult. *Semin Thromb Hemost* 1977;**3**:160–74.

5 George JN, El-Harake MA, Raskob GE. Chronic idiopathic thrombocytopenic purpura. *N Engl J Med* 1994;**331**:1207–11.

6 George JN, Woolf SH, Raskob GE, *et al*. Idiopathic thrombocytopenic purpura: a practice guideline developed by explicit methods for the American Society of Hematology. *Blood* 1996;**88**:3–40.

7 Karpatkin S. Autoimmune thrombocytopenic purpura. *Am J Med Sci* 1971;**261**:127.

8 Bussel JB, Pham LC. Intravenous treatment with gamma globulin in adults with immune thrombocytopenia purpura: review of the literature. *Vox Sang* 1987;**52**:206.

9 Boughton BJ, Chakraverty R, Baglin TP, *et al*. The treatment of chronic idiopathic thrombocytopenia with anti-D (Rho) immunoglobulin: its effectiveness, safety, and mechanism of action. *Clin Lab Haematol* 1988;**10**:275–84.

10 Newman GC, Novoa MV, Fodero EE, *et al*. A dose of 75 mg/kg/d of i.v. anti-D increased the platelet count more rapidly that 50 mg/kg/d in adults with immune thrombocytopenic purpura. *Br J Haematol* 2001;**112**:1076–8.

11 Michel M, Novoa MV, Bussel JB. Intravenous anti-D as a treatment for immune thrombocytopenic purpura (ITP) during pregnancy. *Br J Haematol* 2003;**123**:142–6.

12 Gaines AR. Disseminated intravascular coagulation associated with acute hemoglobinemia or hemoglobinuria following Rh(0)(D) immune globulin intravenous administration for immune thrombocytopenic purpura. *Blood* 2005;**106**:1532–7.

13 Kaplan C, Daffos F, Forestier F, *et al*. Fetal platelet counts in thrombocytopenic pregnancy. *Lancet* 1990;**336**:979–82.

14 Christiaens GCML, Nieuwenhuis HK, Von Dem Borne AEGK, *et al*. Idiopathic thrombocytopenic purpura in pregnancy: a randomized trial on the effect of antenatal low dose corticosteroids on neonatal platelet count. *Br J Obstet Gynaecol* 1990;**97**:893–8.

15 Cook RL, Miller RC, Katz VL, Cefalo RC. Immune thrombocytopenic purpura in pregnancy: a reappraisal of management. *Obstet Gynecol* 1991;**78**:578–83.

16 Scott JR, Rote NS, Cruikshank DP. Antiplatelet antibodies and platelet counts in pregnancies complicated by autoimmune thrombocytopenic purpura. *Am J Obstet Gynecol* 1983;**145**: 932–9.

17 Silver, RM. Management of idiopathic thrombocytopenic purpura in pregnancy. *Am J Obstet Gynecol* 1998;**41**: 436–48.

18 Silver RM, Brand DW, Scott JR. Maternal thrombocytopenia in pregnancy: time for a reassessment. *Am J Obstet Gynecol* 1995;**173**:479–82.

19 Carlos HW, McMillan R, Crosby WH. Management of pregnancy in women with immune thrombocytopenic purpura. *JAMA* 1980;**224**:2756–8.

20 Laros RK, Kagan R. Route of delivery for patients with immune thrombocytopenia. *Am J Obstet Gynecol* 1984;**148**:901–8.

21 American Society of Hematology ITP Practice Guideline Panel. Diagnosis and treatment of idiopathic thrombocytopenic purpura: recommendation of the American Society of Hematology. *Ann Intern Med* 1997;**126**:319–26.

22 Blanchette VS, Chen L, Defreideberg A, *et al*. Alloimmunization to the PLA1 platelet antigen: results of a prospective study. *Br J Haematol* 1990;**74**:209–15.

23 Bussel JB, Zabusky MR, Berkowitz RL, McFarland JG. Fetal alloimmune thrombocytopenia. *N Engl J Med* 1997; **337**:22–6.

24 Dreyfus M, Kaplan C, Verdy E, *et al*. Frequency of immune thrombocytopenia in newborns: a prospective study: immune thrombocytopenia working group. *Blood* 1997;**89**:4402–6.

25 Williamson LM, Hackett G, Rennie J, *et al*. The natural history of fetomaternal alloimmunization to the platelet-specific antigen HPA-1a (PL^{A1}, Zw^a) as determined by antenatal screening. *Blood* 1998;**92**:2280–7.

26 Mueller-Eckhardt C, Kiefel V, Grubert A, *et al*. 347 cases of fetal alloimmune thrombocytopenia. *Lancet* 1989;**1**:363–6.

27 Bussel JB, Skupski DW, McFarland JG. Fetal alloimmune thrombocytopenia: consensus and controversy. *J Matern Fetal Med* 1996;**5**:281–92.

28 Kaplan C, Murphy MF, Kroll H, Waters AH. Feto-maternal alloimmune thrombocytopenia: antenatal therapy with IvIgG and steroids: more questions and answers. European Working Group on Feto-maternal Alloimmune Thrombocytopenia. *Br J Haematol* 1998;**100**:62–5.

29 Paidas MJ, Berkowitz RL, Lynch L, *et al*. Alloimmune thrombocytopenia: fetal and neonatal losses related to cordocentesis. *Am J Obstet Gynecol* 1995;**172**:475–9.

30 Ghidini A, Sepulveda W, Lockwood CJ, Romero R. Complications of fetal blood sampling. *Am J Obstet Gynecol* 1993;**168**:1339–44.

31 Silver RM, Porter TF, Branch DW, *et al*. Neonatal alloimmune thrombocytopenia: antenatal management. *Am J Obstet Gynecol* 1999;**182**:1233–8.

32 Giovangrandi Y, Daffos E, Kaplan C, *et al*. Very early intracranial hemorrhage in alloimmune thrombocytopenia. *Lancet* 1990;**2**: 310.

33 Reznikoff-Etievant MF. Management of alloimmune neonatal and antenatal thrombocytopenia. *Vox Sang* 1988;**5**:193–201.

34 Bussel JB, Berkowitz RL, McFarland JG, *et al*. Antenatal treatment of neonatal alloimmune thrombocytopenia. *N Engl J Med* 1988;**319**:1374–8.

35 Lynch L, Bussel JB, McFarland JG, *et al*. Antenatal treatment of alloimmune thrombocytopenia. *Obstet Gynecol* 1992;**80**:67–71.

15 Inherited and acquired thrombophilias

Michael J. Paidas

Inherited thrombophilias are a heterogeneous group of disorders associated with varying degrees of increased thrombotic risk and adverse pregnancy outcome (APO) [1].

At the present time, the predominant thrombophilic mutations include the factor V Leiden mutation, prothrombin gene mutation G20210A, methylene tetrahydrafolate reductase (MTHFR) C667T, and deficiencies of the natural anticoagulants proteins C and S, and antithrombin. Acquired thrombophilic conditions consist of the antiphospholipid antibody syndrome (APAS), which is a well-characterized acquired thrombophilic condition associated with thrombotic and pregnancy complications [2].

Hemostatic changes in pregnancy

Pregnancy is associated with significant elevations of a number of clotting factors. Fibrinogen concentration is doubled, factors VII, VIII, IX, X, and XII increase 20–1000%, and von Willebrand factor increases 20–1000%, with maximum levels reached at term [3]. Prothrombin and factor V levels remain unchanged while levels of factors XIII and XI decline modestly. The overall effect of these changes is to increase thrombin generating potential. Coagulation activation markers in normal pregnancy are elevated, as evidenced by increased thrombin activity, increased soluble fibrin levels (9.2–13.4 nmol/L), increased thrombin–antithrombin (TAT) complexes (3.1–7.1 µg/L), and increased levels of fibrin D-dimer (91–198 µg/L) [4]. Fifty percent of women had elevated TAT levels (11/22) and 36% of women had elevated levels of D-dimers (9/25) in the first trimester.

During pregnancy there are significant changes in the natural anticoagulant and fibrinolytic systems. Protein S levels significantly decrease in normal pregnancy. Mean protein S free antigen levels have been reported to be 38.9 ± 10.3% and 31.2 ± 7.4% in the second and third trimesters, respectively [5]. The protein S carrier molecule, complement 4B-binding protein, is increased in pregnancy, and is one explanation for the diminished protein S levels in pregnancy. Levels of plasminogen activator inhibitor-1 (PAI-1) increase three- to four-fold during pregnancy; plasma PAI-2 values are low prior to pregnancy and reach concentrations of 160 µg/L at term. Table 15.1 summarizes the relevant pregnancy-associated changes in the hemostatic system. The prothrombotic hemostatic changes are exacerbated by pregnancy-associated venous stasis in the lower extremities resulting from compression of the inferior vena cava and pelvic veins by the enlarging uterus, as well as a hormone-mediated increase in deep vein capacitance secondary to increased circulating levels of estrogen and local production of prostacyclin and nitric oxide.

Substantial changes must occur in local decidual and systemic coagulation, anticoagulant, and fibrinolytic systems to meet the hemostatic challenges of pregnancy, including avoidance of hemorrhage at implantation, placentation, and third stage of labor. In addition to the systemic prothrombotic, anticoagulant, and fibrinolytic changes, there are potent local hemostatic effects in the decidua that occur during pregnancy [6,7]. Progesterone augments perivascular decidual cell tissue factor and PAI-1 expression. Decidual tissue factor is critical in maintaining hemostasis, as evidenced by experiments with transgenic tissue factor knockout mice which have a significant risk of fatal postpartum hemorrhage [8]. It is worthwhile to note that obstetric conditions associated with impaired decidualization (e.g., ectopic and cesarean scar pregnancy, placenta previa, and accreta) are associated with potential lethal hemorrhage.

Inherited thrombophilias

In 1965, Egberg, a Norwegian physician, reported a family with a partial antithrombin deficiency, and in his classic article suggested the term thrombophilia, referring to hereditary or acquired conditions that predispose individuals to thromboembolic events [9]. After the description of antithrombin deficiency, deficiencies of proteins C and S were described

Table 15.1 Hemostatic changes in pregnancy. (After Bremme [3] and Paidas et al. [5].)

Variables (Mean ± SD)	1st Trimester*	2nd Trimester*	3rd Trimester*	Normal Range
Platelet ($\times10^9$/L)	275 ± 64	256 ± 49	244 ± 52	150–400
Fibrinogen (g/L)	3.7 ± 0.6	4.4 ± 1.2	5.4 ± 0.8	2.1–4.2
Prothrombin complex (%)	120 ± 27	140 ± 27	130 ± 27	70–30
Antithrombin (U/mL)	1.02 ± 0.10	1.07 ± 0.14	1.07 ± 0.11	0.85–1.25
Protein C (U/mL)	0.92 ± 0.13	1.06 ± 0.17	0.94 ± 0.2	0.68–1.25
Protein S, total (U/mL)	0.83 ± 0.11	0.73 ± 0.11	0.77 ± 0.10	0.70–1.70
Protein S, free (U/mL)	0.26 ± 0.07	0.17 ± 0.04	0.14 ± 0.04	0.20–0.50
Soluble fibrin (nmol/L)	9.2 ± 8.6	11.8 ± 7.7	13.4 ± 5.2	<15
Thrombin-antithrombin (µg/L)	3.1 ± 1.4	5.9 ± 2.6	7.1 ± 2.4	<2.7
D-dimers (µg/L)	91 ± 24	128 ± 49	198 ± 59	<80
Plasminogen activator inhibitor-1 (AU/mL)	7.4 ± 4.9	14.9 ± 5.2	37.8 ± 19.4	<15
Plasminogen activator inhibitor-2 (µg/L)	31 ± 14	84 ± 16	160 ± 31	<5
Cardiolipin antibodies positive	2/25	2/25	3/23	0
Protein Z (µg/mL)†	2.01 ± 0.76	1.47 ± 0.45	1.55 ± 0.48	
Protein S (%)†		34.4 ± 11.8	27.5 ± 8.4	

* 1st trimester, weeks 12–15; 2nd trimester, week 24; 3rd trimester, week 35.

† First trimester, 0–14 weeks; second trimester, 14–27 weeks; third trimester ≥27 weeks.

Table 15.2 Inherited thrombophilias and their association with venous thromboembolism (VTE) [103].

Thrombophilia	Inheritance	Prevalence in European Pop. (from large cohort studies)	Prevalence in Patients with VTE (range)	Relative Risk or Odds Ratio VTE (95% CI) life-time
FVL (homozy.)	AD	0.07%*	<1%*	80 (22–289)
FVL (heterozy.)	AD	5.3%	6.6–50%	2.7 (1.3–5.6)
PGM (homozy.)	AD	0.02%*	<1%	>80-fold*
PGM (heterozy.)	AD	2.9%	7.5%	3.8 (3.0–4.9)
FVL/PGM (compound heterozy.)	AD	0.17%*	2.0%	20.0 (11.1–36.1)
Hyperhomocysteinemia	AR	5%	<5%	3.3 (1.1–10.0)†
Antithrombin def (<60% activity)	AD	0.2%	1–8%	17.5 (9.1–33.8)
Protein S def Heerlen S460P mutation or free S antigen <55%	AD	0.2%	3.1%	2.4 (0.8–7.9)
Protein C (<60% activity)	AD	0.2%	3–5%	11.3 (5.7–22.3)

AD, autosomal dominant; AR, autosomal recessive; FVL, factor V Leiden; PGM, prothrombin gene mutation G20210A; VTE, venous thromboembolism.

* Calculated based on a Hardy–Weinberg equilibrium.

† Odds ratio (OR) adjusted for renal disease, folate and vitamin B_{12} deficiency, while OR are adjusted for these confounders.

in the 1980s [10,11]. Table 15.2 describes the association between inherited thrombophilias and venous thromboembolism (VTE).

Factor V Leiden

Interest in the thrombophilias significantly grew following the discovery of a relatively common genetic predisposition to clotting. In 1994, Dahlback [12] reported an association between a mutation in the factor V gene and increased thrombotic risk, termed the factor V Leiden (FVL) mutation. The FVL mutation results from a substitution of adenine for guanine at the 1691 position of the 10th exon of the factor V gene, causing an amino acid substitution, namely glutamine for arginine at position 506 in the factor V polypeptide (FV Q506). Factor V then is rendered resistant to cleavage by activated protein C. The frequency of the FVL mutation varies among different ethnic groups. The mutation is present in 5.2% of Caucasians, 1.2% of African-Americans [13], and 5–9% of Europeans, while it is rare in Asian and African populations [14]. The FVL mutation is primarily inherited in an autosomal dominant fashion [15]. Heterozygosity for the FVL mutation is present in 20–40% of nonpregnant patients with thromboembolic disease while homozygosity, the rarer condition, is associated with a significantly higher (>100-fold) risk of thromboembolism [14]. However, in a large, prospective, observational study conducted by the Maternal Fetal Medicine Network, 5188 women were enrolled prior to 15 weeks' gestation: 134 women who were carriers for FVL mutation were compared with 4750 women who were not carriers [16]. There were no significant differences in the rates of either preeclampsia, intrauterine growth restriction (IUGR), fetal deaths, or abruptio placentae between the two groups. The study evaluated only FVL, and it was not designed to evaluate the association of FVL and APO.

Prothrombin gene mutation G20210A

A mutation in the prothrombin gene, prothrombin gene mutation G20210A (PGM) was discovered in 1996, following the identification of the FVL mutation, and was associated with a significantly increased risk of thrombosis and, later on, pregnancy complications [1,17]. The presence of heterozygosity of the PGM mutation range from 2–3% of Europeans and leads to increased (150–200%) circulating levels of prothrombin [14]. It accounted for 17% of thromboembolism in pregnancy in one large case–control study [18]. The actual risk of clotting in an asymptomatic pregnant carrier is approximately 1 in 200 or 0.5%. The rarer condition, homozygosity for PGM, likewise confers a high risk of thrombosis, equal to that of homozygosity for FVL [14].

Protein S

Protein S is a vitamin K-dependent 69,000 molecular weight glycoprotein which has several anticoagulant functions including its activity as a nonenzymatic cofactor to the anticoagulant serine protease activated protein C (APC) [19]. Protein S has a plasma half-life of 42 hours, longer than protein C whose half life is approximately 6–8 hours. Circulating protein S exists in both free (40%) and bound (60%) forms. Plasma protein S is reversibly bound (60%) to C4b-binding protein (C4BP), which serves as a carrier protein for protein S. Protein S also has an APC-independent anticoagulant function in the direct inhibition of the prothrombinase complex. Protein S also inhibits thrombin activatable fibrinolysis inhibitor (TAFI) [20]. Protein S deficiency occurs in 0.03–1.3% of the population, and inheritance is autosomal dominant [21]. Protein S deficiency presents with one of three phenotypes: type I, marked by reduced total and free forms; type II, characterized by normal free protein S levels but reduced APC cofactor activity; and type III, in which there are normal total but reduced free protein S levels. Of note, different mutations have highly variable procoagulant sequelae making it extremely difficult to predict which patients with protein S deficiencies will develop thrombotic sequelae.

Pregnancy is associated with decreased levels of protein S activity and free protein S antigen in most patients [22]. Most normal pregnancies acquire some degree of resistance to APC when measured by the first-generation global assays and tests that measure endogenous thrombin potential [23,24]. Factor X's activation to factor Xa and its involvement in the activation of prothrombin is a central element in the generation of thrombin. It is possible that derangements in the control of factor Xa contribute to adverse prothrombotic sequelae in pregnancy.

Until recently, the significance and degree of the decrease in protein S levels commonly seen in pregnancy had not been adequately evaluated. Paidas *et al.* [5] compared second and third trimester protein S levels in 51 healthy women with a normal pregnancy outcome with 51 healthy women with a poor pregnancy outcome. Protein S levels were significantly lower in the second and third trimesters among patients with APO. A small case–control study performed in subjects from larger, multicenter, prospective study also found lower levels of protein S activity and free antigen in the second and third trimesters [16].

Protein C deficiency

Protein C is a vitamin K-dependent 62,000 molecular weight glycoprotein substrate that is a precursor to a serine protease, APC [25]. Protein C is activated to APC by thrombin in the presence of thrombomodulin (TM) on the surface of endothelial cells. APC with protein S and factor V as cofactors inactivate factors Va and VIIIa. The inactivation of factors Va and VIIIa decreases the generation of thrombin. Deficiencies of protein C result from numerous mutations, although two primary types are recognized: type I, in which both immunoreactive and functionally active protein C levels are reduced; and type II, where immunoreactive levels are normal but activity is reduced [26]. The prevalence of protein C deficiency is 0.2–0.5%, and its inheritance is autosomal dominant.

The reported pregnancy and puerperal risk of thromboembolism with protein C and S deficiencies appears modest, ranging from 5–20%, and may be overstated because of ascertainment biases [26]. Preston *et al.* [27] have reported that the risk of stillbirth is modestly increased with an adjusted odds ratio (OR) of 2.3 (95% confidence interval [CI], 0.6–8.3). The risk of miscarriage appears to be minimal with protein C deficiencies (OR 1.4; 95% CI, 0.9–2.2)], or not significant [26,28].

Antithrombin

Antithrombin (AT), a vitamin K-independent glycoprotein, is a pivotal component of the natural anticoagulant system, acting as a major inhibitor of thrombin and other serine proteases. The anticoagulant effect of heparin occurs via increase of AT's inhibitory activity of thrombin. Deficiency of AT is the most thrombogenic of the inherited thrombophilias, with a 70–90% lifetime risk of thromboembolism [26].

In addition to its thrombin inhibitory properties, AT can also inactivate factors Xa, IXa, VIIa, and plasmin. The anticoagulant activity of AT is increased 5000–40,000-fold by heparin. Deficiencies in AT result from numerous point mutations, deletions, and insertions, and are usually inherited in an autosomal dominant fashion [26]. The two classes of AT deficiency are:

1 Type I, the most common deficiency, is characterized by concomitant reductions in both antigenic protein levels and activity;

2 Type II deficiency, which is characterized by normal antigenic AT levels but decreased activity.

Type II deficiency is further classified by the site of the mutation (e.g., RS, reactive site; HBS, heparin binding site; PE, pleiotropic functional defects). The Type II-HBS variant appears to have the least clinical significance. Because the prevalence of AT deficiency is low, 1 in 1000 to 1 in 5000, it is only present in 1% of patients with thromboembolism. The risk of thrombosis among affected patients is as high as 60% during pregnancy and 33% during the puerperium [26]. Preston et al. [27] reported adjusted OR 1.7 (95% CI, 1.0–2.8) and 5.2 (95% CI, 1.5–18.1) for miscarriage and stillbirth, respectively. However, because of its low prevalence compared with that of fetal loss, preeclampsia, IUGR, and abruption, AT deficiency is rarely the cause of these disorders [29].

Protein Z deficiency

Protein Z is a 62-kDa vitamin K-dependent plasma protein that serves as a cofactor for a protein Z-dependent protease inhibitor (ZPI) of factor Xa [30,31]. Protein Z is critical for regulation of factor Xa activity in addition to tissue factor pathway inhibitor [32–34]. Protein Z increases rapidly during the first months of life followed by slow increases during childhood, with adult levels reached during puberty [35,36]. Protein Z deficiency influences the prothrombotic phenotype in FVL patients, and low plasma protein Z levels have been reported in patients with antiphospholipid antibodies [37,38]. There is a high prevalence of protein Z deficiency in patients with unexplained early fetal loss (10th to 19th weeks) [39]. Gris et al. [40] found an increased risk of fetal loss associated with protein Z deficiency (OR 6.7; 95% CI, 3.1–14.8; $P < 0.001$), and noted that the patients with late fetal loss and recurrent miscarriages had lower protein Z levels.

Paidas et al. [5] found that there was a significant decrease in the protein Z levels in patients ($n = 51$) with a variety of APO, including IUGR, preeclampsia, preterm delivery, and bleeding in pregnancy, compared with women ($n = 51$) with normal pregnancy outcomes (second trimester 1.5 ± 0.4 vs. $2.0 \pm 0.5\,\mu g/$ mL, $P < 0.0001$; third trimester 1.6 ± 0.5 vs. $1.9 \pm 0.5\,\mu g/mL$, $P < 0.0002$) [5].

Protein Z levels at the 20th percentile ($1.30\,\mu g/mL$) were associated with an increased risk of APO (OR 4.25; 95% CI, 1.536–11.759), with a sensitivity of 93% and specificity of 32%. Mean first trimester protein Z level was significantly lower among patients with APO compared with pregnant controls (1.81 ± 0.7 vs. $2.21 \pm 0.8\,\mu g/mL$, respectively; $P < 0.001$). Gris et al. [40] carried out a prospective, randomized trial comparing the low molecular weight heparin (LMWH) enoxaparin (40 mg/day) with low-dose aspirin (100 mg/day) in 160 women with one unexplained fetal loss ($\geq$10th week of gestation) and either FVL, prothrombin 20210, or protein S deficiency. Treatments were started at 8 weeks' gestation. The live birth rate was 86% in the enoxaparin-treated women versus 29% in the aspirin-treated group (OR for live birth with LMWH 15.5; 95% CI, 7–34). Birthweights were higher and there were fewer small for gestational age infants in the enoxaparin group. Gris et al. [40] found that the presence of protein Z deficiency or the presence of protein Z antibodies was more frequently present in cases of treatment failures ($P = 0.20$ and 0.019, respectively) as was the complex of protein Z deficiency positive antiprotein Z antibodies ($P = 0.004$); 15 of the 20 cases led to pregnancy failure, nine being treated with aspirin and six with enoxaparin. Both groups of patients received 5 mg/day folic acid, in addition to aspirin or heparin therapy.

Elevated levels of type 1 plasminogen activator inhibitor

Plasminogen activator inhibitors are serine protease inhibitors, often referred to as serpins (serine protease inhibitors) with diverse functions, including blood coagulation, fibrinolysis, and cell migration [41,42]. PAI-1 and PAI-2 regulate tissue and urokinase type plasminogen activators, respectively (tPA and uPA). tPA and uPA regulate fibrin degradation via the conversion of plasminogen to plasmin, and are also involved in the remodeling of extracellular matrix [43]. PAI-1 and PAI-2 are found in the blood of women with normal pregnancies, and their levels tend to rise with advancing gestation [44]. In preeclamptic patients, the vascular endothelium is responsible for the majority of the elevated PAI-1 plasma levels, with platelets accounting for a smaller proportion [45]. Unlike PAI-1, which is found in a variety of nonpregnant disease states, PAI-2 expression has been identified in a limited number of cells, principally placental trophoblasts, macrophages, and various malignant cell lines [45,46].

It is well known that pregnancy is associated with elevated levels of PAI-1, and higher levels are noted in cases of preeclampsia or IUGR (either during manifestations of the disease process, or shortly prior to their manifestation in the case of preeclampsia). Homozygosity for the 4G/4G mutation in the

PAI-1 gene leads to a three- to fivefold increased level of circulating PAI-1. The significance of the 4G/4G PAI-1 mutation is uncertain. The contribution of this prothrombotic mutation to thromboembolic events has been called into question, as evidenced by the recent review by Francis [47]. A large multicenter study did not find a relationship between any of the inherited thrombophilic conditions and fetal loss, but achieved approximately 30% power to detect a difference [48]. Polymorphisms of the thrombomodulin gene are associated with an increased risk of thrombosis, but the pregnancy implications are unclear at this time [49]. Interestingly, pregnant patients with thrombophilia and subsequent APO have been demonstrated to exhibit a decreased first trimester response to thrombomodulin in an activated partial thromboplastin time (APTT) system [50].

Hyperhomocysteinemia and methylene tetrahydrofolate reductase thermolabile mutant gene mutation (MTHFR C677T)

Homocysteine is generated from the metabolism of the amino acid methionine. It normally circulates in the plasma at concentrations of 5–16 µmol/L. Deficiencies in vitamins B_6, B_{12}, and folic acid can result in elevated levels of homocysteine in the setting of inherited hyperhomocysteinemia. Homocysteine levels can vary with diet, however, and normal levels in pregnancy are slightly lower than nonpregnant values.

Hyperhomocysteinemia can be diagnosed by measuring fasting homocysteine levels by gas chromatography mass spectrometry or other sensitive biochemical means. The disorder is classified into three categories according to the extent of the fasting homocysteine elevation: severe (>100 µmol/L); moderate (25–100 µmol/L), or mild (16–24 µmol/L). Methionine loading can improve diagnostic sensitivity. Severe hyperhomocysteinemia results from an autosomal recessive homozygous deficiency in either cystathionine β-synthase (CBS) (prevalence of 1 in 200,000) or MTHFR. Clinical manifestations of hyperhomocysteinemia include neurologic abnormalities, premature atherosclerosis, and recurrent thromboembolism.

The mild and moderate forms can result from autosomal dominant (heterozygote) deficiencies in CBS (0.3–1.4% of population) or from homozygosity for the 667C-T MTHFR thermolabile mutant, present in 11% of white European populations [26]. Patients with mild or moderate hyperhomocysteinemia are at risk for atherosclerosis, thromboembolism, fetal neural tube defects, and possibly recurrent abortion. There are conflicting data on the link between hyperhomocysteinemia and recurrent spontaneous abortion [51–53]. An older meta-analysis of the association between hyperhomocysteinemia and pregnancy loss prior to 16 weeks suggested a weak association with an OR of 1.4 (95% CI, 1.0–2.0) [54]. The natural history of the MTHFR mutation in pregnancy has not

been well documented. The meta-analysis by Rey [28] concluded that MTHFR was not associated with an increased risk of fetal loss.

Another recent meta-analysis concluded that while FVL and PGM were modestly associated with an increased risk of early pregnancy loss, there was no such association with the MTHFR C677T mutation [55]. Table 15.3 provides epidemiologic data and venous thromboembolic risks associated with various thrombophilic conditions.

Acquired thrombophilia

The well-characterized APAS is defined by the combination of VTE, obstetric complications, and antiphospholipid antibodies (APA) [56]. By definition, APA-related thrombosis can occur in any tissue or organ except superficial veins, while accepted associated obstetric complications include at least one fetal death at or beyond the 10th week of gestation, or at least one premature birth at or before the 34th week, or at least three consecutive spontaneous abortions before the 10th week. All other causes of pregnancy morbidity must be excluded. APA must be present on two or more occasions at least 6 weeks apart, and are immunoglobulins directed against proteins bound to negatively charged surfaces, usually anionic phospholipids [57]. Thus, APAs can be detected by screening for antibodies that:

- Directly bind these protein epitopes (e.g., anti-β_2-glycoprotein-1, prothrombin, annexin V, APC, protein S, protein Z, ZPI, high and low molecular weight kininogens, tPA, factor VII(a), and XII, the complement cascade constituents, C4, and CH, and oxidized low-density lipoproteins antibodies); or
- Are bound to proteins present in an anionic phospholipid matrix (e.g., anticardiolipin and phosphatidylserine antibodies); or
- Exert downstream effects on prothrombin activation in a phospholipid milieu (i.e., lupus anticoagulants) [58].

Venous thrombotic events associated with APA include deep venous thrombosis (DVT) with or without acute pulmonary embolism (APE), while the most common arterial events include cerebral vascular accidents and transient ischemic attacks. At least half of patients with APA have systemic lupus erythematosus (SLE). Anticardiolipin antibodies were associated with an OR of 2.17 (95% CI, 1.51–3.11; 14 studies) for any thrombosis, 2.50 (95% CI, 1.51–4.14) for DVT and APE, and 3.91 (95% CI, 1.14–13.38) for recurrent VTE [59]. Patients with SLE and lupus anticoagulants were at a sixfold greater risk for VTE compared with SLE patients without lupus anticoagulants, while SLE patients with anticardiolipin antibodies had a twofold greater risk of VTE compared with SLE patients without these antibodies. The lifetime prevalence of arterial or venous thrombosis in affected patients with antiphospholipid antibodies is approximately 30%, with an event rate of 1% per

Table 15.3 Anticoagulation to prevent adverse pregnancy outcome in the setting of thrombophilia. (After Paidas *et al.* [1].)

Author	Year	Patients (*n*)	Drug	Patients Studied	Outcome
Riyazi	1998	26	Nadroparin + ASA 80 mg	Thrombophilia + prior preeclampsia or IUGR	Treatment associated with lower rates of preeclampsia/IUGR compared with historic control
Brenner	2000	50	Enoxaparin	Thrombophilia + recurrent fetal loss	Treatment associated higher live birth (75% vs. 20% compared with historic control)
Ogueh	2001	24	Unfractionated heparin	Thrombophilia + IUGR or abruption	No improvement compared with historic control
Kupferminc	2001	33	Enoxaparin + ASA 100 mg	Thrombophilia + preeclampsia or IUGR	Higher birthweight and gestational age at delivery
Grandone	2002	25	Unfractionated heparin or enoxaparin	Thrombophilia + APO	Treatment was associated with lower rates of APO in treated (10%) vs. non-treated (93%)
Paidas	2004	41	Unfractionated or low molecular weight heparin	FVL or PGM + history of fetal loss	Treatment was associated with an 80% reduction in fetal loss (OR 0.21; 95% CI, 0.11–0.39)
Gris	2004	160	Enoxaparin or 100 mg aspirin; Folic acid 5mg	Thrombophilia + fetal loss	Enoxaparin was superior to aspirin 29% patients treated with LDA. 86% treated with enoxaparin had healthy live birth (OR 15.55; 95% CI, 7–34)
Brenner	2004	183	Enoxaparin (40 mg/day or 40 mg b.i.d.)	Thrombophilia + ≥3 losses in the first trimester, or ≥2 losses in the second trimester, or ≥1 loss in the third trimester	Enoxaparin increased the rate of live birth (81.4% vs. 28.2%; $P<0.01$ for 40 mg, 76.5% vs. 28.3%, $P<0.01$ for 80 mg), decreased the rate of preeclampsia (3.4% vs. 7.1%, $P<0.01$ for 40 mg; 4.5% vs. 15.7%, $P<0.01$ for 80 mg), and decreased the rate of abruption (4.4% vs. 14.1%, $P<0.01$ for 40 mg; 3.4% vs. 9.6%, $P<0.1$ for 80 mg)

APO, adverse pregnancy outcome; CI, confidence interval; FVL, factor V Leiden; IUGR, intrauterine growth restriction; LDA, low-dose aspirin; OR, odds ratio; PGM, prothrombin gene mutation G20210A.

year [58]. These antibodies are present in up to 20% of individuals with VTE [60]. A review of 25 prospective, cohort, and case–control studies involving more than 7000 patients observed an OR range for arterial and venous thromboses in patients with lupus anticoagulants of 8.65–10.84 and 4.09–16.2, respectively, and 1–18 and 1–2.51 for anticardiolipin antibodies [58].

There is a 5% risk of VTE during pregnancy and the puerperium among patients with APA despite treatment [61]. Recurrence risks of up to 30% have been reported in APA-positive patients with a prior VTE; thus, long-term prophylaxis is required in these patients. A severe form of APAS is termed catastrophic antiphospholipid syndrome (CAPS), which is defined by potential life-threatening variant with multiple vessel thromboses leading to multiorgan failure [62]. In the Euro-Phospholipid Project Group (13 countries included),

DVT, thrombocytopenia, stroke, pulmonary embolism, and transient ischemic attacks were found in 31.7%, 21.9%, 13.1%, 9.0%, and 7.0%, respectively.

APA are associated with obstetric complications in approximately 15–20% including fetal loss after 9 weeks' gestation, abruption, severe preeclampsia, and IUGR. For lupus anticoagulant-associated fetal loss, reported OR range from 3.0 to 4.8 while anticardiolipin antibodies display a wider range of reported OR of 0.86–20.0 [57]. It is unclear whether APA are also associated with recurrent (three or more) early spontaneous abortions in the absence of stillbirth. Fifty percent or more of pregnancy losses in APA patients occur after the 10th week [63]. Patients with APA more often display initial fetal cardiac activity compared with patients with unexplained first trimester spontaneous abortions without APA (86% vs. 43%; $P<0.01$)

[64]. APA have been commonly found in the general obstetric population, with one survey demonstrating that 2.2% of such patients have either immunoglobulin M (IgM) or IgG anticardiolipin antibodies with most such women having relatively uncomplicated pregnancies [65]. Other factors may have a role in the pathogenesis of APA. Potential mechanism(s) by which APA induce arterial and venous thrombosis as well as adverse pregnancy outcomes include: APA-mediated impairment of endothelial thrombomodulin and APC-mediated anticoagulation; induction of endothelial tissue factor expression; impairment of fibrinolysis and antithrombin activity; augmented platelet activation and/or adhesion; impairment of the anticoagulant effects of the anionic phospholipid binding proteins β_2-glycoprotein-I and annexin V [2,66]. RANDAPA-induction of complement activation has been suggested to have a role in fetal loss with heparin preventing such aberrant activation [67].

Inherited thrombophilia and pregnancy complications

Inherited thrombophilic conditions have been implicated in a variety of obstetric complications, including preeclampsia and related conditions, early and late fetal loss, IUGR, and abruptio placentae.

Preeclampsia

Several studies (mostly case controlled) have evaluated the relationship between heterozygous FVL and severe preeclampsia. FVL was identified in 4.5–26% of patients with severe preeclampsia, eclampsia, or HELLP (hemolysis, elevated liver enzymes, and low platelet count) syndrome [1,68–72]. The systematic review by Alfirevic *et al.* [29] suggested a positive association between FVL and preeclampsia and/or eclampsia (OR 1.6; 95% CI, 1.2–2.1). The PGM was identified in up to 9.1% of cases, whereas protein S deficiency was reported in 5–25% of cases [1,68,70,72]. While the preponderance of the studies evaluating severe preeclampsia show a positive association with inherited thrombophilias, there is also evidence demonstrating no association. In a study by Livingston *et al.* [72], maternal and fetal genetic thrombophilias (FVL, MTHFR, PGM) were compared in 110 patients with severe preeclampsia and 97 normotensive patients with healthy outcomes. There were no differences in the rate of FVL (4.4 vs. 4.3%), MTHFR (9.6 vs. 6.3%), or PGM (0 vs. 1.1%) between the two groups. Similar findings were noted in white (*n*=47) and African-American (*n*=63) women, and in those with early or late onset severe preeclampsia. In addition, there were no differences in the frequency of the studied genetic thrombophilias in cord blood in severe preeclampsia and normotensive groups.

Paidas *et al.* [5] found that there was a significant decrease in the protein Z levels in patients (*n*=51) with a variety of APO,

including IUGR, preeclampsia, preterm delivery, and bleeding in pregnancy compared with women (*n*=51) with normal pregnancy outcomes (NPO) (second trimester 1.5±0.4 vs. 2.0±0.5 μg/mL, *P* <0.0001; and third trimester 1.6±0.5 vs. 1.9±0.5 μg/mL, *P* <0.0002). Protein Z levels at the 20th percentile (1.30 μg/mL) were associated with an increased risk of APO (OR 4.25; 95% CI, 1.536–11.759) with a sensitivity of 93% and specificity of 32%.

Intrauterine growth restriction

Infante-Rivard *et al.* [73] found rates of 4.5% and 2.5% for FVL and PGM, respectively, when IUGR was defined as less than 10th percentile. In a recent systematic review, FVL and PGM were associated with an increased risk of IUGR: OR 2.7 (95% CI, 1.3–5.5) and 2.5 (95% CI, 1.3–5.0), respectively, in 10 case–control studies [74]. However, in five cohort studies (three prospective, two retrospective), the relative risk was 0.99 (95% CI, 0.5–1.9). The authors concluded that both FVL and PG confer an increased risk of giving birth to an IUGR infant, although this may be driven by small, poor quality studies that demonstrated extreme associations. Prevalence rates ranging from 5–35%, 2.5–15%, and 11–23% were reported for FVL, PGM, and protein S deficiency, respectively [1,75–79]. Alfirevic [29] found a significant association between protein S deficiency and IUGR (OR 10.2; 95% CI, 1.1–91).

Abruptio placentae and thrombophilia

The determination of the relationship between thrombophilias and abruptio placentae (decidual hemorrhage) is difficult because of the limited number of studies and confounding variables, including chronic hypertension, and cigarette and cocaine use. De Vries [76] found that 9/31 (29%) patients with abruption had a protein S deficiency, compared with their general population prevalence of 0.2–2%. The prevalence of FVL, PGM, and protein S deficiency was in the ranges 22–30%, 18–20%, and 0–29%, respectively [1,80].

Fetal loss

In a meta-analysis of 31 studies, Rey *et al.* [28] found that FVL was associated with increased risk of late fetal loss (OR 3.26; 95% CI, 1.82–5.83). Gris *et al.* [81] found a positive correlation between the number of stillbirths and the prevalence of thrombophilias in a study of 232 women with previous late fetal loss (>22 weeks) and 464 controls. Protein S deficiency was found in 9/84 (10.7%) of those with at least two stillbirths, and the presence of FVL was associated with a high risk of fetal loss later than 22 weeks (OR 7.83; 95% CI, 2.83–21.67). Martinelli *et al.* [82] found that the risk of late fetal death (after 20 weeks) was three times higher if the patient was a carrier of either the FVL or PGM mutation. The relative risk of carriers (FVL, PGM) for late fetal loss was 3.2 (1.0–10.9) and 3.3 (1.1–10.3), respectively. Martinelli et al. [83] evaluated recurrent late loss and found that FVL was present in 28.6% of patients with recurrent late loss.

Rey et al. [28] pooled data from nine studies (n=2087), and found a significant association between fetal loss and PGM. PGM was associated with recurrent fetal loss before 25 weeks (n=690 women; OR 2.56; 95% CI, 1.04–6.29) and with nonrecurrent fetal loss after 20 weeks (five studies, n=1299; OR 2.3; 95% CI, 1.09–4.87). The prevalence of PGM is in the range 0–33%, and for protein S deficiency 29–92% [1,70,84,85]. However, Hefler et al. [48] did not find any significant association between FVL, PGM, or protein S deficiency and fetal death (median gestational age 34 weeks, range 20–42 weeks). Rey et al. [28] found that protein S deficiency was associated with nonrecurrent loss after 22 weeks in three studies (n=565; OR 7.39; 95% CI, 1.28–42.83).

Early pregnancy loss and thrombophilia

The association between early pregnancy loss and thrombophilia has also yielded conflicting results. In three recent systematic reviews, the diversity among included studies implies that meta-analyses are performed including heterogeneous studies [28,55,86]. Factors influencing results include: inclusion of isolated or recurrent fetal loss; presence or absence of successful livebirth in obstetric history; gestational age cut-off for evaluation; and inclusion of proper control groups. The typical OR for FVL is 1.67 (95% CI, 1.16–2.40) and for PGM the typical OR is 2.25 (95% CI, 1.20–4.21) [55]. There was no increased risk of loss with MTHFR C677T [55]. Roque et al. [52] reported that the OR for having thrombophilia was actually significantly lower in women with recurrent embryonic losses. The paternal or fetal genetic contribution has not been well studied to date. In a study of 357 couples with a history of three or more pregnancy losses under 12 weeks, the presence of multiple thrombophilic mutations in either partner was associated with a significantly increased risk of pregnancy loss (relative risk 1.9, range 1.2–2.8) [87].

Thrombophilia, prior history of poor pregnancy outcome, and recurrence

For patients who have had a prior APO and harbor an inherited thrombophilic condition such as FVL, the prothrombin gene mutation G20210A, or protein S deficiency, the reported rate of recurrence of APO is high. Martinelli et al. [83] found that of 82 women with late fetal loss, seven had a recurrence, and two of seven had FVL (28.6%). Kupferminc et al. [70,71,88] have consistently reported very high rates of pregnancy complications in women with prior poor obstetric outcomes: 83% of pregnancies in 18 women, 66% of pregnancies in nine multiparous women with PGM, and 77% occurrence of complications in nine multiparous women. In a cohort of 28

patients with thrombophilia (heterozygous PGM and prior APO), Kupferminc et al. [88] reported that seven of 62 pregnancies were normal. According to the meta-analysis by Rey et al. [28], the presence of PGM was associated with recurrent fetal loss before 25 weeks (n=690 women; OR 2.56; 95% CI, 1.04–6.29) and with nonrecurrent fetal loss after 20 weeks (five studies, n=1299; OR 2.3; 95% CI, 1.09–4.87). Rey et al. also found that late fetal loss was associated with FVL mutation (n=1888; OR 3.26; 95% CI, 1.82–5.83), PGM (n=1299; OR 2.30; 95% CI, 1.09–4.87), protein S deficiency (n=878; OR 7.39; 95% CI, 1.28–42.83) but not MTHFR, protein C deficiency, or antithrombin deficiency. Several factors impact studies concerning thrombophilia and pregnancy complications, including the heterogeneity of the populations studied, small sample size, rarity of the endpoint evaluated, number of thrombophilias assayed for, detection methods employed, lack of consistent assessment of fetal thrombophilia status, as well as potential ascertainment biases [55,89]. These limitations have been recently confirmed from two independent studies on fetal genotype [90,91]. Until more large population-based studies are performed, the debate regarding the association between inherited thrombophilias and APO will continue. For example, positive associations between pregnancy complications and thrombophilia may exist, but the association may be driven by small studies with extreme associations [74].

Prevention of adverse pregnancy outcomes in the setting of thrombophilia

Kupferminc et al. [92] treated 33 women with a history of severe preeclampsia, abruptio placenta, IUGR, or fetal demise and a known thrombophilia with LMWH and low-dose aspirin. Treated patients had a higher birthweight and a higher gestational age at delivery than that of the previous pregnancy. Treated pregnancies were not associated with fetal losses or severe preeclampsia. Riyazi et al. [93] found that treatment with LMWH and low-dose aspirin in patients with previous early onset preeclampsia and/or severe IUGR and a thrombophilic disorder resulted in a higher birthweight than patients with a comparable history not receiving this intervention. Paidas et al. [94] evaluated a cohort of patients carrying either FVL or PGM who experienced at least one prior APO. A total of 41 patients (28 with FVL, 13 with PGM) had 158 pregnancies. The 41 heparin-treated pregnancy outcomes were compared with the remaining 117 untreated pregnancies. Antenatal heparin administration was associated with an 80% reduction in APO overall (OR 0.21; 95% CI, 0.11–0.39; P <0.05). This relationship persisted if first trimester losses were excluded (n=111 total pregnancies; OR 0.46; 95% CI, 0.23–0.94; P <0.05). Brenner et al. [95] reported on the LIVE-ENOX Study, a multicenter prospective randomized trial to evaluate the efficacy and safety of two doses of enoxaparin (40 mg/day or

40 mg b.i.d.) in 183 women with recurrent pregnancy loss and thrombophilia. Inclusion criteria were three or more losses in the first trimester, two or more losses in the second trimester, one loss or more in the third trimester. Compared with the patient's historic rates of live birth and pregnancy complications, enoxaparin was significantly associated with an increased rate of live births, decreased rate of preeclampsia, and decreased rate of abruption. Better outcomes were associated with higher dosage.

Gris *et al.* [40] compared administration of low-dose aspirin (100 mg/day) with 40 mg/day enoxaparin from the 8th week of gestation in a cohort of patients with a prior loss after 10 weeks and the presence of heterozygous FVL, PGM, or protein S deficiency. The authors found that 23/80 patients treated with aspirin and 69/80 patients treated with enoxaparin had a successful pregnancy (OR 15.5; 95% CI, 7–34; $P < 0.0001$). Birthweights were higher and there were less small for gestational age infants in the enoxaparin group.

The small size and inadequate study design of the published studies do not permit any firm recommendations regarding the antenatal administration of heparin for the sole indication of the prevention of APO [96]. These authors strongly recommended a randomized trial to address the use of anticoagulation for prevention. According to a recent Cochrane review [97], based upon an extensive literature search for 1966–2004, women with a history of two or more spontaneous losses or one fetal demise without apparent cause other than inherited thrombophilia, only two trials were available for review. The other study besides the Gris trial was the trial reported by Tulppala *et al.* [98] which involved 82 patients, and compared 50 mg aspirin with placebo starting at the time of positive urine pregnancy test, in women with three or more unexplained consecutive losses. No differences were noted in the aspirin compared with the placebo group (relative risk 1.00 [0.78–1.29]). Table 15.3 summarizes the results of studies using anticoagulation to prevent APO in the setting of thrombophilia.

Heparin and aspirin administration is the best strategy for the treatment of recurrent pregnancy loss associated with APAS, according to the Cochrane review of 2002 [99]. This approach has been associated with a 54% reduction in pregnancy loss, and is better than aspirin alone. Steroid administration is associated with an excessive risk of prematurity, and therefore is not recommended as a first-line prevention strategy.

Thrombophilia screening: testing and candidates

The selection of suitable patients for thrombophilia screening and the thrombophilia work-up continues to evolve. At this time, suitable candidates for thrombophilia screening include: history of unexplained fetal loss ≥10 weeks; history of severe preeclampsia/HELLP <36 weeks; history of abruption; history

of IUGR (>5th percentile; personal history of thrombosis; family history of thrombosis). Initial thrombophilia evaluation should include: protein C (functional level); protein S (functional level); AT-III (functional level); factor V Leiden (polymerase chain reaction [PCR]); prothrombin gene mutation 20210A (PCR); lupus anticoagulant; ACA IgG, IgM, IgA, and platelet count. Other commonly ordered screens include: MTHFR C677T mutation; fasting homocysteine level; and β₂-glycoprotein I, IgG, IgM, and IgA. Depending on the clinical scenario, thrombophilia evaluation can be extended to include other tests, such as protein Z, other APA, and the more uncommon factor V mutations, components of the protein C system, and PAI-1 mutation. Another genetic variant worthy of continuing investigation is the angiotensin I converting enzyme (ACE) gene polymorphism. In one study, LMWH was associated with a 74.1% reduction of preeclampsia and 77.5% reduction of fetal growth restriction in a group of women homozygous for the DD ACE polymorphism and a history of preeclampsia [100]. Large prospective studies are needed to address the role of the interaction of thrombophilic conditions in the causation of VTE and APO. A recent meta-analysis and cost-effectiveness study has concluded that universal thrombophilia screening in pregnancy is not useful, but rather a selective approach based upon personal and family history is most advantageous [101].

Management of acquired and inherited thrombophilias: prevention and treatment strategies

Specific management guidelines relating to the management of thromboembolism are provided in another chapter of this book. Before initiating anticoagulation therapy in the setting of active thrombosis, a thrombophilia panel should be obtained. Functional clotting factor testing should be performed well after the cessation of anticoagulant therapy to diagnose a factor deficiency. Table 15.4 summarizes anticoagulant regimens for treatment and prophylactic settings. Patients with highly thrombogenic thrombophilias such as antithrombin deficiency should receive therapeutic anticoagulation throughout pregnancy. The rare patient who is homozygous for the FVL or PGM, or who is a compound heterozygote for these two mutations, require at the minimum prophylactic anticoagulation, and other investigators would recommend therapeutic anticoagulation during pregnancy and the postpartum period.

Pharmacology of anticoagulation in pregnancy

Thromboembolism and APO management continue to present clinical challenges. The available anticoagulant drugs for

Table 15.4 Anticoagulation in pregnancy: indications and dosing.

Indication	Description	Antepartum		Postpartum	
		Therapeutic	Prophylactic	Therapeutic	Prophylactic
VTE current pregnancy		X		See (1)	
High-risk thrombophilia					
FVL homozygous	History of VTE	X		X	
PGM homozygous	or APO (2)				
Antithrombin III deficiency	No history		X		X
Intermediate risk thrombophilia					
Compound heterozygote (FVL/PGM)			X		X
Low-risk thrombophilia					
FVL heterozygous	Prior VTE		X		X
Prothrombin	History of APO (2) but *not* VTE		± X (3)		X (4)

APO, adverse pregnancy outcomes; FVL, factor V Leiden; VTE, venous thromboembolism.

(1) VTE during current pregnancy should receive therapeutic anticoagulation for 20+ weeks during pregnancy, followed by prophylactic therapy for up to 6 weeks postpartum.

(2) APO includes early onset severe preeclampsia, unexplained recurrent abruption, severe intrauterine growth restriction (IUGR), intrauterine fetal demise (>10 weeks) with placental thrombosis or infarction.

(3) Patients with less thrombogenic thrombophilias and histories of APO should be treated prophylactically in the antepartum period if the clinical scenario suggests a high risk for recurrence or if there are other thrombotic risk factors (e.g., obesity, immobilization).

(4) If cesarean delivery or first-degree relative with history of VTE.

(5) Cases of hyperhomocysteinemia unresponsive to folate, vitamin B_6 and vitamin B_{12} therapy.

Unfractionated heparin (UFH)
Initial dose of UFH for acute VTE to keep activated partial thromboplastin time (APTT) 1.5–2.5× control. Thereafter UFH may be given s.q. q8–12 h to keep APTT 1.5–2× control (when tested 6 h after injection) for therapeutic levels.
Prophylactic doses may range from 5000 to 10,000 units s.q. q12 h and can be titrated to achieve heparin levels (by protamine titration assay) of 0.1–0.2 U/mL.

Low molecular weight heparin (LMWH)
Therapeutic doses of enoxaparin (Lovenox®) may start at 1 mg/kg s.q. q12 h. Therapeutic doses should be titrated to achieve antifactor Xa levels of 0.6–1.0 U/mL (when tested 4–6 h after injection).
Prophylactic doses of enoxaparin (Lovenox®) may start at 40 mg s.q. q24 h. Prophylactic doses should be titrated to achieve antifactor Xa levels of 0.1–0.2 U/mL 4 h after injection.
Regional anesthesia is contraindicated within 18–24 h of LMWH and thus LMWH should be converted to UFH at 36 weeks or earlier if clinically indicated.

Postpartum
Heparin anticoagulation (LMWH or UFH) may be restarted 3–6 h after vaginal delivery and 6–8 h after cesarean.
Warfarin anticoagulation may be started postpartum day 1.
Therapeutic doses of LMWH or UFH must be continued for 5 days *and* until the international normalized ratio (INR) reaches therapeutic range (2.0–3.0) for 2 successive days.

Maternal and fetal surveillance
Fetal growth should be monitored every 4–6 weeks beginning at 20 weeks in all patients on anticoagulation.
Nonstress tests and biophysical profiles may be appropriate at 36 weeks or earlier as clinically indicated.

the prevention and treatment of VTE include warfarin, unfractionated heparin (UFH), LMWH, warfarin, factor Xa inhibitors, and direct thrombin inhibitors. However, heparins are the mainstay of therapy in pregnancy. UFH enhances antithrombin activity, increases factor Xa inhibitor activity, and inhibits platelet aggregation. LMWH is generated by chemical or enzymatic manipulation of UFH from a molecular weight of 15,000 Da to 4000–6500 Da. The smaller size impedes its antithrombin but not antifactor Xa effects. Both LMWH and UFH cross the placenta, are considered safe for pregnancy, and are compatible with breastfeeding. Complications associated with heparins include hemorrhage, osteoporosis, and thrombocytopenia. Heparin-induced thrombocytopenia (HIT) occurs in two forms. Type I HIT typically occurs within days of heparin exposure, is self-limited, and is not associated with significant risk of hemorrhage or thrombosis. Type II HIT is an immunoglobulin-mediated syndrome and occurs in the setting of venous or arterial thrombosis, usually 5–14 days following initiation of heparin therapy. Type II HIT can be confirmed by serotonin release assays, heparin-induced platelet aggregation assays, flow cytometry, or solid phase immunoassay.

UFH has a short half-life and is administered subcutaneously or via continuous infusion. Usually, patients receiving UFH require frequent laboratory monitoring and dosage adjustment. LMWH is administered subcutaneously either once or twice daily. It has advantages over UFH including better bioavailability, longer plasma half-life, more predictable pharmacokinetics and pharmacodynamics but LMWH is much more expensive than UFH. A recent review has found that LMWH has a reassuring risk profile, including antenatal bleeding 0.43 (0.22–0.75); postpartum hemorrhage >500 mL 0.94 (0.61–1.37); wound hematoma 0.61 (0.36–0.98); thrombocytopenia 0.11 (0.02–0.32); HIT 0.00 (0.00–0.11); and osteoporosis 0.04 (<0.01–0.20) [102]. Coumarins are vitamin K antagonists that block the generation of vitamin KH2. The latter serves as a cofactor for the post-translational carboxylation of glutamate residues to γ-carboxyglutamates on the N terminal regions of prothrombin and factors VII, IX, and X as well as the anticlotting agents, proteins C and S.

Several other anticoagulants are now available that may have a role in limited circumstances in pregnancy. Danaparoid is another low molecular weight heparinoid and is especially useful in cases of HIT and heparin allergy. Fondaparinux is a synthetic heparin pentasaccharide that complexes with the antithrombin binding site for heparin to permit the selective inactivation of factor Xa but not thrombin. Direct thrombin inhibitors represent another class of anticoagulants. Hirudin is a 65-amino-acid protein derived from the medicinal leech (*Hirudo medicinalis*). It can be used in patients with HIT-2 and is readily available in a recombinant form, lepirudin. Argatroban is a synthetic direct thrombin inhibitor that competitively binds to thrombin's active site, has a short half-life (45 minutes) and is cleared by the liver, making it the direct thrombin inhibitor of choice for patients with renal failure. Bivalirudin is a 20-amino acid synthetic polypeptide analog of hirudin.

For therapeutic dosing of LMWH, the anti-factor Xa level should be maintained at 0.6–1.0 U/mL 4–6 hours after injection (e.g., starting with 1 mg/kg enoxaparin subcutaneously every 12 hours). Again, treatment should continue for 20 weeks and then prophylactic doses given (e.g., 40 mg enoxaparin subcutaneously every 12 or 24 hours, adjusted to maintain antifactor Xa levels at 0.1–0.2 U/mL 4 hours after an injection). Patients with highly thrombogenic thrombophilias require therapeutic anticoagulation throughout pregnancy. Because regional anesthesia is contraindicated within 18–24 hours of LMWH administration, we recommend switching to UFH at 36 weeks or earlier if preterm delivery is expected. If vaginal or cesarean delivery occurs more than 12 hours from prophylactic or 24 hours from therapeutic doses of LMWH, anticoagulation-related problems with delivery are not anticipated. Protamine can partially reverse the anticoagulant effects of LMWH.

Patients with antithrombin deficiency represent the highest thrombogenic risk. Patients with antithrombin deficiency should receive antithrombin concentrate if they experience an acute arterial or venous thromboembolism. Human antithrombin III (AT-III) is available as Thrombate III® (Bayer Healthcare), a sterile, preservative-free, nonpyrogenic, biologically stable, lyophilized preparation of purified human antithrombin III. The baseline antithrombin level is expressed as the percent of the normal level based on the functional AT-III assay. The goal is to increase the antithrombin levels to those found in normal human plasma (around 100%).

Conclusions

Acquired and inherited thrombophilic conditions are associated with maternal thromboembolic events and a variety of APO. Suitable candidates for thrombophilia screening include: history of unexplained fetal loss at 10 weeks or more; history of severe preeclampsia/HELLP at less than 36 weeks; history of abruption; history of IUGR at 5th percentile or less; personal or family history of thrombosis. UFH and LMWH are the mainstay of treatment and prevention strategies to reduce the risk of thrombotic complications. Assessment of risk factors for thromboembolism will optimize treatment and prevention strategies and minimize hemorrhagic complications associated with anticoagulation. An adequate randomized, placebo controlled clinical trial is necessary to determine the optimal prevention strategy to prevent APO, particularly in the setting of inherited thrombophilic conditions. Limited evidence thus far suggests that antepartum prophylactic anticoagulation in the setting of heterozygous FVL or PGM and a prior history of past poor obstetric history improves the chances for success in a future pregnancy.

References

1 Paidas MJ, Ku DH, Langhoff-Roos J, Arkel YS. Inherited thrombophilias and adverse pregnancy outcome: screening and management. *Semin Perinatol* 2005;**29**:150–63.

2 Rand JH, Wu XX, Andree HA, *et al.* Pregnancy loss in the antiphospholipid-antibody syndrome: a possible thrombogenic mechanism. *N Engl J Med* 1997;**337**:154–60.

3 Bremme KA. Haemostatic changes in pregnancy. *Best Pract Res Clin Haematol* 2003;**16**:153–68.

4 Bremme K, Ostlund E, Almqvist I, Heinonen K, Blomback M. Enhanced thrombin generation and fibrinolytic activity in

normal pregnancy and the puerperium. *Obstet Gynecol* 1992;**80**:132–7.

5 Paidas MJ, Ku DW, Lee MJ, *et al.* Protein Z, protein S levels are lower in patients with thrombophilia and subsequent pregnancy complications. *J Thromb Haemost* 2005;**3**:497–501.

6 Schatz F, Lockwood CJ. Progestin regulation of plasminogen activator inhibitor type-1 in primary cultures of the endometrial stromal and decidual cells. *J Clin Endocrinol Metab* 1993;**77**: 621–5.

7 Lockwood CJ, Krikun G, Schatz F. The decidua regulates hemostasis in the human endometrium. *Semin Reprod Endocrinol* 1999;**17**:45–51.

8 Erlich J, Parry GC, Fearns C, *et al.* Tissue factor is required for uterine hemostasis and maintenance of the placental labyrinth during gestation. *Proc Natl Acad Sci USA* 1999;**96**:8138–43.

9 Egeberg O. Inherited antithrombin deficiency causing thrombophilia. *Thromb Diath Haemorrh* 1965;**13**:516–30.

10 Griffin JH, Evatt B, Zimmerman TS, *et al.* Deficiency of protein C in congenital thrombotic disease. *J Clin Invest* 1981;**68**:1370–3.

11 Comp PC, Nixon RR, Cooper DW, *et al.* Familial protein S deficiency is associated with recurrent thrombosis. *J Clin Invest* 1984;**74**:2082–8.

12 Dahlback B. Inherited resistance to activated protein C, a major cause of venous thrombosis, is due to a mutation in the factor V gene. *Haemostasis* 1994;**24**:139–51.

13 Ridker PM, Miletich JP, Hennekens CH, Buring JE. Ethnic distribution of factor V Leiden in 4047 men and women. Implications for venous thromboembolism screening. *JAMA* 1997;**277**:1305–7.

14 Lockwood CJ. Inherited thrombophilias in pregnant patients. *Prenat Neonat Med* 2001;**6**:3–14.

15 Voorberg J, Roeise J, Koopman R, *et al.* Association of idiopathic venous thromboembolism with single point-mutation at Arg 506 of factor V. *Lancet* 1994;**343**: 1535–6.

16 Dizon-Townson D, Miller C, Sibai B, *et al.* The relationship of the factor V Leiden mutation and pregnancy outcomes for mother and fetus. *Obstet Gynecol* 2005;**106**:517–24.

17 Poort SR. A common genetic variation in the 3'-untranslated region of the prothrombin gene is associated with elevated plasma prothrombin levels and an increase in venous thrombosis. *Blood* 1996;**88**:3698–703.

18 Gerhardt A, Eberhard Scharf R, Wilhelm Beckmann M, *et al.* Prothrombin and factor V mutations in women with a history of thrombosis during pregnancy and the puerperium. *N Engl J Med* 2000;**342**:374–80.

19 Dahlback B. Protein S and C4b-binding protein: components involved in the regulation of the protein C anticoagulant pathway. *Thromb Haemost* 1991;**66**:49–61.

20 Mosnier LO, Meijers JCM, Bouma BN. The role of protein S in the activation of TAFI and regulation of fibrinolysis. *Thromb Haemost* 2001;**86**:1035–9.

21 Dykes AC, Walker ID, McMahon AD, *et al.* A study of protein S antigen levels in 3788 healthy volunteers: influence of age, sex and hormone use, and estimate for prevalence of deficiency state. *Br J Haematol* 2001;**113**:636.

22 Comp PC, Thurnau GR, Welsh J, Esmon CT. Functional and immunologic protein S levels are decreased during pregnancy. *Blood* 1986;**68**:881–5.

23 Cumming AM, Tait RC, Fildes S, Yoong A, Keeney S, Hay CRM. Development of resistance to activated protein C during pregnancy. *Br J Haematol* 1995;**90**:725–7.

24 Sugimura M, Kobayashi T, Kanayama N, Terao T. Detection of decreased response to activated protein C during pregnancy by an endogenous thrombin potential-based assay. *Semin Thromb Hemost* 1999;**25**:497–502.

25 Greenberg DL, Davie EW. Blood coagulation factors. In: Colman RW, Hirsh J, Marder VJ, Clowes AW, eds. *Hemostasis and Thrombosis, Basic Principles and Clinical Practice*, 4th edn. Lippincott Williams & Wilkins, 2001.

26 Lockwood CJ. Inherited thrombophilias in pregnant patients: detection and treatment paradigm. *Obstet Gynecol* 2002;**99**:333–41.

27 Preston FE, Rosendaal FR, Walker ID, *et al.* Increased fetal loss in women with heritable thrombophilia. *Lancet* 1996;**348**: 913–6.

28 Rey E, Kahn SR, David M, Shrier I. Thrombophilic disorders and fetal loss: a meta-analysis. *Lancet* 2003;**361**:901–8.

29 Alfirevic Z. How strong is the association between maternal thrombophilia and adverse pregnancy outcome? A systematic review. *Eur J Obstet Gynecol Reprod Biol* 2002;**101**:6–14.

30 Han X, Fiehler R, Broze GJ Jr. Characterization of the protein Z-dependent protease inhibitor. *Blood* 2000;**96**:3049–55.

31 Kemkes-Matthes B, Matthes KJ. Protein Z. *Semin Thromb Hemost* 2001;**5**:551–6.

32 Broze GJ Jr. Protein Z-dependent regulation of coagulation. *Thromb Haemost* 2001;**86**:8–13.

33 Broze GJ Jr. Protein-Z and thrombosis. *Lancet* 2001;**357**:933–4.

34 Han X, Huang ZF, Fiehler R, Broze GJ Jr. The protein Z-dependent protease inhibitor is a serpin. *Biochemistry* 1999;**38**:11073–8.

35 Yurdakok M, Gurakan B, Ozbag E, Vigit S, Dundar S, Kirazli S. Plasma protein Z levels in healthy newborn infants. *Am J Hematol* 1995;**48**:206–7.

36 Miletich JP, Broze GJ Jr. Human plasma protein Z antigen: range in normal subjects and effect of warfarin therapy. *Blood* 1987;**69**:1580–6.

37 Kemkes-Matthes B, Nees M, Kuhnel G, Matzdorff A, Matthes KJ. Protein Z influences the prothrombotic phenotype in factor V Leiden patients. *Thromb Res* 2002;**106**:183–5.

38 McColl MD, Deans A, Maclean P, Tait RC, Greer IA, Walker ID. Plasma protein Z deficiency is common in women with antiphospholipid antibodies. *Br J Haematol* 2003;**120**:913–4.

39 Gris JC, Quere I, Dechaud H, *et al.* High frequency of protein Z deficiency in patients with unexplained early fetal loss. *Blood* 2002;**99**:2606–8.

40 Gris JC, Mercier E, Quere I I, *et al.* Low-molecular-weight heparin versus low-dose aspirin in women with one fetal loss and a constitutional thrombophilic disorder. *Blood* 2004;**103**:3695–9.

41 Hunt LT, Dayhoff MO. A surprising new protein superfamily containing ovalbumin, antithrombin-III, and alpha-1 proteinase inhibitor. *Biochem Biophys Res Commun* 1980;**95**:864–71.

42 Gettins P, Patston PA, Schapira M. Structure and mechanism of action of serpins. *Hematol Oncol Clin North Am* 1992;**6**:1393–408.

43 Andreasen PA, Georg B, Lund LR, Riccio A, Stacey SN. Plasminogen activator inhibitors: hormonally regulated serpins. *Mol Cell Endocrinol* 1990;**68**:1–19.

44 Kruithof EKO, Tran-Thang C, Gudinchet A, *et al*. Fibrinolysis in pregnancy: a study of plasminogen activator inhibitors. *Blood* 1987;**69**:460–6.

45 Gilabert J, Estelles A, Aznar J, *et al*. Contribution of platelets to increased plasminogen activator inhibitor type 1 in severe preeclampsia. *Thromb Haemost* 1990;**63**:361–6.

46 Astedt B, Lecander I, Ny T. The placental type plasminogen activator inhibitor, PAI-2. *Fibrinolysis* 1987;**1**:203–8.

47 Francis CW. Plasminogen activator inhibitor-1 levels and polymorphisms. *Arch Pathol Lab Med* 2002;**126**:1401–4.

48 Hefler L, Jirecek S, Heim K, *et al*. Genetic polymorphisms associated with thrombophilia and vascular disease in women with unexplained late intrauterine fetal death: a multicenter study. *J Soc Gynecol Invest* 2004;**11**:42–4.

49 Weiler H, Isermann BH. Thrombomodulin. *J Thromb Haemost* 2003;**1**:1515–24.

50 Paidas MJ, Ku DH, Lee MJ, Lockwood CJ, Arkel YS. Patients with thrombophilia and subsequent adverse pregnancy outcomes have a decreased first trimester response to thrombomodulin in an activated partial thromboplastin time (APTT) system. *J Thromb Haemost* 2004;**2**:840–1.

51 Foka ZJ, Lambropoulos AF, Saravelos H, *et al*. Factor V leiden and prothrombin G20210A mutations, but not methylenetetrahydrofolate reductase C677T, are associated with recurrent miscarriages. *Hum Reprod* 2000;**15**:458–62.

52 Roque H, Paidas MJ, Funai EF, Kuczynski E, Lockwood CJ. Maternal thrombophilias are not associated with early pregnancy loss. *Thromb Haemost* 2004;**91**:290–5.

53 Murphy RP, Donoghue C, Nallen RJ, *et al*. Prospective evaluation of the risk conferred by factor V Leiden and thermolabile methylenetetrahydrofolate reductase polymorphisms in pregnancy. *Arterioscler Thromb Vasc Biol* 2000;**20**:266–70.

54 Nelen WL, Blom HJ, Steegers EA, *et al*. Hyperhomocysteinemia and recurrent early pregnancy loss: a meta-analysis. *Fertil Steril* 2000;**74**:1196.

55 Langhoff-Roos J, Paidas MJ, Ku DH, Arkel YS, Lockwood CJ. Inherited thrombophilias and early pregnancy loss. In: Mor G, ed. *Immunology of Pregnancy*. Eurekah, UR.

56 Wilson WA, Gharavi AE, Koike T, *et al*. International consensus statement on preliminary classification criteria for definite antiphospholipid syndrome. *Arthritis Rheum* 1999;**42**:1309–11.

57 Galli M, Barbui T. Antiphospholipid antibodies and thrombosis: strength of association. *Hematol J* 2003;**4**:180–6.

58 Galli M, Luciani D, Bertolini G, Barbui T. Anti-beta 2-glycoprotein I, antiprothrombin antibodies, and the risk of thrombosis in the antiphospholipid syndrome. *Blood* 2003;**102**:2717–23.

59 Wahl DG, Guillemin F, de Maistre E, Perret C, Lecompte T, Thibaut G. Risk for venous thrombosis related to antiphospholipid antibodies in systemic lupus erythematosus: a meta-analysis. *Lupus* 1997;**6**:467–73.

60 Garcia-Fuster MJ, Fernandez C, Forner MJ, Vaya A. Risk factors and clinical characteristics of thromboembolic venous disease in young patients: a prospective study. *Med Clin (Barc)* 2004;**123**:217–9.

61 Branch DW, Silver RM, Blackwell JL, Reading JC, Scott JR. Outcome of treated pregnancies in women with antiphospholipid syndrome: an update of the Utah experience. *Obstet Gynecol* 1992;**80**:614–20.

62 Cervera R, Piette JC, Font J, *et al*. Euro-Phospholipid Project Group. Antiphospholipid syndrome: clinical and immunologic manifestations and patterns of disease expression in a cohort of 1,000 patients. *Arthritis Rheum* 2002;**46**:1019–27.

63 Branch DW, Silver RM. Criteria for antiphospholipid syndrome: early pregnancy loss, fetal loss or recurrent pregnancy loss? *Lupus* 1996;**5**:409–13.

64 Rai RS, Clifford K, Cohen H, Regan L. High prospective fetal loss rate in untreated pregnancies of women with recurrent miscarriage and antiphospholipid antibodies. *Hum Reprod* 1995;**10**:3301–4.

65 Lockwood C, Romero R, Feinberg R, Clyne L, Coster B, Hobbins J. The prevalence and biologic significance of lupus anticoagulant and anticardiolipin antibodies in a general obstetric population. *Am J Obstet Gynecol* 1989;**161**:369–73.

66 Field SL, Brighton TA, McNeil HP, Chesterman CN. Recent insights into antiphospholipid antibody-mediated thrombosis. *Baillieres Best Pract Res Clin Haematol* 1999;**12**:407–22.

67 Girardi G, Redecha P, Salmon JE. Heparin prevents antiphospholipid antibody-induced fetal loss by inhibiting complement activation. *Nat Med* 2004;**10**:1222–6.

68 Dekker GA, de Vries JI, Doelitzsch PM, *et al*. Underlying disorders associated with severe early-onset preeclampsia. *Am J Obstet Gynecol* 1995;**173**:1042–8.

69 Dizon-Townson DS, Nelson LM, Easton K, Ward K. The factor V Leiden mutation may predispose women to severe preeclampsia. *Am J Obstet Gynecol* 1996;**175**:902–5.

70 Kupferminc MJ, Eldor A, Steinman N, *et al*. Increased frequency of genetic thrombophilia in women with complications of pregnancy. *N Engl J Med* 1999;**340**:9.

71 Kupferminc MJ, Fait G, Many A, Gordon D, Eldor A, Lessing JB. Severe preeclampsia: high frequency of genetic thrombophilic mutations. *Obstet Gynecol* 2000;**96**:45–9.

72 Livingston JC, Barton JR, Park V, Haddad B, Phillips O, Sibai BM. Maternal and fetal inherited thrombophilias are not related to the development of severe preeclampsia. *Am J Obstet Gynecol* 2001;**185**:153–7.

73 Infante-Rivard C, Rivard GE, Yotov WV, *et al*. Absence of association of thrombophilia polymorphisms with intrauterine growth restriction. *N Engl J Med* 2002;**347**:19–25.

74 Howley HA. Systematic review: FVL or PGM and IUGR. *Am J Obstet Gynecol* 2005;**192**:694–708.

75 Kupferminc MJ, Many A, Bar-Am A, Lessing JB, Ascher-Landsberg J. Mid-trimester severe intrauterine growth restriction is associated with a high prevalence of thrombophilia. *Br J Obstet Gynaecol* 2002;**109**:1373–6.

76 deVries JI. Hyperhomocysteinaemia and protein S deficiency in complicated pregnancies. *Br J Obstet Gynaecol* 1997;**104**:1248–54.

77 Martinelli I. Familial thrombophilia and the occurrence of fetal growth restriction. *Haematologica* 2001;**86**:428–31.

78 Ananth CV, Smulian JC, Vintzileos AM. Incidence of placental abruption in relation to cigarette smoking and hypertensive disorders during pregnancy: a meta-analysis of observational studies. *Obstet Gynecol* 1999;**93**:622–8.

79 Addis A. Fetal effects of cocaine: an updated meta-analysis. *Reprod Toxicol* 2001;**15**:341–69.

80 Facchinetti F, Marozio L, Grandone E, Pizzi C, Volpe A, Benedetto C. Thrombophilic mutations are a main risk factor for placental abruption. *Haemotologica* 2003;**88**:785–8.

81 Gris JC, Quere I, Monpeyroux F, *et al*. Case–control study of the frequency of thrombophilic disorders in couples with late foetal loss and no thrombotic antecedent: the Nimes Obstetricians and Haematologists Study 5 (NOHA5). *Thromb Haemost* 1999;**81**:891–9.

82 Martinelli I, Taioli E, Cetin I, *et al*. Mutations in coagulation factors in women with unexplained late fetal loss. *N Engl J Med* 2000;**343**:1015–8.

83 Martinelli I, Taioli E, Cetin I, Mannucci PM. Recurrent late fetal death in women with and without thrombophilia. *Thromb Haemost* 2002;**87**:358–9.

84 Alonso A, Soto I, Urgelles MF, *et al*. Acquired and inherited thrombophilia in women with unexplained fetal losses. *Am J Obstet Gynecol* 2002;**187**:1337–42.

85 Gonen R, Lavi N, Attias D, *et al*. Absence of association of inherited thrombophilia with unexplained third-trimester intrauterine fetal death. *Am J Obstet Gynecol* 2005;**192**:742–6.

86 Kujovich JL. Thrombophilia and pregnancy complications. *Am J Obstet Gynecol* 2004;**191**:412–24

87 Jivraj S, Rai R, Underwood J, Regan L. Genetic thrombophilic mutations among couples with recurrent miscarriage. *Hum Reprod* 2006; epub Jan 23.

88 Kupferminc MJ, Peri H, Zwang E, Yaron Y, Wolman I, Eldor A. High prevalence of the prothrombin gene mutation in women with intrauterine growth retardation, abruptio placentae and second trimester loss. *Acta Obstet Gynecol Scand* 2000;**79**:963–7.

89 Greer IA. Thrombophilia: implications for pregnancy outcome. *Thromb Res* 2003;**109**:73–81.

90 Stanley-Christian H, Ghidini A, Sacher R, Shemirani M. Fetal genotype for specific inherited thrombophilias is not associated with severe preeclampsia. *J Soc Gynecol Invest* 2005;**12**:198–201.

91 Vefring H, Lie RT, O'Degard R, Mansoor MA, Nilsen ST. Maternal and fetal variants of genetic thrombophilias and the risk of preeclampsia. *Epidemiology* 2004;**15**:317–22.

92 Kupferminc M, Fait G, Many A, *et al*. Low molecular weight heparin for the prevention of obstetric complications in women with thrombophilia. *Hypertens Pregnancy* 2001;**20**:35–44.

93 Riyazi N, Leeda M, de Vries JI, Huijgens PC, van Geijn HP, Dekker GA. Low-molecular-weight heparin combined with aspirin in pregnant women with thrombophilia and a history of preeclampsia or fetal growth restriction: a preliminary study. *Eur J Obstet Gynecol Reprod Biol* 1998;**80**:49–54.

94 Paidas M, Ku DH, Triche E, Lockwood C, Arkel Y. Does heparin therapy improve pregnancy outcome in patients with thrombophilias? *J Thromb Haemost* 2004;**2**:1194–5.

95 Brenner B, Hoffman R, Carp H, Dulitsky M, Younis J. LIVE-ENOX Investigators. Efficacy and safety of two doses of enoxaparin in women with thrombophilia and recurrent pregnancy loss: the LIVE-ENOX study. *J Thromb Haemost* 2005;**3**:227–9.

96 Walker MC, Ferguson SE, Allen VM. Cochrane Review. In: *The Cochrane Library*, Issue 4, 2003.

97 Nisio M, Peters LW, Middeldorp S. Anticoagulants for the treatment of recurrent pregnancy loss in women without antiphospholipid syndrome [Review]. *Cochrane Database Syst Rev* 2005;**2**:CD004734.

98 Tulppala M, Marttunen M, Soderstrom-Anttila V, *et al*. Low-dose aspirin in prevention of miscarriage in women with unexplained or autoimmune related recurrent miscarriage: effect on prostacyclin and thromboxane A_2 production. *Hum Reprod* 1997;**12**:1567–72.

99 Empson M, Lassere M, Craig JC, Scott JR. Recurrent pregnancy loss with antiphospholipid antibody: a systematic review of therapeutic trials. *Obstet Gynecol* 2002;**99**:135–44.

100 Mello G, Parretti E, Fatini C, *et al*. Low-molecular-weight heparin lowers the recurrence rate of preeclampsia and restores the physiological vascular changes in angiotensin-converting enzyme DD women. *Hypertension* 2005;**45**:86–91.

101 Wu O, Robertson L, Langhorne P, *et al*. Oral contraceptives, hormone replacement therapy, thrombophilias and risk of venous thromboembolism: a systematic review: the Thrombosis Risk and Economic Assessment of Thrombophilia Screening (TREATS) study. *Thromb Haemost* 2005;**94**:17–25.

102 Greer IA, Nelson-Percy C. Safety and efficacy of LMWH: thromboprophylaxis and treatment of venous thromboembolism. *Blood* 2005;**106**:401–7.

103 ACOG. Clinical Updates in Women's Health: Thrombosis, Thrombophilia and Thromboembolism in Women. in Press.

16 Pathophysiology and diagnosis of thromboembolic disorders in pregnancy

Christian M. Pettker and Charles J. Lockwood

Complicating 1 in 1000 to 1 in 2000 pregnancies, venous thromboembolism (VTE) is a leading cause of maternal morbidity and mortality [1–9]. Moreover, despite its seemingly low prevalence, pregnancy confers a nearly 10-fold increased risk of VTE in women of childbearing age. The majority of VTE events occur in the antepartum period, with an even distribution across each trimester [1,3,10–12]. However, the risk of VTE is approximately three- to eightfold higher postpartum compared to an equivalent antepartum period [9]. Pulmonary embolism (PE) is the leading cause of maternal mortality, contributing to 19.6% of such deaths, translating into 2.3 pregnancy-related deaths per 100,000 live births [13]. An untreated deep vein thrombosis (DVT) presents a 25% risk of PE, with a mortality rate of approximately 15% if undetected and untreated [14]. On the other hand, if a DVT is promptly diagnosed and treated, the risk of PE is less than 5% and the risk of maternal mortality is less than 1% [15].

From a teleologic perspective, the increased risk of pregnancy-associated VTE reflects local and systemic mechanisms designed to avoid hemorrhage during the astonishing level of maternal uterine vessel disruption that occurs during placentation and the third stage of labor. Appreciation of the thrombotic risk of pregnancy demands knowledge of the sophisticated systems of coagulation and fibrinolysis and their inhibitors.

Physiology of hemostasis

Platelet plug formation

Vasoconstriction and platelet aggregation are the initial controls on hemorrhage following vascular disruption, particularly in arteries. Vasoconstriction limits blood flow to promote platelet plug formation. Vasoconstriction also limits the size of the requisite plug required to obstruct blood flow through the vascular defect. Circulating von Willebrand factor mediates platelet attachment by binding to platelet glycoprotein (GP) GPIb/IX/V receptors and to subendothelial collagen in damaged vessels [16]. Integrins, an alternative set of extracellular matrix adhering receptors on platelet cell membranes, adhere to subendothelial laminin, fibronectin, and vitronectin. Platelet adhesion then triggers calcium-dependent protein kinase C (PKC) activation that induces thromboxane A2 (TXA2) synthesis and platelet granule release. The α-granules contain various clotting factors while dense-granules contain adenosine diphosphate (ADP) and serotonin, which combine with TXA2 to exacerbate vasoconstriction and platelet activation. The latter activates platelet GPIIB/IIIa receptors to promote aggregation by forming interplatelet fibrinogen, fibronectin, and vitronectin bridges [17]. Platelets can also be activated by epinephrine, arachidonic acid, and platelet-activating factor. Platelet aggregation in the setting of intact endothelium is prevented by active blood flow and prostacyclin, nitric oxide, and ADPase.

The coagulation cascade

Platelet-plug aggregation in the absence of fibrin generation is inadequate to control the hemorrhage attendant on significant vascular injury. Thus, adequate hemostasis also requires fibrin plug formation which follows exposure of circulating factor VII to perivascular tissue factor (TF) (Fig. 16.1) [18]. TF is a cell membrane-bound glycoprotein, constitutively expressed by most nonendothelial cells and induced by progesterone in decidualized endometrial stromal cells [18,19]. It is also present in high levels in the amniotic fluid. The latter accounts for the coagulopathy observed in amniotic fluid embolism [20,21]. Following vascular injury, perivascular TF binds circulating factor VII which attaches to negatively charged phospholipids via divalent calcium ions. Factor VII is autoactivated after binding to TF and can be externally activated by thrombin, factors IXa, Xa, or XIIa [18]. (The activated form of clotting factors is denoted by the letter "a" after the Roman numeral.) The TF/VIIa complex can directly activate factor X (Fig. 16.1) or indirectly activate Xa by activating factor

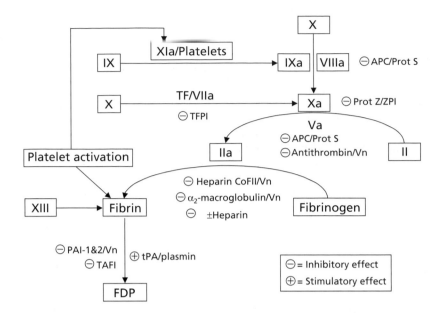

Fig. 16.1 An outline of the mechanisms defining the careful balance of thrombosis and hemostasis versus anticoagulation and fibrinolysis. APC, activated protein C; PAI-1, plasminogen activator inhibitor 1; TF, tissue factor; TFPI, tissue factor pathway inhibitor; TAFI, thrombin activatable fibrinolysis inhibitor; Vn, vitronectin; ZPI, protein Z-dependent protease inhibitor.

IX (IXa) which then complexes with its cofactor, VIIIa, to activate factor X. Factor Xa next complexes with its cofactor, Va, to convert prothrombin (factor II) to thrombin (factor IIa), which converts fibrinogen to fibrin. The cofactors V and VIII are activated by either thrombin or factor Xa. Thrombin, kallikrein-kininogen, and plasmin can each activate factor XII on the surface of platelets (Fig. 16.1). Factor XIIa can activate factor XI, providing another route of factor IX activation. All of these reactions occur on negatively charged phospholipids and require ionized calcium. Ultimately, thrombin cleaves fibrinogen to fibrin monomers which self-polymerize and are cross-linked via thrombin-activated factor XIIIa.

Endogenous anticoagulants

The counterpoint preventing inappropriate activation of the hemostatic system is the anticoagulant system (Fig. 16.1). The TF pathway inhibitor (TFPI) is the first agent in this system and acts on the factor Xa/TF/VIIa complex to inhibit TF-mediated clotting [22]. However, factor XIa can bypass this block and sustain clotting for some time. As a result, additional endogenous anticoagulant molecules are required to avoid thrombosis, including activated protein C, protein S, and protein Z. Thrombin binds thrombomodulin on perturbed endothelial cell membranes producing a conformational change that allows activation of protein C [23]. Activated protein C (APC) also binds to anionic endothelial cell membrane phospholipids or to the endothelial cell protein C receptor (EPCR) to inactivate factors Va and VIIIa [24]. Protein S serves as a cofactor

for both Va and VIIIa inactivation by APC. Protein Z-dependent protease inhibitor (ZPI) can also impede factor Xa activity. When bound to its cofactor, protein Z, the inhibitory activity of ZPI is increased 1000-fold [25].

Serine protease inhibitors (SERPINs), which include heparin cofactor II, α_2-macroglobulin and antithrombin, account for most of the thrombin inhibitory activity of plasma (Fig. 16.1). Antithrombin alone accounts for 80% of plasma antithrombin activity and also inactivates factors IXa, Xa, and Xia [26]. Heparins and vitronectin bind to SERPINs and together augment anticoagulant activity 1000-fold [27,28].

Fibrinolysis

Fibrinolysis is initiated by tissue-type plasminogen activator (tPA), embedded in fibrin, which cleaves plasminogen to generate plasmin. Plasmin, in turn, cleaves fibrin into fibrin degradation products (FDPs), which are often used clinically as indirect measures of fibrinolysis. These FDPs can also inhibit thrombin action, a favorable result when limited, but when generated in excess can contribute to disseminated intravascular coagulation. Inhibitors of fibrinolysis include α_2-plasmin inhibitor and type 1 and 2 plasminogen activator inhibitors (PAI-1 and PAI-2) which inactivate tPA. The endothelium and uterine decidua are primary sources of PAI-1 while the placenta produces PAI-2 [29]. The thrombin-activatable fibrinolysis inhibitor (TAFI) modifies fibrin to render it resistant to inactivation by plasmin [30].

Pathophysiology and risk factors of thrombosis in pregnancy

Risk factors not unique to pregnancy include age over 35 years, obesity, immobility, infection, smoking, nephrotic syndrome, hyperviscosity syndromes, malignancies, trauma, surgery, orthopedic procedures, and a prior history of VTE [31]. Pregnancy-specific risk factors include increased parity, endomyometritis, and cesarean and operative vaginal delivery.

Virchows triad—vascular stasis, hypercoagulability, and vascular trauma—is present in pregnancy. Increases in deep vein capacitance secondary to increased circulating levels of estrogen and endothelial production of prostacyclin and nitric oxide, coupled with compression of the inferior vena cava and pelvic veins by the enlarging uterus, all promote venous stasis [32–34]. Not surprisingly, the incidence of thrombosis is greater in the left than in the right leg [1,11,35].

Changes in decidual and systemic hemostatic systems occur in pregnancy, likely to meet the hemorrhagic challenges poised by implantation, placentation, and the third stage of labor. Decidual TF and PAI-1 expression are increased in response to progesterone, and levels of placental PAI-2, which are negligible prior to pregnancy, increase until term [29,30]. By term, circulating levels of fibrinogen double and levels of factors VII, VIII, IX, X, XII, and von Willebrand factor increase 20–1000% [36,37]. Additionally, levels of protein S decrease by approximately 40%, conferring an overall resistance to APC [36]. Further reductions in free protein S concentrations are seen after cesarean delivery and in the context of infection, accounting for the higher rate of PE in such patients. In general, normalization of these coagulation parameters occurs by 6 weeks postpartum. While these mechanisms generally prevent puerperal hemorrhage, they predispose to thrombosis, a tendency aggravated by maternal thrombophilias.

Vascular trauma occurs in particular at the time of delivery, with the disruption of the placental–uterine interface and the trauma of operative vaginal and cesarean delivery. Cesarean delivery in particular is associated with a ninefold increase in the risk of thromboembolism compared with vaginal delivery [10].

Diagnosis of venous thromboembolism

Deep venous thrombosis

Risk assessment

The signs and symptoms of DVT include erythema, warmth, pain, edema, tenderness, and a palpable cord corresponding to the thrombosed vein. Pain and tenderness may be elicited

upon squeezing the calf muscles ("Homan sign"). The specificity of these findings is less than 50% and the diagnosis of DVT is confirmed by objective testing in only one-third of patients with these signs [38,39]. The differential diagnosis of these signs and symptoms is broad and includes cellulitis, ruptured or strained muscle or tendon, trauma, ruptured popliteal (Baker) cyst, cutaneous vasculitis, superficial thrombophlebitis, and lymphedema. As a result, any patient presenting with these features should be completely evaluated with objective testing.

Clinical features coupled with underlying risk factors should be used to assess the likelihood of DVT in order to improve the diagnostic values of the various tests. This concept guides the diagnostic algorithm outlined for DVT in Fig. 16.2. Wells *et al.* [40,41] have developed an individualized risk model based on specific clinical features and risk factors that may factor into a patient's presentation (Table 16.1). Based on this model, patients are divided into three pretest probabilities: high (≥3), moderate (<3 but >0), and low (= 0), with prevalence of DVT of 85%, 33%, and 5%, respectively. Wells *et al.*'s criteria are the most frequently used pretest evaluation, with a high negative predictive value (median 96%, range 87–100%), although this screening system has not been validated in pregnant patients, and pregnancy itself, given its thrombogenic nature, may add another point to the score [42].

d-dimer assays

The d-dimer assays are useful as both screening tools and initial tests. d-dimers are the products of degradation of fibrin by plasmin, and levels can be elevated in the setting of thrombosis. d-dimer testing employs monoclonal antibodies to d-dimer fragments with the most accurate and reliable tests being two rapid ELISAs (Instant-IA d-dimer, Stago, Asniéres,

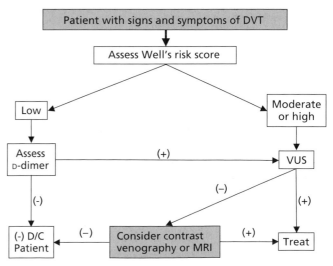

Fig. 16.2 Patient with signs and symptoms of deep vein thrombosis (DVT).

Table 16.1 Deep vein thrombosis (DVT) clinical characteristic score. After Wells *et al.* [40,41].

Risk or Sign	Points
Active cancer	+1
Immobilization (cast, paralysis, paresis)	+1
Bed rest >3 days or surgery within 12 weeks	+1
Local tenderness along deep venous system	+1
Entire leg swollen	+1
Asymmetric calf swelling >3 cm (10 cm below tibial tuberosity)	+1
Pitting edema only in symptomatic leg	+1
Collateral nonvaricose superficial veins	+1
Prior DVT	+1
Alternative diagnosis at least as likely as DVT	−2

France and VIDAS DD, bioMérieux, Marcy-l'Etoile, France) and a rapid whole blood assay (SimpliRED D-dimer, Agen Biomedical, Brisbane, Australia).

While D-dimer testing should not be used as a diagnostic test in place of the imaging modalities [43,44], a recent prospective, randomized study by Wells *et al.* [41] suggests that use of highly accurate D-dimer assay in conjunction with a clinical risk scoring system (Table 16.1) is an effective initial step in excluding DVT in symptomatic patients. This study showed that follow-up with lower extremity venous ultrasound—a test with proven sensitivity—was not necessary in those patients with low pretest probability based on risk scoring and negative D-dimer results. Furthermore, these patients had a very low incidence of subsequent thrombosis. While none of these studies evaluated D-dimer testing in pregnant patients, many factors related to pregnancy as well as the postoperative puerperal state will contribute to high rates of false positive results [45,46]. Thus, D-dimer testing in pregnancy is likely to have a higher negative predictive value given the higher rate of false positive results. For this reason, we suggest that it may have a role in the initial triage of patients with suspected DVT for ruling out disease.

Venous imaging

Intravenous contrast venography has a high sensitivity and specificity for the diagnosis of DVT [47]. It requires injection of a radio-opaque dye into a vein below the site of suspected thrombosis followed by X-rays seeking evidence of intraluminal filling defects. However, contrast venography cannot be performed in up to 20% of patients as a result of technical difficulty and patient intolerance of the test [48] and the risks of radiation and contrast allergy (up to 5%) preclude its use as a screening test in pregnancy [49]. Venous ultrasonography (VUS) with or without color Doppler is the preferred initial imaging modality. It requires sonographic

imaging of the common femoral vein at the inguinal ligament, and then assessment of the other major venous systems of the leg, including the greater saphenous, the superficial femoral, and the popliteal veins to the deep veins of the calf. Pressure is applied to the transducer to determine the compressibility of the vein lumen under duplex and color flow Doppler imaging [38]. The overall sensitivity and specificity of VUS approach 100% for proximal vein thromboses [50] with slightly less efficacy for detecting isolated calf vein DVT (sensitivity 92.5%, specificity 98.7%, and accuracy 97.2%) [51].

Magnetic resonance imaging (MRI) is an excellent, albeit expensive, alternative to VUS, with a sensitivity and specificity approaching 100% for the diagnosis of acute, lower extremity DVT [52]. Further advocating for its use, MRI is even more sensitive and accurate than VUS in the detection of pelvic and calf DVTs. In a prospective trial, MR venography even performed as well as contrast venography [53].

Diagnostic algorithm for suspected DVT

Based on the available data, we propose the diagnostic algorithm in Fig. 16.2 that allows the diagnosis of DVT with highest sensitivity and specificity. We suggest the initial use of the clinical risk score and D-dimer to classify and rule out patients with low pretest probability. When the D-dimer test is unavailable or inappropriate, the testing algorithm should begin with lower extremity compression VUS and the steps followed as outlined.

Pulmonary embolus

Risk assessment

As in DVT, the signs and symptoms of PE are sensitive but not specific. Its clinical hallmarks are tachypnea and tachycardia which are present in up to 90% of affected patients but are nonspecific [54]. Presyncope and syncope are rare, although these signs indicate a massive and potentially fatal embolus [55]. As in DVT, a scoring system can be used to stratify high- and low-risk populations to generate a pretest probability and help with the accuracy of subsequent diagnostic tests. Fedullo and Tapson [55] suggest the system shown in Table 16.2, grouping patients into three risk sets—low (cumulative score <2), intermediate (score 2–6), and high (score >6)—with prevalences of PE of ≤10%, 30%, and ≥70%, respectively [55]. A recent modification of this score is suggested and validated by van Belle *et al.* [56] who categorized patients into those with scores ≤4 ("PE unlikely") or >4 ("PE likely"). As in DVT, these protocols should be applied cautiously in pregnant patients, as they have only been validated in nonpregnant subjects and it is arguable that pregnancy should elevate the risk score even further.

Table 16.2 Pulmonary embolism (PE) clinical characteristic score. After Fedullo and Tapson [55].

Risk or Sign	Points
Clinical signs and symptoms of DVT	+3
Alternative diagnosis deemed less likely than PE	+3
Heart rate >100 beats/min	+1.5
Immobilization or surgery in previous 4 weeks	+1.5
Prior VTE	+1.5
Hemoptysis	+1
Active cancer	+1

DVT, deep vein thrombosis; VTE, venous thromboembolism.

Nonspecific studies

Traditional investigations of patients with suspected PE have included electrocardiogram (ECG), arterial blood gases (ABG), chest X-ray (CXR), and echocardiography. Abnormalities of the ECG may be present in 70–90% of patients with proven PE who do not have underlying cardiopulmonary disease, but these findings are generally nonspecific [57,58]. The classic ECG changes associated with PE are S1, Q3, and inverted T3, but other findings such as nonspecific ST changes, right bundle branch block, or right axis deviation may also be present. These latter findings are usually associated with cor pulmonale and right heart strain or overload, reflective of more serious cardiopulmonary compromise. The Urokinase Pulmonary Embolism Trial found that 26–32% of patients with massive PE had the above ECG changes [57]. A scoring criteria based on ECG changes was proposed by Sreeram *et al.* [59] to aid in the diagnosis of PE with ECG, but this approach has not been validated by prospective studies [60]. A lack of ECG changes should not reassure the physician who has a reasonable suspicion of PE.

The ABG and oxygen saturation have limited value in the assessment for PE, particularly in a pregnant population. Measurements of Po_2 are greater than 80 mmHg in 29% of PE patients less than 40 years old, although in patients over 40 years, only 3% of patients with PE have such values, suggesting that this is a useful test only in older populations and is not likely applicable to pregnancy [61]. In another study, up to 18% of patients with PE had Po_2 measurements of >85 mmHg [54]. The alveolar–arteriolar (A-a) oxygen tension difference appears to be a more useful indicator of disease with A-a gradients of >20 mmHg present in 86% of patients with PE, although up to 6% of patients with APE in this same study had normal gradients [54].

The CXR may be abnormal—with pleural effusion, infiltrates, atelectasis, and elevated hemidiaphragm—in up to 84% of affected patients [54]. Traditional findings of pulmonary infarction such as a wedge-shaped infiltrate ("Hampton hump") or decreased vascularity ("Westermark sign") are rare [47]. The CXR may be valuable in ruling out other causes of hypoxemia, such as pulmonary edema or pneumonia. Thus, while a normal CXR in the setting of dyspnea, tachypnea, and hypoxemia in a patient without pre-existent pulmonary or cardiovascular disease is suggestive of PE, a chest radiograph cannot confirm the diagnosis [47].

PE can create changes consistent with cor pulmonale and right heart strain, occasionally seen on echocardiography. Abnormalities of right ventricular size or function on echocardiogram are seen in 30–80% of patients with PE although similar changes can be seen in exacerbations of chronic obstructive pulmonary disease [62–64]. Typical echocardiographic findings include a dilated and hypokinetic right ventricle or tricuspid regurgitation, in the absence of pre-existing pulmonary arterial or left heart pathology. These findings indicate a large embolus and poor prognosis. Transesophageal echocardiography improves the sensitivity of diagnosing main or right pulmonary artery emboli [65].

Pulmonary arteriography

In the past, intravenous contrast pulmonary arteriography or angiography was considered the gold standard for diagnosis of PE. Given this, it is considered to have a sensitivity and specificity of 100%, although the sensitivity for smaller peripheral lesions decreases from 98% for lobar emboli, to 90% for segmental and 66% for subsegmental emboli [47,66]. Angiography involves venous catheterization through the femoral, basilic, or internal jugular veins and imaging with fluoroscopy with a filling defect on two X-ray views of a pulmonary artery confirming the diagnosis. Of all diagnostic modalities for PE, this technique involves the highest risk, including a 0.5% mortality risk and a 3% complication rate, primarily as a result of the risks of contrast injection and catheter placement, including respiratory failure (0.4%), renal failure (0.3%), cardiac perforation (1%), and groin hematoma requiring transfusion (0.2%) [55,66–68]. Relative contraindications to the procedure include renal failure and significant hemorrhage risk (e.g., disseminated intravascular coagulation or thrombocytopenia), while patients with evidence of cardiopulmonary compromise also pose higher complication risks. Given this, we do not suggest the use of pulmonary arteriography in the initial stages of PE work-up, but rather only after all other available modalities have not effectively ruled out PE in high-risk patients.

D-dimer assays

As with evaluation of DVT, D-dimer is a sensitive, but not specific, test for PE and likely has a role as a screening test in the initial stages of PE work-up in low-risk patients. A negative D-dimer concentration (<500 ng/mL), measured by sensitive enzyme-linked immunosorbent assay (ELISA), is associated with a 95% negative predictive value, but only a 25% specificity, for the diagnosis of PE in nonpregnant patients [47]. A meta-analysis of studies examining the accuracy of D-dimer in the diagnosis of PE in nonpregnant patients showed a sensitivity of 95% (88–100%), specificity of 45% (38–53%), and positive and negative likelihood ratios of 1.74 (1.55–1.91) and 0.11 (0.03–0.39), respectively [69]. The quantitative ELISA assay has a higher sensitivity (98% vs. 82%) but lower specificity (40% vs. 63%) than the whole blood assay [69]. Because of increased concentrations of D-dimer in pregnancy and after surgery, the specificity is likely even better for each test in antepartum and postpartum patients. Thus, a negative D-dimer in a pregnant patient may effectively rule out PE in pregnancy. In conclusion, D-dimer testing, where available and in patients at low risk, may be a high-yield test to rule out PE in pregnancy.

Ventilation–perfusion scanning

In the past, the ventilation–perfusion (V/Q) scan had a critical role in the diagnosis of PE. This test uses comparative imaging of the pulmonary vascular bed and airspaces using intravenous and aerosolized radiolabeled markers [38]. The comparison of the resultant two images allows for differential diagnostic probabilities (high, intermediate, low, or normal). Because the results are reported in probabilities, interpretation relies on pretest risk scoring (similar to that described above) based on the signs, symptoms, and other diagnostic tests. More than 90% of high-risk patients with high-probability V/Q scans have PEs while less than 6% of low-risk patients with low-probability scans have a PE.

The PIOPED (Prospective Investigation of Pulmonary Embolism Diagnosis) study evaluated the accuracy of V/Q scanning in nearly 1000 patients (nonpregnant) with suspected PE [58]. Overall, high-probability V/Q scans correlated with PE in 87.2% of cases; however, only 41% of patients with PE had high-probability scans, yielding a sensitivity of 41% and a specificity of 97%. When patients were classified according to pretest risk, high-probability V/Q results were associated with PE in 95%, 86%, and 56% of high, moderate, and low-risk patients, respectively. Overall, intermediate probability, low probability, and normal scans were associated each with 33.3%, 13.5%, and 3.9% risks of PE, respectively. Accordingly, PE can be present in a substantial proportion of patients with low and intermediate probability results if the pretest risk is high and as many as 44% of low-risk patients with a high probability will not have PE. This emphasizes the importance of pretest risk stratification of the patient undergoing work-up for PE but also points out the limitations of the V/Q scan as a diagnostic modality. In cases of nondiagnostic V/Q results, further tests are necessary to avoid catastrophic consequences of undiagnosed PE or the hazards and inconveniences of unnecessary anticoagulation. In practice, fewer and fewer centers make available V/Q scanning and it is being rapidly displaced by computed tomography (CT) and MRI techniques.

Spiral computed tomographic pulmonary angiography

Spiral computed tomographic pulmonary angiography (spiral CT) scanning has emerged as the primary diagnostic modality for PE. This test uses intravenous contrast injection to visualize the pulmonary vasculature during scanning with highly sensitive multidetector-row CT technology [47]. Sensitivity of this testing is high for large vessel emboli, but limited in small subsegmental vessels or vessels oriented horizontally (e.g., in the right middle lobe). Given its broad diagnostic capabilities, CT can be helpful in detecting nonembolic etiologies for the patient's signs and symptoms, such as pneumonia or pulmonary edema. Comparisons of spiral CT with V/Q scanning for patients with suspected PE shows higher accuracy for the former modality (90% vs. 54%), without any difference in the overall rate of detection of PE for each group [70]. Further meta-analysis of 23 studies showed a very low 3-month rate of subsequent venous thromboembolism and fatal PE after a negative spiral CT (1.4% and 0.51%, respectively) which approximates a negative pulmonary angiogram or a normal or near-normal V/Q scan [71]. Newer technology and thinner CT sections appear to improve the accuracy of spiral CT for diagnosing small-vessel emboli and may reduce overall false negative results to 5% [72].

Magnetic resonance angiography

Magnetic resonance angiography (MRA) uses intravenous gadolinium injection during MRI to visualize the pulmonary vasculature. This modality was initially limited by movement artefact but faster technology and improved capabilities of image acquisition allow for timing to respiratory and cardiac motion ("gating"), allowing it to develop into a powerful tool for diagnosis of PE. Initial studies (in 30 patients) showed a sensitivity and specificity of 100% and 95% and positive and negative predictive values of 87% and 100%, respectively, for MRA in comparison with pulmonary arteriography [73]. However, a prospective study involving 141 patients showed an overall sensitivity of only 77% in comparison with pulmonary angiography, with the sensitivity broken down to 40%, 84%, and 100% for isolated subsegmental, segmental, and central pulmonary emboli, respectively [74]. As MRA does not involve ionizing radiation, it is an appealing alternative to CT scanning and angiography for pregnancy, but further assessment in large trials will prove its ultimate utility as a primary diagnostic modality.

Lower extremity VUS evaluation

Approximately 90% of all pulmonary emboli arise from lower extremity DVTs and among patients with PE, half will have a lower extremity DVT, including 20% of PE patients without signs or symptoms of lower extremity DVT [55]. Thus, in stable high-risk patients in whom V/Q scanning or other non-invasive testing is nondiagnostic or even negative, evaluation of the leg veins for DVT can establish the need for anticoagulation. However, in such cases, a negative VUS study is still associated with a 25% risk of PE, suggesting that further studies are generally needed [75].

Work-up of patients with suspected PE

Evaluation of patients with suspected PE should begin with a pretest risk determination, as described earlier (Table 16.2). A proposed diagnostic algorithm for PE is outlined in Fig. 16.3. This approach incorporates pretest risk assessment and D-dimer testing in the initial triage of patients, as suggested by the work of van Belle *et al.* [56]. Their research involved a large, prospective, observational study of over 3000 nonpregnant patients with clinical suspicion of PE to evaluate the diagnostic value of risk scoring, D-dimer testing, and spiral CT scanning. This algorithm classified risk as either "PE unlikely" (Table 16.2 score ≤4) or "PE likely" (Table 16.2 score >4). Those classified as "unlikely" had D-dimer testing, and PE was ruled out if the D-dimer test result was normal (one-third of patients overall). These patients avoided additional testing, with a rate of subsequent VTE (all nonfatal) of 0.5% in 3 months. All other patients (i.e., "PE likely", plus those initially described as "PE unlikely" with positive D-dimer results) underwent sensitive spiral CT scanning. A PE was considered present or excluded based on the CT results. In the two-thirds of patients requiring spiral CT, a PE was detected in 20.4%, and these patients received treatment. Of the remaining 45.5% of patients in whom the CT angiogram was negative, 95% were not treated and the prevalence of subsequent fatal PE was less than 1%, a risk that is comparable to the

rate of fatal PE after a negative intravenous contrast pulmonary angiogram. This very simple diagnostic paradigm employing a simple clinical assessment, D-dimer testing, and CT angiography may also be an efficient and effective diagnostic approach in pregnancy. However, these results, as well as this use of D-dimer testing and the risk scoring system, have not been validated in pregnancy. The approach described in Fig. 16.3 retains the option of employing traditional pulmonary angiography or MRA imaging in high-risk pregnant patients in whom the spiral CT is negative but where clinical suspicion persists. However, some radiology departments may have sufficient confidence in their spiral CT sensitivity to forgo contrast pulmonary angiography altogether. Consultation with a radiologist before ordering these tests is highly recommended.

In short, there is growing consensus that because of its wide application, high accuracy, and increasing experience, spiral CT scanning should be the initial modality of choice. In patients with concomitant symptoms of DVT, these tests may be delayed following lower extremity VUS examination, as the documentation of lower extremity DVT will require anticoagulation regardless of the pulmonary findings.

Fetal risks of radiation exposure

Fetal ionizing radiation exposure during the work-up of DVT and PE is a concern for the clinician and patient. The American College of Obstetricians and Gynecologists (ACOG) contends that exposure to less than 5 rad is not associated with increases in pregnancy loss or fetal anomalies [76]. However, exposure to doses above 1 rad may create a slightly increased risk of childhood leukemia (from 1 in 3000 baseline to 1 in 2000) [77,78]. Table 16.3 provides the radiation exposure of various radiation modalities. A traditional combination of CXR, V/Q scan, and pulmonary angiography—an extensive work-up

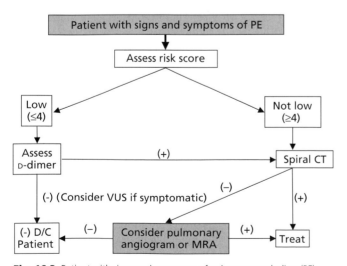

Fig. 16.3 Patient with signs and symptoms of pulmonary embolism (PE).

Table 16.3 Fetal radiation exposure of various ionizing modalities. After Toglia and Weg [6].

Radiological Modality	Fetal Radiation Exposure (rad)
Chest X-ray	<0.01
Venography	
Limited, shielded	<0.05
Full (unilateral), unshielded	0.31
Pulmonary angiography	
Brachial vein	0.05
Femoral vein	0.22–0.37
V/Q scan	
Ventilation scan	0.001–0.019
Perfusion scan	0.006–0.012
Spiral CT	0.013

CT, computed tomography; V/Q, ventilation–perfusion.

nonetheless—exposes the fetus to less than 0.5 rad [6]. The clinician should be aware of these exposure guidelines and thoughtfully use the appropriate tests that will safely provide a diagnosis.

Because of a potential effect of maternal radiographic contrast on the fetal thyroid gland (goiter), hyperthyroidism should be ruled out with fetal heart rate checks in the antepartum period and thyroid function tests in the neonatal period [79]. Ultrasonography has not been associated with any adverse fetal effects. There is also no evidence that MRI, particularly with magnets of ≤1.5 tesla, or gadolinium exposure contributes to any risk to the fetus [79].

Conclusions

Avoidance of hemorrhage and thrombosis presents paradoxical challenges to the pregnant patient. Processes promoting hemostasis and endogenous anticoagulation are held in delicate equipoise, and the adaptations to and conditions of pregnancy predispose the gravid woman to increased risk of thromboembolic disease. Careful evaluation of risk of thromboembolic disease is critical to informing the appropriate steps to take in diagnosis. The knowledge of the pathophysiology of thrombosis helped develop D-dimer testing, an effective test for ruling out venous thromboembolism in nonpregnant patients. Lower extremity VUS and spiral CT scanning, in combination with these initial assessments, are critical tools in the diagnosis of DVT and PE, respectively.

Case presentation 1

A 42-year-old G1 P0 infertility patient is status post-ovulation induction, *in vitro* fertilization, and transfer of three embryos resulting in a triplet gestation. Following several admissions for recurrent severe nausea and vomiting with weight loss she has been resting at home for the past 4 days heavily sedated by her antiemetic regimen. She awakens late at night with left calf and thigh pain. She is seen in her physician's office the following morning. She denies dyspnea and, other than mild calf and posterior thigh tenderness to palpation, has no signs or symptoms of DVT. A venous ultrasound is ordered and she is found to have thrombosis involving the proximal thigh and calf veins. She is begun on therapeutic doses of low molecular weight heparin.

Case presentation 2

A 27-year-old G2 P1 at 27 weeks' gestation complains of left calf pain which she believes began following the development of a painful muscle cramp which awoke her the night before. She is seen in her physician's office and has an unremarkable exam except for bilateral trace lower extremity edema. She is quite healthy, exercises regularly, and has no personal or family history of thrombosis. A D-dimer is ordered which returns negative. She is given instructions to call if the pain worsens or she develops unilateral lower extremity swelling, or dyspnea.

References

1 Ginsberg J, Brill-Edwards P, Burrows R, *et al*. Venous thrombosis during pregnancy: leg and trimester of presentation. *Thromb Haemost* 1992;**67**:519–20.

2 Kierkegaard A. Incidence and diagnosis of deep vein thrombosis associated with pregnancy. *Acta Obstet Gynecol Scand* 1983;**62**:239–43.

3 Rutherford S, Montoro M, McGehee W, Strong T. Thromboembolic disease associated with pregnancy: an 11-year review (SPO Abstract). *Obstet Gynecol* 1991;**164**:286.

4 Simpson E, Lawrenson R, Nightingale A, Farmer R. Venous thromboembolism in pregnancy and the puerperium: incidence and additional risk factors from a London perinatal database. *Br J Obstet Gynaecol* 2001;**108**:56–60.

5 Stein P, Hull R, Jayali F, *et al*. Venous thromboembolism in pregnancy: 21-year trends. *Am J Med* 2004;**117**:121–5.

6 Toglia M, Weg J. Venous thromboembolism during pregnancy. *N Engl J Med* 1996;**335**:108–14.

7 Treffers P, Huidekoper B, Weenink G, Kloosterman G. Epidemiological observations of thrombo-embolic disease during pregnancy and the puerperium, in 56,022 women. *Intl J Gynaecol Obstet* 1983;**21**:327–31.

8 James K, Lohr J, Deshmukh R, Cranley J. Venous thrombotic complications of pregnancy. *Cardiovasc Surg* 1996;**4**:777–82.

9 McColl M, Ramsay J, Tait R, *et al*. Risk factors for pregnancy associated venous thromboembolism. *Thromb Haemost* 1997;**78**:1183–8.

10 Macklon N, Greer I. Venous thromboembolic disease in obstetrics and gynecology: the Scottish experience. *Scott Med J* 1996;**41**:83–6.

11 Bergqvist D, Hedner U. Pregnancy and venous thrombo-embolism. *Acta Obstet Gynecol Scand* 1983;**62**:449–53.

12 Bergqvist A, Bergqvist D, Hallbook T. Deep vein thrombosis during pregnancy: a prospective study. *Acta Obstet Gynecol Scand* 1983;**62**:443–8.

13 Chang J, Elam-Evans L, Berg C, *et al*. Pregnancy-related mortality surveillance, United States, 1991–1999. *MMWR Surveill Summ* 2003;**52**:1–8.

14 Wessler S. Medical management of venous thrombosis. *Annu Rev Med* 1979;**27**:313–9.

15 Vallasanta U. Thromboembolic disease in pregnancy. *Am J Obstet Gynecol* 1965;**93**:142–60.

16 Ruggeri Z, Dent J, Saldivar E. Contribution of distinct adhesive interactions to platelet aggregation in flowing blood. *Blood* 1999;**94**:172–8.

17 Pytela R, Pierschbacher M, Ginsberg M, Plow E, Ruoslahti E. Platelet membrane glycoprotein IIb/IIIa: member of a family of Arg-Gly-Asp-specific adhesion receptors. *Science* 1986;**231**:1559–62.

18 Nemerson Y. Tissue factor and hemostasis. *Blood* 1988;**71**:1–8.

19 Preissner K, de Boer H, Pannekoek H, de Groot P. Thrombin regulation by physiological inhibitors: the role of vitronectin. *Semin Thromb Hemost* 1996;**165**:1335–41.

20 Mackman N. Role of tissue factor in hemostasis, thrombosis, and vascular development. *Arterioscler Thromb Vasc Biol* 2004;**24**:1015–22.

21 Lockwood C, Bach R, Guha A, Zhou X, Miller W, Nemerson Y. Amniotic fluid contains tissue factor, a potent initiator of coagulation. *Am J Obstet Gynecol* 1991;**165**:1335–41.

22 Broze G. The rediscovery and isolation of TFPI. *J Thromb Haemost* 2003;**1**:1671–5.

23 Esmon C. The protein C pathway. *Chest* 2003;**124**(3 Suppl): 26S–32S.

24 Dahlback B. Progress in the understanding of the protein C anticoagulant pathway. *Int J Hematol* 2004;**79**:109–16.

25 Broze G. Protein Z-dependent regulation of coagulation. *Thromb Haemost* 2001;**86**:8–13.

26 Perry D. Antithrombin and its inherited deficiencies. *Blood Rev* 1994;**8**:37–55.

27 Preissner K, Zwicker L, Muller-Berghaus G. Formation, characterization and detection of a ternary complex between protein S, thrombin and antithrombin III in serum. *Biochem J* 1987;**243**:105–11.

28 Bouma B, Meijers J. New insights into factors affecting clot stability: a role for thrombin activatable fibrinolysis inhibitor. *Semin Hematol* 2004;**41**:13–9.

29 Schatz F, Lockwood C. Progestin regulation of plasminogen activator inhibitor type-1 in primary cultures of endometrial stromal and decidual cells. *J Clin Endocrin Metab* 1993;**77**: 621–5.

30 Lockwood C, Krikun G, Schatz F. The decidua regulates hemostasis in the human endometrium. *Semin Reprod Endocrinol* 1999;**17**:45–51.

31 Girling J, de Swiet M. Inherited thrombophilia and pregnancy. *Curr Opin Obstet Gynecol* 1998;**10**:135–44.

32 Wright H, Osborn S, Edmunds D. Changes in the rate of flow of venous blood in the leg during pregnancy, measured with radioactive sodium. *Surg Gynecol Obstet* 1950;**90**:481.

33 Goodrich S, Wood J. Peripheral venous distensibility and velocity of venous blood flow during pregnancy or during oral contraceptive therapy. *Am J Obstet Gynecol* 1964;**90**:740.

34 Macklon N, Greer I, Bowman A. An ultrasound study of gestational and postural changes in the deep venous system of the leg in pregnancy. *Br J Obstet Gynaecol* 1997;**104**:191–7.

35 Hull R, Raskob G, Carter C. Serial impedance plethysmography in pregnant patients with clinically suspected deep-vein thrombosis: clinical validity of negative findings. *Ann Intern Med* 1990;**112**:663–7.

36 Bremme K. Haemostatic changes in pregnancy. *Bailliere's Best Pract Res Clin Haematol* 2003;**16**:153–68.

37 Hellgren M, Blomback M. Studies on blood coagulation and fibrinolysis in pregnancy, during delivery and in the puerperium. *Gynecol Obstet Invest* 1981;**12**:141–54.

38 Hirsh J, Hoak J. Management of deep vein thrombosis and pulmonary embolism: a statement for healthcare professionals from the Council on Thrombosis (in Consultation with the Council on Cardiovascular Radiology), American Heart Association. *Circulation* 1996;**93**:2212–45.

39 Sandler D, Martin J, Duncan J, *et al*. Diagnosis of deep-vein thrombosis: comparison of clinical evaluation, ultrasound, plethysmography, and venoscan with X-ray venogram. *Lancet* 1984;**8405**:716–9.

40 Wells P, Hirsh J, Anderson D, *et al*. A simple clinical model for the diagnosis of deep-vein thrombosis combined with impedance plethysmography: potential for an improvement in the diagnostic process. *J Intern Med* 1998;**243**:15–23.

41 Wells P, Anderson D, Rodger M, *et al*. Evaluation of D-Dimer in the diagnosis of suspected deep-vein thrombosis. *N Engl J Med* 2003;**349**:1227–35.

42 Tamariz L, Eng J, Segal J, *et al*. Usefulness of clinical prediction rules for the diagnosis of venous thromboembolism: a systematic review. *Am J Med* 2004;**117**:676–84.

43 Heim S, Schectman J, Siadaty M, Philbrick J. D-dimer testing for deep venous thrombosis: a metaanalysis. *Clin Chem* 2004;**50**:1136–47.

44 Bounameaux H, de Moerloose P, Perrrier A, Reber G. Plasma measurement of D-dimer as a diagnostic aid in suspected venous thromboembolism: an overview. *Thromb Haemost* 1994;**71**:1–6.

45 Epiney M, Boehlen F, Boulvain M, *et al*. D-dimer levels during delivery and the postpartum. *J Thromb Haemost* 2005;**3**:268–71.

46 Koh S, Pua H, Tay D, Ratnam S. The effects of gynaecological surgery on coagulation activation, fibrinolysis, and fibrinolytic inhibitor in patients with and without ketorolac infusion. *Thromb Res* 1995;**79**:501–14.

47 Tapson V, Carroll B, Davidson B, *et al*. The diagnostic approach to acute venous thromboembolism. Clinical practice guideline. American Thoracic Society. *Am J Respir Clin Care Med* 1999;**160**:1043–66.

48 Heijboer H, Cogo A, Buller H, Prandoni P, ten Cate J. Detection of deep vein thrombosis with impedance plethysmography and real-time compression ultrasonography in hospitalized patients. *Arch Intern Med* 1992;**152**:1901–3.

49 Bockenstedt P. D-dimer in venous thromboembolism. *N Engl J Med* 2003;**349**:1203–4.

50 Kassai B, Boissel J, Cucherat M, Sonie S, Shah N, Leizorovicz A. A systematic review of the accuracy of ultrasound in the diagnosis of deep venous thrombosis in asymptomatic patients. *Thromb Haemost* 2004;**91**:655–66.

51 Gottlieb R, Widjaja J, Tian L, Rubens D, Voci S. Calf sonography for detecting deep venous thrombosis in symptomatic patients: experience and review of the literature. *J Clin Ultrasound* 1999;**27**:415–20.

52 Evans A, Sostman H, Witty L, *et al*. Detection of deep venous thrombosis: prospective comparison of MR imaging and sonography. *J Magn Reson Imaging* 1996;**6**:44–51.

53 Carpenter J, Holland G, Baum R, Owen R, Carpenter J, Cope C. Magnetic resonance venography for the detection of deep venous thrombosis: comparison with contrast venography and duplex Doppler ultrasonography. *J Vasc Surg* 1993;**18**:734–41.

54 Stein P, Terrin M, Hales C, *et al*. Clinical, laboratory, roentgenographic, and electrocardiographic findings in patients with acute pulmonary embolism and no pre-existing cardiac or pulmonary disease. *Chest* 1991;**100**:598–603.

55 Fedullo P, Tapson V. The evaluation of suspected pulmonary embolism. *N Engl J Med* 2003;**349**:1247–56.

56 van Belle A, Buller H, Huisman M, *et al*. Effectiveness of managing suspected pulmonary embolism using an algorithm combining

clinical probability, D-dimer testing, and computed tomography. *JAMA* 2006;**295**:172–9.

57 The Urokinase Pulmonary Embolism Trial. a national cooperative study. *Circulation* 1973;**47**(Suppl II):1–108.

58 Value of the ventilation/perfusion scan in acute pulmonary embolism. Results of the prospective investigation of pulmonary embolism diagnosis (PIOPED). The PIOPED Investigators. *JAMA* 1990;**263**:2653–9.

59 Sreeram N, Cheriex E, Smeets J, Gorgels A, Wellens H. Value of the 12-lead electrocardiogram at hospital admission in the diagnosis of pulmonary embolism. *Am J Cardiol* 1994;**73**: 298–303.

60 Rodger M, Makropoulos D, Turek M, *et al*. Diagnostic value of the electrocardiogram in suspected pulmonary embolism. *Am J Cardiol* 2000;**86**:807–9.

61 Green R, Meyer T, Dunn M, Glassroth J. Pulmonary embolism in younger adults. *Chest* 1992;**101**:1507–11.

62 Come P. Echocardiographic evaluation of pulmonary embolism and its response to therapeutic interventions. *Chest* 1992;**101**:151S–62S.

63 Kasper W, Meinertz T, Kersting F, Lollgen H, Limbourg P, Just H. Echocardiography in assessing acute pulmonary hypertension due to pulmonary embolism. *Am J Cardiol* 1980;**45**:567–72.

64 Gibson N, Sohne M, Buller H. Prognostic value of echocardiography and spiral computed tomography in patients with pulmonary embolism. *Curr Opin Pulm Med* 2005;**11**:380–4.

65 Pruszczyk P, Torbicki A, Pacho R, *et al*. Noninvasive diagnosis of suspected severe pulmonary embolism: transesophageal echocardiography vs spiral CT. *Chest* 1997;**112**:722–8.

66 Stein P, Athanasoulis C, Alavi A, *et al*. Complications and validity of pulmonary angiography in acute pulmonary embolism. *Circulation* 1992;**85**:462–8.

67 Mills S, Jackson D, Older R, Heaston D, Moore A. The incidence, etiologies, and avoidance of complications of pulmonary angiography in a large series. *Radiology* 1980;**136**:295–9.

68 Dalen J, Brooks H, Johnson L, Meister S, Szucs MJ, Dexter L. Pulmonary angiography in acute pulmonary embolism: indications, techniques, and results in 367 patients. *Am Heart J* 1971;**81**:175–85.

69 Stein P, Hull R, Patel K, *et al*. D-dimer for the exclusion of acute venous thrombosis and pulmonary embolism: a systematic review. *Ann Intern Med* 2004;**140**:589–602

70 Cross J, Kemp P, Walsh C, Flower C, Dixon A. A randomized trial of spiral CT and ventilation perfusion scintigraphy for the diagnosis of pulmonary embolism. *Clin Radiol* 1998;**53**:177–82.

71 Moores L, Jackson WJ, Shorr A, Jackson J. Meta-analysis: outcomes in patients with suspected pulmonary embolism managed with computed tomographic pulmonary angiography. *Ann Intern Med* 2004;**141**:866–74.

72 Remy-Jardin M, Remy J, Baghaie F, Fribourg M, Artaud D, Duhamel A. Clinical value of thin collimation in the diagnostic workup of pulmonary embolism. *Am J Roentgenol* 2000;**175**:407–11.

73 Meaney J, Weg J, Chenevert T, Stafford-Johnson D, Hamilton B, Prince M. Diagnosis of pulmonary embolism with magnetic resonance angiography. *N Engl J Med* 1997;**336**: 1422–7.

74 Oudkerk M, van Beek E, Wielopolski P, *et al*. Comparison of contrast-enhanced magnetic resonance angiography and conventional pulmonary angiography for the diagnosis of pulmonary embolism: a prospective study. *Lancet* 2002;**359**:1643–7.

75 Stein P, Hull R, Saltzman H, Pineo G. Strategy for diagnosis of patients with suspected pulmonary embolism. *Chest* 1993;**103**:1553–9.

76 American College of Obstetricians and Gynecologists. *Guidelines for diagnostic imaging during pregnancy*. ACOG Committee Opinion No. 299. 2004.

77 Brent R. The effect of embryonic and fetal exposure to X-ray, microwaves, and ultrasound: counseling the pregnant and nonpregnant patient about these risks. *Semin Oncol* 1989;**16**:347–68.

78 Stewart A, Kneale G. Radiation dose effects in relation to obstetric X-rays and childhood cancers. *Lancet* 1970;**1**:1185–8.

79 Webb J, Thomson H, Morcos S, Members of Contrast Media Safety Committee of European Society of Urogenital Radiology (ESUR). The use of iodinated and gadolinium contrast media during pregnancy and lactation. *Eur J Radiol* 2005;**15**:1234–40.

17 Cardiac disease in pregnancy

Stephanie R. Martin and Michael R. Foley

Advances in diagnosis and treatment of congenital cardiac lesions have led to dramatically improved survival. Consequently, the predominant form of cardiac disease encountered during pregnancy has shifted from primarily rheumatic in origin to congenital heart disease [1–5]. During the mid-1950s, rheumatic heart disease during pregnancy was 16 times more likely than congenital disease. By 1967, this ratio had reversed to 3:1 (congenital:acquired) heart disease during pregnancy [1,2]. According to the National Center for Health Statistics in 2004, the number of patients postponing childbearing beyond 40 years is also growing and is expected to increase the likelihood of other comorbid conditions, including cardiac disease. Despite complicating only 4% of all pregnancies in the USA, a disproportionate number of maternal deaths (10–25%) can be attributed to cardiac disease [6–8]. Intensive care unit (ICU) admissions because of maternal cardiac disease comprise up to 15% of obstetric ICU admissions, yet these patients account for up to 50% of all maternal deaths in the ICU [9–15]. Assessment of the pregnant patient with cardiac disease can be challenging as many common complaints of normal pregnancy such as dyspnea, fatigue, palpitations, orthopnea, and pedal edema mimic symptoms of worsening cardiac disease. Obstetric patients with cardiac disease are susceptible to a number of potential complications resulting from the significant physiologic changes associated with pregnancy and delivery. This chapter outlines the expected hemodynamic and physiologic changes occurring in pregnancy and reviews prognosis and management recommendations for obstetric patients with congenital and acquired cardiac lesions.

Physiologic changes

The adaptations that occur during normal pregnancy place substantial demands on cardiac function. Table 17.1 [16,17] summarizes hemodynamic changes in pregnancy. Numerous physiologic changes develop over the course of pregnancy; however, the greatest impact on a potentially compromised cardiovascular system is a result of four fundamental alterations: increased intravascular volume, decreased systemic vascular resistance, increased cardiac output and hypercoagulability.

During pregnancy, total blood volume and plasma volume increase by approximately 50%. However, the red cell mass rises by only 33%, ultimately resulting in a decreased hemoglobin and hematocrit, as demonstrated in Figs 17.1 and 17.2. The heart is able to accommodate this increase in volume primarily because of decreased systemic vascular resistance. Consequently, systolic and diastolic blood pressures drop during pregnancy, reaching a nadir between 24 and 32 weeks' gestation. Cardiac output increases to 30–50% above prepregnant levels by the end of the third trimester and may increase by an additional 50% in the second stage of labor [16]. Strikingly, half of the increase in cardiac output occurs by 8 weeks' gestation [18]. Profound alterations in the coagulation cascade also occur, including increases in fibrinogen and factor VIII levels, resulting in a thrombophilic state that predisposes patients to the development of thromboembolic complications (Table 17.2). These changes will also impact the findings on various cardiovascular tests as outlined in Table 17.3 [19].

Counseling the patient

Functional status for patients with cardiac disease is commonly classified according to the New York Heart Association (NYHA) classification system as outlined in Table 17.4. The utility of this classification system during pregnancy is limited because it does not address specific lesions. However, as expected, patients with NYHA class I or II have less risk of complications compared with those in class III or IV [4]. In the 1987 edition of *Critical Care Obstetrics*, a guideline was introduced that classified various cardiac abnormalities according to maternal death risk estimates (Table 17.5) [20]. Disorders associated with less than a 1% risk of death were considered minimal risk, moderate risk disorders carried a 5–15% risk of

Measurement	Normal Value	% Change in Pregnancy
Heart rate (beats/min)	71 ± 10	+10–20%
Stroke volume (mL)	73.3 ± 9	+30%
Cardiac output (L/min)	4.3 ± 0.9	+30–50%
Blood volume (L)	5	+20–50%
Systemic vascular resistance (dyne/cm/s)	1530 ± 520	−20%
Mean arterial pressure (mmHg)	86.4 ± 7.5	Not significant
Oxygen consumption (mL/min)	250	+20–30%

Table 17.1 Expected cardiovascular changes in pregnancy. After Clark *et al.* [16] and Elkayam and Gleicher [17].

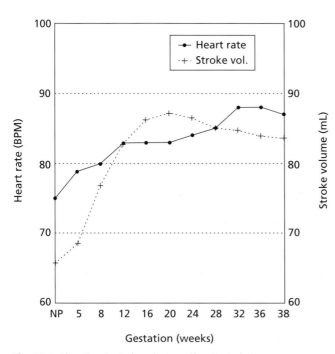

Fig. 17.1 Alterations in stroke volume and heart rate during pregnancy.

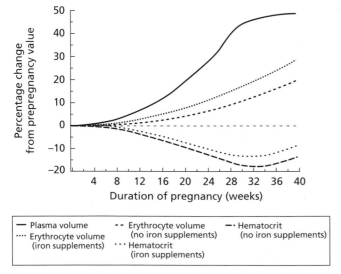

Fig. 17.2 Changes in plasma volume, red cell volume, and hematocrit during pregnancy.

Table 17.2 Clotting factor changes in pregnancy.

Factor II (prothrombin)	Unchanged
Factors VII–X, XII	Increased
Fibrinogen	Increased
Platelets	Unchanged

Table 17.3 Changes in cardiovascular tests during pregnancy. After Gei and Hankins [19].

Cardiovascular Exam	Findings in Pregnancy
Chest X-ray	Apparent cardiomegaly
	Enlarged left atrium
	Increased vascular markings
Electrocardiography	Right axis deviation
	Right bundle branch block
	ST segment depression of 1 mm on left precordial leads
	Q waves in lead III
	T wave inversion in leads III, V2 and V3
Echocardiography	Trivial tricuspid regurgitation
	Pulmonary regurgitation
	Increased left atrial size
	Increased left ventricular end-diastolic dimensions by 6–10%
	Mitral regurgitation
	Pericardial effusion

mortality, and major risk disorders were considered to have a mortality risk in excess of 25%. This classification system certainly provided more information with which to counsel patients; however, the patient's particular history is not taken into consideration. In 1997, Siu *et al.* [21] identified several independent risk factors for cardiac complications such as congestive heart failure, stroke, or arrhythmia, based on a series of 252 pregnant patients with a variety of cardiac diseases. The most significant risk factors for complications include a NYHA class III or IV, cyanosis, history of an arrhythmia, pulmonary vascular disease, ejection fraction of less than 40%, or significant mitral or aortic valve obstruction.

Table 17.4 New York Heart Association (NYHA) functional classification system.

Class I	No limitations of physical activity. Ordinary physical activity does not precipitate cardiovascular symptoms such as dyspnea, angina, fatigue, or palpitations
Class II	Slight limitation of physical activity. Ordinary physical activity will precipitate cardiovascular symptoms. Patients are comfortable at rest
Class III	Less than ordinary physical activity precipitates symptoms that markedly limit activity. Patients are comfortable at rest
Class IV	Patients have discomfort with any physical activity. Symptoms are present at rest

Table 17.5 Maternal mortality associated with pregnancy. After Clark [20].

Group 1—Mortality <1%
Atrial septal defect
Ventricular septal defect
Patent ductus arteriosus
Mitral stenosis: NYHA class I & II
Pulmonic/tricuspid valve disease
Corrected tetralogy of Fallot
Bioprosthetic valve

Group 2—Mortality 5–15%
Group 2A
Mitral stenosis: NYHA class III & IV
Aortic stenosis
Coarctation of aorta without valvular involvement
Uncorrected tetralogy of Fallot
Previous myocardial infarction
Marfan syndrome with normal aorta

Group 2B
Mitral stenosis with atrial fibrillation
Artificial valve

Group 3—Mortality 25–50%
Pulmonary hypertension
 Primary
 Eisenmenger
Coarctation of aorta with valvular involvement
Marfan syndrome with aortic involvement
Peripartum cardiomyopathy with persistent left ventricular dysfunction

NYHA, New York Heart Association.

More recently, in the CARPREG study, Siu *et al.* [22] prospectively evaluated 617 pregnancies complicated by maternal cardiac disease. Four predictors of maternal complications were identified:
1 A history of heart failure, transient ischemic attack, stroke, or arrhythmia;
2 Prepregnancy NYHA class II or above;

Table 17.6 Predicting adverse cardiac events during pregnancy. After Siu *et al.* [22].

Number of risk factors	Risk of adverse event (%)
0	5
1	27
2 or more	75

Risk factors:
 (1) A history of heart failure, transient ischemic attack, stroke or arrhythmia
 (2) Prepregnancy NYHA class III or IV
 (3) Left heart obstruction (mitral or aortic valve stenosis)
 (4) Ejection fraction <40%
Most common adverse events: pulmonary edema, arrhythmias.
NYHA, New York Heart Association.

3 Left heart obstruction (mitral valve area <2 cm², aortic valve area <1.5 cm², peak left outflow gradient >30 mmHg); and
4 Ejection fraction less than 40%.
The risk of maternal complications was directly proportional to the numbers of risk factors identified. Five percent of patients with none of the four predictors developed a complication, whereas the addition of only one risk factor increased the adverse event rate to 27%. The incidence of complications increased to 75% in patients with more than one predictor (Table 17.6) [22]. Pulmonary edema and arrhythmias were the most commonly encountered complications. The route of delivery did not affect the complication rate. Six patients (1%) died secondary to stroke or cardiac decompensation. In the same study, the strongest predictors for neonatal complications were NYHA class II or above, heparin or Coumadin use during pregnancy, smoking, multiple gestation, and left heart obstruction. Twenty percent of the pregnancies in this study delivered small for gestational age infants or delivered prematurely.

In a subsequent study, the same authors prospectively compared 300 pregnant women with cardiac disease with controls, primarily to evaluate neonatal and cardiac outcomes [23]. In this group of patients, 64% had a congenital cardiac lesion, 28% had acquired lesions, and the remaining 8% had dysrhythmias. Forty-one percent of the gravidas had undergone previous surgical interventions. As expected, the rate of miscarriage and neonatal complications such as intraventricular hemorrhage, delivery before 34 weeks' gestation, and neonatal death occurred more commonly in gravidas with cardiac disease compared with controls. However, the addition of risk factors such as smoking, anticoagulant use, and multiple gestations in a patient with cardiac disease further escalated the risk of neonatal complications to twice that of the control group. In this study 17% of patients with cardiac disease had a cardiac complication, 94% of which were caused by cardiac failure or dysrhythmias. In this study, delivery by cesarean section occurred more commonly in patients with cardiac disease (29% vs. 23%), but preeclampsia and hemorrhage developed with equal frequency in patients with and without cardiac disease.

Considering the patient's prior history of cardiac events and evaluation of functional status is important for accurate counseling regarding maternal and fetal risks. However, the greatest risk for maternal mortality continues to be for those patients with coronary artery disease, pulmonary hypertension, endocarditis, cardiomyopathy, and arrhythmias [3,24].

Risk of fetal cardiac abnormalities

Patients with congenital cardiac abnormalities should also be counseled regarding the increased risk of fetal structural cardiac anomalies. This risk is estimated to be between 8.8% and 14.2%, a significant increase above the population risk of 0.08% of live births [25,26]. Paternal cardiac abnormalities also increase the risk of congenital cardiac disease; however, maternal disease poses the greatest risk by up to 3.5 times. Patients with aortic stenosis and ventricular septal defect appear to be at greatest risk for transmission; however, the lesion may be different from that of the parent [27–30]. Therefore, fetal echocardiography is recommended for all patients with a congenital cardiac abnormality. Table 17.7 [31] outlines the risks of congenital cardiac disease by maternal disorder.

Valvular heart disease

Acquired valvular lesions are typically sequelae of rheumatic fever; however, valvular endocarditis secondary to intravenous drug use is not uncommon. During pregnancy, most morbidity and mortality from these lesions is associated with dysrhythmias and congestive failure resulting in pulmonary edema. The degree of risk for the development of complications depends on the specific valve lesion, number of valves involved, and the degree of valvular obstruction, particularly of the mitral and aortic valves. However, pregnancy does not appear to adversely affect long-term sequelae for women with rheumatic heart disease who survive the pregnancy. Tables 17.8 and 17.9 [32] outline the current recommendations for the

prevention of systemic bacterial endocarditis in pregnant patients with valvular abnormalities [33]. Each valvular lesion will be addressed in the sections that follow. Table 17.10 [34] presents a summary of relative maternal and fetal risk in patients with valvular abnormalities.

Mitral stenosis

Congenital mitral stenosis is rare; rheumatic heart disease accounts for the majority of mitral valve disease. In fact, mitral stenosis is the most common rheumatic valvular lesion encountered in pregnancy [35]. The normal mitral valve area is 4–5 cm^2. As the mitral valve orifice diminishes in size, filling of the left ventricle during diastole becomes progressively limited and cardiac output becomes more fixed. In nonpregnant patients, patients are asymptomatic until the valve area falls below 2 cm^2. Moderate mitral stenosis is defined as a valve area measuring between 1 and 1.5 cm^2; less than 1 cm^2 valve area defines severe mitral stenosis [36]. Patients with moderate to severe limitations of the valve area may not tolerate the normal increase in cardiac output, blood volume, and heart rate of pregnancy and should ideally have the valve repaired prior to pregnancy. Patients who remain symptomatic despite conservative management may be candidates for surgical intervention during pregnancy. Case reports of over 100 women describe percutaneous balloon mitral valvuloplasty as a safe and effective procedure during pregnancy [37–39]. Mitral stenosis may be undiagnosed prior to pregnancy and become apparent only when challenged by the normal physiologic changes. These patients may present with atrial fibrillation and/or pulmonary edema as the initial diagnostic clue to underlying mitral stenosis. In a recent series of 80 pregnancies complicated by mitral stenosis, 38% of patients with moderate mitral stenosis (valve area less than 1.5 cm^2) and 67% of patients with severe mitral stenosis (valve area less than 1 cm^2) experienced a cardiac event. However, even patients with mild stenosis experienced complications in 11% of cases. The most common maternal complications were pulmonary edema and arrhythmias, primarily atrial fibrillation and supraventricular tachycardia. A history of prior cardiac events and moderate or severe stenosis were the strongest independent predictors of

Cardiac lesion	Prior affected sibling	Father affected	Mother affected
Tetralogy of Fallot	2.5	1.5	2.6
Aortic coarctation			14.1
Atrial septal defect	2.5	1.5	4.6–11
Ventricular septal defect	3	2	9.5–15.6
Pulmonary stenosis	2	2	6.5
Aortic stenosis	2	3	15–17.9

Table 17.7 Risk of fetal congenital cardiac defects (%). After Lupton *et al.* [31].

Table 17.8 American Heart Association (AHA) and American College of Cardiology (ACC) Task Force recommendations on chemoprophylaxis for bacterial endocarditis. After Dajani *et al.* [32].

	Need for Prophylaxis	
Endocarditis Risk	**Uncomplicated Vaginal Delivery**	**Cesarean Section**
High-risk Prosthetic cardiac valve Prior bacterial endocarditis Complex congenital cyanotic heart disease Surgically constructed shunts	Optional	Not recommended
Moderate-risk Other congenital cardiac malformations Rheumatic heart disease (or other acquired valvular disease) Hypertrophic cardiomyopathy Mitral valve prolapse with leaflet thickening and/or regurgitation	Not recommended	Not recommended
Negligible-risk Mitral valve prolapse without regurgitation Physiologic, functional, or innocent murmurs Previous rheumatic fever without valvular dysfunction	Not recommended	Not recommended

Table 17.9 Antibiotic regimens for genitourinary and gastrointestinal procedures. After Dajani *et al.* [32].

Situation	Regimen
High-risk patients	Ampicillin 2 g IM/IV *plus* gentamicin 1.5 mg/kg (not to exceed 120 mg) within 30 min of starting procedure; 6 h later, ampicillin 1 g IM/IV or amoxicillin 1 g orally
High-risk patients with penicillin allergy	Vancomycin 1 g IV over 1–2 h *plus* gentamicin 1.5 mg/kg IV/IM (not to exceed 120 mg), complete infusion within 30 min of starting procedure
Moderate-risk patients	Amoxicillin 2 g orally 1 h before starting procedure, *or* ampicillin 2 g IM/IV within 30 min of starting procedure
Moderate-risk patients with penicillin allergy	Vancomycin 1 g IV over 1–2 h, complete infusion within 30 min of starting procedure

maternal complications. Sixty percent of patients experience the initial episode of pulmonary edema during the antepartum period, at a mean gestational age of 30 weeks. The most common neonatal complication was prematurity [40].

Management of patients with mitral stenosis should focus on two primary goals: (i) prevention of tachycardia; and (ii) maintenance of left ventricular filling (preload). As the heart rate increases, less time is allowed for the left atrium to adequately empty and fill the left ventricle during diastole. As a result, the left atrium may become overdistended, resulting in dysrhythmias (primarily atrial fibrillation, which will increase the risk of thromboembolic complications), pulmonary edema, or both. Tachycardia is likely to develop as a result of pain, exertion, anxiety, or following the administration of beta-agonists such as terbutaline. Cardiac output can fall dramatically and lead to hypotension and/or sudden onset of pulmonary edema. Tachycardia can be avoided by aggressive pain management and avoidance of exertion during labor. Some patients may require therapy with beta-blockers to maintain heart rate below 90–100 beats/min. During labor, short-acting intravenous beta-blockers, such as esmolol, are recommended instead of longer acting oral agents.

The second major consideration for patients with mitral valve stenosis is maintenance of left ventricular filling (adequate preload). Excessive venous return to the heart (preload) may lead to pulmonary edema and atrial dysrhythmias as a result of overdistension. However, overcoming the obstruction to left ventricular filling depends on high fluid volumes to maintain forward flow. Therefore, the use of diuretics should be carried out cautiously to avoid inadvertent decreases in left ventricular filling and therefore cardiac output. Unlike aortic stenosis, the utility of pulmonary artery catheterization to monitor left ventricular preload is limited as pulmonary

Table 17.10 Classification of valvular heart lesions according to maternal and fetal risks. After Reimold and Rutherford [34].

Low Maternal and Fetal Risks	High Maternal and Fetal Risks	High Maternal Risks
Asymptomatic aortic stenosis with a low mean outflow gradient (<50 mmHg); normal LV systolic function	Severe aortic stenosis with or without symptoms	Ejection fraction <40%
Aortic regurgitation, NYHA class I or II with normal LV function	Aortic regurgitation, NYHA class III or IV	Previous heart failure
Mitral regurgitation, NYHA class I or II, normal LV function	Mitral stenosis, NYHA class II, III or IV	Previous stroke or transient ischemic attack
Mitral valve prolapse with none to moderate mitral regurgitation, normal LV function	Mitral regurgitation, NYHA class III or IV	
Mild to moderate mitral stenosis, no pulmonary hypertension	Aortic or mitral valve disease with pulmonary hypertension	
Mild to moderate pulmonary valve stenosis	Aortic or mitral valve disease with LV dysfunction	
	Maternal cyanosis	
	NYHA class III or IV	

LV, left venticle; NYHA, New York Heart Association.

capillary wedge pressure may reflect a false increase in mean wedge pressure in the setting of mitral stenosis. Epidural anesthetic use is appropriate during labor to minimize tachycardia caused by pain or anxiety and therefore control fluctuations in cardiac output. Care should be taken to avoid sudden decrease in preload caused by abrupt sympathetic blockade from local anesthetics. The use of narcotic agents in the epidural space should be considered as an alternative to local anesthetics for pain relief during labor.

Medical management of these patients involves avoiding tachycardia with activity restriction or beta-blockers when necessary, appropriate treatment of dysrhythmias if present, and careful diuretic use. The section on dysrhythmias addresses anticoagulation issues in patients with atrial fibrillation.

Pulmonic and tricuspid lesions

Pulmonic stenosis is a common congenital lesion; however, in an adult population, isolated pulmonic and tricuspid valvular abnormalities are more commonly brought about by valvular endocarditis from intravenous drug use than by rheumatic heart disease. The physiologic changes of pregnancy are tolerated well by patients with pulmonic or tricuspid valvular abnormalities. Patients with severe pulmonic obstruction (transvalvular pressure gradient exceeding 60 mm) are at highest risk for complications such as right heart failure and if symptomatic may be a candidate for percutaneous valvuloplasty. One study describes a 2.8% risk of congestive heart failure; however, most series indicate maternal and fetal risks are minimal [27,41].

Mitral and aortic regurgitation

Mitral regurgitation is most commonly secondary to mitral valve prolapse in pregnant women [36]. Aortic regurgitation is usually rheumatic in origin. The increased heart rate and decreased systemic vascular resistance that occur normally in pregnancy favor forward flow of blood, therefore both lesions are tolerated quite well in pregnancy. However, patients with long-standing mitral or aortic insufficiency may have left ventricular dysfunction resulting from chronic ventricular dilatation and are therefore at increased risk for complications [42]. The decreased systemic vascular resistance that occurs following epidural placement is generally not problematic; however, it should be undertaken with caution as one death has been reported [43]. Chronic mitral regurgitation may also lead to significant left atrial enlargement which increases the risk for the development of atrial fibrillation. If this occurs, antiarrhythmic therapy is indicated and anticoagulation should be considered.

Mitral valve prolapse

Mitral valve prolapse is present in up to 3% of the general population but may be present in up to 17% of young women, making it one of the most common cardiac issues during pregnancy [44]. Because most women are asymptomatic, the diagnosis is generally made incidentally. The increased blood volume and decreased systemic vascular resistance of pregnancy improve the mitral valve function so patients can be expected to tolerate pregnancy well. Occasionally, symptoms of palpitations will prompt therapy, usually with beta-blockers. The incidence of antepartum and postpartum complications is no different from the general population, therefore no special precautions need to be taken during the pregnancy or labor and delivery. Antibiotic prophylaxis for systemic bacterial endocarditis is not recommended for mitral valve prolapse unless regurgitation is also confirmed [33].

Aortic stenosis

Aortic stenosis can develop as a consequence of rheumatic fever in which case it usually occurs in conjunction with other valvular abnormalities. However, congenital aortic stenosis is quite common, and when identified in younger patients it is usually caused by a bicuspid aortic valve [36]. The hypervolemia and increased cardiac output of pregnancy are well tolerated by patients with mild disease (valve area >1.5 cm^2, peak gradient <50 mmHg). However, as the orifice becomes progressively more stenotic, flow across the valve becomes progressively limited and the velocity of flow increases. This resistance serves as an impediment to increasing cardiac output but is not considered hemodynamically significant until the valve opening is decreased to one-quarter the normal diameter of 3–4 cm^2. These patients may be unable to maintain coronary or cerebral perfusion and can develop angina, myocardial infarction, syncope, or sudden death. Patients with a valve area of less than 1 cm^2, peak gradient of more than 75 mmHg, or an ejection fraction less than 55% have severe disease and should be evaluated for surgical correction, preferably prior to conception [36].

Complications arise in pregnant patients with aortic stenosis primarily as result of the inability to maintain cardiac output. The typical 40–50% increase in cardiac output is unlikely to result in pulmonary edema unless mitral valve disease is coexistent. However, labor and delivery or pregnancy termination is a particularly risky time for these patients. Any factor leading to diminished venous return (preload) will cause an increase in the valvular gradient, difficulty overcoming the obstruction, and ultimately diminished cardiac output. Diminished venous return may result from many common obstetric anesthetic complications including: hypotension resulting from blood loss or intravascular volume depletion; ganglionic blockade from regional anesthesia; or supine vena caval occlusion by the pregnant uterus. Exertion may place additional demands on cardiac output and may lead to coronary artery ischemia or inadequate cerebral perfusion which will manifest as angina, myocardial infarction, syncope, or sudden death. Limitation of physical activity is recommended for patients with severe disease.

Maintenance of adequate venous return and avoidance of exertion will minimize the risk of dangerous decreases in cardiac output. However, these patients are also at risk for the development of pulmonary edema resulting from limitations in the ability to increase cardiac output in response to increasing volume, therefore judicious use of intravenous fluids is recommended. Pulmonary artery catheterization may be indicated in patients with significant aortic stenosis to estimate intravascular volume accurately and guide fluid replacement. Because hypovolemia and decreased venous return present much higher risks for life-threatening complications to the patient than pulmonary edema, pulmonary artery wedge pressures should be maintained in the range of 15–17 mmHg.

Historically, the risk of death in pregnant patients with aortic stenosis has been reported to be as high as 17%. Fortunately, more recent data indicate that patients with aortic stenosis but without coronary artery disease, who receive adequate care, have a minimal risk of dying [41,45]. In one recent series of 49 pregnancies complicated by congenital aortic stenosis, cardiac complications occurred in 6% of patients with severe disease, including one patient who required percutaneous valvuloplasty at 12 weeks' gestation. Prematurity and small for gestational age babies complicated 10% of pregnancies. Fifty percent of patients with severe aortic stenosis required cardiac surgery in the first 4 years after delivery; however, it remains unclear whether the pregnancy negatively impacted the need for surgical intervention [46]. In contrast, in a series of 1000 pregnant women with cardiac disease, 65% of those with moderate or severe aortic stenosis experienced cardiac complications, including one maternal death [47].

Mechanical heart valves

All patients with mechanical heart valves require life-long anticoagulation to decrease the risk of thromboembolic complications. In the nonpregnant population, warfarin is the recommended agent to maintain a target international normalized ratio (INR) between 2.0 and 3.5, depending on the type and location of the valve. Patients with biologic valves do not require anticoagulation beyond the initial 3 months post-replacement unless they also have an additional risk factor for thromboembolic disease such as atrial fibrillation [36].

Recommendations for anticoagulation in pregnant women with mechanical heart valves is among the most controversial and challenging problems in obstetrics. The overall risk of maternal death reported in a recent meta-analysis is 2.9% [48]. The three currently available medications are warfarin, unfractionated heparin (UFH), and low molecular weight heparin (LMWH). Warfarin crosses the placenta and is associated with a risk of fetal malformations including a well-described embryopathy consisting of nasal and limb hypoplasia and epiphyseal stippling. The risk of anomalies appears to be greatest when exposure occurs between 6 and 12 weeks' gestation [49]. Intracranial hemorrhage is also a concern if warfarin is taken during the second and third trimesters and is postulated to be the cause of rare central nervous abnormalities [50]. Spontaneous abortion rates and pregnancy loss rates are more common if warfarin is taken during the pregnancy and are highest (21% and 30%, respectively) if warfarin is taken in the first trimester and continued throughout gestation [48]. While not effective at preventing all thromboembolic complications in pregnant patients with mechanical heart valves, it does appear to be superior to UFH. Warfarin throughout gestation is associated with a 3.9% risk of thromboembolic complications and a 1.8% risk of death. Substituting heparin during the teratogenic period increases the maternal risks to 9.2% incidence of thromboembolic disease and a 4.2% risk of death. Adjusted dose UFH without warfarin use is associated with an ever greater risk of maternal adverse outcomes: 25% risk of thromboembolic issues and 6.7% risk of death.

LMWH is a third alternative for anticoagulation. Like UFH it does not cross the placenta, but the potentially lower risk for osteoporosis and heparin-induced thrombocytopenia, and in particular the longer half-life, offer other advantages for its use [51]. However, it is not only less studied for this indication than warfarin and UFH, but the manufacturer of one LMWH, Lovenox (enoxaparin sodium), recently issued a warning statement against the use of Lovenox for thromboprophylaxis in pregnant patients with prosthetic valves [52]. This statement was issued after two maternal and fetal deaths occurred in patients receiving Lovenox 80 mg twice daily as part of a clinical research trial. According to a recent review article, anti-Xa levels were monitored but not used to adjust dosage; the authors suggest that inadequate dosage of Lovenox may have contributed to the development of thrombi [53]. Prior to the manufacturer's warning, one series of 12 pregnancies managed with empiric Lovenox regimens (1 mg/kg twice daily) reported a thromboembolic event in one patient (8.3%) [54]. The ability to judge the effectiveness of UFH and LMWH in preventing thromboembolic phenomena is complicated by altered pharmacology of these medications in the pregnant patient as a result of increased volume of distribution and alterations in the coagulation cascade [55–57]. These data suggest that monitoring of anticoagulant effect of UFH and LMWH should be accomplished with peak and/or trough anti-Xa measurements instead of utilizing the activated partial thromboplastin time (APTT) (for UFH) or weight-based regimens (for LMWH). Unfortunately, as a result of the statement issued by the manufacturer of Lovenox, the ability to further investigate the effectiveness of LMWH in pregnant patients with mechanical valves is severely hampered by medicolegal concerns.

In 1998, the American College of Cardiology/American Heart Association Task Force on Practice Guidelines through the Committee on Management of Patients with Valvular Heart Disease proposed recommendations for the management of anticoagulation in pregnant patients with mechanical heart valves. These recommendations are summarized in Table 17.11 and do not include a role for LMWH [36]. Other authors have acknowledged the limitations of the available evidence regarding LMWH and have proposed alternative regimens which include three management options:

Table 17.11 American Heart Association (AHA) and American College of Cardiology (ACC) recommendations for the management of anticoagulation in pregnant women with mechanical valve prostheses. After Bonow et al. [36].

Preconception
Evaluation of cardiac functional status and previous cardiac events
Echocardiogram to assess valvular and ventricular function and pulmonary artery pressures
Discussion regarding risks of pregnancy with respect to cardiac status and anticoagulation requirements
Family planning discussion

Conception through completion of first trimester
Change to therapeutic, adjusted-dose unfractionated heparin (titrated to a mid-interval therapeutic PTT or anti-factor Xa level)

Weeks 12–36
Warfarin therapy

Week 36
Discontinue warfarin
Change to unfractionated heparin titrated to a mid-interval therapeutic PTT or anti-factor Xa level

Delivery
Resume heparin therapy 4–6 hours after delivery if no contraindications
Resume warfarin therapy the night after delivery if no contraindications

PTT, partial thromboplastin time.

Table 17.12 Alternative recommendations for the management of anticoagulation in pregnant women with mechanical valve prostheses utilizing low molecular weight heparin (LMWH) [50,53,58,59].

Option 1	UFH throughout gestation to maintain anti-Xa levels >0.3 units/mL or mid-interval APTT > twice control
Option 2	LMWH twice daily throughout gestation to maintain peak (4–6 hours post-injection) anti-Xa levels 0.5–1.5 units/mL and trough levels >0.5–0.7 units/mL
Option 3	Option 1 or 2 above until 12 completed weeks of gestation and resume at 36 weeks, give warfarin to maintain INR 2.5–3.5 between 13 and 36 weeks' gestation

APTT, activated partial thromboplastin time; INR, international normalized ratio; UFH, unfractionated heparin.

1 UFH throughout gestation to maintain anti-Xa levels over 0.3 units/mL or mid-interval APTT more than twice control
2 LMWH twice daily throughout gestation to maintain peak (4–6 hours post-injection) anti-Xa levels 0.5–1.5 units/mL and trough levels more than 0.5–0.7 units/mL
3 Option 1 or 2 above until 12 completed weeks' gestation and resume at 36 weeks, give warfarin to maintain INR 2.5–3.5 between 13 and 36 weeks' gestation [50,53,58,59].
These recommendations are summarized in Table 17.12. The appropriate interval for checking anti-Xa levels is not known.

In a recent review of expert opinion, Seshadri *et al.* [53] recommend weekly anti-Xa levels during the first month of therapy to maintain anti-Xa between 0.5 and 1.0 units/mL. A daily low dose of aspirin is recommended for patients at high risk for thromboembolic disease [36]. Ultimately, the decision regarding an anticoagulation regimen should be made after detailed discussion with the patient regarding the risks and benefits of each regimen to both the patient and the fetus.

Guidelines for management of anticoagulation around the time of cesarean section in these high-risk patients are lacking. In nonpregnant patients with a mechanical valve on Coumadin, the recommendation is to resume Coumadin in the afternoon the day of the procedure if bleeding is controlled. In very high-risk patients with multiple risk factors such as hypercoagulable state, previous thromboembolism, and mechanical mitral valve, UFH is discontinued 6 hours preoperatively and resumed within 24 hours postoperatively and overlapped with warfarin until the INR is more than 2 [36]. Cesarean section is recommended if the patient requires delivery before warfarin can be discontinued in order to minimize the risk of fetal hemorrhagic complications.

Congenital cardiac abnormalities

Aortic coarctation

Aortic coarctation is a narrowing of the caliber of the aorta, usually distal to the left subclavian artery, which occurs in 6–8% of patients with congenital heart disease [60]. The presence of a significant blood pressure gradient between the upper and lower extremities (>20 mmHg) usually prompts evaluation for repair which is accomplished surgically or with balloon angioplasty. Long-term survival following repair of aortic coarctation is quite good; however, the risks of recoarctation, aortic aneurysm, dissection, and rupture persist. Occasionally, patients will remain undiagnosed into adulthood (native coarctation).

While early reports of pregnancy in women with coarctation indicated mortality rates of 9.5%, more recent data suggest that pregnancy in women with a corrected or native coarctation is likely to be more successful [61,62]. Associated cardiac defects commonly coexist with coarctation and may include bicuspid aortic valve in 51–57%, congenital aortic valvular stenosis in 12%, septal defects, and patent ductus arteriosus [63,64]. Intracranial aneurysms also occur with greater frequency in patients with aortic coarctation compared with the general population (10% vs. 2%). Preeclampsia is reported to complicate 2–22% of pregnancies in patients with coarctation [63–65].

In a large series studying pregnancy following coarctation repair, 98 pregnancies in 54 women ended in a live birth without significant maternal complications. The cesarean delivery rate was 6% with only one cesarean performed for a perceived maternal cardiovascular risk. Data on arm–leg blood pressure gradients or echocardiographic measurements were not available. Interestingly, the median gestational age at delivery was 40 weeks [64]. In a recent series of 118 pregnancies in women with repaired and native coarctation, one maternal death resulting from aortic dissection was reported [63]. The patient had Turner syndrome and conceived twins through *in vitro* fertilization. During pregnancy she had no evidence of hypertension; however, she expired suddenly at 36 weeks because of an acute aortic dissection at a site apart from the previous repair. The remaining patients tolerated pregnancy well with good neonatal outcomes. Patients with significant coarctation were more likely to be hypertensive during pregnancy compared with those without significant coarctation (58% vs. 11%). The presence of hypertension in this group strongly suggested the presence of a significant coarctation. Delivery was accomplished by cesarean section in 36% of patients, primarily for perceived maternal cardiovascular risk (82%). No difference was seen in maternal and neonatal outcomes between patients with repaired versus native coarctation in this cohort.

Concerns about the risk of aortic or intracranial aneurysm rupture and aortic dissection have prompted some physicians to recommend elective cesarean delivery. Coarctation of the aorta is associated with inherent abnormalities of the aorta which predispose patients for rupture, dilatation, and dissection [66]. Other risk factors for rupture or dissection include Turner syndrome, bicuspid aortic valve, and aortic dilatation [67,68]. Most patients will be able to have a successful vaginal delivery with careful management of pain using narcotic epidural anesthesia, control of blood pressure fluctuations, maintaining adequate cardiac preload, and minimizing valsalva efforts at delivery.

Ventricular septal defect

Although isolated ventricular septal defects (VSDs) account for approximately 15–20% of congenital cardiac abnormalities, most will close spontaneously in the first 2 years of life, making it an uncommonly encountered lesion in the pregnant patient [69]. Moderate to large-sized defects that remain unclosed or persist to adulthood may result in secondary pulmonary hypertension or congestive heart failure. Although blood flow across the shunt is usually left-to-right, reversal may occur and result in Eisenmenger syndrome, which is addressed in a later section. Isolated VSDs and corrected VSDs do not appear to increase the risk of adverse outcomes during pregnancy [70]. However, echocardiography should be considered in a patient with a history of a VSD, repaired or unrepaired, to exclude underlying pulmonary hypertension which would substantially increase the risk of life-threatening complications [71,72].

Atrial septal defect

Atrial septal defects (ASDs) do not appear to substantially increase the risk of pregnancy and are usually well tolerated [73]. Even if unrepaired, complications such as arrhythmias and pulmonary hypertension generally do not occur during the childbearing years [74]. Paradoxical embolism, presenting as a stroke, has been described during pregnancy and is possible in any patient with an intracardiac shunt [75,76].

Patent ductus arteriosus

Patent ductus arteriosus (PDA) is a commonly encountered lesion in neonates, particularly premature neonates. However, it is generally repaired in childhood and is therefore very unusual during pregnancy. The pregnancy outcome following repair does not appear to be negatively impacted [77]. However, patients with a large unrepaired PDA may develop secondary pulmonary hypertension and potentially Eisenmenger syndrome.

Eisenmenger syndrome

Unrepaired congenital intracardiac shunts such as a VSD, ASD or PDA lead to chronic overperfusion of the pulmonary vasculature. Over time, pulmonary hypertension results and may become significant enough to reverse the direction of flow across the shunt. This reversal of shunt flow to right-to-left defines Eisenmenger syndrome. Correction of the septal defect or patent ductus before the development of pulmonary hypertension prevents Eisenmenger syndrome. Once established, the only surgical alternative is a heart-lung transplant. Thirty-two percent of heart-lung transplants are performed for pulmonary hypertension secondary to congenital cardiac defects, making it the leading indication [78].

The deaths are attributed primarily to worsening hypoxia as a result of the normal physiologic changes of pregnancy. Increased blood volume and lower right ventricular filling pressures that result from decreased systemic vascular resistance place increased demands on the right ventricle and may precipitate right heart failure if unable to overcome the elevated pulmonary pressures. The decreased systemic vascular resistance in pregnancy lowers the peripheral resistance relative to the pulmonary resistance, increasing the likelihood of shunt reversal and worsening hypoxia and cyanosis. Hypoxia in turn will lead to pulmonary vasoconstriction and further increase pulmonary artery pressures. The thrombophilic state induced by pregnancy also predisposes patients to thromboembolic phenomena, another common cause of death in Eisenmenger syndrome.

Although Eisenmenger syndrome may be a common cause of pulmonary hypertension in young women, it remains a rare complication of pregnancy. Therefore, the available data on outcomes, optimal route of delivery, and anesthetic risks are limited. The maternal mortality rate in Eisenmenger syndrome is estimated at 30–40% [79–81]. In the most recent review of 73 patients with Eisenmenger syndrome, overall mortality was 36%, essentially unchanged in the past two decades [80]. Isolated VSD was the most common cardiac shunt (38%), followed by ASD (18%), and PDA (9%). Of the 26 patients who died, 88.5% died in the postpartum period, on average within 5 days of delivery. Patients diagnosed late or admitted to the hospital at later gestational ages were at much greater risk of death. Other factors historically associated with increased mortality include operative delivery, severe pulmonary hypertension, and multiparity. In this large series, the route of delivery did not appear to impact mortality rates.

Because of the high maternal mortality rates, patients with Eisenmenger syndrome should be counseled to avoid pregnancy, and if pregnant to consider termination. In ongoing pregnancies, therapies should be directed at minimizing cardiac demands, maximizing oxygenation, and avoiding excessive declines in systemic vascular resistance. Patients should be hospitalized at the end of the second trimester prophylactically, anticoagulated, and given supplemental oxygen. More recently, studies have utilized selective pulmonary artery vasodilators such as inhaled nitric oxide and IV epoprostenol (prostacyclin) during pregnancy with favorable results [82–84]. Regional anesthetics must be used cautiously to avoid decreases in systemic vascular resistance and ventricular filling that may precipitate reversal of shunt flow and cyanosis. However, recent studies suggest that the cautious use of slow-onset epidural anesthetics may be associated with lower mortality rates than general anesthesia for cesarean section delivery [80,85]. Similarly, avoidance of hypotensive events at any time during gestation, but particularly during labor and delivery, is extremely important.

Accurate assessment of pulmonary artery pressures may be a challenge in many patients. Echocardiographic assessment of pulmonary artery pressures has been shown to be less accurate in the pregnant patient and pulmonary artery catheters have been associated with higher complication rates in Eisenmenger syndrome [86,87].

Ebstein anomaly

Ebstein anomaly is a congenital cardiac defect characterized by an apical displacement of the septal leaflet of the tricuspid valve. Tricuspid regurgitation is always present, leading to right atrial dilatation. Right outflow tract obstruction can occur secondary to a fixed anterior leaflet of the tricuspid valve. ASD or patent foramen ovale coexists in 50% of cases. Twenty-five percent will have an accessory conduction pathway such as the Wolff–Parkinson–White syndrome [88]. Because it accounts for only 1% of all congenital cardiac disease, Ebstein anomaly is uncommonly encountered during pregnancy [89–91]. Pregnancy appears to be well tolerated in patients with Ebstein anomaly. In a series of 44 patients with 111 pregnancies, the live birth rate was 76% with no maternal complications reported [90]. Prematurity (21%) and congenital cardiac abnormalities (6%) were the most common neonatal issues.

Transposition of the great vessels

Complete transposition of the great vessels (TOGV) is uncommon during pregnancy. If uncorrected at birth, mortality rates approach 90% in the first year of life. Long-term survival rates are also diminished, with a reported 70–80% survival at 20–30 years post-repair [92]. The most common corrective procedure for complete TOGV performed on patients currently of childbearing age is the atrial switch (Mustard) procedure in which blood is surgically redirected through the atria [88]. Right ventricular dysfunction and dysrhythmias such as atrial flutter are commonly encountered in patients who survive into adulthood. The most significant issue reported in a recent series of 28 pregnancies in 16 women with a prior Mustard operation was irreversible right ventricular dysfunction despite the fact that pregnancy itself was tolerated well [93]. Other studies confirm the low risk of maternal mortality in 22 pregnant patients with a history of a Mustard or Rastelli operation, but do not address right ventricular function [94,95]. In one case, however, pregnancy termination was deemed necessary because of maternal deterioration.

Tetralogy of Fallot

Tetralogy of Fallot refers to the cyanotic complex of VSD, overriding aorta, right ventricular hypertrophy, and pulmonary stenosis. Most patients with tetralogy of Fallot undergo surgical correction in infancy and can expect excellent long-term survival rates [96]. Twenty years after surgical correction, approximately 10–15% will develop significant complications including pulmonary insufficiency which leads to right-sided heart failure and arrhythmias [97].

Most series report no adverse maternal events in pregnancy following surgical correction [98–100]. However, in a recent series of 50 pregnancies in 29 women with corrected tetralogy of Fallot, 12% of pregnancies were complicated by an arrhythmia or right-sided heart failure. Those patients with severe pulmonary regurgitation appear to be at greatest risk for these complications [101].

Marfan syndrome

Marfan syndrome is an autosomal, dominantly inherited, connective tissue disorder which leads to defective fibrillin, an important component of all connective tissues. Therefore patients have a 50% chance of passing the disorder to their children. The defective fibrillin results in cardiovascular, ocular, and musculoskeletal abnormalities; 80% of patients have adverse cardiac effects [102]. Classic Marfan syndrome is estimated to occur in 4–6 in 100,000 people. Patients with Marfan syndrome have a shortened life expectancy (mean 32 years) and more than 90% succumb to cardiac complications such as aortic dissection or rupture [103]. The weakened aortic media allows for progressive aortic dilatation which increases the risk of rupture. The hemodynamic changes of pregnancy place additional stress on a dilated aorta and place the patient at further risk of rupture.

Four population-based studies have been published which include a total of 107 women followed through 274 pregnancies [104–107]. The overall live birth rate was 80%, and 3.3% of patients experienced an aortic dissection. One percent of patients died as a result of aortic dissection. The degree of aortic dilatation appears to correlate directly with degree of risk for aortic dissection and rupture. Patients with an aortic root diameter more than 4.5 cm appear to be at greatest risk for aortic dissection and rupture. However, the exact threshold at which pregnancy termination should be advised is unclear. European guidelines recommend discouraging pregnancy if the aortic root is ≥4.0 cm whereas the Canadian guidelines recommend ≥4.5 cm as the threshold [105,107,108]. Elective replacement should be considered for patients with an aortic root diameter ≥4.7 cm although rupture and aneurysm at the repair site have been described.

It is important to assess the aortic root diameter preconception if possible, to provide the patient with information regarding pregnancy risks. Echocardiography should be performed regularly throughout gestation (every 4–8 weeks) to assess for evidence of worsening aortic dilatation. Beta-blockers have been shown to improve long-term outcomes and should be continued throughout gestation [109]. Vaginal delivery is acceptable if pain is adequately managed with epidural anesthesia and valsalva maneuvers are avoided. Cesarean delivery has been recommended by some in patients with an aortic root ≥4.5 cm [108].

Peripartum cardiomyopathy

Peripartum cardiomyopathy (PPCM) is defined by the development of heart failure in the last month of pregnancy or within 5 months of delivery in the absence of an identifiable cause or pre-existing heart disease. Additional specific criteria for diagnosing PPCM include evidence of left ventricular systolic dysfunction as demonstrated by classic echocardiographic criteria: ejection fraction less than 45%, shortening fraction less than 30%, and left ventricular end-diastolic dimension more than $2.7 \, cm/m^2$ body surface area [110]. Table 17.13 summarizes these diagnostic criteria.

Table 17.13 Criteria for diagnosis of peripartum cardiomyopathy. From Pearson et al. [110]

Classic

Development of cardiac failure in last month or within 5 months postpartum

Absence of an identifiable cause for cardiac failure

Absence of recognizable heart disease prior to last month of pregnancy

Additional

Left ventricular systolic dysfunction demonstrated by classic echocardiographic criteria: ejection fraction <45%, shortening fraction <30%, and left ventricular end-diastolic dimension >2.7 cm/m^2 body surface area

The exact incidence of this disease remains unknown; fortunately, PPCM is relatively rare, occurring in only 1 in 5000 births [111]. Historically, mortality rates have been reported as high as 56%; however, more recent studies suggest mortality rates may be closer to 9% [111,112]. Despite this, PPCM accounts for 8% of all maternal deaths and is one of the few causes of maternal mortality that is rising [111,113]. Forty-eight percent of patients who succumb to PPCM will die in the first 6 weeks postpartum. Fifty percent of PPCM deaths occur in the ensuing 1 year postpartum. African-American race increases risk of death from PPCM by more than sixfold [112].

Classic risk factors for PPCM include multiparity, advanced maternal age, multifetal gestation (fourfold increased risk), preeclampsia, hypertension, and African-American race. The etiology of peripartum cardiomyopathy has not been definitively determined; however, the most current available evidence suggests a viral myocarditis. One study reported endomyocardial biopsies consistent with myocarditis in 76% of patients [114]. Evidence of autoantibodies against cardiac tissue proteins in patients with PPCM also supports a role for an autoimmune phenomenon.

Once PPCM is diagnosed, management is focused on reducing cardiac preload with diuretic therapy (e.g., furosemide), reducing cardiac afterload with vasodilators (e.g., hydralazine, nitroglycerin, nitroprusside), and improving cardiac contractility with inotropic agents (e.g., dobutamine, digoxin). Diuresis should be undertaken cautiously in patients who are still pregnant at the time of diagnosis. Overly aggressive fluid loss may result in decreased uterine perfusion and fetal compromise. Afterload reduction decreases the pressure against which the heart must pump and is important to improve cardiac output in a failing heart. Stimulating cardiac output with inotropic agents is often necessary and will also improve uterine perfusion. Dobutamine (a selective beta$_1$-agonist and inotropic vasodilator) offers the advantage of selective decrease in systemic vascular resistance, but is primarily used as short-term therapy. Digoxin is useful for prolonged inotropic support but may require significantly higher doses and

more frequent dosing intervals in pregnant patients to achieve therapeutic levels. Dysrhythmias such as atrial fibrillation may occur as cardiac chamber distension worsens. Angiotensin-converting enzyme (ACE) inhibitors and angiotensin receptor blockers (ARBs) are a standard part of heart failure management in nonpregnant patients but should not be used in pregnant women. Beta-blocker therapy to reduce myocardial oxygen requirement may also be used if cardiac output does not improve satisfactorily with preload and afterload reduction. Therapeutic anticoagulation with UFH or LMWH should be considered to prevent thromboembolic events, especially in patients with arrhythmia or markedly depressed ejection fractions. Coumadin may be used in postpartum patients and is compatible with breastfeeding. The risk of thrombus formation increases as the severity of ventricular dilatation increases. Figure 17.3 outlines the approach to the patient with PPCM.

For pregnant patients diagnosed with PPCM, delivery poses particular concerns. In general, there is no evidence to suggest that cesarean section is beneficial and should be reserved for the usual obstetric indications. With careful monitoring, regional anesthesia is acceptable in patients with cardiomyopathy and has an important role in controlling pain, minimizing maternal effort, and reducing cardiac work. An assisted third stage should be considered if contractions are of insufficient force to deliver the fetus without maternal pushing efforts. In the immediate postpartum period, decompensation may occur as fluid is redistributed from the uteroplacental unit into the intravascular spaces. Approximately half of patients will demonstrate significant improvement in left ventricular function following delivery [115].

The prognosis for patients with PPCM is poor if left ventricular function does not normalize within 6 months postpartum. In this group of patients, mortality rates approach 85% by 5 years [115,116]. Death usually results from arrhythmias, thromboembolic phenomena, or progressive heart failure. Recent studies suggest that recovery of left ventricular function can be expected in 41–54% of patients [117,118]. However, predicting which patients are most likely to experience recovery has been a challenge. Normalization of left ventricular function is significantly more likely in patients with an initial ejection fraction more than 30% [117]. Other markers of ventricular size and function at initial diagnosis may also predict those who are less likely to recover. Left ventricular end-diastolic dimension greater than 6 cm and a fractional shortening value less than 20% predict a threefold higher chance of poor ventricular recovery [118]. Four to 6% of patients will undergo cardiac transplantation for failing to improve within 6 months postpartum.

Recurrent peripartum cardiomyopathy has been well described, even in patients whose left ventricular function has apparently returned to normal. This may be because of deficient contractile reserve, which may be demonstrated in response to a dobutamine challenge [119]. One author has

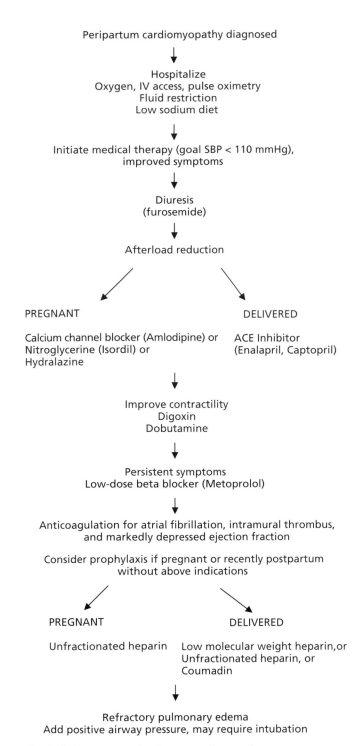

Peripartum cardiomyopathy diagnosed

↓

Hospitalize
Oxygen, IV access, pulse oximetry
Fluid restriction
Low sodium diet

↓

Initiate medical therapy (goal SBP < 110 mmHg),
improved symptoms

↓

Diuresis
(furosemide)

↓

Afterload reduction

PREGNANT

Calcium channel blocker (Amlodipine) or
Nitroglycerine (Isordil) or
Hydralazine

DELIVERED

ACE Inhibitor
(Enalapril, Captopril)

↓

Improve contractility
Digoxin
Dobutamine

↓

Persistent symptoms
Low-dose beta blocker (Metoprolol)

↓

Anticoagulation for atrial fibrillation, intramural thrombus,
and markedly depressed ejection fraction

Consider prophylaxis if pregnant or recently postpartum
without above indications

PREGNANT

Unfractionated heparin

DELIVERED

Low molecular weight heparin, or
Unfractionated heparin, or
Coumadin

↓

Refractory pulmonary edema
Add positive airway pressure, may require intubation

Fig. 17.3 Management of peripartum cardiomyopathy.

reported no adverse events in four pregnancies in patients with a history of PPCM [120]. In contrast, Elkayam *et al*. [121] recently detailed outcomes in 35 ongoing pregnancies in women with a history of PPCM. Even in patients with apparently normal cardiac function at the onset as measured by an ejection fraction more than 50%, cardiac symptoms occurred in 6% and 17% exhibited deteriorating cardiac function during

gestation. This deterioration persisted after delivery in 9% but no deaths occurred. Those with evidence of compromised left ventricular performance (ejection fraction less than 50%) suffered significant complications during gestation, with cardiac symptoms developing in 50%, deterioration of cardiac function in 33%, persistent decompensation in 42%, and death in 25% of women in this group. Other authors have reported similar findings in smaller case series [118,122]. Therefore, women with a history of PPCM and evidence of incomplete left ventricular recovery should be counseled to avoid pregnancy. However, even women with apparent recovery remain at high risk for cardiac complications in subsequent pregnancies.

Acute myocardial infarction

Acute myocardial infarction (AMI) occurring during pregnancy and the puerperium is rare, affecting approximately 1 in 35,000 gravidas [123]. However, the incidence can be expected to increase as more women postpone childbearing into the fourth and fifth decades of life, when risk factors for coronary artery disease are more prevalent. In fact, a recent population-based study of AMI in pregnancy 1991–2000 demonstrated an increasing incidence across the decade [123]. In this study of 151 patients, the mortality rate of AMI during pregnancy was 7.3%, significantly lower than reported in previous studies [124–126]. The three strongest predictors of AMI in this study were chronic hypertension, advancing maternal age, and diabetes. Sixty-six percent of the AMIs occurred in women older than 30 years. Only 21% of AMIs were diagnosed intrapartum; the remainder was evenly divided between the antepartum and postpartum periods but no deaths occurred postpartum. Patients diagnosed with an AMI intrapartum had the highest mortality rate and were more likely to have severe preeclampsia and eclampsia. Myocardial infarction occurring before or after labor was more likely to be related to diabetes, coronary artery disease, and lipid disorders [123].

Despite the lower mortality rate, these findings are similar to a 1996 review which described the pregnancy outcomes of 125 pregnant patients diagnosed with myocardial infarction [126]. The majority of myocardial infarctions occurred in women older than 33 years and during the third trimester of pregnancy. In this study, the maternal death rate was 21% and overall fetal mortality rate was 13%. Atherosclerotic disease was identified in 43% of patients, coronary thrombus in 21%, and apparently normal coronary arteries in 29%.

The acute treatment of AMI in pregnancy should adhere to the same management principles as the nonpregnant patient: administer supplemental oxygen, 325 mg aspirin, narcotic analgesia, nitroglycerin, heparin, and beta-blockers. The use of fibrinolytic agents during pregnancy (almost exclusively for the treatment of pulmonary emboli) has been associated with an increased rate of maternal hemorrhagic

Table 17.14 *Continued.*

Drug (Safety in Pregnancy)	Dose	Uterine Blood Flow (UBF)	Fetal Effects
Antiarrhythmic agents			
Lidocaine (B)	1 mg/kg bolus; repeat ½ bolus at 10 min as needed ×4; infusion at 1–4 mg/min; total dose 3 mg/kg	No effect	Not teratogenic Rapidly crosses placenta
Procainamide (C)	100 mg over 30 min, then 2–6 mg/min infusion Total dose 17 mg/kg		
Quinidine (C)	15 mg/kg over 60 min, then 0.02 mg/kg/min infusion		
Bretylium (C)	5 mg/kg IV bolus, then 1–2 mg/min infusion	↓ UBF	Unknown
Phenytoin (D)	300 mg IV, then 100 mg every 5 min to a total of 1000 mg	No effect	Teratogenic "Fetal hydantoin syndrome"
Amiodarone (D)	5 mg/kg IV over 3 min, then 10 mg/kg/day		Teratogenic Transient bradycardia Prolonged QT
AV node blocking agents			
Adenosine	6 mg IV bolus over 1–3 s, followed by 20 mL saline bolus; may repeat at 12 mg in 1–2 min ×2	↑ or ↓ UBF	No known adverse fetal effects
Verapamil	As stated above		
Beta-blockers	As stated above		
Digoxin	As stated above		

ents have been reported, abundant data exist on the use of these medications to prevent graft rejection in pregnant renal transplant recipients. In general, patients can be reassured that the neonatal risks posed by these medications are minimal. Azathioprine has been associated with neonatal immunosuppression when used at high doses; however, current protocols utilize much lower doses and adverse neonatal events have not been reported. Animal studies suggested that mycophenolate mofetil may be associated with higher rates of congenital anomalies. Data in human pregnancies are very limited [136].

Case presentation

A 30-year-old, gravida 4, para 3 at 34 weeks' gestation by last menstrual period presents complaining of shortness of breath and contractions. She has had no prenatal care during this pregnancy. The patient appears short of breath and anxious. Her blood pressure is 134/78 mmHg, and her pulse is irregular at 100–110 beats/min. Respiratory rate is 26/min.

She is admitted to the hospital for evaluation and management. An ECG demonstrates atrial fibrillation and chest X-ray confirms pulmonary edema. Arterial blood gas on 40% Fio_2 reveals pH 7.48, Pao_2 60, Pco_2 27, HCO_3^- 18, O_2 saturation 90%, consistent with hypoxemia and respiratory alkalosis. An ultrasound confirms an intrauterine gestation measuring 33 weeks with normal amniotic fluid volume. Fetal heart rate tracing is reactive with occasional late decelerations.

Diuresis is accomplished with furosemide while oxygen supplementation by face mask is continued to maintain oxygen saturations above 95%. Digoxin is started to control atrial fibrillation and prophylactic subcutaneous heparin is begun. An echocardiogram reveals mitral stenosis with a mean valve area of 1.2 cm² , left atrial enlargement, as well as mild aortic, mitral, and tricuspid insufficiency, consistent with rheumatic valvular disease.

Amniocentesis is performed; fetal lung maturity is confirmed and the decision made to proceed with delivery. Epidural is placed to control pain and therefore minimize tachycardia. A continuous esmolol drip is started to maintain maternal heart rate below 90–100 beats/min.

Oxytocin induction of labor was begun and the patient progressed to complete dilatation. Persistent variable decelerations developed, a low-vacuum assisted vaginal delivery was accomplished with delivery of a viable 2600-g infant with Apgars 7[1], 9[5]. Postpartum, the patient continued to improve, with resolution of pulmonary edema and control of atrial fibrillation. She was discharged home on postpartum day 4 on digoxin. Outpatient follow-up with cardiology was arranged for consideration of surgical correction of the stenotic mitral valve.

References

1 Ullery JC. The management of pregnancy complicated by heart disease. *Am J Obstet Gynecol* 1954;**67**:834–66.

2 Szekely P, Turner R, Snaith L. Pregnancy and the changing pattern of rheumatic heart disease. *Br Heart J* 1973;**35**: 1293–303.

3 De SM. Maternal mortality from heart disease in pregnancy. *Br Heart J* 1993;**69**:524.

4 Hsieh TT, Chen KC, Soong JH. Outcome of pregnancy in patients with organic heart disease in Taiwan. *Asia Oceania J Obstet Gynaecol* 1993;**19**:21–7.

5 Chalupczak P, Kolasinska-Kloch W, Jach R, Basta A. Pregnancy in patients with heart disease. *Clin Exp Obstet Gynecol* 2004;**31**:271–3.

6 Berg CJ, Atrash HK, Koonin LM, Tucker M. Pregnancy-related mortality in the United States, 1987–1990. *Obstet Gynecol* 1996;**88**:161–7.

7 Hogberg U, Innala E, Sandstrom A. Maternal mortality in Sweden, 1980–1988. *Obstet Gynecol* 1994;**84**:240–4.

8 Koonin LM, Atrash HK, Lawson HW, Smith JC. Maternal mortality surveillance, United States, 1979–1986. *MMWR CDC Surveill Summ* 1991;**40**:1–13.

9 El-Solh AA, Grant BJ. A comparison of severity of illness scoring systems for critically ill obstetric patients. *Chest* 1996;**110**:1299–304.

10 Loverro G, Pansini V, Greco P, Vimercati A, Parisi AM, Selvaggi L. Indications and outcome for intensive care unit admission during puerperium. *Arch Gynecol Obstet* 2001;**265**:195–8.

11 Mabie WC, Sibai BM. Treatment in an obstetric intensive care unit. *Am J Obstet Gynecol* 1990;**162**:1–4.

12 Mahutte NG, Murphy-Kaulbeck L, Le Q, Solomon J, Benjamin A, Boyd ME. Obstetric admissions to the intensive care unit. *Obstet Gynecol* 1999;**94**:263–6.

13 Naylor DF Jr, Olson MM. Critical care obstetrics and gynecology. *Crit Care Clin* 2003;**19**:127–49.

14 Tang LC, Kwok AC, Wong AY, Lee YY, Sun KO, So AP. Critical care in obstetrical patients: an eight-year review. *Chin Med J (Engl)* 1997;**110**:936–41.

15 Zeeman GG, Wendel GD, Jr., Cunningham FG. A blueprint for obstetric critical care. *Am J Obstet Gynecol* 2003;**188**:532–6.

16 Clark SL, Cotton DB, Lee W, et al. Central hemodynamic assessment of normal term pregnancy. *Am J Obstet Gynecol* 1989;**161**:1439–42.

17 Elkayam U, Gleicher N. Hemodynamics and cardiac function during normal pregnancy and the puerperium. In: Elkayam U, Gleicher N, eds. *Cardiac Problems in Pregnancy*, 3rd edn. New York: Wiley-Liss, 1998; 3–19.

18 Capeless EL, Clapp JF. Cardiovascular changes in early phase of pregnancy. *Am J Obstet Gynecol* 1989;**161**:1449–53.

19 Gei AF, Hankins GD. Cardiac disease and pregnancy. *Obstet Gynecol Clin North Am* 2001;**28**:465–512.

20 Clark SL. Structural cardiac disease in pregnancy. In: Clark SL, Cotton DB, Phelan JP, eds. *Critical Care Obstetrics*. Oradell, N.J.: Medical Economics Books, 1987; 92.

21 Siu SC, Sermer M, Harrison DA, et al. Risk and predictors for pregnancy-related complications in women with heart disease. *Circulation* 1997;**96**:2789–94.

22 Siu SC, Sermer M, Colman JM, et al. Prospective multicenter study of pregnancy outcomes in women with heart disease. *Circulation* 2001;**104**:515–21.

23 Siu SC, Colman JM, Sorensen S, et al. Adverse neonatal and cardiac outcomes are more common in pregnant women with cardiac disease. *Circulation* 2002;**105**:2179–84.

24 Dye TD, Gordon H, Held B, Tolliver NJ, Holmes AP. Retrospective maternal mortality case ascertainment in West Virginia, 1985 to 1989. *Am J Obstet Gynecol* 1992;**167**: 72–6.

25 Montana E, Khoury MJ, Cragan JD, Sharma S, Dhar P, Fyfe D. Trends and outcomes after prenatal diagnosis of congenital cardiac malformations by fetal echocardiography in a well defined birth population, Atlanta, Georgia, 1990–1994. *J Am Coll Cardiol* 1996;**28**:1805–9.

26 Rose V, Gold RJ, Lindsay G, Allen M. A possible increase in the incidence of congenital heart defects among the offspring of affected parents. *J Am Coll Cardiol* 1985;**6**:376–82.

27 Whittemore R, Hobbins JC, Engle MA. Pregnancy and its outcome in women with and without surgical treatment of congenital heart disease. *Am J Cardiol* 1982;**50**:641–51.

28 Driscoll DJ, Michels VV, Gersony WM, et al. Occurrence risk for congenital heart defects in relatives of patients with aortic stenosis, pulmonary stenosis, or ventricular septal defect. *Circulation* 1993;**87**(Suppl):I114–20.

29 Presbitero P, Somerville J, Stone S, Aruta E, Spiegelhalter D, Rabajoli F. Pregnancy in cyanotic congenital heart disease: outcome of mother and fetus. *Circulation* 1994;**89**:2673–6.

30 Teerlink JR, Foster E. Valvular heart disease in pregnancy: a contemporary perspective. *Cardiol Clin* 1998;**16**:573–98, x.

31 Lupton M, Oteng-Ntim E, Ayida G, Steer PJ. Cardiac disease in pregnancy. *Curr Opin Obstet Gynecol* 2002;**14**: 137–43.

32 Dajani AS, Taubert KA, Wilson W, et al. Prevention of bacterial endocarditis: recommendations by the American Heart Association. *JAMA* 1997;**277**:1794–801.

33 Dajani AS, Taubert KA, Wilson W, et al. Prevention of bacterial endocarditis: recommendations by the American Heart Association. *Clin Infect Dis* 1997;**25**:1448–58.

34 Reimold SC, Rutherford JD. Clinical practice. Vulvular heart disease in pregnancy. *N Engl J Med* 2003;**349**:52–9.

35 Clark SL, Phelan JP, Greenspoon J, Aldahl D, Horenstein J. Labor and delivery in the presence of mitral stenosis: central hemodynamic observations. *Am J Obstet Gynecol* 1985;**152**: 984–8.

36 Bonow RO, Carabello B, de LA Jr, et al. Guidelines for the management of patients with valvular heart disease: executive summary. A report of the American College of Cardiology/ American Heart Association Task Force on Practice Guidelines (Committee on Management of Patients with Valvular Heart Disease). *Circulation* 1998;**98**:1949–84.

37 Iung B, Cormier B, Elias J, *et al*. Usefulness of percutaneous balloon commissurotomy for mitral stenosis during pregnancy. *Am J Cardiol* 1994;73:398–400.

38 Kalra GS, Arora R, Khan JA, Nigam M, Khalillulah M. Percutaneous mitral commissurotomy for severe mitral stenosis during pregnancy. *Catheter Cardiovasc Diagn* 1994;33:28–30.

39 Sivadasanpillai H, Srinivasan A, Sivasubramoniam S, *et al*. Long-term outcome of patients undergoing balloon mitral valvotomy in pregnancy. *Am J Cardiol* 2005;95: 1504–6.

40 Silversides CK, Colman JM, Sermer M, Siu SC. Cardiac risk in pregnant women with rheumatic mitral stenosis. *Am J Cardiol* 2003;91:1382–5.

41 Hameed A, Karaalp IS, Tummala PP, *et al*. The effect of valvular heart disease on maternal and fetal outcome of pregnancy. *J Am Coll Cardiol* 2001;37:893–9.

42 Sheikh F, Rangwala S, DeSimone C, Smith HS, O'Leary AM. Management of the parturient with severe aortic incompetence. *J Cardiothorac Vasc Anesth* 1995;9:575–7.

43 Alderson JD. Cardiovascular collapse following epidural anaesthesia for Caesarean section in a patient with aortic incompetence. *Anaesthesia* 1987;42:643–5.

44 Savage DD, Devereux RB, Garrison RJ, *et al*. Mitral valve prolapse in the general population. 2. Clinical features: the Framingham Study. *Am Heart J* 1983;106:577–81.

45 Lao TT, Sermer M, MaGee L, Farine D, Colman JM. Congenital aortic stenosis and pregnancy: a reappraisal. *Am J Obstet Gynecol* 1993;169:540–5.

46 Silversides CK, Colman JM, Sermer M, Farine D, Siu SC. Early and intermediate-term outcomes of pregnancy with congenital aortic stenosis. *Am J Cardiol* 2003;91:1386–9.

47 Avila WS, Rossi EG, Ramires JA, *et al*. Pregnancy in patients with heart disease: experience with 1000 cases. *Clin Cardiol* 2003;26:135–42.

48 Chan WS, Anand S, Ginsberg JS. Anticoagulation of pregnant women with mechanical heart valves: a systematic review of the literature. *Arch Intern Med* 2000;160:191–6.

49 Hall JG, Pauli RM, Wilson KM. Maternal and fetal sequelae of anticoagulation during pregnancy. *Am J Med* 1980;68:122–40.

50 Ginsberg JS, Hirsh J, Turner DC, Levine MN, Burrows R. Risks to the fetus of anticoagulant therapy during pregnancy. *Thromb Haemost* 1989;61:197–203.

51 Weitz JI. Low-molecular-weight heparins. *N Engl J Med* 1997;337:688–98.

52 Aventis Pharmaceuticals Inc. Lovenox injection [package insert]. Bridgewater, NJ; 2002.

53 Seshadri N, Goldhaber SZ, Elkayam U, *et al*. The clinical challenge of bridging anticoagulation with low-molecular-weight heparin in patients with mechanical prosthetic heart valves: an evidence-based comparative review focusing on anticoagulation options in pregnant and nonpregnant patients. *Am Heart J* 2005;150:27–34.

54 Rowan JA, McCowan LM, Raudkivi PJ, North RA. Enoxaparin treatment in women with mechanical heart valves during pregnancy. *Am J Obstet Gynecol* 2001;185:633–7.

55 Raschke RA, Guidry JR, Foley MR. Apparent heparin resistance from elevated factor VIII during pregnancy. *Obstet Gynecol* 2000;96:804–6.

56 Whitfield LR, Lele AS, Levy G. Effect of pregnancy on the relationship between concentration and anticoagulant action of heparin. *Clin Pharmacol Ther* 1983;34:23–8.

57 Olson JD, Arkin CF, Brandt JT, *et al*. College of American Pathologists Conference XXXI on laboratory monitoring of anticoagulant therapy: laboratory monitoring of unfractionated heparin therapy. *Arch Pathol Lab Med* 1998;122: 782–98.

58 Bates SM, Greer IA, Hirsh J, Ginsberg JS. Use of antithrombotic agents during pregnancy: the Seventh ACCP Conference on Antithrombotic and Thrombolytic Therapy. *Chest* 2004;126(Suppl):627S–44S.

59 Klein LL, Galan HL. Cardiac disease in pregnancy. *Obstet Gynecol Clin North Am* 2004;31:429–59; viii.

60 Hoffman JI, Kaplan S. The incidence of congenital heart disease. *J Am Coll Cardiol* 2002;39:1890–900.

61 Deal K, Wooley CF. Coarctation of the aorta and pregnancy. *Ann Intern Med* 1973;78:706–10.

62 Goodwin JF. Pregnancy and coarctation of the aorta. *Lancet* 1958;1:16–20.

63 Beauchesne LM, Connolly HM, Ammash NM, Warnes CA. Coarctation of the aorta: outcome of pregnancy. *J Am Coll Cardiol* 2001;38:1728–33.

64 Vriend JW, Drenthen W, Pieper PG, *et al*. Outcome of pregnancy in patients after repair of aortic coarctation. *Eur Heart J* 2005;26:2173–8.

65 Saidi AS, Bezold LI, Altman CA, Ayres NA, Bricker JT. Outcome of pregnancy following intervention for coarctation of the aorta. *Am J Cardiol* 1998;82:786–8.

66 Niwa K, Perloff JK, Bhuta SM, *et al*. Structural abnormalities of great arterial walls in congenital heart disease: light and electron microscopic analyses. *Circulation* 2001;103:393–400.

67 Bonderman D, Gharehbaghi-Schnell E, Wollenek G, Maurer G, Baumgartner H, Lang IM. Mechanisms underlying aortic dilatation in congenital aortic valve malformation. *Circulation* 1999;99:2138–43.

68 Lin AE, Lippe B, Rosenfeld RG. Further delineation of aortic dilation, dissection, and rupture in patients with Turner syndrome. *Pediatrics* 1998;102:e12.

69 Myung K, Park MD, eds. *Pediatric Cardiology for Practitioners*, 4th edn. St. Louis: Mosby, 2002.

70 Schaefer G, Arditi LI, Solomon HA, Ringland JE. Congenital heart disease and pregnancy. *Clin Obstet Gynecol* 1968;11:1048–63.

71 Gilman DH. Caesarean section in undiagnosed Eisenmenger's syndrome. Report of a patient with a fatal outcome. *Anaesthesia* 1991;46:371–3.

72 Jackson GM, Dildy GA, Varner MW, Clark SL. Severe pulmonary hypertension in pregnancy following successful repair of ventricular septal defect in childhood. *Obstet Gynecol* 1993;82(Suppl):680–2.

73 Neilson G, Galea EG, Blunt A. Congenital heart disease and pregnancy. *Med J Aust* 1970;1:1086–8.

74 Perloff JK. Congenital heart disease and pregnancy. *Clin Cardiol* 1994;17:579–87.

75 Daehnert I, Ewert P, Berger F, Lange PE. Echocardiographically guided closure of a patent foramen ovale during pregnancy after recurrent strokes. *J Interv Cardiol* 2001;14:191–2.

76 Kozelj M, Novak-Antolic Z, Grad A, Peternel P. Patent foramen ovale as a potential cause of paradoxical embolism in the postpartum period. *Eur J Obstet Gynecol Reprod Biol* 1999;**84**:55–7.

77 Actis Dato GM, Cavaglia M, Aidala E, *et al*. Patent ductus arteriosus: follow-up of 677 operated cases 40 years later. *Minerva Cardioangiol* 1999;**47**:245–54.

78 Trulock EP, Edwards LB, Taylor DO, *et al*. The Registry of the International Society for Heart and Lung Transplantation: Twentieth Official adult lung and heart-lung transplant report, 2003. *J Heart Lung Transplant* 2003;**22**:625–35.

79 Gleicher N, Midwall J, Hochberger D, Jaffin H. Eisenmenger's syndrome and pregnancy. *Obstet Gynecol Surv* 1979;**34**:721–41.

80 Weiss BM, Zemp L, Seifert B, Hess OM. Outcome of pulmonary vascular disease in pregnancy: a systematic overview from 1978 through 1996. *J Am Coll Cardiol* 1998;**31**:1650–7.

81 Yentis SM, Steer PJ, Plaat F. Eisenmenger's syndrome in pregnancy: maternal and fetal mortality in the 1990s. *Br J Obstet Gynaecol* 1998;**105**:921–2.

82 Goodwin TM, Gherman RB, Hameed A, Elkayam U. Favorable response of Eisenmenger syndrome to inhaled nitric oxide during pregnancy. *Am J Obstet Gynecol* 1999;**180**: 64–7.

83 Lust KM, Boots RJ, Dooris M, Wilson J. Management of labor in Eisenmenger syndrome with inhaled nitric oxide. *Am J Obstet Gynecol* 1999;**181**:419–23.

84 Geohas C, McLaughlin VV. Successful management of pregnancy in a patient with eisenmenger syndrome with epoprostenol. *Chest* 2003;**124**:1170–3.

85 Martin JT, Tautz TJ, Antognini JF. Safety of regional anesthesia in Eisenmenger's syndrome. *Reg Anesth Pain Med* 2002;**27**: 509–13.

86 Devitt JH, Noble WH, Byrick RJ. A Swan-Ganz catheter related complication in a patient with Eisenmenger's syndrome. *Anesthesiology* 1982;**57**:335–7.

87 Penning S, Robinson KD, Major CA, Garite TJ. A comparison of echocardiography and pulmonary artery catheterization for evaluation of pulmonary artery pressures in pregnant patients with suspected pulmonary hypertension. *Am J Obstet Gynecol* 2001;**184**:1568–70.

88 Webb GD, Smallhorn JF, Therrien J, Redington AN. Congenital heart disease. In: Zipes DP, Libby P, Bonow RO, Braunwald E, eds. *Braunwald's Heart Disease: A Textbook of Cardiovascular Medicine*, 7th edn. Saunders, 2005.

89 Waickman LA, Skorton DJ, Varner MW, Ehmke DA, Goplerud CP. Ebstein's anomaly and pregnancy. *Am J Cardiol* 1984;**53**:357–8.

90 Donnelly JE, Brown JM, Radford DJ. Pregnancy outcome and Ebstein's anomaly. *Br Heart J* 1991;**66**:368–71.

91 Connolly HM, Warnes CA. Ebstein's anomaly: outcome of pregnancy. *J Am Coll Cardiol* 1994;**23**:1194–8.

92 Wilson NJ, Clarkson PM, Barratt-Boyes BG, *et al*. Long-term outcome after the mustard repair for simple transposition of the great arteries: 28-year follow-up. *J Am Coll Cardiol* 1998;**32**:758–65.

93 Guedes A, Mercier LA, Leduc L, Berube L, Marcotte F, Dore A. Impact of pregnancy on the systemic right ventricle after a Mustard operation for transposition of the great arteries. *J Am Coll Cardiol* 2004;**44**:433–7.

94 Clarkson PM, Wilson NJ, Neutze JM, North RA, Calder AL, Barratt-Boyes BG. Outcome of pregnancy after the Mustard operation for transposition of the great arteries with intact ventricular septum. *J Am Coll Cardiol* 1994;**24**:190–3.

95 Lao TT, Sermer M, Colman JM. Pregnancy following surgical correction for transposition of the great arteries. *Obstet Gynecol* 1994;**83**:665–8.

96 Murphy JG, Gersh BJ, Mair DD, *et al*. Long-term outcome in patients undergoing surgical repair of tetralogy of Fallot. *N Engl J Med* 1993;**329**:593–9.

97 Therrien J, Marx GR, Gatzoulis MA. Late problems in tetralogy of Fallot: recognition, management, and prevention. *Cardiol Clin* 2002;**20**:395–404.

98 Singh H, Bolton PJ, Oakley CM. Pregnancy after surgical correction of tetralogy of Fallot. *Br Med J (Clin Res Ed)* 1982;**285**:168–70.

99 Nissenkorn A, Friedman S, Schonfeld A, Ovadia J. Fetomaternal outcome in pregnancies after total correction of the tetralogy of Fallot. *Int Surg* 1984;**69**:125–8.

100 Lewis BS, Rogers NM, Gotsman MS. Successful pregnancy after repair of Fallot's tetralogy. *S Afr Med J* 1972;**46**:934–6.

101 Meijer JM, Pieper PG, Drenthen W, *et al*. Pregnancy, fertility, and recurrence risk in corrected tetralogy of Fallot. *Heart* 2005;**91**:801–5.

102 Child AH. Marfan syndrome: current medical and genetic knowledge: how to treat and when. *J Card Surg* 1997;**12**(Suppl):131–5.

103 Lalchandani S, Wingfield M. Pregnancy in women with Marfan's Syndrome. *Eur J Obstet Gynecol Reprod Biol* 2003;**110**:125–30.

104 Lipscomb KJ, Smith JC, Clarke B, Donnai P, Harris R. Outcome of pregnancy in women with Marfan's syndrome. *Br J Obstet Gynaecol* 1997;**104**:201–6.

105 Meijboom LJ, Vos FE, Timmermans J, Boers GH, Zwinderman AH, Mulder BJ. Pregnancy and aortic root growth in the Marfan syndrome: a prospective study. *Eur Heart J* 2005;**26**:914–20.

106 Pyeritz RE, McKusick VA. The Marfan syndrome: diagnosis and management. *N Engl J Med* 1979;**300**:772–7.

107 Rossiter JP, Repke JT, Morales AJ, Murphy EA, Pyeritz RE. A prospective longitudinal evaluation of pregnancy in the Marfan syndrome. *Am J Obstet Gynecol* 1995;**173**:1599–606.

108 Expert consensus document on management of cardiovascular diseases during pregnancy. *Eur Heart J* 2003;**24**:761–81.

109 Shores J, Berger KR, Murphy EA, Pyeritz RE. Progression of aortic dilatation and the benefit of long-term beta-adrenergic blockade in Marfan's syndrome. *N Engl J Med* 1994;**330**:1335–41.

110 Pearson GD, Veille JC, Rahimtoola S, *et al*. Peripartum cardiomyopathy: National Heart, Lung, and Blood Institute and Office of Rare Diseases (National Institutes of Health) workshop recommendations and review. *JAMA* 2000;**283**:1183–8.

111 Tidswell M. Peripartum cardiomyopathy. *Crit Care Clin* 2004;**20**:777–88; xi.

112 Whitehead SJ, Berg CJ, Chang J. Pregnancy-related mortality due to cardiomyopathy: United States, 1991–1997. *Obstet Gynecol* 2003;**102**:1326–31.

113 Chang J, Elam-Evans LD, Berg CJ, *et al*. Pregnancy-related mortality surveillance: United States, 1991–1999. *MMWR Surveill Summ* 2003;**52**:1–8.

114 Midei MG, DeMent SH, Feldman AM, Hutchins GM, Baughman KL. Peripartum myocarditis and cardiomyopathy. *Circulation* 1990;**81**:922–8.

115 Demakis JG, Rahimtoola SH, Sutton GC, *et al*. Natural course of peripartum cardiomyopathy. *Circulation* 1971;**44**:1053–61.

116 Sutton MS, Cole P, Plappert M, Saltzman D, Goldhaber S. Effects of subsequent pregnancy on left ventricular function in peripartum cardiomyopathy. *Am Heart J* 1991;**121**:1776–8.

117 Elkayam U, Akhter MW, Singh H, *et al*. Pregnancy-associated cardiomyopathy: clinical characteristics and a comparison between early and late presentation. *Circulation* 2005;**111**: 2050–5.

118 Chapa JB, Heiberger HB, Weinert L, Decara J, Lang RM, Hibbard JU. Prognostic value of echocardiography in peripartum cardiomyopathy. *Obstet Gynecol* 2005;**105**:1303–8.

119 Lampert MB, Weinert L, Hibbard J, Korcarz C, Lindheimer M, Lang RM. Contractile reserve in patients with peripartum cardiomyopathy and recovered left ventricular function. *Am J Obstet Gynecol* 1997;**176**:189–95.

120 Sutton MS, Cole P, Plappert M, Saltzman D, Goldhaber S. Effects of subsequent pregnancy on left ventricular function in peripartum cardiomyopathy. *Am Heart J* 1991;**121**: 1776–8.

121 Elkayam U, Tummala PP, Rao K, *et al*. Maternal and fetal outcomes of subsequent pregnancies in women with peripartum cardiomyopathy. *N Engl J Med* 2001;**344**:1567–71.

122 Sliwa K, Forster O, Zhanje F, Candy G, Kachope J, Essop R. Outcome of subsequent pregnancy in patients with documented peripartum cardiomyopathy. *Am J Cardiol* 2004;**93**:1441–3; A10.

123 Ladner HE, Danielsen B, Gilbert WM. Acute myocardial infarction in pregnancy and the puerperium: a population-based study. *Obstet Gynecol* 2005;**105**:480–4.

124 Badui E, Enciso R. Acute myocardial infarction during pregnancy and puerperium: a review. *Angiology* 1996;**47**: 739–56.

125 Hankins GD, Wendel GD Jr, Leveno KJ, Stoneham J. Myocardial infarction during pregnancy: a review. *Obstet Gynecol* 1985;**65**:139–46.

126 Roth A, Elkayam U. Acute myocardial infarction associated with pregnancy. *Ann Intern Med* 1996;**125**:751–62.

127 Upshaw CB Jr. A study of maternal electrocardiograms recorded during labor and delivery. *Am J Obstet Gynecol* 1970;**107**:17–27.

128 Gowda RM, Khan IA, Mehta NJ, Vasavada BC, Sacchi TJ. Cardiac arrhythmias in pregnancy: clinical and therapeutic considerations. *Int J Cardiol* 2003;**88**:129–33.

129 Hameed AB, Foley MR. Cardiac disease in pregnancy. In: Foley MR, Strong TH Jr, Garite TJ, eds. *Obstetric Intensive Care Manual*, 2nd edn. McGraw-Hill, 2004: 96–112.

130 Schroeder JS, Harrison DC. Repeated cardioversion during pregnancy. Treatment of refractory paroxysmal atrial tachycardia during 3 successive pregnancies. *Am J Cardiol* 1971;**27**:445–6.

131 Natale A, Davidson T, Geiger MJ, Newby K. Implantable cardioverter-defibrillators and pregnancy: a safe combination? *Circulation* 1997;**96**:2808–12.

132 Jaffe R, Gruber A, Fejgin M, Altaras M, Ben-Aderet N. Pregnancy with an artificial pacemaker. *Obstet Gynecol Surv* 1987;**42**:137–9.

133 Scott JR, Wagoner LE, Olsen SL, Taylor DO, Renlund DG. Pregnancy in heart transplant recipients: management and outcome. *Obstet Gynecol* 1993;**82**:324–7.

134 Kim KM, Sukhani R, Slogoff S, Tomich PG. Central hemodynamic changes associated with pregnancy in a long-term cardiac transplant recipient. *Am J Obstet Gynecol* 1996;**174**:1651–3.

135 Greenberg ML, Uretsky BF, Reddy PS, *et al*. Long-term hemodynamic follow-up of cardiac transplant patients treated with cyclosporine and prednisone. *Circulation* 1985;**71**:487–94.

136 Armenti VT, Radomski JS, Moritz MJ, Gaughan WJ, McGrory CH, Coscia LA. Report from the National Transplantation Pregnancy Registry (NTPR): outcomes of pregnancy after transplantation. *Clin Transpl* 2003;131–41.

137 Branch KR, Wagoner LE, McGrory CH, *et al*. Risks of subsequent pregnancies on mother and newborn in female heart transplant recipients. *J Heart Lung Transplant* 1998;**17**:698–702.

18 Renal disease in pregnancy

John Hayslett

Physiologic changes in pregnancy

Renal disease in pregnancy may threaten fetal development as well as the health of the mother. To identify possible pathologic alterations in renal function during pregnancy it is important to recognize the physiologic changes that occur in normal pregnancy. Normal pregnancy is associated with a unique set of parameters associated with cardiovascular and renal function. In human pregnancy, there is a marked expansion of the extracellular fluid volume as a result of peripheral vasodilatation that begins by 8 weeks' gestation and continues until term. This vascular change is associated with a cumulative retention of 500–700 mEq sodium and 1.5-fold increase in plasma volume [1]. Cardiac output increases 50%, with a similar rise in blood flow to other visceral organs [2]. The cause of the vascular dilatation may be secretion of relaxin a hormone related to the insulin family of hormones, by the placenta [3]. The administration of relaxin in physiologic doses causes cardiovascular changes in experimental animals which simulate changes in human gestation. Additional sources of vasodilatation include increased endothelial prostacyclin and nitric oxide production.

Despite the gestationally induced expansion of the vascular system, diastolic blood pressure falls slightly in the second trimester. Pregnancy-associated sodium retention most likely results from the action of aldosterone. The plasma concentration of aldosterone rises 4–6 times above normal levels during gestation to achieve levels of 80–100 ng/dL [4]. Studies in normal gravidas indicate that the concentration of aldosterone in pregnancy is under dynamic control, dependent on the volume of the extracellular fluid [5]. Despite the high circulating levels of aldosterone, metabolism of potassium remains unaffected.

Renal blood flow increases by approximately 80% from conception until term. Correspondingly, glomerular filtration rates increase 30–50% by the second trimester. In normal gravidas the filtration rate remains stable from 20 weeks until term.

However, in healthy ambulatory women a modest decrease in filtration occurs near term because of fluid collection in the lower extremities [6]. Studies in experimental animals and in pregnant women demonstrate that this remarkable rise in filtration rate correlates with the increase in glomerular plasma flow [7]. In one report the glomerular filtration rate in the third trimester averaged 140–160 mL/min compared with 105 mL/min in the same women when not pregnant [6]. Because of the increase in glomerular filtration rate and expansion of extracellular fluid volume, the concentration of plasma creatinine is reduced from the average of 0.67 ± 0.2 mg/dL in non-pregnant women to 0.5 ± 0.1 mg/dL in pregnancy [1]. A useful role of thumb is that a plasma concentration of creatinine of more than 0.8 mg/dL should raise suspicion of renal insufficiency.

Pregnancy also induces changes in water metabolism that include a fall in the osmostat from 280 mOsm/kg to approximately 270 mOsm/kg and parallel changes in the thirst threshold [8]. The level of serum sodium declines 3–4 mEq as a consequence. Furthermore, studies show that the metabolic clearance of vasopressin is accelerated approximately fourfold as a result of the production of placental vasopressinase, an enzyme that rapidly cleaves and degrades circulating vasopressin [9]. Maximum levels of the enzyme are achieved after 22 weeks' gestation. However, plasma levels of vasopressin are normal because of the compensatory increased production of vasopressin. The ability to concentrate urine, and alternatively to excrete a water load during normal pregnancy, is unchanged compared with the nongravid state [9].

Some women fail to compensate fully for the degradation of vasopressin or have excess levels of vasopressinase near term, and consequently develop diabetes insipidus [10]. Under these circumstances, copious dilute urine results in hypernatremia which may result in cerebral injury in both the mother and fetus. In both conditions, diabetes insipidus is associated with intense thirst when patients are conscious and have access to water. Both conditions occur in late pregnancy when vasopressinase levels are highest. If diabetes insipidus is brought about by an occult central form that is unmasked by pregnancy, then treatment with vasopressin will concentrate urine and stem the loss of free water. These patients usually experience recurrences in subsequent pregnancies. In contrast, if diabetes insipidus is caused by excess vasopressinase, vasopressin will not correct the urinary concentration defect. However, treatment with the vasopressin analog dDAVP, which is not degraded by vasopressinase, will promptly result in a concentrated urine. This condition is termed "transient diabetes insipidus of pregnancy" and will usually not recur in subsequent pregnancies.

Pregnancy also alters renal tubular function. Studies show that the fractional excretion of glucose, small peptides, and amino acids is increased during pregnancy [11]. In some women, glucosuria occurs in the absence of an elevation of blood glucose level. The appearance of glucosuria therefore requires evidence of glucose intolerance from measurements of blood glucose before a patient can be labeled a diabetic. In addition, protein excretion in pregnancy can increase twofold above nonpregnant levels and can reach values of 250 mg/24 hours [12]. Taken together, these observations indicate that there is a generalized reduction in the absorption of nonelectrolyte solutes by the proximal tubule during pregnancy.

These insights into the physiologic alterations that occur in normal pregnancy indicate that a different scale of values must be considered in determining normal renal function when renal disease and/or insufficiency is suspected. In instances where the level of renal function requires monitoring during pregnancy, glomerular filtration rate should be measured. In early pregnancy, the filtration rate can be estimated from a 24-hour urine collection. In late pregnancy, however, the glomerular filtration rate should be measured with the hydrated gravida lying on her left side during at least two consecutive measured periods of approximately 1 hour to avoid underestimation of filtration because of sequestered fluid in the lower extremities.

Renal disease in pregnancy

Renal disease in pregnancy, as in nonpregnant individuals, can be caused by primary disease or secondarily by a systemic disease. In the evaluation of a patient with signs of renal disease, the first consideration is whether renal disease predates conception or occurs *de novo* during gestation. If there is no evidence of preceding disease, the second consideration is whether renal disease began before or after 20 weeks' gestation because preeclampsia rarely occurs before that time. This algorithm is important to establish a working diagnosis of renal disease and usually requires scrutiny of the past medical history and laboratory results in the early period of gestation. Regardless of the type of renal disease, the clinical signs of injury are recognized by two nonexclusive presentations: proteinuria and renal insufficiency.

Proteinuria

Proteinuria is defined as total protein excretion of more than 300 mg/24 hours, and usually denotes renal disease. It is helpful to classify renal disease on the basis of the major site of injury to the kidney; that is, as primary injury to the glomerulus or primary injury to the renal tubules and interstitium. Both types of injury can result in proteinuria, but excretion rates of more than 2.0 g/24 hours usually indicate a glomerular disease. Patients with proteinuria excretion of less than 3.0 g/24 hours are usually asymptomatic. In contrast, rates of more than 3.0 g/24 hours may cause the nephrotic syndrome which is symptomatic because excess retention of sodium and water results in dependent edema. The nephrotic syndrome is defined as proteinuria of more than 3.0 g/24 hours and a serum albumin level less than 3 g/dL. Edema does not occur in the absence of hypoalbuminemia, but in its presence patients exhibit a lower capacity to excrete sodium. Under that condition, edema formation will occur if sodium intake exceeds the maximum capacity for sodium excretion.

The nephrotic syndrome in pregnancy can be caused by pre-existing renal disease or renal disease that develops *de novo* (e.g., preeclampsia). Several analyses have concluded that the presence of nephrotic syndrome resulting from renal diseases, in the absence of significant renal insufficiency and/or significant hypertension, does not seem to affect the natural course of renal disease or fetal survival [13]. Regarding maternal complications, however, severe edema near term can cause or aggravate hypertension and complicate delivery because of vulva edema. It has been reported that preeclampsia is the most common cause for *de novo* nephrotic syndrome in pregnancy, and when that occurs the preeclampsia is regarded as severe [14].

Measurement for urine protein prior to 20 weeks' gestation can be of great value when pregnancies are complicated by the presence of proteinuria at later stages of gestation. The distinction between underlying renal disease and preeclampsia is important because it affects clinical management. The aim in patients with renal disease is usually term delivery, while patients with preeclampsia are delivered when the fetus is mature.

The management of nephrotic syndrome should aim to reduce edema formation to a level that allows comfort during ambulation. The dietary intake of sodium should be limited to 1.5 g sodium/day (approximately 60 mEq) to reduce new edema formation. Frequently, bed rest in a lateral recumbent position will suffice to mobilize pre-existing edema by promoting an increase in the excretion of sodium. In general, the use of diuretic agents has been discouraged because of the possibility that reduction of extracellular fluid volume could decrease blood flow to the placenta. However, when diuretics are required to reduce intractable edema, therapy should aim only to reduce excessive edema at a slow rate of approximately

0.5–1.0 kg/day with a loop diuretic, while a low sodium diet is maintained. If treatment on a chronic basis is needed, diuretic therapy should be administered on an alternate day schedule to avoid a reduction of plasma volume and electrolyte disturbances. A written record of daily weights, taken by the patient, is highly recommended. Diuretics should not be administered to patients with preeclampsia because this condition is characterized by a reduction in circulating plasma volume.

Renal insufficiency

Renal insufficiency in pregnancy can occur with or without proteinuria. A serum creatinine of 0.8 mg/dL or more is indicative of renal insufficiency [1]. The clinical severity of renal insufficiency in pregnancy is usually classified by the level of the serum creatinine at the first antepartum visit, as mild (>0.8 to ≤1.4 mg/dL), moderate (>1.4 to ≤2.5 mg/dL), and severe (>2.5 mg/dL).

Information related to maternal complications and pregnancy outcomes in women with pre-existing renal disease is derived from retrospective observations. The first of several large studies of women with mild renal disease, creatinine ≤1.4 mg/dL, showed that complications were infrequent and usually resolved spontaneously, especially when hypertension was absent or mild, as shown in Table 18.1 [15]. The incidence of hypertension in the third trimester (48% vs. 28%) and nephrotic syndrome (41% vs. 29%) is greater with moderate and severe than mild disease (Table 18.1). Approximately one-quarter of gravidas experienced a new onset of hypertension or aggravation of previous hypertension, and less than 20% also experienced reversible reductions in renal function. However, proteinuria, when resulting from glomerular disease, usually tends to progress to a nephrotic range by the third trimester [16]. Table 18.2 outlines pregnancy outcomes in patients with serum creatinine values above and below 1.4 mg/dL. These studies suggest that pregnancy did not alter the natural course of the underlying mild renal disease.

Regarding pregnancy outcome in mothers with moderate and severe renal disease, the overall live birth rate was 93%, with a perinatal mortality rate of 7.3% (stillbirths and neonatal deaths) [16]. Obstetric complications include a preterm delivery rate of 59% and growth restriction rate of 37% [16]. In addition, renal function decreased during pregnancy and 6 weeks postpartum in nearly half of this group, and in most cases was irreversible. In 23% of this subgroup (10% of the total series) there was a rapid decline to end-stage renal failure within 6 months after delivery. The risk of a rapid decline in glomerular filtration rates was highest in patients with an initial antepartum serum creatinine of more than 2.0 mg/dL, as shown in Fig. 18.1. In summary, patients with severe renal disease, especially when the serum creatinine is above 2.0 mg/dL, are at risk for severe maternal complications that may not be reversible and a high incidence of obstetric complications.

Most patients with renal insufficiency exhibit chronic hypertension and require blood pressure control during gestation. It has been difficult to determine whether the high rate of fetal growth restriction and preterm deliveries were related to hypertension per se, its treatment, or some factor specifically related to renal insufficiency. The National High Blood Pressure Education Program Working Group Report, published in 1990, indicated that women with chronic hypertension are at risk for "preeclampsia, perinatal morbidity and death, and the possibility of deterioration of renal function" [17]. This report suggested the continuation of antihypertensive agents, using the same antihypertensive agents that were shown to be effective before conception, except for angiotensin-converting enzyme (ACE) inhibitors and angiotensin receptor blockers

Table 18.1 New maternal complications during pregnancy in primary renal disease with preserved and moderately severe renal function.

	Cr ≤ 1.4 mg/dL*	Cr > 1.4 mg/dL[†]
Number of pregnancies	121	82
Reduction in GFR (pregnancy and postpartum)	16%	43%
Exacerbation or *de novo* onset of hypertension	28%	48%
Significant proteinuria	29%	41%

Cr, creatinine; GFR, glomerular filtration rate.
* Katz *et al*. [15].
[†] Jones and Hayslett [16].

Table 18.2 Obstetric complications in primary renal disease with preserved and moderately severe renal function.

	Cr ≤ 1.4 mg/dL*	Cr > 1.4 mg/dL[†]	General population in USA[‡]
Number of pregnancies	121	82	
Preterm (<37 weeks)	20%	59%	11%
Growth restriction (<10th percentile)	24%	37%	10%
Birthweight	2693 ± 878 g	2239 ± 839 g	2800 g
Stillbirths	5%	5%	0.7%
Neonatal deaths	4.9%	2%	0.7%
Infant survival	89%	91%	98.6%

Cr, creatinine.
* Katz *et al*. [15].
[†] Jones and Hayslett [16].
[‡] Cunningham *et al*. [20].

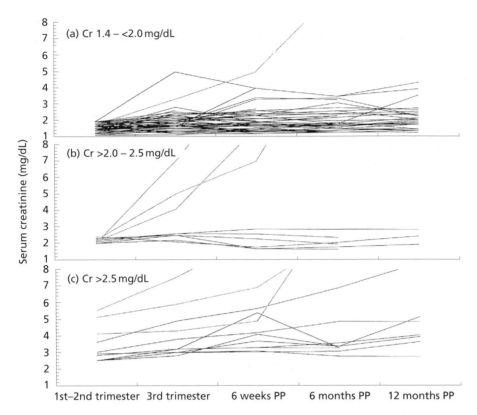

Fig. 18.1 Serum creatinine concentrations in women with primary renal disease during and after pregnancy, according to concentration measured early in gestation. Dashed lines represents women who had a pregnancy progression-related decline in renal function and subsequent end-stage disease within 1 year postpartum (PP). Data are stratified according to the serum creatinine at the onset of gestation: (a) ≤2.0 mg/dL; (b) 2.0–2.4 mg/dL; and (c) >2.5 mg/dL. (From Jones and Hayslett [16].)

(ARB) because they are fetotoxic. Subsequently, studies showed that blood pressure levels above normal in patients with chronic renal disease are a major factor promoting progressive decline in renal function [18]. It seems likely that pregnant women with chronic renal insufficiency would be highly vulnerable to accelerated renal injury because of the renal vascular dilatation that characterizes pregnancy. We therefore favor blood pressure control sufficient to maintain normal values.

Methyldopa has been favored by the obstetric community because of the proven demonstration of safety for the fetus. Unfortunately, this agent is not as potent as some of the newer categories of antihypertensive drugs. Despite the lack of evidence based on scientific studies that affirm the effectiveness and safety of newer agents, beta-adrenergic blocking agents, such as labetolol and calcium-channel blockers, are used widely and appear to be safe [19]. Both categories can be employed by either oral or parenteral routes and therefore can be used for outpatient management and hypertensive crises.

On the basis of these accounts of the course of pregnancy in women with pre-existing primary renal disease, there is now better information on this group to assess risk for maternal complications and the likelihood of achieving a favorable pregnancy outcome. It should be remembered, however, that these data were derived from centers with high-risk pregnancy specialists and infant intensive care units.

Management

Women with renal disease are best managed at a tertiary hospital under the coordinated care of a maternal-fetal specialist and a nephrologist. Initial laboratory tests should include a database that aids in early detection of renal loss and provides a basis for comparison during the course of pregnancy:

1 Serum creatinine concentration and its time clearance if the baseline creatinine value is 0.8 mg/dL or more.

2 Albumin, and cholesterol concentration.

3 Electrolytes, urine analysis, screening bacterial culture, and a 24-hour urine collection for protein excretion.

Biweekly prenatal visits should be scheduled until week 32 and weekly thereafter. Serum creatinine and quantitative urinary excretion of protein should be performed at least every 6 weeks.

Case presentation 1

During her first pregnancy, a 24-year-old woman developed the nephrotic syndrome in the third month of gestation, in the setting of otherwise good health. Renal function and blood pressure were normal. The administration of prednisone induced a complete remission of the nephrotic syndrome, which was then maintained until a term delivery. A subsequent renal biopsy confirmed the diagnosis of minimal change disease. In a second pregnancy 1 year later, a relapse of the nephrotic syndrome occurred in the second month of gestation. To spare the patient exposure to steroid therapy for 7 months, the patient was managed conservatively with a low sodium diet and an intermittent diuretic, which minimized but did not eliminate edema. Following a term delivery the patient was treated with short-term high-dose prednisone therapy which resulted in long-term cure.

This case illustrates the usual good pregnancy outcome when the nephrotic syndrome occurs as a primary renal disease in the absence of renal insufficiency and significant hypertension.

Case presentation 2

A 29-year-old woman was referred to the maternal-fetal medicine section because of renal insufficiency with a serum creatinine of 1.7 mg/dL and the nephrotic syndrome, characterized by the protein excretion of 3.5 g/24 hours and a serum albumin concentration of 2.6 g/dL. Blood pressure was normal but anemia (Hct 27%) required treatment with Epogen or erythropoietin therapy. Edema formation was controlled with a low sodium diet and intermittent use of a diuretic to reduce but not eliminate dependent edema. The course of pregnancy was uneventful and ended with a term delivery.

This case illustrates the usual good pregnancy outlook of pregnancies characterized by moderate renal insufficiency and normal blood pressure or mild hypertension.

Case presentation 3

A 29-year-old nulliparous woman was referred to the maternal-fetal medicine section because of chronic hypertension and renal insufficiency. Renal insufficiency had been present for at least 3 years and the serum creatinine level had been stable at 2.0 mg/dL for approximately 6 months before the onset of pregnancy. A renal biopsy before pregnancy had identified the renal disease as being caused by focal and segmental glomerular nephritis and severe scarring. Hypertension was reasonably controlled with medication. The serum creatinine rose progressively from week 18 to week 33, from 2.2 to 4.8 mg/dL, when an intrauterine death occurred. The patient required renal replacement therapy with dialysis approximately 2 months after the termination of pregnancy and ultimately a successful renal transplantation.

This case illustrates the poor outcome that often occurs when pregnancy is associated with severe renal insufficiency.

References

1 Lindheimer MD, Katz AI. The kidney in pregnancy. *N Engl J Med* 1970;**283**:1095–7.
2 Davison JM, Dunlop W. Renal hemodynamics and tubular function normal human pregnancy. *Kidney Int* 1980;**18**:152–61.
3 Baylis C. Relaxin may be the "elusive" renal vasodilatory agent of normal pregnancy. *Am J Kidney Dis* 1999;**34**:1142–4; discussion 1144–5.
4 Weinberger MH, Kramer NJ, Petersen LP, Cleary RE, Young PC. Sequential changes in the renin–angiotensin–aldosterone systems and plasma progesterone concentration in normal and abnormal human pregnancy. *Perspect Nephrol Hypertens* 1976;**5**:263–9.
5 Bay WH, Ferris TF. Factors controlling plasma renin and aldosterone during pregnancy. *Hypertension* 1979;**1**:410–5.
6 Davison JM, Hytten FE. Glomerular filtration during and after pregnancy. *J Obstet Gynaecol Br Commonw* 1974;**81**:588–95.
7 Roberts M, Lindheimer MD, Davison JM. Altered glomerular permselectivity to neutral dextrans and heteroporous membrane modeling in human pregnancy. *Am J Physiol* 1996;**270**:F338–43.
8 Davison JM, Shiells EA, Philips PR, Lindheimer MD. Serial evaluation of vasopressin release and thirst in human pregnancy. Role of human chorionic gonadotrophin in the osmoregulatory changes of gestation. *J Clin Invest* 1988;**81**:798–806.
9 Davison JM, Sheills EA, Barron WM, Robinson AG, Lindheimer MD. Changes in the metabolic clearance of vasopressin and in plasma vasopressinase throughout human pregnancy. *J Clin Invest* 1989;**83**:1313–8.
10 Durr JA, Hoggard JG, Hunt JM, Schrier RW. Diabetes insipidus in pregnancy associated with abnormally high circulating vasopressinase activity. *N Engl J Med* 1987;**316**:1070–4.
11 Davison JM, Hytten FE. The effect of pregnancy on the renal handling of glucose. *Br J Obstet Gynaecol* 1975;**82**:374–81.
12 Davison JM. The effect of pregnancy on kidney function in renal allograft recipients. *Kidney Int* 1985;**27**:74–9.
13 Strauch BS, Hayslett JP. Kidney disease and pregnancy. *Br Med J* 1974;**4**:578–82.
14 Fisher KA, Luger A, Spargo BH, Lindheimer MD. Hypertension in pregnancy: clinical-pathological correlations and remote prognosis. *Medicine (Baltimore)* 1981;**60**:267–76.
15 Katz AI, Davison JM, Hayslett JP, Singson E, Lindheimer MD. Pregnancy in women with kidney disease. *Kidney Int* 1980;**18**: 192–206.
16 Jones DC, Hayslett JP. Outcome of pregnancy in women with moderate or severe renal insufficiency [see comments]. *N Engl J Med* 1996;**335**:226–32. [Erratum appears in *N Engl J Med* 1997;**336**:739.]
17 National High Blood Pressure Education Program Working Group report on high blood pressure in pregnancy. *Am J Obstet Gynecol* 1990;**163**:1691–712.
18 Zucchelli P, Gaggi R, Zuccala A. Angiotensin converting enzyme inhibitors and calcium antagonists in the progression of renal insufficiency. *Contrib Nephrol* 1992;**98**:116–24.
19 Sibai BM. Treatment of hypertension in pregnant women. *N Engl J Med* 1996;**335**:257–65.
20 Cunningham FG, MacDonald PC, Gant NF, *et al.* (eds). *Williams Obstetrics*, 20th edn. Stamford, CT: Appleton & Lange, 1997: Chapter 1.

19 Pregnancy in transplant patients

James R. Scott

Chronic renal failure or end-stage renal disease affects over 20 million people in the USA alone. These patients have only two treatment options for survival: dialysis or a kidney transplant. Kidney transplantation leads to a longer life than dialysis, restores many patients to near normal lifestyles, and is cost effective for the health care system. The donor kidney is surgically placed extraperitoneally in the recipient's iliac fossa. The procedure is accomplished by anastomosing the donor renal artery to the proximal end of the divided hypogastric artery and the donor renal vein to the external iliac vein as illustrated in Fig. 19.1(a) or anastomosing the donor renal artery directly to the external iliac artery as shown in Fig. 19.1(b). The donor ureter is then attached to the recipient's bladder by ureteroneocystostomy. Transplantation has also evolved as the treatment of choice or only option for many women of reproductive age with end-stage liver, heart, and lung disease.

It has been almost 50 years since the first child was born to a renal allograft recipient, and women with virtually all types of organ transplants have now had successful pregnancies. Nevertheless, it is clear that these are high-risk pregnancies that require expert obstetric care [1]. All transplant patients have underlying medical disorders that can adversely affect pregnancy outcome. Problems can occur unpredictably, and each organ has its own specific issues. This combination of factors presents a unique management challenge to the obstetrician. There are no randomized trials that have investigated pregnancy management options for transplant patients, but a great deal has been learned through experience.

Prepregnancy assessment and counseling

Preconception counseling is indicated for all female transplant recipients at the pretransplant evaluation and before a pregnancy is attempted [1]. Any woman contemplating pregnancy should be in good health with no evidence of graft rejection (Table 19.1). Serious medical problems such as diabetes mellitus, cardiovascular or pulmonary disease, recurrent infec-

tions, and major side-effects from immunosuppressive drugs may make pregnancy inadvisable. The ideal time for pregnancy is between 2 and 5 years after transplantation when allograft function has stabilized and immunosuppressive medication has been reduced to moderate doses. An assessment of the patient's family and spouse support as well as a tactful but honest discussion of her life expectancy and potential pregnancy problems is important. The medical literature and media tend to be overly optimistic about pregnancy outcomes and long-term prognosis, which tend to give patients unrealistic expectations. Long-term organ allograft survival rates are not 100%, and the transplant recipient may not live to raise her child to adulthood.

Antepartum care

Kidney transplantation is the prototype, but prenatal care is similar with essentially all other organ allografts. Early diagnosis of pregnancy is important, and a first trimester ultrasound examination is essential to establish an accurate date of delivery. Antenatal management should be meticulous with frequent prenatal visits and serial assessment of maternal allograft function and prompt diagnosis and treatment of infections, anemia, hypertension, and preeclampsia. Nausea and vomiting or hyperemesis gravidarum can lead to decreased absorption and inadequate immunosuppression. Close fetal surveillance for preterm labor is necessary, and the known risk for fetal growth restriction is monitored by serial ultrasound examinations.

The incidence of intraepithelial and invasive cancer of the genital tract in patients taking immunosuppressive drugs is increased, and regular Papanicolaou (Pap) tests and screening for malignancies are vital components of clinical care [2]. Skin cancer is the most common malignancy and affects the majority of patients eventually, with 30–70% of patients developing squamous cell carcinoma, melanoma, and basal cell carcinoma within 20 years [3].

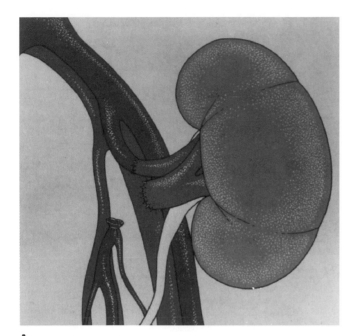

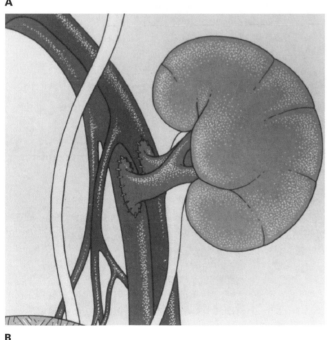

Fig. 19.1 (a,b) Technique of renal transplantation. (From Garovoy *et al.* [40] with permission.)

Table 19.1 Factors associated with optimum pregnancy outcome in transplant patients. Pregnancies outside these guidelines need to be evaluated on a case-by-case basis.

Good general health and prognosis
No evidence of rejection in the past year
Serum creatinine <1.5 mg/dL
Stable immunosuppressive regimen
No or minimal hypertension and proteinuria
Spouse and family support
Established medical compliance

Some patients have become Rh-sensitized from the allograft, and commonly acquired viral infections such as cytomegalovirus (CMV), herpes genitalis (HSV), human papillomavirus (HPV), human immunodeficiency virus (HIV), and hepatitis B (HBV) and hepatitis C (HCV) pose a risk for both the mother and her fetus. The transplanted graft is a source of CMV, and patients typically receive prophylaxis against CMV for 1–3 months postoperatively when the risk for infection is highest. The greatest risk of congenital infection in the fetus is with primary CMV infection during pregnancy, but recurrent CMV infection in immunosuppressed women has also caused congenital CMV in the infant [4]. HBV and HCV are usually acquired through dialysis and blood transfusions prior to transplantation. Hepatitis B immunoglobulin (HBIG) and HBV vaccine should be given to the newborn and are 90% effective in preventing chronic hepatitis. Acyclovir as prophylaxis or treatment of HSV can be used safely during pregnancy.

Immunosuppressive agents

Obstetricians are not usually familiar with this class of drugs, but it is important that they understand their impact on pregnancy and the potential side-effects. Most maintenance antirejection regimens in transplant patients include combinations of daily corticosteroids, azathioprine, cyclosporine, and, more recently, tacrolimus. However, new agents continually become available, and multiple drug regimens are common.

Lack of information about the teratogenic effects of some of these drugs is a serious practical problem for the obstetrician. Available data are insufficient to determine the teratogenic risk in human pregnancy of therapy with mycophenolate mofetil or muromonab-CD3, both now widely used in transplant patients. Other new antimetabolites also raise substantial theoretical concern because rapidly dividing cells in the embryo may be susceptible to damage by these inhibitors of DNA and RNA synthesis. The potential fetal risks for each drug as presently categorized by the US Food and Drug Administration are shown in Table 19.2.

Prednisone is the usual maintenance corticosteroid used in transplant patients, and intravenous glucocorticoids are used

Urinary tract infections are particularly common in kidney transplant patients, with up to a twofold increase in the incidence of pyelonephritis. Asymptomatic bacteruria should be treated for 2 weeks with follow-up urine cultures, and suppressive doses of antibiotics may be needed for the rest of the pregnancy. Other bacterial and fungal infections associated with immunosuppression include endometritis, wound infections, skin abscesses, and pneumonia, often with unusual organisms.

Table 19.2 Classification of fetal risk for immunosuppressive drugs used in transplantation. Category A, controlled studies, no risk; Category B, no evidence of risk in humans; Category C, risk cannot be ruled out, Category D, positive evidence of risk; Category X, contraindicated in pregnancy.

	Pregnancy Category
Corticosteroids (prednisone)	B
Azathioprine (Imuran)	D
Cyclosporine (Sandimmun, Neoral, SangCya)	C
Tacrolimus (Prograf)	C
Sirolimus (Rapamune)	C
Mycophenolate mofetil (CellCept)	C
Antithymocyte globulin (ATGAM, ATG, Thymoglobulin)	C
Muromonab-CD3 (Orthoclone OKT3)	C
Basilizimab (Simulect)	B
Daclizumab (Zenapax)	C
Leflunomide (Avara)	X

to treat acute rejection reactions. Because prednisone is largely metabolized by placental 11-hydroxygenase to the relatively inactive 11-keto form, the fetus is exposed to only 10% of the maternal dose of the active drug. Most patients are maintained on moderate doses of prednisone (10–30 mg/day) which are relatively safe with few fetal effects.

Azathioprine, and its more toxic metabolite 6-mercaptopurine, is a purine analog whose principal action is to decrease delayed hypersensitivity and cellular cytotoxicity. The primary maternal hazards of azathioprine administration are an increased risk of infection and neoplasia. Maternal liver toxicity and bone marrow supression have occurred but usually resolve with a decrease in dosage. Between 64% and 90% of azathioprine crosses the placenta in human pregnancies, but the majority is the inactive form thiouric acid. Classification of azathioprine as Category D is based largely on two early series which reported an incidence of congenital anomalies of 9% and 6.4% [5,6]. No specific pattern has emerged, and experience has shown that azathioprine is not associated with more congenital malformations than seen in the normal population [7–12].

Cyclosporine, a fungal metabolite whose major inhibitory effect is on T-cell-mediated responses by preventing formation of interleukin-2 (IL-2), is a calcineurin inhibitor. It became a standard component of most immunosuppressant regimens. The drug has a propensity for nephrotoxicity and hypertension. Other side-effects include hirsutism, tremor, gingival hyperplasia, hyperuricemia, viral infections, hepatotoxicity, and an increased risk for neoplasia such as lymphomas. Cyclosporine readily crosses the placenta, but there is no evidence of teratogenicity in the human [7–12].

Tacrolimus is a macrolide that has become widely used in solid organ transplantation, replacing some of the older immunosuppressant agents. There are currently over 90,000 transplant recipients being treated with tacrolimus in the USA, and it is prescribed to the majority of new kidney and liver transplant recipients worldwide [7–12]. There is an increase in glucose intolerance and new onset diabetes mellitus among recipients treated with tacrolimus, but control of blood glucose levels can usually be achieved by decreasing the dosage. Nephrotoxicity and hyperkalemia develops in many patients, and neurotoxicities such as headache, tremor, changes in motor function, mental status, or sensory function have also been described. Cord blood concentrations are approximately 50% of maternal levels; there has been no proven association with congenital malformations [13–16].

New classes of immunosuppressant agents are becoming available, but less is known about their teratatogenic potential or safety during pregnancy [15]. Sirolimus is an orally administered macrolide that inhibits cytokine-stimulated T-lymphocyte activation and proliferation. The major adverse effects have been hypercholesterolemia, hypertriglyceridemia, thrombocytopenia, and leukopenia. Basilizimab and dacliximab are genetically engineered "humanized" mouse IgG1 antibodies that block the IL-2 receptor. Lefluomide is a pyrimidine synthesis inhibitor of dihydroorotate dehydrogenase which is required for the biosynthesis of pyrimidines, and therefore of DNA, and RNA. It has teratogenic and fetotoxic effects in animal studies, and 7/90 babies from full-term pregnancies have been born with congenital malformations [17,18].

Kidney transplant patients

Approximately 1 in 20 women of childbearing age with a functioning renal allograft becomes pregnant [19–21], and it is estimated that more than 15,000 pregnancies have now occurred (Fig. 19.2). Many women have now had more than one pregnancy, and some have successfully delivered twins and triplets. One of our patients has had five live births with no deleterious effect on the kidney [22].

If preconception graft function is adequate as evidenced by a plasma creatinine of less than 1.5 mg/dL, the pregnancy can be expected to progress normally until near term. The transplanted kidney usually functions satisfactorily during gestation, but most patients do not have the increased glomerular filtration rate (GFR) seen in normal pregnant women. GFR instead typically decreases during the third trimester. Proteinuria also occurs in 40% of renal transplant patients in the third trimester, but this characteristically resolves postpartum. If there are no signs of preeclampsia, this proteinuria requires no specific treatment.

In contrast, pregnancy is almost always more complicated in patients with elevated creatinine levels or chronic rejection episodes [23]. Deterioration of renal function, rejection, and even maternal death have occurred. Rejection is characterized by fever, oliguria, deteriorating renal function, enlargement of the

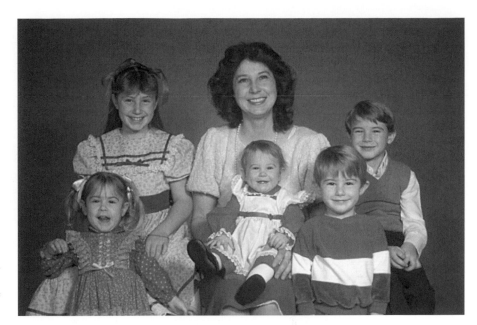

Fig. 19.2 Renal transplant recipient with her five children all born after her transplant. These pregnancies were all managed at the University of Utah Medical Center.

kidney, and tenderness to palpation. This diagnosis can be difficult because the findings overlap with other disorders such as pyelonephritis, preeclampsia, and nephrotoxicity from immunosuppressant drugs. Nevertheless, it is crucial to establish the diagnosis of rejection before initiating additional antirejection therapy. Imaging studies such as ultrasound are useful to detect changes in the kidney indicative of rejection. If the diagnosis is still unclear, renal biopsy is sometimes necessary.

Chronic hypertension and preeclampsia are the most common complications in these patients and contribute to the increase in preterm births, fetal growth restriction, and perinatal death [19–22]. Hypertension is present in at least half of these pregnancies, and almost one-third develop preeclampsia. In a transplant patient with a blood pressure greater than 140/90 mmHg, antihypertensive medications should be continued during pregnancy. However, angiotensin-converting enzyme (ACE) inhibitors should not be used because of adverse effects on the fetus including oligohydramnios, pulmonary hypoplasia, and long-lasting neonatal anuria. Calcium-channel blockers are the preferred agents, and an additional beneficial effect appears to be in countering the vasoconstrictive effect of cyclosporine. Preeclampsia should be anticipated, and the management is the same as with nontransplant patients.

Other organ transplant patients

Pancreas

Whole or segmental cadaveric pancreas transplantation, usually combined with kidney transplantation, is now a treatment option for patients with juvenile onset insulin-

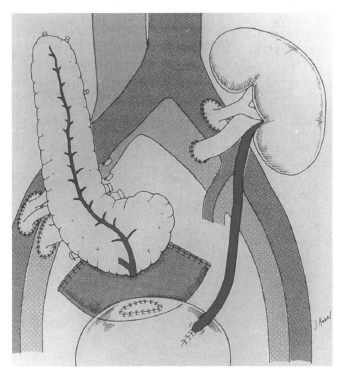

Fig. 19.3 Combined pancreas–kidney transplantation with duodenal segment technique. (From Sollinger and Knechtle [41] with permission.)

dependent (type I) diabetes mellitus. One-year graft survival rate is approximately 80%, with a 5-year graft survival rate of 60%. The 10-year probability of insulin independence is approximately 90% if the patient has a functioning graft at 5 years [24]. Most cases of pancreas transplantation are performed in patients who already have or will receive a kidney allograft at the same time they receive the pancreas (Fig. 19.3).

Although renal transplantation allows diabetic women to become pregnant, immunosuppression adds to the complexity of management [24,25]. Because many issues are the same, antepartum and intrapartum management is similar to kidney transplant patients. However, the diabetogenic effects of pregnancy, corticosteroids, cyclosporine, and other immunosuppressive drugs can all lead to or aggravate hyperglycemia, macrosomia, and other sequela in pancreas transplant patients. Euglycemia should be achieved preconception, and glucose tolerance testing (GTT) is warranted prior to 20 weeks. If hypoglycemia is present, diet and insulin therapy should be instituted at that time. If the GTT screen is normal, it should be repeated at 24–28 weeks as with any pregnant patient. Most pancreas transplant patients have maintained euglycemia throughout pregnancy and labor, but complications have included osteoporosis, fractures, diabetic neuropathy, chronic vascular insufficiency, maternal death, stillbirth, neonatal hypocalcemia, and hypoglycemia.

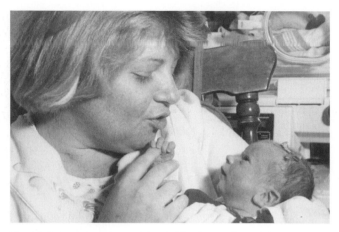

Fig. 19.4 Heart transplant recipient holding her newborn, delivered at the University of Utah Medical Center 6 years after transplant. (From *Am J Transplant* 2005:7 with permission.)

Liver

Improvements in immunosuppressant drug therapy and surgical techniques have resulted in longer life expectancy and many pregnancies have been reported in women with liver allografts [26–28]. Currently, 11% of all patients receiving liver transplants are women of reproductive age, and an additional 15% are younger patients who will survive beyond the childbearing age. Of particular concern is HCV, because it is the most common indication for liver transplantation, and the rate of maternal–fetal transmission is unknown. Clinical signs suggestive of liver rejection are fever, right upper quadrant pain, leukocytosis, and elevated serum bilirubin and aminotransferase levels. Because these tests are nonspecific, suspected graft rejection needs biopsy confirmation. Most rejection episodes can be managed by adjusting the drug regimen. Maternal complications have included elevated liver function tests, rejection, recurrent hepatitis, decreased renal function, urinary tract infection, adrenal insufficiency, and endometritis [26–28]. There is also an increased rate of fetal growth restriction; preeclampsia; hemolysis, elevated liver enzymes, and low platelet count (HELLP) syndrome; premature rupture of membranes; preterm birth; and neonatal infections. These complications are in part dependent on maternal health before pregnancy, and management is similar to that in renal transplant patients.

Heart

More than 5000 women in North America have undergone heart transplants at a current rate of more than 500 per year (Fig. 19.4). The transplanted heart must adapt to the physiologic changes of pregnancy. Arrhythmias may be present, and the denervated heart may not respond to some vasopressors in a predictable way. Only direct acting vasoactive drugs have an effect, and the transplanted heart may be more sensitive to beta-adrenergic agonists because of an increase in beta receptors [29].

One-third of patents have tricuspid regurgitation 1 year post-transplant, and it may worsen with the increased blood volume associated with pregnancy. Almost one-third of cardiac transplant patients have atherosclerotic coronary vessel stenosis by 3 years after the transplant and up to 50% have atherosclerosis at 5 years [30]. Because myocardial ischemia does not cause chest pain as there is no afferent innervation, paroxysmal dyspnea may be the only presenting symptom. Maternal graft rejection episodes occur in 20–30% of pregnancies, but most are not clinically evident and are diagnosed by routine surveillance biopsies. These biopsies are obtained from the right ventricle guided by either fluoroscopy or echocardiography [31]. Rejection episodes are usually successfully managed by increasing the immunosuppression regimen. The increased incidence of hypertension, preeclampsia, prematurity, and low birthweights are similar to that of other transplant patients [31,32]. It is well to involve an anesthesiologist to formulate a well-organized plan for labor and delivery because these patients have an increased sensitivity to hypovolemia and catecholamines.

Lung

The most frequent indications for heart-lung or lung transplants are congenital heart disease with Eisenmenger syndrome, primary pulmonary hypertension, and, less commonly, cystic fibrosis and emphysema [33–35]. One-year survival rate for heart-lung recipients is 63%, and this decreases to approximately 40% at 5 years. In addition to the management issues related to heart transplant patients, there are specific issues to be considered in the pregnant lung transplant recipient. Diagnosing chronic rejection of the lung allograft may be challenging, but one of the first symptoms is often a mild cough with subsequent deterioration in pulmonary function. During the transplant, there is a loss of pulmonary innervation, bronchial arterial supply, and pulmonary lymphatics. This denervation leads to compromise of the cough reflex and difficulty protecting the airway. Decreased lung compliance may result in a persistent alveolar–arterial oxygen gradient. Pulmonary edema is a definite possibility in these patients, and excess intravenous hydration should be avoided. Two patients have died postpartum from complications of obliterative bronchiolitis.

Intrapartum management

The timing of delivery is often dependent on events such as premature labor, premature ruptured membranes, or severe preeclampsia. The extraperitoneal location of the transplanted kidney in the iliac fossa usually does not interfere with vaginal delivery (Fig. 19.5). There are no particular contraindications to induction, labor, or vaginal delivery in organ graft recipients. Because of an increased susceptibility to infection, vaginal examinations should be kept to a minimum and artificial rupture of membranes and internal monitoring performed only when specifically indicated.

Cesarean delivery should be based on accepted obstetric indications. Operative deliveries in these patients are managed with prophylactic antibiotics and additional glucocorticoids, and require strict asepsis and careful attention to hemostasis.

A lower midline vertical incision provides the greatest exposure and avoids the region of the transplanted kidney. A low transverse uterine incision is almost always possible, but the obstetrician should be aware of the anatomic alterations associated with the transplanted kidney to avoid inadvertent damage to the blood supply, urinary drainage, or bladder damage.

Obstetric emergencies

Acute emergencies may arise in pregnant transplant patients with severe consequences that require aggressive management and intensive care. These are best managed in a tertiary setting where the transplant surgeon, obstetrician, nephrologist, and other subspecialists and intensivists can work together. Most difficult is severe and chronic rejection or allograft vasculopathy with loss of graft function which threatens the life of the mother and fetus. Renal allograft patients with deteriorating function may have to be placed back on dialysis therapy for the remainder of the pregnancy, and other organ recipients need a variety of supportive measures or retransplantation. Sepsis and overwhelming infections are also a constant threat in these women, and patients have died of meningitis, pneumonia, gastroenteritis, HCV and HBV, and AIDS [8–12,20,21]. With the high incidence of hypertension and preeclampsia, it is not surprising that HELLP syndrome, stroke and eclampsia have occurred [8–12,20,21]. Other causes of morbidity that have required emergent surgery include rupture of renal vessel anastomosis, mechanical obstruction of the ureter, antepartum bleeding, uterine rupture, small

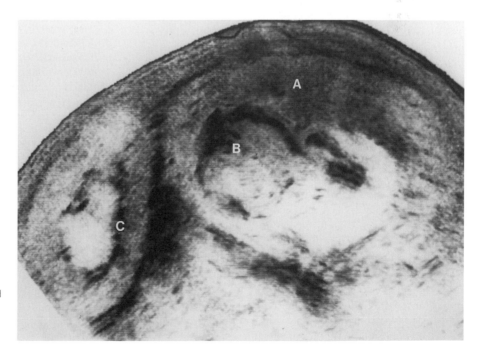

Fig. 19.5 Transverse sonogram at 22 weeks' gestation below the level of the iliac crest showing: anterior placenta (A), fetal trunk (B), and mild hydronephrosis of the transplanted kidney (C) . (From Norton and Scott [42] with permission.)

bowel injury at cesarean delivery, severe postpartum hemorrhage, abdominal wound dehiscence, and pelvic abscess [3,20].

The baby

All immunosuppressive drugs cross the placental barrier and diffuse into the fetal circulation. Because there is no convincing evidence that prednisone, azathioprine, cyclosporine, or tacrolimus produce congenital abnormalities in the human fetus, they are the drugs of choice during pregnancy. Other than fetal growth restriction and preterm birth, most offspring born to these mothers have had relatively uncomplicated neonatal courses. Mothers are usually empirically advised against breastfeeding, but the dosage of immunosuppressive drugs detected in breastmilk and delivered to the infant is small. Breastfeeding in these patients should no longer be viewed as absolutely contraindicated [1].

Most neonates have progressed normally through childhood [36,37]. Concerns have recently been raised about the possibility of delayed adverse effects in adulthood such as later development of fertility problems, autoimmune disorders, and neoplasia [37–39]. Thus, it is important that all offspring exposed to these agents have long-term follow-up.

Case presentation

This 26-year-old primigravida underwent heart transplantation for idiopathic dilated cardiomyopathy and intractable congestive heart failure. When she conceived 4 years after the transplant, she was receiving conventional doses of cyclosporine, azathioprine, and prednisone.

The patient was followed from 7 weeks' gestation with frequent antepartum visits and serial sonograms for fetal growth. Right-heart catheterizations and cardiac biopsies showed stable cardiac function throughout pregnancy. The pregnancy progressed normally until 33 weeks. At that time, she developed pruritus, slight icterus, and a blood pressure of 130/90 mmHg. Admission laboratory tests were normal except for a hematocrit of 28.5%, platelet count 99,000/μL, alkaline phosphatase 12 mg/dL, lactic dehydrogenase 345 mg/dL, and total bilirubin 2.8 mg/dL. Despite bed rest, her blood pressure gradually rose to 150/100 mmHg, and she developed proteinuria. A diagnosis of preeclampsia was made, and labor was induced at 34 weeks' gestation. The patient delivered a healthy 2500-g female infant.

Over the first 4 postpartum days, the mother had three intermittent episodes of sudden vaginal bleeding, which were treated with uterine massage, intravenous oxytocin, intramuscular prostaglandin $F_{2\alpha}$, uterine curettage, and blood transfusions. Persistent uterine bleeding on the fifth postpartum day prompted an abdominal hysterectomy. The uterus contained an unusual arteriovenous malformation which was most likely unrelated to her heart transplant. She had an uneventful postoperative course and her infant did well.

The patient developed coronary artery arteriosclerosis and gradual compromise of cardiac function over the next decade. She was otherwise in relatively good health except for chronic vulvar condylomata unresponsive to multiple therapeutic regimens. At age 35, 14 years after her transplant and 9 years after her delivery, a vulvar biopsy revealed invasive vulvar carcinoma which was treated with a radical vulvectomy and bilateral inguinal lymphadenectomy. One year later, her allograft vasculopathy was progressing and she was hospitalized and treated for an acute myocardial infarction and a pulmonary embolism. She was again admitted to the intensive care unit 3 weeks later with herpes encephalitis, where she developed acute tachycardia, severe hypoxia despite intubation, rapidly deteriorated, and expired. She is survived by her husband and her daughter, who is now 14 years old.

This case illustrates short- and long-term problems that commonly occur in transplant patients of reproductive age.

References

1 McKay DB, Josephson MA. Reproduction and transplantation: report on the consensus conference on reproductive issues and transplantation. *Am J Transplant* 2005;**5**:1592–9.
2 Dantal J, Soulillou J-P. Immunosuppressive drugs and the risk of cancer after organ transplantation. *N Engl J Med* 2005;**352**:1271–3.
3 Hampton T. Skin cancer's ranks rise. Immunosuppression to blame. *JAMA* 2005;**294**:1476–80.
4 Perinatal viral and parasitic infections. *ACOG Pract Bull* 2000;**20**:1–5.
5 Penn I, Makowski EL, Harris P. Parenthood following renal transplantation. *Kidney Int* 1980;**18**:221–33.
6 Registration Committee of the European Dialysis and Transplant Association. Successful pregnancies in women treated by dialysis and kidney transplantation. *Br J Obstet Gynaecol* 1980;**87**:839–45.
7 Rizzoni G, Ehrich JHH, Broyer M. Successful pregnancies in women on renal replacement therapy: Report from the EDTA Registry. *Nephrol Dial Transplant* 1992;**7**:279–87.
8 Lau RJ, Scott JR. Pregnancy following renal transplantation. *Clin Obstet Gynecol* 1985;**23**:339–50.
9 Bumgardner GL, Matas AJ. Transplantation and pregnancy. *Transplant Rev* 1992;**6**:139–62.
10 Armenti VT, Moritz MJ, Radomski JS, *et al.* Pregnancy and transplantation. *Graft* 2000;**3**:59–63.
11 Kallen B, Westgren M, Aberg A, Olaussen PO. Pregnancy outcome after maternal organ transplantation in Sweden. *Br J Obstet Gynaecol* 2005;**112**:904–9.
12 Sims CJ. Organ transplantation and immunosuppressive drugs. *Clin Obstet Gynecol* 1991;**34**:100–11.
13 Pirsch JD, Miller J, Deierhoi MH, Vincenti D, Filo RS. A comparison of tacrolimus (FK506) and cyclosporine for immunosuppression after cadaveric renal transplantation. FK506 kidney transplant study group. *Transplantation* 1997;**63**:977–83.

14 Kainz A, Harabacz I, Cowlrick IS, Gadgil D, Hagiwara D. Review of the course and outcome of 100 pregnancies in 84 women treated with tacrolimus. *Transplantation* 2000;**70**:1718–21.

15 Vincenti F. A decade of progress in kidney transplantation. *Transplantation* 2004;**77**:S52–61.

16 Miller J, Mendez R, Pirsch JD, Jensik SC. Safety and efficacy of tacrolius in combination with mycophenolate mofetil (MMF) in cadaveric renal transplant recipients. FK506/MMF dose ranging kidney transplant study group. *Transplantation* 2000;**69**:875–80.

17 DeSantis M, Straface G, Cavaliere A, Carducci B, Caruso A. Paternal and maternal exposure to leflunomide: pregnancy and neonatal outcome. *Ann Rheum Dis* 2005;**64**:1096–7.

18 Ostensen M. Disease specific problems related to drug therapy in pregnancy. *Lupus* 2004;**13**:746–50.

19 Winkler ME, Niessart S, Ringe B, Pichlmayr R. Successful pregnancy in a patient after liver transplantation maintained on FK 506. *Transplantation* 1993;**56**:751.

20 Alston PK, Kuller JA, McMahon MJ. Pregnancy in transplant recipients. *Obstet Gynecol Surv* 2001;**56**:289–95.

21 Norton PA, Scott JR. Gynecologic and obstetric problems in renal allograft recipients. In: Buchsbaum H, Schmidt J, eds. *Gynecologic and Obstetric Urology*, 3rd edn. Philadelphia, PA: WB Saunders, 1993: 657–74.

22 Scott JR. Pregnancy in transplant recipients. In: Coulam CB, Faulk WP, McIntyre JA, eds. *Immunology and Obstetrics*. WW Norton Co. 1992: 640–4.

23 Scott JR, Branch DW, Kochenour NK, Larkin RM. The effect of repeated pregnancies on renal allograft function. *Transplantation* 1986;**42**:694–5.

24 Davidson JM. Towards long-graft survival in renal transplantation in pregnancy. *Nephrol Dial Transplant* 1995;**10**:85–9.

25 Sutherland DER, Gruessner A. Long-term function (>5 years) of pancreas grafts from the International Pancreas Transplant Registry database. *Transplant Proc* 1995;**27**:2977.

26 Barrou BM, Gruessner AC, Sutherland DER, Gruessner RWG. Pregnancy after pancreas transplantation in the cyclosporine era: report from the International Pancreas Transplant Registry. *Transplantation* 1998;**65**:524–7.

27 Casele HL, Laifer SA. Pregnancy after liver transplantation. *Semin Perinatol* 1998;**22**:149–55.

28 Armenti VT, Wilson GA, Radomski JS, Moritz MJ, McGrory CH, Coscia LA. Report from the National Transplantation Pregnancy Registry (NTPR). Outcomes of pregnancy after transplantation. In: Cecka JM, Terasaki, PI (eds). *Clinical Transplants*. Los Angeles, CA: UCLA Immunogenetics Center, 1999: 111–9.

29 Camann WR, Goldman GA, Johnson MD, Moore J, Greene M. Cesarean delivery in a patient with a transplanted heart. *Anesthesiology* 1989;**71**:618–20.

30 Uretsky BF, Murali S, Reddy PS, *et al*. Development of coronary disease in cardiac transplant patients receiving immunosuppressive therapy with cyclosporine and prednisone. *Circulation* 1987;**76**:827–34.

31 Scott JR, Wagoner LE, Olsen SL, Taylor DO, Renlund DG. Pregnancy in heart transplant recipients. Management and outcome. *Obstet Gynecol* 1993;**82**:324–7.

32 Branch KR, Wagoner LE, McGrory CH, *et al*. Risks of subsequent pregnancies on mother and newborn in female heart transplant recipients. *J Heart Lung Transplant* 1998;**17**:698–702.

33 Parry D, Hextall A, Banner N, Robinson V, Yacoub M. Pregnancy following lung transplantation. *Transplant Proc* 1997;**29**:629.

34 Trouche V, Ville Y, Fernandez H. Pregnancy after heart or heart-lung transplantation: a series of 10 pregnancies. *Br J Obstet Gynaecol* 1998;**105**:454–8.

35 Rigg CD, Bythell VE, Bryson MR, Halshaw J, Davidson JM. Caesarean section in patients with heart-lung transplants: a report of three cases and review. *Int J Obstet Anesth* 2000;**9**:125–32.

36 Willis FR, Findlay CA, Gorrie MJ, Watson MA, Wilkinson AG, Beattie TJ. Children of renal transplant recipient mothers. *J Pediatr Child Health* 2000;**36**:230–5.

37 Scott JR. Development of children born to mothers with connective tissue diseases. *Lupus* 2002;**11**:655–60.

38 Classen BJ, Shevach EM. Evidence that cyclosporine treatment during pregnancy predisposes offspring to develop autoantibodies. *Transplantation* 1991;**51**:1052–7.

39 Scott, JR, Branch DW, Holman J. Autoimmune and pregnancy complications in the daughter of a kidney transplant patient. *Transplantation* 2002;**73**:815–6.

40 Garovoy MR, Vincenti F, Amend WJC, *et al*. *Renal Transplantation, the Modern Era*. New York: Gower Medical, 1987.

41 Sollinger HW, Knechtle SJ. The current status of combined kidney-pancreas transplantation. In: Sabiston DC, ed. *Textbook of Surgery, Update 6*. Philadelphia: WB Saunders, 1990.

42 Norton PA, Scott JR. Gynecologic and obstetric problems in renal allograft recipients. In: Buchsbaum H, Schmidt J, eds. *Gynecologic and Obstetric Urology*, 3rd edn. Philadelphia: WB Saunders, 1993.

20

Gestational diabetes mellitus

Deborah L. Conway

Normal pregnancy is a state of insulin resistance. To spare glucose for the developing fetus, the placenta produces several hormones that antagonize insulin and shifts the principal energy source from glucose to ketones and free fatty acids [1,2]. Most pregnant women maintain normal blood glucose levels despite the increased insulin resistance through enhanced insulin production and release by the pancreas, both in the basal state, and in response to meals.

Gestational diabetes mellitus (GDM) is a state of carbohydrate intolerance that develops or is first recognized during pregnancy. In some women, β-cell production of insulin cannot keep pace with the resistance to insulin produced by the diabetogenic hormones from the placenta. The prevalence of GDM in the USA is 2–5%, and is proportional to the prevalence of type 2 diabetes in the population under examination, because they share a similar pathophysiology [3]. It is the most common medical complication of pregnancy, and it is clearly linked to several maternal and fetal complications including: fetal macrosomia with operative delivery and birth trauma [4]; preeclampsia and hypertensive disorders [5]; metabolic complications in the neonate including hypoglycemia, hypocalcemia, and hyperbilirubinemia [6]; prematurity and perinatal mortality [7–10].

Screening for diabetes in pregnancy

Rigorous identification and effective treatment of women with diabetes minimize the occurrence of pregnancy complications that can result from maternal hyperglycemia. Most experts agree that all pregnant women should undergo screening for GDM. However, "screening" does not necessarily involve universal laboratory testing for hyperglycemia. In risk factor-based screening, women who meet all criteria listed in Table 20.1 are deemed "low-risk" for GDM, and may forego laboratory glucose testing. In a retrospective comparison, over 18,000 women were screened for GDM with the 1-hour 50-g glucose challenge test (GCT) [11]. If only those with risk factors had

undergone laboratory testing, just 3% of women with GDM would have been undetected. However, in this population, only 10% of women were "low risk" by all criteria, and thus able to forego the 1-hour GCT. Therefore, in clinical settings with a high burden of GDM and type 2 diabetes, a risk factor-based screening algorithm is unlikely to be either cost or time efficient.

The most commonly employed cut-off value for the GCT is 140 mg/dL, which results in an approximately 15% test positive rate. By reducing the cut-off to 130 mg/dL, the sensitivity of the test (i.e., the proportion of women with GDM who have a "positive" screen) improves to nearly 100%, at the expense of specificity [12]. In a low-risk population (i.e., one with a low burden of type 2 diabetes), the actual number of extra cases identified with this increase in sensitivity is greatly outweighed by the number of false positive screens between 130 and 140 mg/dL. Conversely, in a high-risk population in which type 2 diabetes is common, the number missed by using the higher cut-off may be unacceptable. Therefore, the population characteristics should be taken into consideration when selecting the appropriate cut off for gestational diabetes screening.

For women at low risk for GDM, screening should occur between 24 and 28 weeks, because insulin resistance during pregnancy increases as a function of increasing gestational age until approximately 32 weeks' gestation. Women who are at high risk should be tested upon entry to prenatal care. Women at high risk for GDM include those with GDM, macrosomia, stillbirth, or congenital anomaly in a prior pregnancy, those with a first-degree relative with type 2 diabetes, as well as women with polycystic ovarian syndrome or a history of glucose intolerance or "pre-diabetes" prior to the current pregnancy.

After a positive screening test result is obtained, a diagnostic 3-hour glucose tolerance test (GTT) should be performed. This test involves a 100-g glucose load after a fasting plasma glucose level is drawn. Plasma glucose levels are then obtained at 1, 2, and 3 hours post-glucose load. Several recent studies have shown no difference in GTT results with or without carbohydrate "loading" in the days prior to the test [13–15]. There are two different sets of values commonly used that define a

Table 20.1 Criteria for avoiding laboratory screening for gestational diabetes. All criteria must be met for a patient to be considered "low-risk" and glucose testing avoided. (From American Diabetes Association [47] with permission.)

Age less than 25 years
Not a member of an ethnic group with an increased prevalence of type 2 DM
Body mass index of ≤25
No prior history of glucose intolerance (GDM, DM, IGT, or IFG)
No prior history of obstetric outcomes associated with GDM (macrosomia, stillbirth, malformations)
No known diabetes in a first-degree relative

DM, diabetes mellitus; GDM, gestational diabetes mellitus; IFG, impaired fasting glucose; IGT, impaired glucose tolerance.

Table 20.2 Diagnostic thresholds for gestational diabetes using the 3-hour 100-g glucose tolerance test.

Time	ADA/Carpenter & Coustan Thresholds* [16] (mg/dL)	NDDGThresholds* [17] (mg/dL)
Fasting	95	105
1-hour	180	190
2-hour	155	165
3-hour	140	145

ADA, American Diabetes Association; NDDG, National Diabetes Data Group.
* If two or more values *meet or exceed* these thresholds, the diagnosis of gestational diabetes is made.

positive result. According to the recommendations by the American Diabetes Association's Fourth International Workshop Conference on Gestational Diabetes, the Carpenter and Coustan modification of O'Sullivan and Mahan's original values should be used [16]. These values are more stringent than the values cited by the National Diabetes Data Group (NDDG) (Table 20.2) [17].

The precise thresholds above which all diabetes-related morbidity occurs, and below which none does, are not likely to be determined. However, evidence exists that lack of treatment of milder forms of gestational glucose intolerance result in increased rates of GDM-related morbidity, particularly excessive fetal growth. In the Toronto Tri-Hospital Study [18], women with "borderline" GDM (meeting Carpenter and Coustan criteria, but not NDDG criteria) were not treated, and had more than twice the rate of macrosomia as women with completely normal glucose testing (28% vs. 13%). Similarly, women with one abnormal value using the higher NDDG criteria also have increased rates of overgrown infants [19].

Therapeutic modalities in gestational diabetes

Medical management of GDM aims to optimize glycemic control to prevent or minimize the complications associated with the disease, while avoiding ketosis and poor nutrition. A multidisciplinary approach (involving obstetricians, perinatologists, dietitians, diabetes educators, internists, and endocrinologists) is essential to management. Diet, exercise, patient education, and, if need be, medical therapies should be utilized.

The cornerstone of care of a pregnancy complicated by diabetes is diet. Medical nutrition therapy for GDM is aimed at optimizing metabolic outcomes, and improving health by encouraging healthy food choices while addressing personal and cultural preferences and providing adequate energy and nutrients for optimal pregnancy outcomes [20]. Elements of dietary therapy include total calorie allocation, calorie distribution, and nutritional component management. Total daily calorie intake is based on ideal body weight, with overweight and obese women allocated fewer kilocalories per kilogram of prepregnancy body weight than normal and underweight women. For example, overweight and obese women can be given approximately 25 kcal/kg, up to a total of 2800–3000 kcal/day. Women with normal prepregnancy body mass index (BMI) receive approximately 30 kcal/kg, with a minimum intake of 1800 kcal/day. These calories are typically distributed between three meals and two to four snacks during the day. Smaller, more frequent meals lead to better satiety, improved compliance with the diet, and reduced magnitude of postprandial peaks.

Postprandial glucose measurements are directly influenced by the amount of carbohydrate in the consumed food. A traditional diet for diabetics typically contains 55–60% carbohydrate. Major *et al.* [21] described their success with a diet containing 40–42% carbohydrate. Compared with a 45–50% carbohydrate diet, mild carbohydrate restriction resulted in improved glycemic control, less need for insulin, and fewer large-for-gestational age infants.

Exercise is another key component in diabetic care. Cardiovascular exercise reduces insulin resistance [22]. Fasting and postprandial glucose levels are lower in women with GDM who exercise, possibly avoiding the need for insulin treatment in some women [23,24]. The physiologic and anatomic constraints of pregnancy should be taken into consideration when counseling pregnant women about exercise.

There is no established standard as to how frequently glucose levels should be checked in patients with GDM. The goal of monitoring is to identify whether or not glycemic targets are being met. Commonly used targets include fasting values below 95 mg/dL and 2-hour postprandial values below 120 mg/dL [25]. Alternatively, 1-hour postprandial values may be used, with a target below 130–140 mg/dL. Many experts recommend daily monitoring with a meter that has built-in memory, so that results can be verified, analyzed, and reviewed with the patient during clinic visits. Langer *et al.* [26] have demonstrated the benefits of an "intensified" approach to care of diabetes during pregnancy. One essential component of this regimen is frequent daily readings (seven times per day) that provide information on the effectiveness of the current treatment regimen. Using this intensified approach, rates of macrosomia, shoulder dystocia, cesarean delivery, and neonatal hypoglycemia were reduced compared with those women monitored less frequently with weekly fasting and 2-hour postprandial readings.

One randomized trial suggested that monitoring postprandial glucose determinations was more effective than preprandial values in managing women with GDM on insulin [27]. The group randomized to postprandial readings had significantly less fetal overgrowth, fewer cesarean deliveries for cephalopelvic disproportion, and less neonatal hypoglycemia, compared with women who checked their glucose levels before meals. Although postprandial readings are superior to preprandial readings, they have not been shown to be superior to a combination of pre- and post-meal readings. Results from continuous blood glucose monitors in "well-controlled" nonpregnant type 2 diabetics revealed unrecognized hypoglycemic episodes in 80% of patients, and postprandial hyperglycemia after 57% of all meals [28].

Ultimately, some women with GDM will not be able to meet glycemic targets with diet therapy alone and will require medical intervention with insulin or a hypoglycemic agent. This can usually be determined once dietary therapy has been in place for 2 weeks [29]. Insulin dosage is calculated according to body weight, starting in the range of 0.7–1.0 units/kg of current body weight, usually given in the form of short- and intermediate-acting human insulin, in split doses. Two-thirds of the total calculated dose is given with breakfast and one-third in the evening. A sample calculation is provided in Fig. 20.1. The pregnant diabetic demonstrates both insulin resistance and relative insulin deficiency; thus, it is typical to require large doses of insulin to achieve adequate glycemic control [30]. It is important to remember that with advancing gestational age, the patient will become more insulin resistant, and therefore insulin requirements will increase. The insulin dose can be adjusted as frequently as every 3–4 days and can be increased 10–20% depending on the corresponding values obtained from patient monitoring.

Another treatment option for women who are not adequately controlled on diet alone is the sulfonylurea drug glyburide. In the past, there was concern over transplacental passage of sulfonylurea drugs leading to fetal and neonatal hypoglycemia. Studies using human placental models demonstrated that the transplacental passage of glyburide is negligible [31]. In a randomized trial comparing insulin with glyburide in 404 women with GDM, no differences were found between groups in terms of mean maternal blood glucose, large for gestational age infants, macrosomia (greater than 4000 g), lung complications, hypoglycemia, or cord blood insulin levels. In addition, no glyburide could be detected in the cord blood of infants born to women treated with that agent [32]. The criteria we use for consideration of glyburide therapy are the following: gestational age 11–33 weeks; fasting glucose on 3-hour GTT less than 110 mg/dL [33]; and no known allergy to sulfa-containing drugs. For women who do not meet these criteria, we recommend insulin. The initial dose of glyburide is usually 2.5 mg, given in the morning if daytime control is required or at bedtime if fasting hyperglycemia is present. The dosage can be adjusted upward by 2.5–5 mg on a weekly basis, to a maximum of 20 mg/day (10 mg b.i.d.). Although maternal hypoglycemia is a potential complication of glyburide therapy, it occurs less often than in insulin-treated women [32].

Antenatal testing

Documenting fetal well-being during the antepartum period is important for any woman whose pregnancy is complicated by pregestational diabetes (White class B or higher). However, there is no unified opinion regarding the need for antepartum fetal assessment in women with well-controlled, uncomplicated pre-existing and gestational diabetes [34]. The American College of Obstetricians and Gynecologists (ACOG) recommends that antenatal testing be performed on all pregestational diabetics, gestational diabetics with poor glycemic control, or gestational diabetics with another pregnancy complication such as hypertension or abnormal fetal growth [25]. The method of testing (e.g., nonstress testing, biophysical

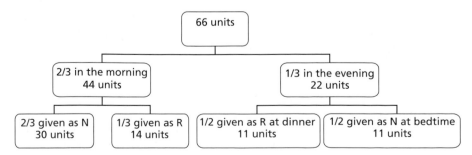

Fig. 20.1 Sample initial insulin dose calculation. Current patient weight: 94 kg (207 lb). Total daily insulin (0.7 units/kg): 0.7 × 94 kg = 66 units. N, insulin NPH; R, insulin regular.

profile) is left to the discretion of the provider, guided by local practice. In addition, all women with GDM should be instructed to perform fetal kick counts daily, beginning in the third trimester, and to notify her care provider promptly if fetal movements are diminished.

Delivery: when to deliver, how to deliver

Timing of delivery is a delicate balance in a pregnancy complicated by diabetes. Once term has been reached, ongoing pregnancy exposes the fetus to the risk of stillbirth and continued *in utero* growth that may make delivery more risky. On the other hand, needless intervention places women at risk for the complications associated with long labors and operative deliveries. Very few prospective trials have been undertaken with regard to optimizing delivery outcomes in diabetics. What has been consistently shown is that the cesarean delivery rate is higher in diabetics than in nondiabetics [35], even when skilled antenatal care has achieved near normal rates of fetal overgrowth [18].

An additional consideration in the optimal timing of delivery is that infants of diabetic mothers may have delayed pulmonary maturity and are at increased risk of respiratory distress syndrome (RDS). Poorly controlled diabetes is associated with fetal pulmonary immaturity, but the risk in well-controlled pregnancies parallels that of a nondiabetic population [36]. Other investigators have found that the risk of RDS becomes equal to that of nondiabetic pregnancies at 38.5 weeks [37]. In a study by Piper *et al.* [36], no cases of RDS occurred after 37 weeks' gestation, despite "immature" results on the amniotic fluid tests for fetal lung maturity. Lung maturity testing in the setting of diabetes might only be necessary if early delivery is considered, if glucose control has been very poor, or if gestational age is uncertain. Furthermore, tests for lung maturity should only be obtained in cases where delay in delivery is prudent even if the test is negative.

Indications for delivery at any time after 37–38 weeks include: inability to achieve adequate glucose control; poor compliance with visits or prescribed treatment; prior stillbirth; and presence of chronic hypertension. Women with well-controlled GDM, good compliance with care, and an appropriately grown fetus are allowed to enter spontaneous labor, until 40–41 weeks' gestation is reached. Kjos *et al.* [38] studied a similar approach in women with Class A2 and B diabetes, comparing it to labor induction at 38 weeks in a randomized trial. Expectant management prolonged gestation by 1 week, and resulted in a doubling in the rate of macrosomic infants. The women managed expectantly had a similar cesarean delivery rate to those induced at 38 weeks, although half of the expectant management group underwent labor induction. The most frequent indication for induction was abnormal antepartum testing.

Macrosomia and shoulder dystocia occur more frequently in pregnancies complicated by diabetes than in the general obstetric population. Based on the observation that most cases of shoulder dystocia in diabetic women occur when birthweight is above 4000 g [39], we recommend cesarean delivery without a trial of labor to women with an estimated fetal weight above 4250 g who have diabetes. By implementing this practice, our shoulder dystocia rate in diabetic women has been reduced by 80%, and shoulder dystocia rates among macrosomic infants (birthweight over 4000 g) fell from 19% to 7% after implementing this practice. There was a small but significant increase in the cesarean delivery rate [40]. We use a threshold of 4250 g to account for ultrasound error, so that operative intervention is not overused. Shoulder dystocia remains most often an unpredictable and unpreventable obstetric emergency. ACOG recomends that planned cesarean delivery to prevent shoulder dystocia may be considered for suspected fetal macrosomia with estimated fetal weight exceeding 4500 g in women with diabetes [41].

Postpartum

Gestational diabetes may be the first warning of inherent insulin resistance. Women with GDM need to have glucose tolerance reassessed in the postpartum period. The most commonly used assessment method is the 2-hour GTT identifying both impaired glucose tolerance and overt diabetes. Twenty to thirty percent of women will have abnormal values when tested early in the postpartum period [42–45]. Kjos *et al.* [43] found that 10% will have impaired glucose tolerance and 9% will have frank diabetes when testing took place 5–8 weeks after delivery. The factors that increased risk for abnormal GTT postpartum included: diagnosis of GDM at an earlier gestational age, higher glucose values on GTT during pregnancy, increased age, increased parity, increased BMI, and increased birthweight. All of these risk factors suggest a higher degree of insulin resistance.

The importance of postpartum testing cannot be understated. Within 5–6 years after a pregnancy complicated with GDM, up to 50% of women will have type 2 diabetes [46]. Early identification of impaired glucose tolerance affords the opportunity to institute therapeutic measures such as exercise, diet, and weight control, perhaps preventing progression to diabetes. Identification and treatment of overt diabetes early in the course of the disease offers the best opportunity to delay or avoid the micro- and macrovascular complications associated with the disease.

Case presentation

A 27-year-old woman, G2 P1001, at 12 weeks' gestation presents for initial prenatal care. She denies a history of

GDM. Her first child, born by uncomplicated spontaneous vaginal delivery, weighed 4100 g at 38 weeks' gestation. Her records indicate that the 3-hour GTT performed at 25 weeks in her first pregnancy had the following values: fasting 96 mg/dL, 1-hour 191 mg/dL, 2-hour 152 mg/dL, 3-hour 122 mg/dL. Her mother and her older sister have type 2 diabetes mellitus.

A 50-g GCT is performed with her initial prenatal laboratory tests, and it is abnormal. A 3-hour GTT performed at 13 weeks' gestation is normal (96/177/148/125). However, repeat testing at 25 weeks reveals she has GDM (99/202/168/141). In initiating treatment, she is prescribed medical nutrition therapy which provides 40–45% carbohydrates, 30–35% protein, and 25% fat. Total energy supplied is calculated to be 2500 kcal/day, based on her prepregnancy weight of 100 kg (BMI 35 obese, 25 kcal/kg). She is instructed to perform self-monitored blood glucose readings. After 1 week of therapy, her fasting glucose levels are consistently above 95 mg/dL, and more than 50% of her postprandial glucose values are also above target range. Insulin is initiated, but despite increasing doses over the subsequent weeks, she remains poorly controlled as term approaches. Her fundal height at 38 weeks measures 41 cm, and an ultrasound reveals a fetal weight estimate of 4600 g, with a head circumference : abdominal circumference ratio of 0.85. Given these findings, in the setting of poorly controlled GDM, the patient is counseled about and accepts a cesarean delivery. The infant's birth weight is 4450 g, and the neonatal course is complicated by hypoglycemia that requires intravenous glucose infusion.

At the time of the postpartum visit, a 2-hour GTT is obtained and indicates impaired glucose tolerance (Fasting 97 mg/dL, 2-hour 178 mg/dL). Lifestyle modifications are recommended to prevent progression to type 2 diabetes mellitus, and annual screening for diabetes is suggested.

References

1 Felig P. Maternal and fetal fuel homeostasis in human pregnancy. *Am J Clin Nutr* 1973;**26**:998–1005.

2 Beicher SG, Sullivan JB, Freinkel N. Carbohydrate metabolism in pregnancy. *N Engl J Med* 1964;**271**:866.

3 Engelgau MM, Herman WH, Smith PJ, German RR, Aubert RE. The epidemiology of diabetes and pregnancy in the US, 1988. *Diabetes Care* 1995;**18**:1029–33.

4 Ballard JL, Rosenn B, Khoury JC, Miodovnik M. Diabetic fetal macrosomia: significance of disproportionate growth. *J Pediatr* 1993;**122**:115–9.

5 Garner PR, D'Alton ME, Dudley DK, Huard P, Hardie M. Preeclampsia in diabetic pregnancies. *Am J Obstet Gynecol* 1990;**163**:505–8.

6 Mimouni F, Tsang RC, Hertzberg VS, Miodovnik M. Polycythemia, hyopmagnesemia, and hypocalemia in infants of diabetic mothers. *Am J Dis Child* 1986;**140**:798–800.

7 Mimoumi F, Miodovnik M, Siddiqi TA, Khoury J, Tsang RC. Perinatal asphyxia in infants of insulin-dependent diabetic mothers. *J Pediatr* 1988;**113**:345–53.

8 Mimoumi F, Miodovnik M, Siddiqi TA, Berk MA, Wittekind C, Tsang RC. High spontaneous premature labor rate in insulin-dependent diabetic pregnant women: an association with poor glycemic control and urogenital infection. *Obstet Gynecol* 1988;**72**:175–80.

9 Robert MF, Neff RK, Hubbell JP, Taeusch HW, Avery ME. Association between maternal diabetes and the respiratory-distress syndrome in the newborn. *N Engl J Med* 1976;**294**:357–60.

10 Weintrob N, Karp M, Hod M. Short- and long-range complications of offspring of diabetic mothers. *J Diabetes Complications* 1996;**10**:294–301.

11 Danilenko-Dixon DR, Van Winter JT, Nelson RL, Ogburn PL Jr. Universal versus selective gestational diabetes screening: application of 1997 American Diabetes Association recommendations. *Am J Obstet Gynecol* 1999;**181**:798–802.

12 Coustan DR, Widness JA, Carpenter MW, Rotondo L, Pratt DC, Oh W. Should the fifty-gram one-hour glucose screening test for gestational diabetes be administered in the fasting or fed state? *Am J Obstet Gynecol* 1986;**154**:1031–5.

13 Crowe SM, Mastrobattista JM, Monga M. Oral glucose tolerance test and the preparatory diet. *Am J Obstet Gynecol* 2000;**182**: 1052–4.

14 Entrekin K, Work B, Owen J. Does a high carbohdrate preparatory diet affect the 3-hour oral glucose tolerance test in pregnancy? *J Matern Fetal Med* 1998;**7**:68–71.

15 Harlass FE, McClure GB, Read JA, Brady K. Use of a standard preparatory diet for the oral glucose tolerance test. Is it necessary? *J Reprod Med* 1991;**36**:147–50.

16 Carpenter MW, Coustan DR. Criteria for screening tests for gestational diabetes. *Am J Obstet Gynecol* 1982;**144**:768–73.

17 National Diabetes Data Group. Classification and diagnosis of diabetes mellitus and other categories of glucose intolerance. *Diabetes* 1979;**28**:1039–57.

18 Naylor CD, Sermer M, Chen E, Sykora K. Cesarean delivery in relation to birth weight and gestational glucose tolerance: pathophysiology or practice style? *JAMA* 1996;**275**:1165–70.

19 Langer O, Brustman L, Anyaegbunam A, Mazze R. The significance of one abnormal glucose tolerance test value on adverse outcome in pregnancy. *Am J Obstet Gynecol* 1987;**157**:758–63.

20 American Diabetes Association. Nutrition principles and recommendations in diabetes. *Diabetes Care* 2004;**27**(Suppl 1): S36–S46.

21 Major CA, Henry MJ, De Veciana M, Morgan MA. The effects of carbohydrate restriction in patients with diet-controlled gestational diabetes. *Obstet Gynecol* 1998;**91**:600–4.

22 Horton ES. Exercise in the treatment of NIDDM. Applications for GDM? *Diabetes* 1991;**40**(Suppl 2):175–8.

23 Jovanovic-Peterson L, Durak EP, Peterson CM. Randomized trial of diet versus diet plus cardiovascular conditioning on glucose levels in gestational diabetes. *Am J Obstet Gynecol* 1989;**161**:415–9.

24 Artal R, Wiswell R, Romem Y. Hormonal responses to exercise in diabetic and nondiabetic pregnant patients. *Diabetes* 1985;**34**(Suppl 2):78–80.

25 ACOG Practice Bulletin Number 30. *Gestational Diabetes*. September, 2001.

26 Langer O, Rodriquez DA, Xenakis EM, McFarland MB, Berkus MD, Arrendondo F. Intensified versus conventional management of gestational diabetes. *Am J Obstet Gynecol* 1994;**170**:1036–47.

27 de Veciana M, Major CA, Morgan MA, *et al*. Postprandial versus preprandial glucose monitoring in women with gestational diabetes mellitus requiring insulin therapy. *N Engl J Med* 1995;**333**:235–46.

28 Hay LC, Wilmshurst EG, Fulcher G. Unrecognized hypo- and hyperglycemia in well-controlled patients with type 2 diabetes mellitus: the results of continuous glucose monitoring. *Diabetes Technol Ther* 2003;**5**:19–26.

29 McFarland MB, Langer O, Conway DL, Berkus MD. Dietary therapy for gestational diabetes: how long is long enough? *Am J Obstet Gynecol* 1999;**93**:978–82.

30 Langer O, Anyaegbunam A, Brustman L, Guidetti D, Mazze R. Gestational diabetes: insulin requirements in pregnancy. *Am J Obstet Gynecol* 1987;**157**:669–75.

31 Elliot BD, Langer O, Schenker S, Johnson RF. Insignificant transfer of glyburide occurs across the human placenta. *Am J Obstet Gynecol* 1991;**165**:807–12.

32 Langer O, Conway DL, Berkus MD, Xenakis EM, Gonzales O. A comparison of glyburide and insulin in women with gestational diabetes mellitus. *N Engl J Med* 2000;**343**:1134–8.

33 Conway DL, Gonzales O, Skiver D. Use of glyburide for the treatment of gestational diabetes: the San Antonio experience. *J Matern Fetal Neonatal Med* 2004;**15**:173–7.

34 Landon MB, Vickers S. Fetal surveillance in pregnancy complicated by diabetes mellitus: is it necessary? *J Matern Fetal Neonatal Med* 2002;**12**:413–6.

35 Jacobson JD, Cousins L. A population-based study of maternal and perinatal outcome in patients with gestational diabetes. *Am J Obstet Gynecol* 1989;**161**:981–6.

36 Piper JM, Xenakis EM, Langer O. Delayed appearance of pulmonary maturation markers is associated with poor glucose control in diabetic pregnancies. *J Matern Fetal Med* 1998;**7**:148–53.

37 Kjos SL, Walther FJ, Montoro M, Paul RH, Diaz F, Stabler M. Prevalence and etiology of respiratory distress in infants of diabetic mothers: predictive value of fetal lung maturation tests. *Am J Obstet Gynecol* 1990;**163**:898–903.

38 Kjos SL, Henry OA, Montoro M, Buchanan TA, Mestman JH. Insulin-requiring diabetes in pregnancy: a randomized trial of active induction of labor and expectant management. *Am J Obstet Gynecol* 1993;**169**:611–5.

39 Langer O, Berkus MD, Huff RW, Samueloff A. Shoulder dystocia: should the fetus weighing greater than or equal to 4000 grams be delivered by cesarean section? *Am J Obstet Gynecol* 1991;**165**:831–7.

40 Conway DL, Langer O. Elective delivery of infants with macrosomia in diabetic women: reduced shoulder dystocia versus increased cesarean deliveries. *Am J Obstet Gynecol* 1998;**178**:922–5.

41 ACOG Practice Bulletin Number 40. Shoulder dystocia November 2002.

42 Catalano PM, Vargo KM, Bernstein IM, Amini SB. Incidence and risk factors associated with abnormal postpartum glucose tolerance in woman with gestational diabetes. *Am J Obstet Gynecol* 1991;**165**:914–9.

43 Kjos SL, Buchanan TA, Greenspoon JS, Montoro M, Bernstein GS, Mestman JH. Gestational diabetes mellitus: the prevalence of glucose intolerance and diabetes mellitus in the first two months postpartum. *Am J Obstet Gynecol* 1990;**163**:93–8.

44 Damm P, Kuhl C, Bertelsen A, Molsted-Pedersen L. Predictive factors for the development of diabetes in women with previous gestational diabetes mellitus. *Am J Obstet Gynecol* 1992;**167**:607–12.

45 Conway DL, Langer O. Effects of new criteria for type 2 diabetes on the rate of postpartum glucose intolerance in women with gestational diabetes. *Am J Obstet Gynecol* 1999;**181**:610–4.

46 Kjos SL, Peters RK, Xiang A, Henry OA, Montoro M, Buchanan TA. Predicting future diabetes in Latino women with gestational diabetes: utility of early postpartum glucose tolerance testing. *Diabetes* 1995;**44**:586–91.

47 American Diabetes Association. Gestational diabetes mellitus. *Diabetes Care* 2004;**27**(Suppl 1):S88–S90.

21 Diabetes mellitus

George Saade

As more women with diabetes are contemplating pregnancy and more women are delaying pregnancy, health care providers should expect to see more pregnant women with pregestational as well as gestational diabetes. Management of these women should follow accepted guidelines in order to decrease maternal and perinatal morbidity and mortality. To that effect, the central goal is to decrease the risk for congenital anomalies secondary to preconception hyperglycemia, as well as to shepherd the pregnant woman through pregnancy in order to reach term without maternal complications such as preeclampsia, or fetal complications such as uteroplacental insufficiency, antepartum stillbirth, intrapartum hypoxemia, macrosomia, birth injury, and postnatal hypoglycemia. This can be achieved by a combination of frequent glucose monitoring, dietary and pharmacologic interventions, diligent fetal surveillance, appropriate timing of delivery, and judicious choice of delivery route. The time-honored method of managing the pregnant diabetic patient has been by means of elective premature delivery at some arbitrary date—usually between 36 and 38 weeks' gestation—in an attempt to prevent fetal demise. With advances in antepartum fetal monitoring and improved techniques for determining fetal maturity, however, management can now be varied to suit the individual patient. More diabetic patients can be brought to term, and perinatal mortality rates from stillbirth, prematurity, and birth injury can be markedly reduced. It is important that the obstetrician who occasionally manages diabetic patients becomes familiar with the uses and limitations of some of the newer methods now practiced in large obstetric services that deliver many diabetic patients. This chapter concentrates on the pregestational diabetic patient. For discussion of gestational diabetes, see Chapter 20.

At present, the leading cause of perinatal mortality in pregnancies complicated by insulin-dependent diabetes mellitus is congenital malformation. The risk of major malformations in such pregnancies is increased three- to fourfold over the 2–3% incidence noted in the general population. There is increasing evidence that these anomalies are a result of marked alterations in maternal glycemic control during the critical period of fetal embryogenesis, at 5–8 weeks' gestation. Patients whose diabetes is poorly regulated are also at greater risk for a spontaneous abortion. There is a direct correlation between maternal glycosylated hemoglobin (hemoglobin A_{1C}) levels and the risk for spontaneous abortion and fetal anomalies [1]. In one study, the risks of spontaneous abortion and major malformations were 12.4% and 3.0%, respectively, with first-trimester hemoglobin A_{1C} ≤9.3%, vs. 37.5% and 40%, respectively, with hemoglobin A_{1C} >14.4% [2]. Preconception care in diabetic women is associated with fewer maternal hospitalizations, less use of neonatal intensive care, and a reduction in major congenital anomalies and perinatal deaths [3]. The aim should be to maintain hemoglobin A_{1C} less than 7%. For this reason, treatment of the woman with insulin-dependent diabetes who is considering a pregnancy should be initiated before conception [4]. In addition, the preconception patient should be placed on 4 mg/day folic acid supplementation in order to reduce the risk for neural tube defect. Thorough evaluation should be made to detect evidence of maternal retinopathy, nephropathy, or coronary artery disease. For the most recent classification and diagnostic criteria for pregestational diabetes, refer to the Report of the Expert Committee of the American Diabetes Association [5]. The American College of Obstetricians and Gynecologists (ACOG) has also issued a recent Technical Bulletin addressing pregestational diabetes [6].

Initial evaluation

For women with previously diagnosed diabetes, it is important to take a careful history and perform a physical examination as soon as pregnancy is diagnosed, paying special attention to the following:

1 Careful dating of the pregnancy by history and physical signs.

Table 21.1 White's classification of diabetes in pregnancy.

Class A₁
Abnormal glucose tolerance test with normal fasting capillary (95 mg/dL) and postprandial (120 mg/dL) glucose levels
Controlled with diet alone

Class A₂
Abnormal glucose tolerance test with abnormal fasting or postprandial glucose levels
Treated with diet and insulin

Class B
Insulin-treated diabetic
Onset over age 20 years
Duration less than 10 years
No vascular disease or retinopathy

Class C
Insulin-treated diabetic
Onset between ages 10 and 20 years
Duration between 10 and 20 years
Background retinopathy

Class D
Insulin-treated diabetic
Onset under age 10
Duration more than 20 years
Background retinopathy

Class F
Diabetic nephropathy

Class H
Cardiac disease

Class R
Proliferative retinopathy

2 Classification of the diabetic patient, using White's criteria (Table 21.1).
3 Progress and outcome of any previous pregnancies.
4 Careful funduscopic examination for the presence of retinopathy.
5 Findings of urinalysis and culture, as well as 24-hour urine collection for creatinine clearance and protein.
6 Baseline blood pressure measurement, electrocardiogram (ECG), and thyroid function tests.
7 Baseline glycosylated hemoglobin measurement.
8 Thorough instruction about insulin dosage, importance of adhering to the prescribed diet, and home glucose monitoring.

Regulating maternal glycemia

Careful control of maternal glucose levels significantly improves perinatal outcome. Except during brief periods after meals, these levels should normally remain below 100 mg/dL. Maternal hyperglycemia and rapid fluctuations in blood glucose produce similar changes in the fetal compartment. Fetal hyperglycemia leads to β-cell hyperplasia and hyperinsulinemia. Also, there is a significant correlation between maternal glucose levels and subsequent adiposity in the infant. Ketoacidosis at any time during pregnancy may lead to death *in utero*. Management of diabetic ketoacidosis includes aggressive fluid and electrolyte replacement, in addition to insulin administration.

Maintenance of euglycemia depends not only on diligent regulation of diet and insulin, but also on strict attention to physical activity and stress. Capillary glucose levels of 60–140 mg/dL throughout the day should be the objective of therapy. Patients should eat three meals and three snacks each day, adding up to 30–35 cal/kg of ideal body weight. This regimen permits a total weight gain of approximately 25 lb.

The most successful regimen of insulin administration usually includes two injections daily of both NPH and regular insulin. The amount of NPH insulin given in the morning generally exceeds that of regular insulin by a 2:1 ratio. In the evening, equal amounts of NPH and regular insulin are given. If several fasting or postprandial glucose levels are not acceptable (usually more than one-third of values), insulin doses are increased by 20%. Several days are then allowed to pass before further changes are made. The use of other insulin types or administration (e.g., short- or long-acting, insulin pump), as well as oral hypoglycemic agents, should be individualized and reserved for special circumstances [7]. Limited evidence suggest that diabetic women who continue oral hypoglycemics when they become pregnant are at higher risk for complications [8]. During labor, a continuous insulin infusion is best to stabilize maternal glucose levels and reduce neonatal hypoglycemia. The goal is to maintain hourly glucose levels at less than 110 mg/dL.

Glycemic control cannot be accurately assessed by random blood glucose determinations or by testing urine specimens for glucose. The patient should be taught to assess her capillary glucose levels by using glucose oxidase-impregnated reagent strips with a blood glucose reflectance meter. Determinations should be made in the fasting state, and 2 hours after meals. Measurements made before lunch, dinner, and bedtime may also be helpful. The goal of therapy is to maintain capillary whole-blood glucose levels as close to normal as possible, including a fasting glucose level of 95 mg/dL or less, premeal values of 100 mg/dL or less, 1-hour postprandial levels of 140 mg/dL or less, and 2-hour postprandial values of 120 mg/dL or less. When using a meter, it is imperative to determine whether it tests whole blood, serum, or plasma, as results may vary (plasma levels approximately 10 mg/dL higher than whole blood). A blood glucose sample drawn 80 minutes after breakfast correlates well with the mean amplitude of glycemic excursions throughout the day.

A useful parameter for assessing control over previous weeks and months is hemoglobin A_{1c}, a minor variant of hemoglobin A, produced by the addition of a single glucose moiety to the terminal valine of the beta-chain. This glycosylated hemoglobin is synthesized throughout the red blood cell's life cycle in amounts that reflect the degree of chronic hyperglycemia present. Levels correlate significantly with mean fasting glucose, mean daily glucose, and highest daily glucose values. In normal pregnancy, glycosylated hemoglobin declines during the first and second trimesters, returning to baseline levels at term. To convert the hemoglobin A_{1c} level to the mean glucose level, one can use the "rule of 8s." A hemoglobin A_{1c} level of 8% reflects a mean glucose level of 180 mg/dL in most laboratories. Each change of 1% in the hemoglobin A_{1c} value indicates a change of 30 mg/dL in mean glucose. There is a direct correlation between maternal third trimester hemoglobin A_{1c} levels and increased birthweight [9]. Hemoglobin A_{1c} should be checked every trimester.

The insulin requirement postpartum decreases dramatically (usually by 50%). Type 1 diabetics are at increased risk for postpartum thyroiditis. Therefore a high index of suspicion should be maintained.

Management during pregnancy

During the second trimester, a careful search for the presence of fetal malformations is performed by obtaining a maternal serum alpha-fetoprotein level at 16 weeks, a targeted ultrasound at 18 weeks, and fetal echocardiography at 20 weeks [10]. In addition, the rate of uterine growth, development of early signs of preeclampsia, and incidence of infection of the urinary tract or other sites are closely monitored.

By accurately assessing fetal health and maturity, clinicians can prevent intrauterine deaths while safely prolonging pregnancy to avoid the hazards of iatrogenic prematurity. Antepartum heart rate testing using the nonstress test (NST) twice weekly has proved to be a reliable index of fetal well-being in a metabolically stable patient [11]. Daily maternal assessment of fetal activity is a valuable screening test.

At 28 weeks, daily maternal assessment of fetal activity is begun. Twice weekly NSTs are ordered at 32 weeks, or earlier if there are other maternal or fetal complications (e.g., hypertension, growth restriction) [12]. A nonreactive NST must be followed by a biophysical profile or contraction stress test. Timing of delivery should be individualized and depends on glycemic control, presence of associated maternal complications, and fetal status [13]. The goal is to achieve at least 38 weeks' gestation as long as these tests of fetal well-being are reassuring. If, at 38 weeks, the cervix is favorable, there is no macrosomia, phosphatidylglycerol is present, and the presenting part is cephalic, labor is induced. If the cervix is unfavorable and the fetus is not macrosomic, it appears reasonable to wait as long as fetal activity is normal and antepartum heart rate testing is reassuring.

Finally, in order to avoid birth injury from fetal macrosomia, a liberal attitude toward cesarean section (CS) should be employed in such cases. Sonographic assessment of estimated fetal weight and growth of the abdominal circumference are of value in detecting fetal macrosomia. If the estimated fetal weight exceeds 4500 g, delivery by elective CS should be considered at approximately 38 weeks after presence of amniotic fluid phosphatidylglycerol is documented [14]. Ideally, the pregnant diabetic patients should not go beyond 40 weeks' gestation.

Case presentation

A 30-year-old gravida 4, para 3 was first seen at 18 weeks' gestation. Her past obstetric history included the vaginal delivery of a 4100-g baby boy, who suffered a fractured humerus in the process. The patient's mother had diabetes mellitus. Plasma glucose was obtained 1 hour after a 50-g oral glucose load and was found to be 175 mg/dL. A 3-hour oral glucose tolerance test (OGTT) was then ordered. The results were as follows: fasting, 110 mg/dL; 1 hour, 243 mg/dL; 2 hours, 176 mg/dL; and 3 hours, 154 mg/dL. Pregestational diabetes was suspected.

The patient was started on a 2200-calorie diet with strict avoidance of concentrated sweets. Fasting and postprandial capillary glucose determinations were obtained daily. The fasting values ranged from 100 to 110 mg/dL, so she was started on split-dose insulin. Fetal growth was normal, and the patient remained normotensive. Antepartum fetal evaluation was initiated with twice weekly nonstress testing initiated at 32 weeks. Her glucose levels remained within the acceptable range. At 40 weeks, the estimated fetal weight was 4600 g. A cesarean section was performed. A 2-hour OGTT performed at 6 weeks postpartum confirmed diabetes.

References

1 Kitzmiller JL, Buchanan TA, Kjos S, *et al*. Preconception care of diabetes, congenital malformations, and spontaneous abortions. *Diabetes Care* 1996;**19**:514–41.

2 Greene MF, Hare JW, Cloherty JP, Benacerraf BR, Soeldner JS. First-trimester hemoglobin A1 and risk for major malformation and spontaneous abortion in diabetic pregnancy. *Teratology* 2002;**65**:97–101.

3 Korenbrot CC, Steinberg A, Bender C, Newberry S. Preconception care: a systematic review. *Matern Child Health J* 2002;**6**:75–88.

4 American Diabetes Association. Preconception care of women with diabetes. *Diabetes Care* 2004;**27**(Suppl 1):S76–8.

5 Expert Committee on the Diagnosis and Classification of Diabetes Mellitus. American Diabetes Association. Report of the Expert

Committee on the Diagnosis and Classification of Diabetes Mellitus. *Diabetes Care*, 2003;**26**(Suppl 1):January.

6 ACOG. *Pregestational Diabetes Mellitus*. ACOG Practice Bulletin 60, March 2005.

7 Siebenhofer A, Plank J, Berghold A, *et al*. Short acting insulin analogues versus regular human insulin in patients with diabetes mellitus. Cochrane Metabolic and Endocrine Disorders Group. *Cochrane Database Syst Rev* 2006;**2**:CD003287.

8 Hughes RC, Rowen JA. Pregnancy in women with Type 2 diabetes: who takes metformin and what is the outcome? *Diabet Med* 2006;**23**:318–22.

9 Widness JA, Schwartz HC, Thompson D, *et al*. Glycohemoglobin (HbA$_{1c}$): a predictor of birth weight in infants of diabetic mothers. *J Pediatr* 1978;**92**:8.

10 Albert TJ, Landon MB, Wheller JJ, *et al*. Prenatal detection of fetal anomalies in pregnancies complicated by insulin-dependent diabetes mellitus. *Am J Obstet Gynecol* 1996;**174**: 1424–8.

11 Landon MB, Langer O, Gabbe SG, *et al*. Fetal surveillance in pregnancies complicated by insulin-dependent diabetes mellitus. *Am J Obstet Gynecol* 1992;**167**:617–21.

12 Gabbe SG, Graves CR. Management of diabetes mellitus complicating pregnancy. *Obstet Gynecol* 2003;**102**: 857–68.

13 Boulvain M, Stan C, Irion O. Elective delivery in diabetic pregnant women. Cochrane Pregnancy and Childbirth Group. *Cochrane Database Syst Rev* 2006;2:CD000451.

14 ACOG. *Macrosomia*. ACOG Practice Bulletin 22, November 2000.

Maternal hypothyroidism and hyperthyroidism

Brian Casey

Hypothyroidism

Overview

Hypothyroidism complicates 1–3 in 1000 pregnancies. Women with overt hypothyroidism are at an increased risk for complications such as early pregnancy failure, preeclampsia, placental abruption, low birthweight, and stillbirth [1,2]. Treatment of women with hypothyroidism has been associated with improved pregnancy outcomes. *Subclinical hypothyroidism* affects 2–3% of pregnant women [3,4], and has recently been implicated in impaired neurologic development in offspring [5], as well as an increase in pregnancy complications such as preterm birth and fetal death [4,6]. However, there have been no randomized clinical trials confirming the efficacy of early pregnancy treatment and/or screening for subclinical hypothyroidism and this topic remains an area of controversy.

The most common cause of primary hypothyroidism in pregnancy is chronic autoimmune thyroiditis (Hashimoto thyroiditis). This is a painless inflammation with progressive enlargement of the thyroid gland which is characterized by diffuse lymphocytic infiltration, fibrosis, parenchymal atrophy, and eosinophilic change. Other important causes of primary hypothyroidism include endemic iodine deficiency and a history of either ablative radioiodine therapy or thyroidectomy. Secondary hypothyroidism is pituitary in origin. For example, Sheehan syndrome resulting from prior obstetric hemorrhage is characterized by pituitary ischemia and necrosis, with subsequent deficiencies in some or all pituitary responsive hormones. Other etiologies of secondary hypothyroidism include lymphocytic hypophysitis and a history of a hypophysectomy. Tertiary or hypothalamic hypothyroidism is very rare.

Presentation

Clinical hypothyroidism is often characterized by vague, nonspecific signs or symptoms which are insidious in onset. Initial symptoms include fatigue, constipation, cold intolerance, and muscle cramps. These may progress to insomnia, weight gain, carpal tunnel syndrome, hair loss, voice changes, and intellectual slowness. The presence of an enlarged thyroid gland is dependent upon the etiology of hypothyroidism. Specifically, women in areas of endemic iodine deficiency and those with Hashimoto thyroiditis are much more likely to have a goiter. Other signs of hypothyroidism include periorbital edema, dry skin, and prolonged relaxation phase of deep tendon reflexes. The diagnosis of clinical hypothyroidism during pregnancy is especially difficult because many of the signs or symptoms listed above may be attributed to the pregnancy itself. For example, pregnancy is accompanied by moderate enlargement of the thyroid gland from hyperplasia of glandular tissue and increased vascularity. By definition, *subclinical hypothyroidism* occurs in asymptomatic women whose thyroid-stimulating hormone (TSH) concentration is above the statistically defined upper limit of normal while their serum free thyroxine (fT_4) concentration is within its reference range [3].

Diagnosis

The diagnosis of hypothyroidism is generally established by an elevated serum TSH and a low serum fT_4. If the free thyroxine concentration is low in the presence of a normal or depressed TSH, then pituitary (central) hypothyroidism should be suspected. The nonpregnancy reference ranges for serum TSH and fT_4 concentration are 0.4–4.5 mIU/L and 0.7–1.8 ng/dL, respectively. During pregnancy, maternal serum chorionic gonadotropin (hCG) peaks at approximately 10 weeks' gestation and has some thyroid stimulating activity as a result of its structural homology with TSH. This results in a decrease in the maternal serum TSH and a modest increase in fT_4 during the first trimester [7]. These physiologic changes confound the laboratory diagnosis of hypothyroidism during pregnancy and underscore the need for gestational age-specific TSH and possibly fT_4 thresholds. Such TSH thresholds have been established from a large population-based screening study of pregnant women in Dallas (Table 22.1) [8]. From these data, the upper limit of the statistically defined normal range for TSH (97.5th percentile) in the first half of pregnancy

Table 22.1 Thyroid-stimulating hormone (TSH) value thresholds according to gestational age. Reprinted with permission from Dashe JS, Casey BM, Wells CE, McIntire DD, Byrd W, Leveno KJ, Cunningham FG. Thyroid-stimulating hormone in singleton and twin pregnancy: importance of gestational age-specific reference ranges. *Obstet Gynecol* 2005;**106**:753–7. Lippincott Williams & Wilkins [8].

Gestational age (weeks)	*n*	2.5th percentile	50th percentile	97.5th percentile
6	368	0.23	1.36	4.94
7	742	0.14	1.21	5.09
8	936	0.09	1.01	4.93
9	1037	0.03	0.84	4.04
10	982	0.02	0.74	3.12
11	888	0.01	0.76	3.65
12	754	0.01	0.79	3.32
13	684	0.01	0.78	4.05
14	606	0.01	0.85	3.33
15	559	0.02	0.92	3.40
16	456	0.04	0.92	2.74
17	398	0.02	0.98	3.32
18	352	0.17	1.07	3.48
19	318	0.22	1.07	3.03
20	327	0.25	1.11	3.20
21	317	0.28	1.21	3.04
22	298	0.26	1.15	4.09
23	285	0.25	1.08	3.02
24	261	0.34	1.13	2.99
25	261	0.30	1.11	2.82
26	237	0.20	1.07	2.89
27	223	0.36	1.11	2.84
28	218	0.30	1.03	2.78
29	188	0.31	1.07	3.14
30	188	0.20	1.07	3.27
31	172	0.23	1.06	2.81
32	170	0.31	1.07	2.98
33	152	0.31	1.20	5.25
34	152	0.20	1.18	3.18
35	160	0.30	1.20	3.41
36	144	0.33	1.31	4.59
37	147	0.37	1.35	6.40
38	141	0.23	1.16	4.33
39	166	0.57	1.59	5.14
≥40	312	0.38	1.68	5.43

was 3.0 mU/L. Moreover, if population-specific medians for TSH were determined for each trimester, these data indicate that the upper limit of TSH during the first trimester should be 4.0 multiples of the median (MoM) for singleton gestations and 3.5 MoM for twins. The upper limit for TSH in the second and third trimesters for both singleton and twin gestations should be 2.5 MoM [8]. Similar gestational age-specific fT_4 thresholds have not been established and use of nonpregnant fT_4 thresholds for diagnosis of thyroid dysfunction is acceptable. Even though pregnancy is associated with significant shifts in free thyroxine, overall, fT_4 levels remain within the nonpregnancy reference range [7]. Finally, it may be helpful to confirm the presence of either antimicrosomal or antithyroglobulin antibodies in cases where autoimmune thyroiditis is suspected. Specifically, the presence of antithyroid antibodies may identify a population of women at a particular risk for pregnancy complications or progression to symptomatic disease. For example, in one recent study, more than 47% of women who tested positive for thyroid peroxidase antibodies early in pregnancy developed postpartum thyroid dysfunction [9].

Management and treatment

The goal of treatment for pregnant women with overt hypothyroidism is clinical and biochemical euthyroidism. Levothyroxine sodium is the treatment of choice for routine management of hypothyroidism. Starting doses usually range from 1.6 to 1.8 μg/kg/day. Serum TSH is then measured at 6 week intervals and thyroxine is adjusted by 25- to 50-μg increments. Women who have hypothyroidism at the time of conception should have a serum TSH evaluated at their first prenatal visit. An increased requirement for thyroid replacement in hypothyroid women during pregnancy has been demonstrated [10]. Because of the risks for early pregnancy failure and the potential for neurodevelopmental impairment in offspring, some have recommended that hypothyroid women increase levothyroxine dose by 30% when pregnancy is confirmed [10]. However, this practice has not been shown to be beneficial and thyroid treatment is probably best guided through evaluation of thyroid function studies. Therefore, it is recommended that serum TSH be measured at least each trimester during pregnancy. Notably, several drugs may interfere with levothyroxine absorption (e.g., cholestyramine, ferrous sulfate, aluminum hydroxide in antacids) or its metabolism (e.g., phenytoin, carbamazepine, and rifampin).

Treatment of women with *subclinical hypothyroidism* is controversial. A report has linked subclinical hypothyroidism during pregnancy with subsequent neurodevelopmental complications in offspring [5]. This has prompted several national organizations to recommend treatment of subclinical hypothyroidism to restore the TSH to the reference range [11]. Importantly, however, there are no published intervention trials assessing the safety or efficacy of screening and treatment to improve neuropsychologic performance in such offspring. Currently, routine screening and treatment of subclinical hypothyroidism during pregnancy is not recommended by the American College of Obstetricians and Gynecologists [12].

Follow-up

After completion of pregnancy, the levothyroxine dose should be restored to the prepregnancy value and a TSH should be checked 6–8 weeks postpartum. Breastfeeding is not contraindicated in women treated for hypothyroidism. Levothyroxine is excreted into breastmilk but levels are too low to alter thyroid function in the infant or to interfere with neonatal thyroid screening programs [13]. Periodic monitoring of hypothyroidism with an annual serum TSH concentration is advised because of the impact of changing weight and age on thyroid function. Women with *subclinical hypothyroidism*, particularly those with thyroid autoantibodies, are at an increased risk for developing clinical disease within 5 years. While treatment of these women is not recommended, yearly evaluation for the development of clinically apparent disease is recommended.

Hyperthyroidism

Overview

Hyperthyroidism complicates approximately 1–2 in 1000 pregnancies. The overwhelming cause of hyperthyroidism during pregnancy is Graves disease or autoimmune thyrotoxicosis. Pregnant women with hyperthyroidism are at increased risk for congestive heart failure, thyroid storm, preterm labor, preeclampsia, fetal growth restriction, and perinatal mortality. Treatment of hyperthyroid women to achieve adequate metabolic control will result in improved pregnancy outcomes. However, overtreatment may result in maternal or fetal hypothyroidism. *Gestational transient thyrotoxicosis* (GTT) is 10 times more prevalent than Graves disease and may be caused by the elevated hCG values typically observed with hyperemesis gravidarum. *Subclinical hyperthyroidism* effects 1.7% of pregnant women and has only recently been introduced into clinical practice because of the development of extremely sensitive serum TSH assays. Subclinical hyperthyroidism is not associated with any adverse maternal pregnancy outcomes [14]. Treatment of the latter two clinical entities has not been shown to be beneficial.

Graves disease is an organ-specific autoimmune process whereby thyroid-stimulating autoantibodies attach to and activate TSH receptors. Other less common causes include toxic multinodular goiter, subacute thyroiditis, adenoma, or iodine-induced thyrotoxicosis. Thyrotropin receptor activation by hCG, which has some cross-reactivity with TSH, explains the biochemical and occasional clinical findings of thyrotoxicosis in women with hyperemesis gravidarum and gestational trophoblastic decrease.

Presentation

As with hypothyroidism, clinical features of hyperthyroidism can be easily confused with physiologic symptoms of pregnancy. Suggestive complaints or findings include nervousness, heat intolerance, palpitations, goiter, failure to gain weight or weight loss, and exophthalmos. *GTT* usually occurs in women with hyperemesis gravidarum. *Subclinical hyperthyroidism* defined as a serum TSH concentration below the statistically defined lower limit of normal with a serum concentration of fT_4 within the reference range, is typically identified in asymptomatic women.

Diagnosis

In women with a depressed serum TSH level (<0.4 mIU/L), clinical hyperthyroidism is confirmed by an elevation in fT_4 (>1.8 ng/dL) concentration. As is true for the diagnosis of hypothyroidism, one must consider the impact of pregnancy on TSH and possibly fT_4 (Table 22.1). Rarely, hyperthyroidism is caused by abnormally high serum triiodothyronine values (T_3 *thyrotoxicosis*). In women with depressed TSH yet normal fT_4, evaluation of fT_3 or free T_3 index may explain a patient's hypermetabolic symptoms. Also, evaluation of TSH receptor antibodies may be helpful in evaluation of women with Graves disease to identify those at risk for delivery of an infant with fetal or neonatal hyperthyroidism.

Management and treatment

Thyrotoxicosis during pregnancy can nearly always be controlled by thioamide drugs and treatment has been associated with improved pregnancy outcomes [15,16]. Some clinicians prefer propylthiouracil because it inhibits peripheral conversion of T_4 to T_3 and it crosses the placenta less readily than methimazole. Methimazole used in early pregnancy has also been associated with esophageal and choanal atresia as well as aplasia cutis [17–20]. Transient leukopenia occurs in approximately 10% of women treated with thioamides, but this does not require cessation of therapy. In approximately 0.2%, agranulocytosis develops suddenly, is not dose related, and, because of its acute onset, serial leukocyte counts during therapy are not helpful. Rather, if fever or sore throat develops, patients should be instructed to discontinue medication immediately and report for a complete blood count.

The dose of propylthiouracil is empirical, and the American Thyroid Association recommends an initial daily dose of 100–600 mg for propylthiouracil or 10–40 mg for methimazole [21]. Women with overt hyperthyroidism diagnosed during pregnancy may require a higher initial dose between 300 and 450 mg/day. The starting daily dose of methimazole is

20–40 mg. The goal of therapy is clinical euthyroidism with free thyroxine in the upper range of normal. The median time to normalization of thyroid function tests is 6–8 weeks, but TSH levels may remain suppressed beyond normalization of fT_4. Once euthyroidism is achieved, serial measurement of TSH and fT_4 during each trimester is recommended.

There is currently no convincing evidence that *subclinical hyperthyroidism* should be treated in nonpregnant individuals [22]. In fact, it should be considered contraindicated during pregnancy because maternal antithyroid drugs cross the placenta and may cause fetal thyroid suppression. There are other alternatives for treatment of overt hyperthyroidism which are rarely undertaken during pregnancy. For example, although thyroidectomy is typically reserved for treatment outside of pregnancy, pregnant women who cannot adhere to medical therapy or in whom therapy is toxic may benefit from surgical management [23]. Ablative radioactive iodine is contraindicated in pregnancy as it can cause fetal thyroid destruction.

Thyroid storm

Thyroid storm or heart failure are rare and acute life-threatening exacerbations of thyrotoxicosis. Women with thyroid storm classically present with fever, tachycardia, nausea, diarrhea, dehydration, and delirium or coma. Treatment of thyrotoxic storm or heart failure is similar and should be carried out in an intensive care setting. Specific treatment consists of 1 g propylthiouracil (PTU) given orally or crushed and placed through a nasogastric tube. PTU is continued in 200-mg doses every 6 hours. An hour after initial PTU dosing, iodide is given to inhibit thyroid release of T_3 and T_4. It is given every 8 hours intravenously as 500–1000 mg sodium iodide; or it can be given orally as five drops of supersaturated solution of potassium iodide (SSKI) or as 10 drops of Lugol solution every 8 hours. With a history of iodine-induced anaphylaxis, lithium carbonate, 300 mg every 6 hours, is given instead. Dexamethasone can be used to further block peripheral conversion of T_4 to T_3 and may be given intravenously as 2 mg every 6 hours for a total of four doses. Beta-blocker therapy such as propranolol, labetalol, and esmolol to control tachycardia have all been used successfully intrapartum.

Follow-up

Women with Graves disease should be followed closely after delivery because recurrence or aggravation of symptoms is not uncommon in the first few months postpartum. Asymptomatic women should have a TSH and fT_4 performed approximately 6 weeks postpartum. Both PTU and methimazole are excreted in breastmilk; however, PTU less so than methimazole. PTU is largely protein bound and does not seem to pose a significant risk to the breastfed infant. Methimazole has been found in breastfed infants of treated women in amounts sufficient to cause thyroid dysfunction; however, at low doses

(10–20 mg/day) methimazole does not appear to pose a major risk to the nursing infant [24]. The American Academy of Pediatricians considers both compatible with breastfeeding [25].

Postpartum thyroiditis

Transient autoimmune thyroiditis has been identified in up to 10% of women during the first year after childbirth [26,27]. The likelihood of developing postpartum thyroiditis antedates pregnancy and is related to increasing serum levels of thyroid autoantibodies. Women with high antibody titers in early pregnancy are most commonly affected [28]. In clinical practice, postpartum thyroiditis is infrequently diagnosed because it typically develops months after delivery and has vague and nonspecific symptoms. These include depression, carelessness, and memory impairment [29]. Risk factors other than antithyroid antibodies include previous thyroid dysfunction or a family history of thyroid or other autoimmune disease. For example, 25% of women with type 1 diabetes develop postpartum thyroid dysfunction [30].

There are two recognized clinical phases of postpartum thyroiditis. Between 1 and 4 months after delivery, approximately 4% of all women develop transient thyrotoxicosis from excessive release of hormone caused by glandular disruption [31]. The onset is abrupt, and a small, painless goiter is commonly found. Fatigue and palpitations are the most common complaints in women with early postpartum thyroiditis. Antithyroid medications such as thioamides are typically ineffective and approximately two-thirds of these women spontaneously return to a euthyroid state. Between 4 and 8 months postpartum, 2–5% of women develop hypothyroidism [26,32]. However, hypothyroidism can even develop within 1 month of the onset of thyroiditis. Thyromegaly and other symptoms are common and more prominent than during the thyrotoxic phase. Thyroxine replacement is recommended for at least 6–12 months. Importantly, women who experience either type of postpartum thyroiditis have an approximately 30% risk of developing permanent hypothyroidism [33,34].

Case presentation

A 32-year-old woman who was previously diagnosed with hypothyroidism and currently taking 100 μg levothyroxine presented for prenatal care at 12 weeks' gestation. At that time her TSH was 7.8 mU/L and her fT_4 was 0.54 ng/dL. Her levothyroxine dose was increased to 125 μg and thyroid function testing was planned for 4 weeks hence. Repeat thyroid studies were as follows: TSH 2.3 mU/L and fT_4 1.0 ng/dL. Normal ranges for TSH and fT_4 were 0.4–4.5 mU/L and 0.7–1.8 ng/dL, respectively. Further thyroid function testing was performed at 24 weeks' gestation (TSH 1.8 mU/L, and fT_4 1.1 ng/dL) and 32 weeks' gestation (TSH 2.2 mU/L and fT_4 0.9 ng/dL). No further change in therapy was prescribed.

During a routine prenatal care visit at 37 weeks' gestation she was found to have a blood pressure of 144/98 mmHg. Laboratory evaluation revealed an aspartate amino-transferase (AST) of 92 U/L, a platelet count of 236×10^3/L and 3+ proteinuria. A labor induction for severe preeclampsia with magnesium sulfate seizure prophylaxis was initiated. Hydralazine was given during the intrapartum period for severe hypertension. A cesarean delivery for fetal distress was performed. The infant weighed 3205 g and Apgar scores were 7 and 9 at 1 and 5 minutes, respectively. There was no evidence of placental abruption. The postpartum course was further complicated by a postpartum hemorrhage with a total estimated blood loss of 2000 mL for which the patient received a blood transfusion. Upon discharge, she was instructed regarding the safety of breastfeeding while taking levothyrox-ine and to resume taking 100 µg levothyroxine each day. Repeat thyroid function testing was scheduled for 6 weeks postpartum.

References

1 Davis LE, Leveno KJ, Cunningham FG. Hypothyroidism complicating pregnancy. *Obstet Gynecol* 1988;**72**:108.

2 Leung AS, Millar LK, Koonings PP, Montoro M, Mestman JH. Perinatal outcome in hypothyroid pregnancies. *Obstet Gynecol* 1993;**81**:349–53.

3 Surks MI, Ortiz E, Daniels GH, *et al.* Subclinical thyroid disease, scientific review and guidelines for diagnosis and management. *JAMA* 2004;**291**:228–38.

4 Casey BM, Dashe JS, Wells CE, *et al.* Pregnancy outcomes in women with subclinical thyroid insufficiency. *Obstet Gynecol* 2005;**105**:239–45.

5 Haddow JE, Palomaki GE, Allan WC, *et al.* Maternal thyroid deficiency during pregnancy and subsequent neuropsychological development of the child. *N Engl J Med* 1999;**341**:1549–55.

6 Allan WC, Haddow JE, Palomaki GE, *et al.* Maternal thyroid deficiency and pregnancy complications: implications for population screening. *J Med Screen* 2000;**7**:127–30.

7 Glinoer D, de Nayer P, Bourdoux P, *et al.* Regulation of maternal thyroid during pregnancy. *J Clin Endocrinol Metab* 1990;**71**: 276–87.

8 Dashe JS, Casey BM, Wells CE, *et al.* Thyroid-stimulating hormone in singleton and twin pregnancy: importance of gestational age-specific reference ranges. *Obstet Gynecol* 2005;**106**:753–7.

9 Lucas A, Pizarro E, Granada ML, *et al.* Postpartum thyroiditis: epidemiology and clinical evolution in a nonselected population. *Thyroid* 2000;**10**:71.

10 Premawardhana LD, Parkes AB, John R, Harris B, Lazarus JH. Thyroid peroxidase antibodies in early pregnancy: utility for prediction of postpartum thyroid dysfunction and implications for screening. *Thyroid* 2004;**14**:610–5.

11 Alexander EK, Marqusee E, Lawrence J, Jarolim P, Fischer GA, Larsen PR. Timing and magnitude of increases in levothyroxine requirements during pregnancy in women with hypothyroidism. *N Engl J Med* 2004;**351**:241–9.

12 Gharib H, Tuttle RM, Baskin HJ, Fish LH, Singer PA, McDermott MT. Consensus Statement No 1. Subclinical Thyroid Dysfunction: A joint statement on management from the American Association of Clinical Endocrinologists, the American Thyroid Association, and the Endocrine Society. *Thyroid* 2005;**15**:24–8.

13 American College of Obstetricians and Gynecologists. *Thyroid disease in pregnancy*. ACOG Practice Bulletin Number 37, August 2002.

14 Franklin R, O'Grady C, Carpenter L. Neonatal thyroid function: comparison between breast-fed and bottle-fed infants. *J Pediatr* 1985;**106**:124–6.

15 Casey BM, Dashe JS, Wells CE, McIntire DD, Leveno KJ, Cunningham FG. Subclinical hyperthyroidism and pregnancy outcomes. *Obstet Gynecol* 2006;**107**:337–41.

16 Davis LE, Lucas MJ, Hankins GD, Roark ML, Cunningham FG. Thyrotoxicosis complicating pregnancy. *Am J Obstet Gynecol* 1989;**160**:63–70.

17 Millar KJ, Wing DA, Leung AS, Koonings PP, Montoro MN, Mestman JH. Low birth weight and preeclampsia in pregnancies complicated by hyperthyroidism. *Obstet Gynecol* 1994;**84**:946–9.

18 Jansson R, Dahlberg PA, Karlsson FA. Postpartum thyroiditis. *Bailliere's Clin Endocrinol Metab* 1988;**2**:619–35.

19 Muller AF, Drexhage HA, Berghout A. Postpartum thyroiditis and autoimmune thyroiditis in women of childbearing age: recent insights and consequences for antenatal and postnatal care. *Endo Rev* 2001;**22**:605–30.

20 Premawardhana LD, Parkes AB, Ammari F, *et al.* Postpartum thyroiditis and long-term thyroid status: prognostic influence of thyroid peroxidase antibodies and ultrasound echogenicity. *J Clin Endocrinol Metab* 2000;**85**:71–5.

21 Milham S Jr, Elledge W. Maternal methimazole and congenital defects in children. *Teratology* 1972;**5**:125.

22 Clementi M, Di Gianantonio E, Pelo E, Manni I, Basile RT, Tenconi R. Methimazole embryopathy: delineation of the phenotype. *Am J Med Genet* 1999;**83**:43–6.

23 Di Gianantino E, Schaefer C, Mastroiacovo P, *et al.* Adverse effects of prenatal methimazole exposure. *Teratology* 2001;**64**:262–6.

24 Mandel S, Cooper D. The use of antithyroid drugs in pregnancy and lactation. *J Clin Endocrinol Metab* 2001;**86**:2354–9.

25 Singer PA, Cooper DS, Levy EG, *et al.* Treatment guidelines for patients with hyperthyroidism and hypothyroidism. *JAMA* 1995;**273**:808–12.

26 Woeber KA. Observations concerning the natural history of subclinical hyperthyroidism. *Thyroid* 2005;**15**:687–91.

27 Davison S, Lennard TWJ, Davison H, *et al.* Management of a pregnant patient with Graves' disease complicated by thionamide-induced neutropenia in the first trimester. *Clin Endocrinol* 2001;**54**:559.

28 Cooper DS. Antithyroid drugs: to breast-feed or not to breast-feed. *Am J Obstet Gynecol* 1987;**157**:234–5.

29 Committee on Drugs American Academy of Pediatricians. 2001;**108**:776–89.

30 Amino N, Tada H, Hidaka Y, Izumi Y. Postpartum autoimmune thyroid syndrome. *Endocr J* 2000;**47**:645–55.

31 Dayan CM, Daniels GH. Chronic autoimmune thyroiditis. *N Engl J Med* 1996;**335**:99–107.

32 Pearce EN, Farwell AP, Braverman LE. Thyroiditis. *N Engl J Med* 2003;**348**:2646–55.

33 Hayslip CC, Baker JR Jr, Wartofsky L, Klein TA, Opsahl MS. Burman KD. Natural killer cell activity and serum autoantibodies in women with postpartum thyroiditis. *J Clin Endocrinol Metab* 1988;**66**:1089–93.

34 Alvarez-Marfany M, Roman SH, Drexler AJ, Robertson C, Stagnaro-Green A. Long-term prospective study of postpartum thyroid dysfunction in women with insulin dependent diabetes mellitus. *J Clin Endocrinol Metab* 1994;**79**:10–6.

23 Asthma

Michael Schatz

Recent data suggest that asthma affects 4–8% of pregnant women [1], making it probably the most common, potentially serious, medical problem to complicate pregnancy. Moreover, the prevalence of asthma during pregnancy appears to be increasing [1]. Although data have been conflicting, the largest recent studies [2–4] have suggested that maternal asthma increases the risk of perinatal mortality, preeclampsia, preterm birth, and low birthweight infants. More severe asthma is associated with increased risks [3,5], while better controlled asthma is associated with decreased risks [6–9]. The course of asthma may also change during pregnancy; some women improve while others worsen [10]. This chapter reviews the definition and diagnosis of asthma and the interrelationships between asthma and pregnancy as a prelude to discussing the management of asthma in pregnant women.

Definition of asthma

Asthma is an inflammatory disease of the airways that is associated with reversible airway obstruction and airway hyperreactivity to a variety of stimuli. Although the cause of asthma is unknown, a number of clinical triggering factors exist, including viral infections, allergens, exercise, sinusitis, reflux, weather changes, and stress.

Airway obstruction in asthma can be produced by varying degrees of mucosal edema, bronchoconstriction, mucus plugging, and airway remodeling. In acute asthma, these changes can lead to ventilation–perfusion imbalance and hypoxia. Although early acute asthma is typically associated with hyperventilation and hypocapnea, progressive acute asthma can cause respiratory failure with associated carbon dioxide retention and acidosis.

Effect of pregnancy on the course of asthma

Clinical observations

A contemporary meta-analysis of 14 studies evaluating the effect of pregnancy on the course of asthma which included 1658 patients came to the conclusion that asthma severity improves in one-third of women, worsens in one-third of women, and remains unchanged in one-third of women [10]. However, a more recent and critical review of the literature found only three studies of 54 women that were prospective, enrolled women before the third trimester, and assessed their patients with objective measures of asthma severity or validated severity scales [11]. Asthma appears to be more likely to worsen during pregnancy in women with more severe asthma before becoming pregnant [12].

The course of asthma may vary by stage of pregnancy. The first trimester is generally well-tolerated in asthmatics, with infrequent acute episodes [12–14]. Increased symptoms and more frequent exacerbations have been reported to occur between weeks 17 and 36 of gestation [12–14]. In contrast, asthmatic women in general tend to experience fewer symptoms and less frequent asthma exacerbations during weeks 37–40 of pregnancy than during any earlier 4-week gestational period [13,14]. These studies suggest that the first trimester and the last month of pregnancy are relatively free of asthma exacerbations and that the second and earlier third trimester have more potential for increased asthma symptoms.

The variable effect of pregnancy on the course of asthma appears to be more than just random fluctuation in the natural history of the disease, because pregnancy-associated changes revert toward the prepregnancy state by 3 months postpartum [13]. It is also of interest that the course of asthma is often consistent in an individual woman during successive pregnancies [13,15].

Mechanisms

The mechanisms responsible for the altered clinical course of asthma during pregnancy are unknown and represent a fertile area for additional research. There are multiple biochemical and physiologic changes during pregnancy that could potentially ameliorate or exacerbate gestational asthma [16]. However, it is not clear which, if any, of these factors are actually important in determining the course of asthma during pregnancy.

There are additional factors that may contribute to the clinical course of asthma during pregnancy. Pregnancy may be a source of stress for many women, and this stress can aggravate asthma. Adherence to therapy can change during pregnancy with a corresponding change in asthma control. Most commonly observed is decreased adherence as a result of a mother's concerns about the safety of medications for the fetus.

Physician reluctance to treat may also affect the severity of asthma during pregnancy. A recent surveillance study identified 51 pregnant women and 500 nonpregnant women presenting to the emergency department with acute asthma [17]. Although asthma severity appeared to be similar in the two groups based on peak flow rates, pregnant women were significantly less likely to be treated with systemic steroids in the emergency department (44% vs. 66%) and significantly less likely to be discharged on oral steroids (38% vs. 64%). Presumably related to this undertreatment, pregnant women were three times more likely than nonpregnant women to report an ongoing exacerbation 2 weeks later ($P=0.02$).

Infections during pregnancy can certainly affect the course of gestational asthma. Some degree of decrease in cell-mediated immunity may make the pregnant patient more susceptible to viral infections, and upper respiratory tract infections have been reported to be the most common precipitants of severe asthma during pregnancy [15]. Sinusitis, a known asthma trigger, has been shown to be six times more common in pregnant compared with nonpregnant women [18]. In addition, pneumonia has been reported to be greater than five times more common in asthmatic than nonasthmatic women during pregnancy [19].

Finally, changes in specific immunoglobulin E (IgE) or environmental exposure may influence the gestational asthma course. Most pregnant asthmatic patients are atopic. A positive correlation between levels of specific IgE against cockroach antigen and gestational asthma severity was recently described in pregnant inner city women [20].

Effect of asthma on pregnancy

Clinical observations

Controlled studies that have evaluated outcomes of pregnancy in asthmatic compared with nonasthmatic women have been comprehensively reviewed [21]. The largest single study [3] described the outcomes of pregnancy in 36,985 women identified as having asthma in either the Swedish Medical Birth Registry and/or the Swedish Hospital Discharge Registry. These outcomes were compared with the total of 1.32 million births that occurred in the Swedish population during the years of the study (1984–95). Significantly increased rates of preeclampsia (odds ratio [OR] 1.15), perinatal mortality (OR 1.21), preterm births (OR 1.15), and low birthweight infants (OR 1.21), but not congenital malformations (OR 1.05), were found in the pregnancies of asthmatic versus control women. The risks appeared to be greater in patients with more severe asthma. In contrast to older studies and database studies, more recent prospective cohort studies [22–24] have not generally reported increased risks of perinatal complications in the pregnancies of women with asthma, suggesting either a previous ascertainment bias or that prospective asthma management may reduce perinatal risks. In addition to fetal morbidity and mortality, severe asthma during pregnancy may be a cause of maternal mortality [25].

Mechanisms

Definition of the mechanism(s) of maternal asthma's adverse effect on pregnancy outcomes reported in some studies should allow institution of optimal intervention strategy. Mechanisms postulated to explain these increased perinatal risks have included:

1 Hypoxia and other physiologic consequences of poorly controlled asthma;

2 Medications used to treat asthma; and

3 Demographic or pathogenic factors *associated with* asthma but not actually caused by the disease or its treatment.

The latter would imply that asthma and adverse perinatal outcomes may share the same underlying pathogenetic mechanism (such as a predisposition to inflammation) or demographic associations (such as smoking), but that inadequately controlled asthma or asthma treatment is not causally related to the adverse perinatal outcome [25]. Data supporting specific mechanisms for the most common specific adverse outcomes have been recently reviewed [21,25]. The published data do not fully define the mechanism(s) of maternal asthma's potential adverse effects on pregnancy and the infant reported in some studies. Available information, however, suggests that inadequate asthma control, as defined by symptoms [26,27], pulmonary function [8,9], or acute exacerbations [6,7], may be the most remedial factor and supports the important generalization that adequate asthma control during pregnancy is important in improving maternal–fetal outcome. Oral corticosteroids have also been associated with increased risks of preeclampsia [28,29] and prematurity [5,26,30] in pregnant asthmatic women. However, whether this represents a drug effect, an effect of inadequately controlled asthma, or a marker for common pathogenesis factors associated with more severe asthma is not clear from the data.

Diagnosis of asthma during pregnancy

Many patients with asthma during pregnancy will already have a physician diagnosis of asthma. A new diagnosis of asthma is usually suspected on the basis of typical symptoms—wheezing, chest tightness, cough, and associated shortness of breath—which tend to be episodic or at least fluctuating in intensity and are typically worse at night. Identification of the characteristic triggers described above further supports the diagnosis. Wheezing may be present on auscultation of the lungs, but the absence of wheezing on auscultation does not exclude the diagnosis. The diagnosis is ideally confirmed by spirometry which shows a reduced forced expiratory volume in 1 second (FEV_1; <80% predicted) with an increase in FEV_1 of 12% or more after an inhaled short-acting bronchodilator.

It is sometimes difficult to demonstrate reversible airway obstruction in patients with mild or intermittent asthma. Although methacholine challenge testing may be considered in nonpregnant patients with normal pulmonary function to confirm asthma, such testing is not recommended during pregnancy. Thus, therapeutic trials of asthma therapy should generally be used during pregnancy in patients with possible but unconfirmed asthma. Improvement with asthma therapy supports the diagnosis, which can then be confirmed postpartum with additional testing if necessary.

The most common differential diagnosis is dyspnea of pregnancy, which may occur in early pregnancy in approximately 70% of women. This dyspnea is differentiated from asthma by its lack of association with cough, wheezing, or airway obstruction.

Management

The National Asthma Education and Prevention Program (NAEPP) first published guidelines on the management of asthma during pregnancy in 1993 [31], and an update on pharmacologic treatment was published in 2005 [32]. The guidelines describe the management of asthma during pregnancy in four categories:
1 Assessment and monitoring;
2 Control of factors contributing to severity;
3 Patient education; and
4 Pharmacologic therapy.

Assessment and monitoring

Once the diagnosis of asthma is considered confirmed, the next step is assessment of severity (in patients not already on controller medications) or assessment of control (in patients already on controller medications). Severity is assessed in untreated patients based on the frequency of daytime and night-time symptoms and pulmonary function (ideally spirometry, minimally peak flow rate) (Table 23.1). Based on this severity assessment, controller therapy is initiated (if indicated).

In treated patients (either initially or with follow-up), it is important to determine whether their asthma is controlled. At a minimum this entails achievement of mild intermittent symptom and pulmonary function status: daytime symptoms no more than 2 days per week, interference with sleep no more than 2 days per month, and pulmonary function >80% predicted. In addition, well-controlled asthma includes no limitation of activity, including exercise, and no acute exacerbations [31].

Patients with persistent asthma should be monitored monthly for asthma control. This is in part because, as described above, the course of asthma changes in approximately two-thirds of women during pregnancy. Home peak flow monitoring should be considered for patients with moderate to severe asthma, especially for those who have difficulty perceiving signs of worsening asthma.

Because asthma has been associated with intrauterine growth restriction and preterm birth in some studies, pregnancy dating should be established accurately by first trimester ultrasound where possible [32]. All patients should be instructed to be attentive to fetal activity. The intensity of antenatal testing of fetal well-being should be considered on the basis of the severity and control of the asthma as well as other high-risk features of the pregnancy that may be present [32]. Evaluation of fetal activity and growth by serial ultrasounds should be considered for women:
1 Who have suboptimally controlled asthma;
2 With moderate to severe asthma (starting at 32 weeks); or
3 Who are recovering from a severe asthma exacerbation [32].

Control of factors contributing to asthma severity

Identifying and avoiding asthma triggers can lead to improved maternal well-being with less need for medications. In previously untested patients, *in vitro* tests (RAST, ELISA) should be performed to identify relevant allergens, such as mite, animal dander, mold, and cockroach, for which specific environmental control instructions can be given. Smokers must be encouraged to discontinue smoking, and all patients should try to avoid exposure to environmental tobacco smoke and other potential irritants as much as possible. Effective allergen immunotherapy can be continued during pregnancy, but risk–benefit considerations do not generally favor beginning immunotherapy during pregnancy [31].

Sinusitis and reflux are relatively common comorbidities during pregnancy that may exacerbate asthma. A high index

Table 23.1 Stepwise approach for managing asthma during pregnancy in patients not on controllers [32].

Clinical Features Before Treatment			Medications Required to Maintain Long-Term Control
	Symptoms/Day	**PEFR or *FEV*₁**	
	Symptoms/Night		**Daily Medications**

Step 4 Severe persistent	Continual Frequent	≤60%	• Preferred treatment:
			  ○ High-dose inhaled corticosteroid
			    and
			  ○ Long-acting inhaled beta₂-agonist
			    and, if needed,
			  ○ Corticosteroid tablets or syrup long term (2 mg/kg/day, generally not to exceed 60 mg/day) (Make repeat attempts to reduce systemic corticosteroid and maintain control with high-dose inhaled corticosteroid)
			• Alternative treatment:
			  ○ High-dose inhaled corticosteroid
			    and
			  ○ Sustained release theophylline to serum concentration of 5–12 µg/mL

Step 3 Moderate persistent	Daily >1 night/week	>60–<80%	• Preferred treatment:
			  either
			  ○ Low-dose inhaled corticosteroid and long-acting beta₂-agonist
			    or
			  ○ Medium-dose inhaled corticosteroid
			  If needed (particularly in patients with recurring severe exacerbations):
			  ○ Medium-dose inhaled corticosteroid and long acting inhaled beta₂-agonist
			• Alternative treatment:
			  ○ Low-dose inhaled corticosteroid and either theophylline or leukotriene receptor antagonist.
			  If needed:
			  ○ Medium-dose inhaled corticosteroid and either theophylline or leukotriene receptor antagonist

Step 2 Mild persistent	>2 days/week but <daily >2 nights/month	>80%	• Preferred treatment: ○ Low-dose inhaled corticosteroid • Alternative treatment (listed alphabetically): cromolym, leukotriene receptor antagonist *or* sustained-release theophylline to serum concentration of 5–12 µg/mL
Step 1 Mild intermittent	≤2 days/week ≤2 nights/month	≥80%	• No daily medication needed • Severe exacerbations may occur, separated by long periods of normal lung function and no symptoms. A course of systemic corticosteroid is recommended

*FEV*₁, forced expiratory volume in 1 second; PEFR, peak expiratory flow rate.

of suspicion should be maintained for sinusitis, for which symptoms and signs during pregnancy may be subtle [18]. Although reflux is common during pregnancy and may not require pharmacologic treatment, reflux treatment should be considered in patients with difficult to control asthma during pregnancy or those with very symptomatic reflux symptoms.

Patient education

Pregnant women should have access to information about asthma in general as well as regarding the interrelationships between asthma and pregnancy. Controlling asthma during pregnancy is important for the well-being of the fetus as well as for the mother's well-being, and the pregnant woman must understand that it is safer to be treated with asthma medications than it is to have uncontrolled symptoms, reduced pulmonary function, or exacerbations. She should also understand how she can reduce her exposure to or otherwise control the asthma triggers that contribute to her asthma severity.

The pregnant woman should be instructed regarding optimal inhaler technique, and she should be asked to demonstrate this technique to assure its correctness. The pregnant patient must be able to recognize symptoms of worsening asthma and know what to do about them. She should be given an individualized action plan that defines:

1 Maintenance medication;

2 Symptoms (and possibly peak flow levels) that indicate exacerbations;

3 Rescue therapy and increases in maintenance medications in response to her level of exacerbation; and

4 How and when to contact her asthma clinician for uncontrolled symptoms.

Pharmacologic therapy

Asthma medicines are classified into two types: relievers and long-term controllers. Relievers provide quick relief of bronchospasm and include short-acting beta-agonists (albuterol is preferred during pregnancy, 2–4 puffs every 3–4 hours when required) and the anticholinergic bronchodilator ipratropium (generally used as second-line therapy for acute asthma—see below). Long-term control medications are described in Table 23.2. Inhaled corticosteroids (Table 23.3) are the most effective controller asthma medications.

Chronic asthma

Patients with intermittent asthma do not need controller therapy. In patients with persistent asthma not already on controller therapy, it should be initiated as shown in Table 23.1. Controller therapy should be progressed in steps (Table 23.4) until adequate control is achieved, as defined above. Once control is achieved and sustained for several months, a step down to less intensive therapy is encouraged for nonpregnant patients to identify the minimum therapy necessary to maintain control. Although a similar step-down approach can be considered for pregnant patients, stepping down in therapy should be undertaken cautiously and gradually to avoid compromising the patient's asthma control [32]. For some patients it may be prudent to postpone attempts to reduce therapy that

Table 23.2 Long-term control medications for asthma during pregnancy (after [32]).

Medication	Dosage Form	Adult Dose	Use During Pregnancy
Inhaled corticosteroids	See Table 23.3		First-line controller therapy
Systemic corticosteroids		Short course "burst" to achieve	Burst therapy for severe
Methylprednisolone	2,4,8,16,32 mg tablets	control: 40–60 mg/day as	acute symptoms
Prednisolone	5 mg tablets, 5 mg/mL, 15 mg/mL	single or divided doses for	Maintenance therapy for
Prednisone	1, 2.5, 5, 10, 20, 50 mg tablet	3–10 days	severe asthma
	5 mg/mL, 5 mg/5 mL	7.5–60 mg/day in a single dose	uncontrolled by other
		in AM or q.o.d., taper to	means
		lowest effective dose	
Long-acting beta-agonists			Add-on therapy in patients
Salmeterol	DPI 50 µg/blister	1 blister q 12 hours	not controlled by low–
Formoterol	DPI 12 µg/single-use capsule	1 capsule q 12 hours	medium-dose inhaled
			corticosteroids
Cromolyn	MDI 1 mg/puff	2–4 puffs t.i.d.–q.i.d.	Alternative therapy for mild
	Nebulizer 20 mg/ampule	1 ampule t.i.d.–q.i.d.	persistent asthma
Leukotriene receptor anagonists			Alternative therapy for persistent asthma in
Montelukast	10 mg tablets	10 mg q HS	patients who have shown
Zafirlukast	10 or 20 mg tablets	20 mg b.i.d.	good response prior to pregnancy
Theophylline	Liquids, sustained-release tablets, and capsules	400–800 mg/day to achieve serum concentration of 5–12 µg/mL	Alternative therapy for persistent asthma during pregnancy

Table 23.3 Estimated comparative daily adult dosages for inhaled corticosteroids [32].

Drug	Low Daily Dose (µg)	Medium Daily Dose (µg)	High Daily Dose (µg)
Beclomethasone HFA 40 or 80 µg/puff	80–240	240–480	>480
Budesonide DPI 200 µg/inhalation	200–600	600–1200	>1200
Flunisolide 250 µg/puff	500–1000	1000–2000	>2000
Fluticasone			
MDI: 44, 110, 250 µg/puff	88–264	264–660	>660
DPI*: 50,100,or 250 µg/inhalation	100–300	300–600	>600
Triamcinolone acetonide 100 µg/puff	400–1000	1000–2000	>2000

* Also available combined with salmeterol (50 µg/inhalation) at 100, 250, or 500 µg/inhalation.

Table 23.4 National Asthma Education and Prevention Program (NAEPP) recommendations for preferred step therapy for persistent asthma during pregnancy [32].

STEP ONE
Low-dose inhaled corticosteroids*

STEP TWO
Medium-dose inhaled corticosteroids*
or
Low-dose inhaled corticosteroids*
+ Long-acting beta-agonist[†]

STEP THREE
Medium-dose inhaled corticosteroids*
+ Long-acting beta-agonist[†]

STEP FOUR
High-dose inhaled corticosteroids*
+ Long-acting beta-agonist[†]

STEP FIVE
High-dose inhaled corticosteroids*
+ Long-acting beta-agonist[†]
+ Oral corticosteroids at lowest effective dose

* Budesonide is the preferred inhaled corticosteroid during pregnancy because of availability of more reassuring human gestational safety data.
[†] Salmeterol is the preferred long-acting beta-agonist during pregnancy because of longer availability in the USA.

is effectively controlling the woman's asthma until after the infant's birth [32].

Inhaled corticosteroids are the mainstay of controller therapy during pregnancy. Because it has the most published reassuring human gestational safety data, budesonide is considered the preferred inhaled corticosteroid for asthma during pregnancy. It is important to note that no data indicate that the other inhaled corticosteroid preparations are unsafe. Therefore, inhaled corticosteroids other than budesonide may be continued in patients who were well-controlled by these agents prior to pregnancy, especially if it is thought that changing formulations may jeopardize asthma control. Based

on longer duration of availability in the USA, salmeterol is considered the long-acting beta-agonist of choice during pregnancy. As described in Table 23.2, the following drugs are considered by the NAEPP to be alternative, but not preferred, treatments for persistent asthma during pregnancy: cromolyn, because of decreased efficacy compared with inhaled corticosteroids; theophylline, primarily because of increased side-effects compared with alternatives; and leukotriene receptor antagonists, because of the availability of minimal published human gestational data for these drugs. Although oral corticosteroids have been associated with possible increased risks during pregnancy, such as oral clefts [33] and preeclampsia and prematurity as described above, if needed during pregnancy, they should be used because these risks are less than the potential risks of severe uncontrolled asthma, which include maternal mortality, fetal mortality, or both.

Acute asthma

A major goal of chronic asthma management is the prevention of acute asthmatic episodes. When increased asthma does not respond to home therapy, expeditious acute management is necessary for both the health of the mother and that of the fetus.

As a result of progesterone-induced hyperventilation, normal blood gases during pregnancy reveal a higher P_{O_2} (100–106 mmHg) and a lower P_{CO_2} (28–30 mmHg) than in the nonpregnant state. The changes in blood gases that occur secondary to acute asthma during pregnancy will be superimposed on the "normal" hyperventilation of pregnancy. Thus, a $P_{CO_2} > 35$ or a $P_{O_2} < 70$ associated with acute asthma will represent more severe compromise during pregnancy than will similar blood gases in the nongravid state.

The recommended pharmacologic therapy of acute asthma during pregnancy is summarized in Table 23.5 [32]. Intensive fetal monitoring as well as maternal monitoring is essential. In addition to pharmacologic therapy, supplemental oxygen (initially 3–4 L/min by nasal cannula) should be administered, adjusting F_{IO_2} to maintain at $P_{O_2} \geq 70$ and/or O_2

Table 23.5 National Asthma Education and Prevention Program (NAEPP) Recommendations for the pharmacologic management of acute asthma during pregnancy (after [32]).

1 *Initial therapy*

A FEV_1 or PEFR ≥ 5% predicted or personal best
   1 Short-acting inhaled beta$_2$-agonist by metered dose inhaler or nebulizer, up to three doses in first hour
   2 Oral systemic corticosteroid if not immediate response or if patient recently took oral systemic corticosteroid

B FEV_1 or PEFR < 50% predicted or personal best (severe exacerbation)
   1 High-dose short-acting inhaled beta$_2$-agonist by nebulization every 20 minutes or continuously for 1 hour plus inhaled ipratropium bromide
   2 Oral systemic corticosteroid

2 *Repeat assessment*

A Moderate exacerbation (FEV_1 or PEFR 50–80% predicted or personal best, moderate symptoms)
   1 Short-acting inhaled beta$_2$-agonist every 60 minutes
   2 Oral systemic corticosteroid (if not already given)
   3 Continue treatment 1–3 hours, provided there is improvement

B Severe (FEV_1 or PEFR < 50% predicted or personal best, severe symptoms at rest)
   1 Short-acting inhaled beta$_2$-agonist hourly or continuously plus inhaled ipratropium bromide
   2 Systemic corticosteroid (if not already given)

3 *Response and disposition*

A Good (FEV_1 or PEFR ≥ 70% predicted or personal best, no distress, response sustained 60 minutes after last treatment). Discharge home

B Incomplete (FEV_1 or PEFR ≥ 50% predicted or personal best but <70%, mild or moderate symptoms). Individualize decision regarding discharge home versus admit to hospital ward

C Poor (FEV_1 or PEFR < 50% predicted or personal best, Pco_2 > 42 mmHg, severe symptoms, drowsiness, confusion). Admit to hospital intensive care

FEV_1, forced expiratory volume in 1 second; PEFR, peak expiratory flow rate.

saturation by pulse oximetry >95%. Intravenous fluids (containing glucose if the patient is not hyperglycemic) should also be administered, initially at a rate of at least 100 mL/hour.

Systemic corticosteroids (approximately 1 mg/kg) are recommended for patients who do not respond well (FEV_1 or peak expiratory flow rate [PEFR] ≥70% predicted) to the first beta-agonist treatment as well as for patients who have recently taken systemic steroids and for those who present with severe exacerbations (FEV_1 or PEFR ≤50% predicted). Patients with good responses to emergency therapy (FEV_1 or PEFR ≥70% predicted) can be discharged home, generally on a course of oral corticosteroids. Inhaled corticosteroids should also be continued or initiated upon discharge until review at medical follow-up. Hospitalization should be considered for patients with an incomplete response (FEV_1 or PEFR ≥ 50% but <70% predicted). Admission to an intensive care unit should be considered for patients with persistent FEV_1 or PEFR < 50% predicted, Pco_2 > 42 or sensorium changes.

Management during labor and delivery

Asthma medications should be continued during labor and delivery. If systemic corticosteroids have been used in the previous 4 weeks, then stress-dose steroids (e.g., 100 mg hydrocortisone every 8 hours i.v.) should be administered during labor and for the 24-hour period after delivery to prevent maternal adrenal crisis [31].

Prostaglandin E_2 or E_1 can be used for cervical ripening, the management of spontaneous or induced abortions, or postpartum hemorrhage [32]. However, 15-methyl-PGF$_2$-alpha and methylergonovine can cause bronchospasm [32]. There is no contraindication to the use of oxytocin for postpartum hemorrhage [31]. Magnesium sulfate and beta-adrenergic agents, which are bronchodilators, can be used to treat preterm labor [32]. Indomethacin can induce bronchospasm in the aspirin-sensitive patient and thus must be avoided in such patients [32].

Epidural anesthesia has the additional benefit of reducing oxygen consumption and minute ventilation during labor [32]. If a general anesthetic is necessary, preanesthetic use of atropine and glycopyrrolate may provide bronchodilatation [31]. Ketamine is the agent of choice for induction of anesthesia because it decreases airway resistance and can prevent bronchospasm [31]. Low concentrations of halogenated anesthetics are recommended as inhalation anesthetic agents in pregnant asthmatic patients because they also cause bronchodilatation [31].

Conclusions

Asthma is a common medical problem during pregnancy. Optimal diagnosis and management of asthma during pregnancy should maximize maternal and fetal health.

Case presentation

The patient is a 23-year-old GII PI woman who is seen during her first trimester for asthma while she is pregnant. Her asthma was first diagnosed at age 15. She has not been hospitalized for asthma, but did require an emergency department visit for asthma 6 months previously. She was worse during her prior pregnancy 2 years ago. She is currently having daily asthma symptoms, nocturnal symptoms twice a week, and using her albuterol inhaler 3–4 times per day. She was given a steroid inhaler, but was afraid to use it while she was pregnant. She has noticed that cleaning the house triggers her asthma. She has had a cat at home for 1 year, has been worse over this time period, but does not think the cat affects her asthma. She has had some daily sneezing and nasal congestion since childhood, which she considers mild. She does not smoke cigarettes, has not been previously evaluated for allergies, and denies any other significant medical history.

Auscultation of the lungs was normal, and examination of the nose revealed mild mucosal edema. Spirometry showed an FEV_1 of 70% predicted. The diagnostic impression was moderate persistent asthma with a probable mite and dander allergy component and mild allergic rhinitis. The initial plan included education regarding asthma and pregnancy, an allergy evaluation (*in vitro* tests), environmental control instructions based on the testing, initiation of inhaled budesonide with instructions on inhaler technique, provision of a symptom-based home action plan, and scheduled follow-up in 1 month.

References

1 Kwon HL, Belanger K, Bracken MB. Asthma prevalence among pregnant and childbearing-aged women in the United States: estimates from national health surveys. *Ann Epidemiol* 2003;**13**:317–24.

2 Demissie K, Breckenridge MB, Rhoads GG. Infant and maternal outcomes in the pregnancies of asthmatic women. *Am J Respir Crit Care Med* 1998;**158**:1091–5.

3 Kallen B, Rydhstroem H, Aberg A. Asthma during pregnancy: a population based study. *Eur J Epidemiol* 2000;**16**:167–71.

4 Wen SW, Demissie K, Liu S. Adverse outcomes in pregnancies of asthmatic women: results from a Canadian population. *Ann Epidemiol* 2001;**11**:7–12.

5 Perlow JH, Montgomery D, Morgan MA, Towers CV, Porto M. Severity of asthma and perinatal outcome. *Am J Obstet Gynecol* 1992;**167**:963–7.

6 Greenberger, Patterson R. The outcome of pregnancy complicated by severe asthma. *Allergy Proc* 1988;**9**:539–43.

7 Jana N, Vasishta K, Saha SC, Khunnu B. Effect of bronchial asthma on the course of pregnancy, labour and perinatal outcome. *J Obstet Gynaecol* 1995;**21**:227–3.

8 Schatz, M, Zeiger RS, Hoffman CP, *et al*. Intrauterine growth is related to gestational pulmonary function in pregnant asthmatic women. *Chest* 1990;**98**:389–92.

9 Schatz M, Dombrowski MP, Wise R, *et al*. Spirometry is related to perinatal outcomes in pregnant asthmatic women. *Am J Obstet Gynceol* 2006;**194**:120.

10 Juniper EF, Newhouse MT. Effect of pregnancy on asthma: a systematic review and meta-analysis. In: Schatz M, Zeiger RS, Claman HN, (eds). *Asthma and Immunological Diseases in Pregnancy and Early Infancy*. New York: Marcel-Dekker, 1998: 401–27.

11 Kwon HL, Belanger K, Bracken MB. Effect of pregnancy and stage of pregnancy on asthma severity: a systematic review. *Am J Obstet Gynecol* 2004;**190**:1201–10.

12 Gluck JC, Gluck PA. The effects of pregnancy on asthma: a prospective study. *Ann Allergy* 1976;**37**:164–8.

13 Schatz M, Harden K, Forsythe A, *et al*. The course of asthma during pregnancy, post-partum, and with successive pregnancies: a prospective analysis. *J Allergy Clin Immunol* 1988;**81**:509–17.

14 Stenius-Aarniala BSM, Hedman J, Teramo KA. Acute asthma during pregnancy. *Thorax* 1996;**51**:411–4.

15 Williams DA. Asthma and pregnancy. *Acta Allergol* 1967;**22**:311–23.

16 Gluck JC, Gluck PA. The effect of pregnancy on the course of asthma. *Immunol Allergy Clin N Am* 2000;**20**:729–43.

17 Cydulka RK, Emerman CL, Schreiber D, Molander KH, Woodruff PG, Camargo C. Acute asthma among pregnant women presenting to the emergency department. *Am J Respir Crit Care Med* 1999;**160**:887–92.

18 Sorri M, Hartikanen-Sorri A-L, Karja J. Rhinitis during pregnancy. *Rhinology* 1980;**18**:83–6.

19 Munn MB, Groome LJ, Atterbury JL, *et al*. Pneumonia as a complication of pregnancy. *J Matern Fetal Med* 1999;**8**:151–4.

20 Henderson CE, Ownby DR, Trumble A, DerSimonian R, Kellner LH. Predicting asthma severity from allergic sensitivity to cockroaches in pregnant inner city women. *J Reprod Med* 2000;**45**:341–4.

21 Murphy VE, Gibson PG, Smith R, Clifton VL. Asthma during pregnancy: mechanisms and treatment implications. *Eur Respir J* 2005;**25**:731–50.

22 Schatz M, Zeiger RS, Hoffman CP, *et al*. Perinatal outcomes in the pregnancies of asthmatic women: a prospective controlled analysis. *Am J Respir Crit Care Med* 1995;**151**:1170–4.

23 Stenius-Aarniala BSM, Hedman J, Teramo KA. Acute asthma during pregnancy. *Thorax* 1996;**51**:411–4.

24 Dombrowski MP, Schatz M, Wise R, *et al*. Asthma during pregnancy. *Obstet Gynecol* 2004;**103**:5–12.

25 Schatz M, Dombrowski M. Outcomes of pregnancy in asthmatic women. *Immunol Allergy Clin North Am* 2000;**20**:715–27.

26 Bracken MB, Triche EW, Belanger K, *et al.* Asthma symptoms, severity, and drug therapy: a prospective study of effects on 2205 pregnancies. *Obstet Gynecol* 2003;**102**:739–52.

27 Triche EW, Saftlas AF, Belanger K, *et al.* Association of asthma diagnosis, severity, symptoms, and treatment with risk of preeclampsia. *Obstet Gynecol* 2004;**104**: 585–93.

28 Schatz M, Zeiger RS, Harden K, *et al.* The safety of asthma and allergy medications during pregnancy. *J Allergy Clin Immunol* 1997;**100**:301.

29 Martel M-J, Rey E, Beauchesne M-F, *et al.* Use of inhaled corticosteroids during pregnancy and risk of pregnancy-induced hypertension: nested case–control study. *Br Med J* 2005;**330**:230–5.

30 Schatz M, Dombrowski MP, Wise R. The relationship of asthma medication use to perinatal outcomes. *J Allergy Clin Immunol* 2004;**113**:1040–5.

31 National Asthma Education Program Report of the Working Group on Asthma and Pregnancy. *Management of asthma during pregnancy.* NIH Publication 93-3279A, September 1993.

32 National Asthma Education and Prevention Program Working Group Report on Managing Asthma During Pregnancy. *Recommendations for pharmacologic treatment.* Update 2004. NIH Publication 05-5236, March 2005.

33 Park-Wyllie L, Mazzotta P, Pastuszak A, *et al.* Birth defects after maternal exposure to corticosteroids: prospective cohort study and meta-analysis of epidemiological studies. *Teratology* 2000;**62**:385–92.

24 Epilepsy

Page B. Pennell

Epilepsy is a chronic brain disorder of various etiologies characterized by recurrent unprovoked seizures. A seizure is caused by paroxysmal abnormal cerebral neuronal discharges. Clinical manifestations are stereotyped episodic alterations in behavior or perception. Epilepsy can begin at any age of life, and two-thirds of cases are idiopathic. The prevalence is approximately 0.64% in the USA [1]. Epilepsy is the most common neurologic disorder that requires continuous treatment during pregnancy and antiepileptic drugs (AEDs) are one of the most frequent chronic teratogen exposures [2,3]. Over 1 million women with epilepsy in the USA are in their active reproductive years and give birth to over 24,000 infants each year. However, it is estimated that the total number of children in the USA exposed *in utero* to AEDs is nearly two times that amount with the emergence of AED use for other illnesses including headache, chronic pain, and mood disorders [4]. Many of the principles outlined below of AED use during pregnancy can be extrapolated to women with any disorder treated with these agents. Although some of the other disorders may allow for discontinuation of the AEDs during pregnancy, unlike most epilepsy cases, pregnancies are often not identified until after organogenesis occurs.

The vast majority of women with epilepsy will have a normal pregnancy with a favorable outcome, but there are increased maternal and fetal risks compared with the general population. Careful management of any pregnancy in a woman with epilepsy is essential to minimize these risks, ideally beginning with preconceptional planning. The initial visit between the physician and a woman with epilepsy of childbearing age should include a discussion about family planning. Topics should include effective birth control, the importance of planned pregnancies with AED optimization and folate supplementation prior to conception, obstetric complications, and teratogenicity of AEDs versus the risks of seizures during pregnancy. The goal is effective control of maternal seizures with the least risk to the fetus.

Birth control for women on antiepileptic drugs

Many of the AEDs induce the hepatic cytochrome P450 system, the primary metabolic pathway of the sex steroid hormones. This leads to rapid clearance of steroid hormones and may allow ovulation in women taking oral contraceptives or other hormonal forms of birth control [5,6]. The 1998 guidelines by the American Academy of Neurology recommend a dose of 50 µg estradiol or its equivalent for 21 days of each cycle when using oral contraceptive agents with the enzyme-inducing AEDs [7]. This is still not entirely adequate protection against pregnancy, and a back-up barrier method is recommended. Table 24.1 lists effects of the individual AEDs on hormonal contraceptive agents [6,8,9]. The newer transdermal patch and vaginal ring formulations also have higher failure rates with these AEDs.

Fetal anticonvulsant syndrome

Offspring of women with epilepsy on AEDs are at an increased risk for intrauterine growth restriction, minor anomalies, major congenital malformations, cognitive dysfunction, microcephaly, and infant mortality [10,11]. The term "fetal anticonvulsant syndrome" is used to include various combinations of these findings and has been described with virtually all of the AEDs [12,13].

Minor anomalies

Minor anomalies are defined as structural deviations from the norm that do not constitute a threat to health. Minor anomalies affect 6–20% of infants born to women with epilepsy, an approximately 2.5-fold increased rate compared to the general population [14]. Minor anomalies seen in infants of mothers on AEDs include distal digital and nail hypoplasia and the

Table 24.1 Antiepileptic drug (AED) effects on hormonal contraceptive agents.

Lowers Hormone Levels	No Significant Effects
Phenobarbital	Ethosuximide
Phenytoin	Valproate
Carbamazepine	Gabapentin
Primidone	Lamotrigine
Topiramate	Tiagabine
Oxcarbazepine	Levetiracetam
	Zonisamide

Table 24.2 Major malformations in infants of women with epilepsy.

	General Population (%)	Infants of Women with Epilepsy (%)
Congenital heart	0.5	1.5–2
Cleft lip/palate	0.15	1.4
Neural tube defect	0.06	1–3.8 (VPA)
		0.5–1 (CBZ)
Urogenital defects	0.7	1.7

CBZ, carbamazepine; VPA, valproic acid.

Table 24.3 Relative timing and developmental pathology of certain malformations [68,77].

Tissues	Malformations	Postconceptional Age (Days)
CNS	Neural tube defect	28
Heart	Ventricular septal defect	42
Face	Cleft lip	36
	Cleft maxillary palate	47–70

CNS, central nervous system.

midline craniofacial anomalies, including broad nasal bridge, ocular hypertelorism, epicanthal folds, short upturned nose, altered lips, and low hairline [14,15].

Major congenital malformations

The reported major congenital malformation (MCM) rates in the general population vary between 1.6% and 3.2% [16], and women with a history of epilepsy but not on AEDs show similar MCM rates. The average MCM rates among all AED exposures vary between 3.1% and 9%, or approximately two- to threefold higher than the general population. Reported MCM rates in monotherapy exposures are 2.3–7.8%, while AED polytherapy exposures carry an average MCM rate of 6.5–18.8% [13]. Monotherapy use of AEDs is preferred to polytherapy during pregnancy and should be achieved during the preconception planning phase [14]. Previous guidelines recommended use of monotherapy during pregnancy with the AED that best controlled that individual's seizure types [7,17]. However, data recently released from several ongoing pregnancy registries illuminate that there are significant differential risks for MCM among the various AED monotherapy regimens.

MCMs most commonly associated with AED exposure include congenital heart disease, cleft lip/palate, urogenital defects, and neural tube defects (Table 24.2) [13,14]. The congenital heart defects can involve almost any structural abnor-

mality and the urogenital defects commonly involve glandular hypospadias. The neural tube defects (NTD) are usually lower defects, but tend to be severe open defects frequently complicated by hydrocephaly and other midline defects [18]. Some studies have identified spina bifida aperta (an open defect with failure of the neural tube to close over the spinal cord) as the NTD most commonly associated with valproic acid (VPA) or carbamazepine (CBZ) exposure. The abnormal neural tube closure usually occurs between the third and fourth weeks of gestation. By the time most women realize they are pregnant, it is too late to make medication adjustments to avoid malformations (Table 24.3).

AED monotherapies during pregnancy

Although features of the fetal anticonvulsant syndrome have been described in association with virtually all of the AEDs, there are some notable differences in the likelihood of specific malformations with the different AEDs [13,19].

A comparison between two cohorts highlighted differences in fetal MCM with changes in prescribing practices over time [18]. The older cohort (1972–79) had more women taking phenobarbital, primidone, and phenytoin; the newer cohort (1981–85) represented more monotherapy with VPA or CBZ. The features of the older cohort were congenital heart defects, facial clefts, and minor anomalies. The MCM identified most frequently with the newer cohort were NTD and glandular hypospadias. The relative risk (RR) for NTD with valproate is at least 20 times the general population [20]. One analysis pooling data from five prospective studies suggested that the absolute risk with valproate monotherapy may be as high as 3.8% for NTD, and that offspring of women receiving >1000 mg/day valproate were especially at increased risk [21].

Recent prospective data from the North American AED Pregnancy Registry is available for phenobarbital, valproic acid, and lamotrigine. Of 77 women receiving phenobarbital monotherapy, five of the infants had confirmed major malformations (6.5%; 95% confidence interval [CI] 2.1–14.5%). Major malformations in exposed infants included one cleft lip and palate and four heart defects [22].

In first-trimester VPA monotherapy exposures ($n=149$), major birth defects occurred in 10.7% of infants, compared with 1.6% in external control infants (RR to controls 7.3; 95% CI, 4.4–12.2). Birth defects included cardiac anomalies, NTD, hypospadias, polydactyly, bilateral inguinal hernia, dysplastic kidney, and equinovarus club foot [23]. Perhaps more relevant to the prescribing physician is the relative risk compared to the internal comparison group. The internal comparison group was the major congenital malformation rate (2.9%) of three other AED monotherapy regimens; the relative risk of VPA for malformations compared to this group was 4.0 (95% CI, 2.1–7.4).

The UK Epilepsy and Pregnancy Register has collected prospective, full outcome data on 3607 cases [24]. Comparisons between monotherapy regimens revealed a statistically significant increased MCM rate for pregnancies exposed to valproate (6.2%; 95% CI, 4.6–8.2%) compared to those exposed to carbamazepine (2.2%; 1.4–3.4%; adjusted odds ratio [OR] 2.97; $P < 0.001$). Although a lower MCM rate was identified for pregnancies exposed to lamotrigine (3.2%; 95% CI, 2.1–4.9), adjusted OR 0.59 compared to the valproate group was not statistically significant ($P = 0.064$) [24]. The Australian Pregnancy Registry has enrolled over 800 women [25,26]. Significantly greater risk for MCM on VPA monotherapy was demonstrated (17.1%) compared to other AED monotherapy exposures (2.4%) and no AED exposures (2.5%). The MCM rate increased with increasing VPA dosage ($P < 0.05$) with a MCM rate of more than 30% for doses of more than 1100 mg/day. Other MCM rates reported were phenytoin 4.7%, CBZ 4.5%, and lamotrigine 5.6% for monotherapy exposures. The consistent findings of these large prospective pregnancy registries scattered across different regions of the world reveal a consistent pattern of amplified risk for the development of MCM in pregnancies exposed to VPA.

The newer generation of AEDs consists of a large number of structurally diverse compounds, most of which have demonstrated teratogenic effects in preclinical animal experiments and MCM in offspring of women on these AEDs. With the possible exception of lamotrigine, none have sufficient human pregnancy experience to assess their safety or teratogenicity. The reported rates for MCM with lamotrigine use during the first trimester are consistently moderately low across several studies, varying between 2.0% and 3.2% [24,27,28]. The reported MCM rate for lamotrigine use from the North American Pregnancy Registry was 2.7% (95% CI, 1.5–4.3%), but a significantly increased risk for nonsyndromic cleft lip and palate was noted [27].

Prenatal screening

Women on AEDs during pregnancy should be encouraged to undergo adequate prenatal screening to detect any fetal MCM. Adequate prenatal screening includes a combination of mater-nal serum alpha-fetoprotein at 15–20 weeks and expert detailed structural ultrasound at 16–20 weeks and fetal echocardiography at 20–22 weeks [7,17]. Ideally, the latter should be performed by a perinatologist. Amniocentesis (with measurements of amniotic fluid alpha-fetoprotein and acetylcholinesterase) is not performed routinely but should be offered if these tests are equivocal, increasing the sensitivity for detection of NTD to greater than 99%. If the patient's weight gain and fundal growth do not appear appropriate, serial sonography should be performed to assess fetal size and amniotic fluid volume [17].

Neurodevelopmental outcome

Studies investigating cognitive outcome in children of women with epilepsy report an increased risk of mental deficiency, affecting 1.4–6% of children of women with epilepsy, compared to 1% of controls [10,29,30]. Verbal scores on neuropsychometric measures may be selectively more involved [4]. A variety of factors contribute to the cognitive problems of children of mothers with epilepsy, but AEDs appear to have a role [4].

Studies of particular AEDs have reported that the child's level of IQ is negatively correlated with *in utero* exposure to VPA [31,32], primidone [33], phenobarbital [34], phenytoin [32,35], CBZ [32,36,37], polytherapy [31–33,38], and seizures [39]. Exposure during the last trimester may actually be the most detrimental [34].

Several studies have suggested a notably higher risk of VPA for the neurodevelopment of children exposed *in utero*, often with lower verbal IQ scores [31,38,40,41]. Additionally, greater than five convulsive seizures during pregnancy had a negative effect on verbal IQ [41]. The findings of increased risk for neurodevelopmental consequences with polytherapy, VPA exposure, and with frequent convulsive seizures should be considered by the prescribing physician and included in the discussion with women with epilepsy.

Microcephaly has been associated with *in utero* AED exposure [10,11], and most often with polytherapy, phenobarbital, and primidone [42]. The risk of epilepsy in children of women with epilepsy is higher (RR 3.2) compared to controls [43]. Interestingly, this same increased risk has not been demonstrated for children of fathers with epilepsy.

Mortality

Fetal death (fetal loss at more than 20 weeks' gestation) is another increased risk for women with epilepsy. Reported stillbirth rates vary between 1.3% and 14.0% compared to rates of 1.2–7.8% for women without epilepsy [10]. Perinatal death rates are also up to twofold higher for women with epilepsy (1.3–7.8%) compared to controls (1.0–3.9%) [10]. Spontaneous abortion (<20 weeks' gestation) figures vary considerably [7,44,45].

Potential mechanisms

The causes of the "anticonvulsant embryopathy" are likely multifactorial. However, recent studies have supported the anticonvulsant drugs as the most significant offending factor, more so than actual traits carried by mothers with epilepsy, environmental factors, or possibly even seizures during pregnancy [46–48]. Observational studies have reported that infants whose mothers had a history of epilepsy but took no AEDs during pregnancy do not have a higher frequency of these abnormalities compared to control infants [47], including abnormalities of cognitive function [48].

Teratogenecity by AEDs is likely mediated by several mechanisms, including antifolate effects and reactive intermediates of AEDs. Almost all AEDs are associated with folate deficiency or interference with folate metabolism [49–51]. Although the beneficial effects of folic acid supplementation are clear for lowering the risk of NTD in women without epilepsy [52,53], it is not as clear in women with epilepsy on AEDs. However, all women with epilepsy of childbearing potential should be placed on a minimum of folate supplementation of at least 0.4 mg/day [7]. Some authors recommend as much as 4–5 mg/day supplemental folate for women on AEDs [54–56].

Seizures during pregnancy

The effect of pregnancy on seizure frequency is variable. Approximately 20–33% of patients will have an increase in their seizures, 7–25% a decrease in seizures, and 50–83% will experience no significant change [57–60].

The physiologic changes and psychosocial adjustments that accompany pregnancy can alter seizure frequency, including changes in sex hormone concentrations, changes in AED metabolism, sleep deprivation, and new stresses. Noncompliance with medications is common during pregnancy and is in large part because of the strong message that any drugs during pregnancy are harmful to the fetus. Teratogenic effects of AEDs are well-described, but risks to the fetus are often exaggerated or misrepresented. Proper education about the risks of AEDs versus the risks of seizures can be very helpful in assuring compliance during pregnancy.

Generalized tonic–clonic seizures (GTCS) can cause maternal and fetal hypoxia and acidosis [10,61]. After a single GTCS, fetal intracranial hemorrhages [62], miscarriages, and still-births have been reported [49]. A single brief tonic–clonic seizure has been shown to cause depression of fetal heart rate for more than 20 minutes [63], and longer or repetitive tonic–clonic seizures are incrementally more hazardous to the fetus as well as the mother. Status epilepticus is an uncommon complication of pregnancy, but when it does occur it carries a high maternal and fetal mortality rate [64].

It is not as clear what the effects of nonconvulsive seizures are on the developing fetus. Many types of seizures can cause trauma, which can result in ruptured fetal membranes with an increased risk of infection, premature labor, and even fetal death [15]. If the woman is still having seizures, restrictions from driving and climbing heights should be reinforced with her, with special emphasis on the risk to the fetus.

Antiepileptic drug management

Management of AEDs during pregnancy can be complex. Clearance of virtually all of the AEDs increases during pregnancy, resulting in a decrease in serum concentrations (Table 24.4) [65]. Clearance of most of the AEDs normalizes

AED	Reported Increases in Clearance (%)	Reported Decreases in Total Concentrations (%)	Reported Decreases in Free Concentrations (%)
LTG	65–230	50–75	50
PHT	20–100	55–61	18–31
CBZ	0–20	0–42	0–28
PB	–	55	50
PRM	–	55	–
Derived PB	–	70	–
VPA	35–183	50	(25–30)*
ESX	–	Inconsistent decreases	–

Table 24.4 Alterations of antiepileptic drug (AED) clearance and/or concentrations during pregnancy (after Pennell [65]).

CBZ, carbamazepine; ESX, ethosuximide; LTG, lamotrigine; PB, phenobarbital; PHT, phenytoin; PRM, primidone; VPA, valproic acid.

* Free concentrations of VPA decrease during the first two trimesters, but then normalize or increase by delivery.

Table 24.5 Physiologic changes during pregnancy: effects on drug disposition (after Pennell [65]).

Parameter	Consequences
↑ Total body water, extracellular fluid	Altered drug distribution
↑ Fat stores	↓ Elimination of lipid soluble drugs
↑ Cardiac output	↑ Hepatic blood flow leading to ↑ elimination
↑ Renal blood flow and glomerular flow rate	↑ Renal clearance of unchanged drug
Altered cytochrome P450 activity	Altered systemic absorption and hepatic elimination
↓ Maternal albumin	Altered free fraction; increased availability of drug for hepatic extraction

gradually over the first 2–3 postpartum months. Lamotrigine metabolism, however, undergoes an exaggerated increase throughout pregnancy, and quickly converts back to baseline clearance within the first few weeks postpartum [66,67].

Several physiologic factors contribute to the decline in AED levels during pregnancy (Table 24.5). The greater extent of increased lamotrigine clearance during pregnancy probably reflects its distinctive metabolic pathway of glucuronidation. The changes in AED levels during pregnancy can vary widely and are not predictable for an individual. The ratio of free to bound drug may increase during pregnancy for many of the older AEDs, but the amount of free AED still usually declines [65]. The optimal approach to monitoring AED levels during pregnancy is one that measures free levels of any AED that is highly or moderately protein-bound [7]. Total levels are sufficient for AEDs that are minimally protein-bound. The ideal AED (free) level(s) need to be established for each individual patient prior to conception, and should be the level at which seizure control is the best possible for that patient without debilitating side-effects. Levels should be obtained at least at baseline prior to conception and repeated at the beginning of each trimester and again in the last 4 weeks of pregnancy [7,17]. Some authors recommend monthly monitoring given the possibility of rapid and unpredictable decreases in AED levels in an individual patient [65,68].

Obstetric complications

Women with epilepsy have an increased risk of certain obstetric complications. There is an approximate twofold increased risk of vaginal bleeding, hyperemesis gravidarum, anemia, eclampsia, abruptio placentae, preterm delivery, and the need for induced labor, interventions during labor, and/or cesarean delivery [10,69].

Neonatal vitamin K deficiency

Many of the AEDs can inhibit vitamin K transport across the placenta [10,70–72]. Infant mortality from this hemorrhagic disorder is very high at more than 30% and is usually a result of bleeding in the abdominal and pleural cavities leading to shock. Therefore, guidelines recommend prophylactic treatment with vitamin K_1 administered orally as 10 mg to the mother during the last month of pregnancy and 1 mg i.m./i.v. administered to the newborn at birth [7]. If the woman has not received supplemental vitamin K_1 prior to labor onset, then she should receive parenteral vitamin K_1. If two of the neonate's coagulation factors fall below 5% of normal values, intravenous fresh frozen plasma needs to be administered.

Labor and delivery

The majority of women with epilepsy will not experience seizures during labor and delivery. Reports of women with seizures during labor and the first 24 hours postpartum are 2%, but may be as high as 12.5% of women with primary generalized epilepsy syndromes [73,74]. Sleep deprivation may provoke seizures and obstetric anesthesia may be used to allow for some rest prior to delivery if sleep deprivation has been prolonged. The specific analgesic meperidine should be avoided because of its potential to lower seizure threshold.

During a prolonged labor, oral absorption of AEDs may be erratic and any emesis will confound the problem. Phenobarbital, (fos)phenytoin, and VPA can be given intravenously at the same maintenance dosage. Convulsive seizures and repeated seizures during labor should be treated promptly with parenteral lorazepam (1–4 mg) or valium (5–10 mg) [73]. Benzodiazepines can cause neonatal respiratory depression, decreased heart rate, and maternal apnea if given in large doses, and these potential side-effects need to be monitored closely. Administration of another, longer acting AED is controversial because of the inhibitory effects on myometrial contractions [73]. If convulsive seizures occur, oxygen should be administered to the patient and she should be placed on her left side to increase uterine blood flow and decrease the risk of maternal aspiration [17]. Prompt cesarean delivery should be performed when repeated GTCS cannot be controlled during labor or when the mother is unable to cooperate during labor because of impaired awareness during repetitive absence or complex partial seizures [73,74].

Postpartum care

Most of the AED levels gradually increase after delivery and plateau by 10 weeks postpartum. AED levels may need to be followed closely during this postpartum period [7]. Lamotrigine levels, however, increase immediately and plateau within 2–3 weeks postpartum. Adjustments in lamotrigine dosage may need to be made on an anticipatory basis beginning within the first few days after delivery [75].

Perinatal lethargy, irritability, and feeding difficulties have been attributed to intrauterine exposure to benzodiazepines and barbiturates, and breastfeeding on these medications may prolong sedation and feeding problems. However, most infants of women with epilepsy can successfully breastfeed without complications. The concentrations of the different AEDs in breastmilk are considerably less than those in maternal serum (Table 24.6). The infant's serum concentration is determined by this factor as well as the AED elimination half-life in neonates, which is usually more prolonged than that in adults [65]. The benefits of breastfeeding are believed to outweigh the small risk of adverse effects of AEDs [7,76]. The parents should be advised to watch for signs of increased lethargy to a degree that interferes with normal growth and development.

Conclusions

Improving maternal and fetal outcomes for women with epilepsy involves effective preconceptional counseling and

Table 24.6 Antiepileptic drug (AED) exposure through breastmilk (after Pennell [65]).

AED	Breast Milk/Maternal Concentration	Adult Half-Life	Neonate Half-Life
CBZ	0.4–0.6	8–25	8–28
PHT	0.18–0.4	12–50	15–105
PB	0.36–0.6	75–126	45–500
ESX	0.8–0.9	32–60	32–40
PRM	0.7–0.9	4–12	7–60
VPA	0.01–0.10	6–18	30–60
LTG	0.5–0.6	–	–
TPM	0.69–0.86	–	–
ZNS	0.41–0.93	63	61–109
LEV	3.09	–	–

CBZ, carbamazepine; ESX, ethosuximide; LEV, levetiracetam; LTG, lamotrigine; PB, phenobarbital; PHT, phenytoin; PRM, primidone; TPM, topiramate; VPA, valproic acid; ZNS, zonisamide.

preparation. The importance of planned pregnancies with effective birth control should be emphasized, with consideration of the effects of the enzyme-inducing AEDs on lowering efficacy of hormonal contraceptive medications.

Before pregnancy occurs, the patient's diagnosis and treatment regimen should be reassessed. Once the diagnosis of epilepsy is confirmed, it is important to verify whether that individual patient continues to need medications and whether she is on the most appropriate AED to balance control of her seizures against teratogenic risks. For most women with epilepsy, withdrawal of all AEDs prior to pregnancy is not a realistic option. In the vast majority of cases requiring continued AED therapy, monotherapy at the lowest effective dose should be employed. If large daily doses are needed, then frequent smaller doses or extended-release formulations may be helpful to avoid high peak levels. Some of the newest information about differential risks between AEDs should also be considered. The woman's AED regimen should be optimized and folate supplementation should begin prior to pregnancy. Given that 50% of pregnancies are unplanned in the USA, folate supplementation should be encouraged in all women of childbearing age on any AED and for any indication. Dosing recommendations vary between 0.4 and 5 mg/day.

If a woman with epilepsy presents after conception on a single AED that is effective, her medication should usually not be changed. Exposing the fetus to a second agent during a cross-over period of AEDs only increases the teratogenic risk, and seizures are more likely to occur with any abrupt medication changes. If a woman is on polytherapy, it may be possible to switch safely to monotherapy. Maintaining seizure control during pregnancy is important, and monitoring of serum AED levels can help achieve that goal.

Prenatal screening can detect major malformations in the first and second trimesters. Vitamin K_1 is given as 10 mg/day orally during the last month of pregnancy, followed by 1 mg i.m./i.v. to the newborn [7].

Although women on AEDs for epilepsy, or for other indications, have increased risks for maternal and fetal complications, these risks can be considerably reduced with effective preconceptional planning and careful multidisciplinary management during pregnancy and the postpartum period.

Case presentation

The patient is a 32-year-old, G1P0, right-handed white female who had a closed head injury with loss of consciousness in 1988 during a motor vehicle accident. Five years later, she developed her first seizure, which presented as an aura followed by a generalized tonic–clonic (grand mal) seizure. Her second seizures occurred in 1994, with similar semiology. She was diagnosed with epilepsy and started on phenytoin. Two years later, because of interference with birth control pills, her phenytoin was switched to 500 mg VPA p.o. b.i.d. of the extended-release formulation. She had no further grand mal seizures but still had occasional auras with dizziness and wave-like vision once per year. The patient stopped her birth control in 2005 with eager anticipation of pregnancy. She was not counseled about specific risks of her medication and was not on any vitamin supplementation.

The patient presented to our clinic at 17 weeks' gestation for a second opinion regarding her epilepsy management in the setting of recent ultrasound diagnosis of MCM, including meningomyelocele, severe hydrocephalus, and heart calcifications. Folic acid at 4 mg/day and a prenatal vitamin were prescribed. She was referred to a fetal maternal medicine specialist and chose to undergo therapeutic dilatation and evacuation. She returned to neurology clinic 6 weeks later. The patient and her husband were given information on specific reported risks of MCM for lamotrigine monotherapy compared to valproate monotherapy. A gradual cross-over of her medication from VPA to lamotrigine was prescribed. A baseline, trough lamotrigine serum concentration measurement 1 month after the transition to lamotrigine monotherapy was ordered. She was counseled to wait until 6 months after the cross-over was complete before trying to conceive again, to assure medication tolerability and efficacy.

References

1 Hauser WA, Hersdorffer DC. *Epilepsy: Frequency, Causes, and Consequences*. Landover, MD: Epilepsy Foundation of America, 1990.

2 Holmes LB. The teratogenecity of anticonvulsant drugs: a progress report. *J Med Genet* 2002;**39**:245–7.

3 Fairgrieve SD, Jackson M, Jonas P, *et al*. Population based, prospective study of the care of women with epilepsy in pregnancy. *Br Med J* 2000;**321**:674–5.

4 Meador KJ, Zupanc ML. Neurodevelopmental outcomes of children born to mothers with epilepsy. *Cleve Clin J Med* 2004;**71**(Suppl 2):S38–41.

5 Janz D, Schmidt D. Anti-epileptic drugs and failure of oral contraceptives. *Lancet* 1974;**1**:113.

6 Guberman A. Hormonal contraception and epilepsy. *Neurology* 1999;**53**(Suppl 1):S38–40.

7 Report of the Quality Standards Subcommittee of the American Academy of Neurology. Practice parameter: management issues for women with epilepsy (summary statement). *Neurology* 1998;**51**:944–8.

8 Krauss G, Brandt J, Campbell M, Plate C, Summerfield M. Antiepileptic medication and oral contraceptive interactions: a national survey of neurologists and obstetricians. *Neurology* 1996;**46**:1534–9.

9 Rosenfeld W, Doose D, Walker S, Nayak R. Effect of topiramate on the pharmacokinetics of an oral contraceptive containing norethindrone and ethinyl estradiol in patients with epilepsy. *Epilepsia* 1997;**38**:317–23.

10 Yerby MS. Quality of life, epilepsy advances, and the evolving role of anticonvulsants in women with epilepsy. *Neurology* 2000;**55**:21–31.

11 Hvas C, Henriksen T, Ostergaard J, Dam M. Epilepsy and pregnancy: effect of antiepileptic drugs and lifestyle on birthweight. *Br J Obstet Gynaecol* 2000;**107**:896–902.

12 Arpino C, Brescianini S, Robert E, *et al*. Teratogenic effects of antiepileptic drugs: use of an international database on malformations and drug exposure (MADRE). *Epilepsia* 2000;**41**:1436–43.

13 Pennell PB. Pregnancy in women who have epilepsy. *Neurol Clin* 2004;**22**:799–820.

14 Morrell M. Guidelines for the care of women with epilepsy. *Neurology* 1998;**51**(Suppl 5):S21–7.

15 Yerby M, Devinsky O. Epilepsy and pregnancy. In: Devinsky O, Feldmann E, Hainline B, eds. *Advances in Neurology: Neurological Complications of Pregnancy*. New York: Raven Press, 1994: 45–63.

16 Honein MA, Paulozzi LJ, Cragan JD, Correa A. Evaluation of selected characteristics of pregnancy drug registries. *Teratology* 1999;**60**:356–64.

17 Committee on Educational Bulletins of the American College of Obstetricians and Gynecologists. Seizure disorders in pregnancy. *Int J Gynecol Obstet* 1997;**56**:279–86.

18 Lindhout D, Meinardi H, Meijer J, Nau H. Antiepileptic drugs and teratogenesis in two consecutive cohorts: changes in prescription policy paralleled by changes in pattern of malformations. *Neurology* 1992;**42**(Suppl 5):94–110.

19 Barrett C, Richens A. Epilepsy and pregnancy: Report of an Epilepsy Research Foundation Workshop. *Epilepsy Res* 2003;**52**:147–87.

20 Lindhout D, Schmidt D. *In utero* exposure to valproate and neural tube defects. *Lancet* 1986;**2**:1392–3.

21 Samren E, van Duijn C, Koch S, *et al*. Maternal use of antiepileptic drugs and the risk of major congenital malformations: a joint European prospective study of human teratogenesis asssociated with maternal epilepsy. *Epilepsia* 1997;**38**:981–90.

22 Holmes LB, Wyszynski DF, Lieberman E. The AED (antiepileptic drug) pregnancy registry: a 6-year experience. *Arch Neurol* 2004;**61**:673–8.

23 Wyszynski DF, Nambisan M, Surve T, Alsdorf RM, Smith CR, Holmes LB. Increased rate of major malformations in offspring exposed to valproate during pregnancy. *Neurology* 2005;**64**:961–5.

24 Morrow J, Russell A, Guthrie E, *et al*. Malformation risks of antiepileptic drugs in pregnancy: a prospective study from the UK Epilepsy and Pregnancy Register. *J Neurol Neurosurg Psychiatry* 2006;**77**:193–8.

25 Vajda FJ, O'Brien TJ, Hitchcock A, Graham J, Lander C. The Australian registry of anti-epileptic drugs in pregnancy: experience after 30 months. *J Clin Neurosci* 2003;**10**:543–9.

26 Vajda F, O'Brien T, Hitchcock A, Graham J, Lander C. The Australian registry of anti-epileptic drugs in pregnancy: multivariate logistic regression analysis demonstrating an increased risk for valproate, with a dose dependent relationship. *Epilepsia* 2002.

27 Holmes LB, Wyszynski DF, Baldwin EJ, Habecker E, Glassman LH, Smith CR. Increased risk for non-syndromic cleft palate among infants exposed to lamotrigine during pregancy. Birth Defects Research (Part A): Clinical and Molecular Teratology. 2006. Ref Type: Abstract

28 Sabers A, Dam M, Rogvi-Hansen B, *et al.* Epilepsy and pregnancy: lamotrigine as main drug used. *Acta Neurol Scand* 2004;**109**:9–13.

29 Leavitt A, Yerby M, Robinson N, Sells C, Erickson D. Epilepsy in pregnancy: developmental outcome of offspring at 12 months. *Neurology* 1992;**42**(Suppl 5):141–3.

30 Ganstrom M, Gaily E. Psychomotor development in children of mothers with epilepsy. *Neurology* 1992;**42**(Suppl 5):144–8.

31 Adab N, Jacoby A, Smith D, Chadwick D. Additional educational needs in children born to mothers with epilepsy. *J Neurol Neurosurg Psychiatry* 2001;**70**:15–21.

32 Dean J, Hailey H, Moore S, Lloyd D, Turnpenny P, Little J. Long-term health and neurodevelopment in children exposed to antiepileptic drugs before birth. *J Med Genet* 2002;**39**:251–9.

33 Koch S, Titze K, Zimmerman R, Schroder M, Lehmkuhl U, Rauh H. Long-term neuropsychological consequences of maternal epilepsy and anticonvulsant treatment during pregnancy for school-age children and adolescents. *Epilepsia* 1999;**40**:1237–43.

34 Reinisch J, Sanders S, Mortensen E, Rubin D. *In utero* exposure to phenobarbital and intelligence deficits in adult men. *JAMA* 1995;**724**:1518–25.

35 Vanoverloop D, Schnell R, Harvey E, Holmes L. The effects of prenatal exposure to phenytoin and other anticonvulsants on intellectual function at 4 to 8 years of age. *Neurotoxicol Teratol* 1992;**14**:329–35.

36 Ornoy A, Cohen E. Outcome of children born to epileptic mothers treated with carbamazepine during pregnancy. *Arch Dis Child* 1996;**75**:517–20.

37 Matalon S, Schechtman S, Goldzweig G, Ornoy A. The teratogenic effect of carbamazepine: a meta-analysis of 1255 exposures. *Reprod Toxicol* 2002;**16**:9–17.

38 Adab N, Tudor-Smith C, Vinten J, Winterbottom J. A systematic review of long-term developmental outcomes in children exposed to antiepileptic drugs *in utero*. *Epilepsia* 2002;**43**(Suppl 7):230–1.

39 Leonard G, Andermann E, Ptito A. Cognitive effects of antiepileptic drug therapy during pregnancy on school-age offspring [Abstract]. *Epilepsia* 1997;**38**(Suppl 3):170.

40 Gaily E, Kantola-Sorsa E, Hiilesmaa V, *et al.* Normal intelligence in children with prenatal exposure to carbamazepine. *Neurology* 2004;**62**:28–32.

41 Vinten J, Adab N, Kini U, Gorry J, Gregg J, Baker GA. Neuropsychological effects of exposure to anticonvulsant medication *in utero*. *Neurology* 2005;**64**:949–54.

42 Battino D, Kaneko S, Andermann E, *et al.* Intrauterine growth in the offspring of epileptic women: a prospective multicenter study. *Epilepsy Res* 1999;**36**:53–60.

43 Annegers J, Hauser W, Elveback L, Anderson V, Kurland L. Congenital malformations and seizure disorders in the offspring of parents with epilepsy. *Int J Epidemiol* 1978;**7**:241–7.

44 Yerby M, Cawthon M. Fetal death, malformations and infant mortality in infants of mothers with epilepsy. *Epilepsia* 1996;**37**(Suppl 5):98.

45 Yerby M, Collins S. Teratogenecity of antiepileptic drugs. In: Engel J, Pedley T, eds. *Epilepsy, a Comprehensive Textbook.* Philadelphia, PA: Lippincott-Raven, 1997: 1195–203.

46 Canger R, Battino D, Canerini M, *et al.* Malformations in offspring of women with epilepsy: a prospective study. *Epilepsia* 1999;**40**:1231–6.

47 Holmes LB, Harvey EA, Coull BA, *et al.* The teratogenicity of anticonvulsant drugs. *N Engl J Med* 2001;**344**:1132–8.

48 Holmes LB, Rosenberger PB, Harvey EA, Khoshbin S, Ryan L. Intelligence and physical features of children of women with epilepsy. *Teratology* 2000;**61**:196–202.

49 Zahn CA, Morrell MJ, Collins SD, Labiner DM, Yerby MS. Management issues for women with epilepsy: a review of the literature. *Neurology* 1998;**51**:949–56.

50 Dansky L, Rosenblatt D, Andermann E. Mechanisms of teratogenesis: folic acid and antiepileptic therapy. *Neurology* 1992;**42**:32–42.

51 Wegner C, Nau H. Alteration of embryonic folate metabolism by valproic acid during organogenesis: implications for mechanisms of teratogenesis. *Neurology* 1992;**42**(Suppl 5):17–24.

52 Botto L, Moore C, Khoury M, Erickson J. Medical progress: neural-tube defects. *N Engl J Med* 1999;**341**:1509–19.

53 MRC Vitamin Study Research Group. Prevention of neural-tube defects: results of the Medical Research Council Vitamin Study. *Lancet* 1991;**338**:131–7.

54 Nambisan M, Wyszynski DF, Holmes LB. No evidence of a protective effect due to periconceptional folic acid (PCFA) intake on risk for congenital anomalies in the offspring of mothers exposed to antiepileptic drugs (AEDs). *Birth Defects Res* 2003;**67**:5.

55 Hernandez-Diaz S, Werler M, Walker A. Folic acid antagonists during pregnancy and the risk of birth defects. *N Engl J Med* 2000;**343**:1608–14.

56 American College of Obstetricians and Gynecologists. *Seizure disorders in pregnancy.* ACOG Education Bulletin 1996; No. 231.

57 Devinsky O, Yerby M. Women with epilepsy. *Neurol Clin* 1994;**12**:479–95.

58 Gee K, McCauley L, Lan N. A putatative receptor for neurosteroids on the GABA receptor complex: the pharmacological properties and therapeutic potential of epalons. *Crit Rev Neurobiol* 1995;**9**:205–7.

59 Cantrell D. Epilepsy and pregnancy: a study of seizure frequency and patient demographics. *Epilepsia* 1997;**38**(Suppl 8):231.

60 Yerby M, Collins S. Pregnancy and the mother. In: Engel J, Pedley T, eds. *Epilepsy, A Comprehensive Textbook.* Philadelphia, PS: Lippincott-Raven, 1997: 2027–35.

61 Stumpf D, Frost M. Seizures, anticonvulsants, and pregnancy. *Am J Dis Child* 1978;**132**:746–8.

62 Minkoff H, Schaffer R, Delke I, Grunevaum A. Diagnosis of intracranial hemorrhage *in utero* after a maternal seizure. *Obstet Gynecol* 1985;**65**(Suppl):22S–24S.

63 Teramo K, Hiilesmaa V, Bardy A, *et al.* Fetal heart rate during a maternal grand mal epileptic seizure. *J Perinat Med* 1979;**7**:3–5.

64 Teramo K, Hiilesmaa V. Pregnancy and fetal complications in epileptic pregnancies: review of the literature. In: Janz D, Bossi L, Dam M, *et al.* eds. *Epilepsy, Pregnancy and the Child.* New York: Raven Press, 1982: 53–9.

65 Pennell PB. Antiepileptic drug pharmacokinetics during pregnancy and lactation. *Neurology* 2003;**61**(Suppl 2):S35–S42.

66 Pennell P, Montgomery J, Clements S, Newport D. Lamotrigine clearance markedly increases during pregnancy. *Epilepsia* 2002;**43**(Suppl 7):234.

67 Tran TA, Leppik IE, Blesi K, Sathanandan ST, Remmel R. Lamotrigine clearance during pregnancy. *Neurology* 2002;**59**:251–5.

68 Yerby MS. Clinical care of pregnant women with epilepsy: neural tube defects and folic acid supplementation. *Epilepsia* 2003;**44**:33–40.

69 Fonager K, Larsen H, Pedersen L, Sorensen HT. Birth outcomes in women exposed to anticonvulsant drugs. *Acta Neurol Scand* 2000;**101**:289–94.

70 Howe A, Oakes D, Woodman P, Webster W. Prothrombin and PIVKA-II levels in cord blood from newborn exposed to anticonvulsants during pregnancy. *Epilepsia* 1999;**40**: 980–4.

71 Srinivasan G, Seeler RA, Tiruvury A, *et al.* Maternal anticonvulsant therapy and hemorrhagic disease of the newborn. *Obstet Gynecol* 1982;**59**:250–2.

72 Nelson KB, Ellenber JH. Maternal seizure disorder, outcomes of pregnancy, and neurologic abnormalities in the children. *Neurology* 1982;**32**:1247–54.

73 Delgado-Escueta A, Janz D. Consensus guidelines: preconception counseling, management, and care of the pregnant woman with epilepsy. *Neurology* 1992;**42**:149–60.

74 Katz JM, Devinsky O. Primary generalized epilepsy: a risk factor for seizures in labor and delivery? *Seizure* 2003;**12**:217–9.

75 Pennell PB, Newport DJ, Stowe ZN, Helmers SL, Montgomery JQ, Henry TR. The impact of pregnancy and childbirth on the metabolism of lamotrigine. *Neurology* 2004;**62**:292–5.

76 Pschirrer E, Monga M. Seizure disorders in pregnancy. *Obstet Gynecol Clin* 2001;**28**:601–11.

77 Moore K. *The Developing Human: Clinically Oriented Embryology*, 4th edn. Philadelphia, PA: WB Saunders, 1988.

25 Chronic hypertension

C. Kevin Huls and Dinesh M. Shah

Hypertensive disorders of pregnancy are one of the most serious complications in pregnancy because of the potential to cause serious maternal and perinatal morbidity and mortality. Although a substantial number of hypertensive patients have relatively good outcomes, difficulty in differentiating between various hypertensive conditions, inability to predict which patients are at highest risk, and variability in the progression of preeclampsia make these disorders the greatest challenge of clinical medicine in obstetrics.

Diagnosis and classification

Chronic hypertension in pregnancy is diagnosed if there is a sustained elevation of arterial blood pressure of 140/90 mmHg or greater prior to the 20th week of gestation, or if hypertension existed prior to pregnancy [1]. The diagnosis of chronic hypertension in pregnancy may be missed because of the decline in blood pressure as a result of the vascular relaxation of pregnancy. As a result of this, chronic hypertension may be diagnosed as gestational hypertension in the third trimester. Chronic hypertension should be suspected if first-trimester diastolic pressures are in the 80s, in a multiparous patient, or in a patient with a family history of chronic hypertension. Patients who develop hypertension in more than one pregnancy most likely have chronic hypertension [2,3]. The rates of adverse perinatal and maternal outcomes increase when preeclampsia develops in a patient with underlying hypertension [4]. Patients with preeclampsia, in general, have a greater risk of cardiovascular mortality later in life [5]. Associated conditions involving the kidneys, such as systemic lupus erythematosus and diabetes mellitus, help make the diagnosis of secondary hypertension.

Classification

Although during pregnancy hypertension is commonly classified as mild (≥140/90 mmHg) or severe (≥160/110 mmHg), chronic hypertension in pregnancy can be categorized as mild, moderate, or severe depending on the absolute level of blood pressure with or without evidence of end-organ damage. The High Blood Pressure Council has recommended that blood pressure be taken in the sitting position after 10 minutes of rest. Diastolic measurement is the pressure at Korotkoff phase V, when the sound disappears [1]. If automated blood pressure monitors are used, the diastolic pressure will be between the fourth and fifth Korotkoff sounds. Uterine size and compression of the inferior vena cava and aorta are factors (especially in the supine position) that alter blood pressure readings as the uterus enlarges.

Preconceptional therapy guidelines

Preconceptional counseling is important for the woman who has chronic hypertension. It is important to establish baseline data on this patient, and to teach her self-blood pressure monitoring prior to conception. Medication should be changed to one acceptable during pregnancy. If she is taking diuretics, their dosage should gradually be diminished and preferably eliminated prior to conception. Angiotensin-converting enzyme (ACE) inhibitors and angiotensin receptor blockers are associated with renal anomalies, and both are associated with renal failure which may not be reversible, which is why these are contraindicated after the first trimester [6,7].

Evaluation

When hypertension is present or suspected, additional testing should be carried out based on clinical considerations. If a practitioner has not had extensive experience with hypertension during pregnancy, consultative advice should be sought from a subspecialist (i.e., maternal fetal medicine).

Reasonable assessment for all patients may include urinalysis for protein and microscopic examination for sediment, especially if significant proteinuria is detected by the dipstick method. A 24-hour collection for total protein and creatinine clearance should be performed early in the pregnancy for patients with overt hypertension. We suggest repeating this around 26–28 weeks' gestation to define a new baseline, because of pregnancy-associated increase in renal blood flow which may physiologically increase proteinuria. Such an increase, if proportionate to increased glomerular filtration rate, should be interpreted as a physiologic change. This assists the practitioner's management if superimposed preeclampsia develops later in gestation. An assessment of complete blood count with platelet count should be performed.

Other tests to consider are based on clinical presentation. Consideration should be given to the possibility of systemic lupus erythematosus in patients with proteinuria disproportionate to the degree of hypertension, and one should check antinuclear antibodies (ANA) and anti double-stranded DNA. Generally, the presence of diabetes mellitus is known, but in patients with proteinuria this should remain a consideration. If the hypertension is severe and gestation is less than 20 weeks, one should check serum electrolytes to evaluate for hyperaldosteronism or consider evaluation for a molar pregnancy. Cushing syndrome is rare and difficult to evaluate during pregnancy. If hypertension is paroxysmal, has frequent "crisis," or is associated with anxiety, a 24-hour collection of urine for vanillylmandelic acid, metanephrines, or unconjugated catecholamines should be performed to identify pheochromocytoma. A toxicology screen should be obtained in all patients with severe and/or accelerated hypertension to examine for cocaine use.

If the hypertension has been present for several years, additional consideration should be given to ordering an electrocardiogram, echocardiogram, or ophthalmologic examination. For patients with an elevated creatinine, a renal ultrasound may be occasionally useful. A young woman with severe hypertension may also require Doppler flow studies or magnetic resonance angiography to evaluate for renal artery stenosis, but this is generally detected before the patient has seen the obstetrician.

Differential diagnosis

Pre-existing hypertension should be suspected in the absence of proteinuria and other corroborative laboratory findings of preeclampsia, family history of hypertension, obesity, multiparity, or other diseases known to affect the kidney. One should review medical records from prior health care visits to ascertain prepregnancy blood pressure measurements.

Pre-existing hypertension, secondary to renal disease should be suspected when proteinuria is disproportionate to the degree of hypertension, especially when the patient is multiparous or presents with hypertension prior to 34 weeks [8].

Forty-three percent of multiparous women presenting with preeclampsia had renal biopsies showing evidence of pre-existing renal parenchymal or vascular disease [9]. Of women with preeclampsia diagnosed prior to 34 weeks, 70% had laboratory or renal biopsy evidence of pre-existing renal disease [10].

Therapy during pregnancy

Home blood pressure monitoring permits the patient to be her own advocate and further reinforces the control of her environmental situation. Home blood pressure data is preferable, and correct calibration should be confirmed. Self-monitoring can reduce the use of antihypertensives and the need for hospitalization [11,12].

Bed rest has been suggested as therapy for women who have chronic hypertensive diseases of pregnancy. Uterine blood flow is increased when the woman is in the left lateral recumbent position.

Antihypertensive therapy should be considered when the diastolic blood pressure exceeds 90 mmHg in the office, or 84 mmHg on home monitoring. The National High Blood Pressure Education Program Working Group on High Blood Pressure in Pregnancy recommends that therapy should be initiated or increased if the systolic blood pressure exceeds 150–160 mmHg or the diastolic pressure exceeds 100–110 mmHg. A table of commonly used antihypertensive medications is included for reference (Table 25.1).

Antihypertensive therapy has not been shown to improve fetal condition or to prevent preeclampsia [13], probably because appropriate studies have not been conducted to answer these questions. However, such therapy controls acceleration of blood pressure and should help prevent maternal stroke from uncontrolled hypertension. The drug of choice in the past was methyldopa in divided doses. It is important to note that a side-effect of methyldopa is elevation of liver enzymes in a small number of patients. Labetalol is an alternative medication that has alpha-adrenergic and central beta-blocking effects. Other beta-blocking medications do not have this dual effect, which may explain why these other beta-blockers are associated with intrauterine growth restriction [14].

In recent years, calcium-channel blockers, such as nifedipine, have come into use. The effect of calcium-channel blockade is vasodilatation and it may have a salutary effect on the uterine blood flow similar to the effect on renal blood flow. Oral hydralazine is a rather mild vasodilator and may be associated with lupus-like reaction. Diuretics should be considered only as adjuvant therapy and preferably infrequently used. These should be reserved for patients with excessive fluid retention and for fluid overload. We would not recommend diuretic use for leg edema of pregnancy.

Table 25.1 Antihypertensive medications for chronic hypertension.

	Doses	Important Side-effects	Comment
Methyldopa	250 mg b.i.d. to 500 mg q.i.d.	Lethargy, fever, hepatitis, hemolytic anemia, positive Coombs test	Centrally acting alpha-agonist
Labetalol	100 mg b.i.d. to 800 mg t.i.d.; maximum dose 2400 mg/day	Flushing, headache; other beta-blocking agents may lead to decreased placental perfusion	Beta-blocker with alpha-blocking activity
Nifedipine	30 mg XL q.d. to 60 mg XL b.i.d.; maximum dose 120 mg/day	Headache, tachycardia, hypotension; avoid use in women >40 years of age or coronary artery disease	Calcium-channel blocker
Thiazide diuretics	12.5–25 mg/day	May be harmful in volume contracted states such as preeclampsia; initial effect is to decrease plasma volume	Limit use to fluid overload only
Hydralazine	5–10 mg i.v.	May cause fetal distress; flushing, headache, tachycardia, lupus syndrome	Vasodilator used in hypertensive emergencies

b.i.d., twice a day; q.d., every day; t.i.d., three times a day; XL extended release.

All the drugs probably cross the placenta and enter the fetal circulation. The aforementioned antihypertensive drugs have not been known to cause birth defects. Antihypertensive medication that works through the renin–angiotensin system is associated with congenital renal anomalies and is contraindicated.

One should avoid using two antihypertensives of the same class whenever a patient needs more than one agent to control the hypertension. This is most likely to occur for agents acting on the adrenergic system (e.g., avoid combining methyldopa with labetalol). It is better to use a vasodilator such as nifedipine as a second agent.

Antepartum fetal evaluation

Careful dating of gestation is important. Intrauterine growth restriction is usually not seen until after 30–32 weeks' gestation in the majority of patients with mild hypertension not requiring pharmacotherapy. Antepartum fetal evaluation should include sonography for the establishment of gestational age and then serial ultrasound to diagnose intrauterine growth restriction. Serial sonograms should be performed as clinically indicated, generally at 4-week intervals. If interval growth is not appropriate or estimated fetal weight is below the tenth percentile, umbilical artery Doppler velocimetry should be assessed.

Twice-weekly antenatal testing, consisting of nonstress tests or biophysical profiles, and weekly amniotic fluid assessment should begin at 32 weeks in patients with moderate or severe hypertension and for all patients receiving pharmacotherapy. Patients should be instructed on performing fetal movement assessment at home. It is generally recommended that patients assess fetal movement by counting the number of perceived movements that occur in 1 hour, or the length of time required for 10 movements.

Indications for delivery

Most pregnant patients with mild chronic hypertension remain stable. Delivery should be considered whenever any of the following exist:

1 Superimposed preeclampsia of any severity at term.

2 Severe preeclampsia or eclampsia at any gestational age.

3 Evidence of fetal compromise, low biophysical profile, persistently non-reactive nonstress test (NST) or repetitive decelerations at any gestational age.

4 Documentation of fetal lung maturity.

5 Moderate or severe chronic hypertension at or beyond 37–38 weeks' gestation.

Generally, the patient should not be permitted to go beyond term, and often delivery prior to the 38th week of gestation is necessary. Chronic hypertension is associated with a doubling in the rate of abruptio placentae. Among those with mild chronic hypertension, their risk for abruption is 0.7–1.4%, but increases to 5–10% for women with severe hypertension [13].

If the patient develops preeclampsia, hospitalization and early delivery may be indicated. Expectant management in selected cases of severe preeclampsia prior to 34 weeks' gestation may be considered to maximize perinatal outcome, within the bounds of maternal safety. Stable patients may be delivered before 37 weeks after documentation of fetal lung maturity. Expert opinion suggests that pregnancy in patients with chronic hypertension should not be allowed to advance beyond 40 weeks.

Postpartum follow-up

Women who have chronic hypertension usually do well during pregnancy, although 5–10% with severe hypertension have major catastrophic events [13]. Many of these women have completed their childbearing and can be offered a permanent form of contraception. Oral contraceptives are not contraindicated and can be prescribed postpartum; a barrier form of contraception is an alternative. Long-term follow-up includes monitoring of blood pressure and appropriate laboratory studies to address long-term cardiovascular health.

Case presentation

A physician must be diligent when evaluating hypertension during pregnancy. The initial steps in diagnostic evaluation require careful consideration of the clinical history of the patient.

A 40-year-old G3P2 presented to her physician in the second trimester with systolic blood pressures 130–140 mmHg and diastolic measurements of 90–100 mmHg. A 24-hour urine collection revealed 351 mg/24 hours of protein and creatinine clearance of 162 mL/min. The remaining laboratory findings were in the accepted normal range of reference for the laboratory. Because she had evidence of end-organ damage, antihypertensive medications were started.

The patient had persistent hypertension and proteinuria that would suggest preeclampsia. However, she also had hypertension in a prior pregnancy. This should raise suspicion that her hypertension is related to essential hypertension. She subsequently presented at 37 weeks with an increase in her blood pressure despite antihypertensive medication and 930 mg protein in 24 hours. Labor was induced. She stopped her medication during the postpartum period and 12

weeks after delivery still had blood pressures greater than 140/90 mmHg. She should be followed by a primary care physician for long-term management of hypertension and to address her cardiovascular health.

References

1 Report of the National High Blood Pressure Education Program Working Group on High Blood Pressure in Pregnancy. *Am J Obstet Gynecol* 2000;**183**:S1–S22.

2 Chesley LC. Remote prognosis after eclampsia. *Perspect Nephrol Hypertens* 1976;**5**:31–40.

3 Chesley SC, Annitto JE, Cosgrove RA. The remote prognosis of eclamptic women. Sixth periodic report. *Am J Obstet Gynecol* 1976;**124**:446–59.

4 Sibai BM, Lindheimer M, Hauth J, *et al.* Risk factors for preeclampsia, abruptio placentae, and adverse neonatal outcomes among women with chronic hypertension. *N Engl J Med* 1998;**339**:667–71.

5 Funai EF, Friedlander Y, Paltiel O, *et al.* Long-term mortality after preeclampsia. *Epidemiology* 2005;**16**:206–15.

6 Martinovic J, Benachi A, Laurent N, *et al.* Fetal toxic effects and angiotensin-II-receptor antagonists. *Lancet* 2001;**358**:241–2.

7 Piper JM, Ray WA, Rosa FW. Pregnancy outcome following exposure to angiotensin-converting enzyme inhibitors. *Obstet Gynecol* 1992;**80**:429–32.

8 Browne JC, Veall N. The maternal placental blood flow in normotensive and hypertensive women. *J Obstet Gynaecol Br Emp* 1953;**60**:141–7.

9 Fisher KA, Luger A, Spargo BH, Lindheimer MD. Hypertension in pregnancy: clinical-pathological correlations and remote prognosis. *Medicine (Baltimore)* 1981;**60**:267–76.

10 Ihle BU, Long P, Oats J. Early onset pre-eclampsia: recognition of underlying renal disease. *Br Med J (Clin Res Ed)* 1987;**294**:79–81.

11 Rayburn WF, Zuspan FP, Piehl EJ. Self-monitoring of blood pressure during pregnancy. *Am J Obstet Gynecol* 1984;**148**:159–62.

12 Symonds EM. Bed rest in pregnancy. *Br J Obstet Gynaecol* 1982;**89**:593–5.

13 Sibai BM. Chronic hypertension in pregnancy. *Obstet Gynecol* 2002;**100**:369–77.

14 Bayliss H, Churchill D, Beevers M, Beevers DG. Antihypertensive drugs in pregnancy and fetal growth: evidence for "pharmacological programming" in the first trimester? *Hypertens Pregnancy* 2002;**21**:161–74.

26 Systemic lupus erythematosus

Benjamin Hamar and Edmund Funai

Systemic lupus erythematosus (SLE) is a chronic autoimmune disorder characterized by periods of disease flares and remissions. It is a heterogeneous disorder with a variety of clinical and laboratory manifestations. It can follow a relatively benign course, affecting only the skin and musculoskeletal system, or be more aggressive with life-threatening involvement of vital organs such as the kidney and brain.

Epidemiology

The prevalence of SLE varies with the population studied but is generally 5–125 per 100,000 and affects approximately 1% of pregnancies [1]. The lifetime risk of a woman developing SLE is 1 in 700, with a peak incidence at age 30 [2]. Lupus affects women 3–10 times as often as men and disproportionately affects African-Americans and Hispanics [2,3].

Etiology

There is no known etiology for SLE. However, genetic linkage studies in the chromosome 1q41-42 region provide evidence to support a genetic predisposition or causal relationship, although the exact mechanism is unknown [4]. Efforts to determine the specific genes responsible for development of SLE are underway in several laboratories across the country. It is clear that multiple genes are involved, many likely related to pathways of B- and T-cell biology and immune clearance mechanisms.

Pathogenesis

Autoantibodies in SLE have a key role in mediating many of the disease effects. Lupus anticoagulant and other antiphospholipid antibodies (APA) increase the risk for thrombosis [5]. Renal damage is secondary to immune complex deposition, complement activation, and inflammation and subsequent fibrosis [3].

Placentas from women with SLE demonstrate characteristic changes: reduction in size, placental infarctions, intraplacental hemorrhage, deposition of immunoglobulin and complement, and thickening of the trophoblast basement membrane [6,7]. These changes appear to be responsible for many of the effects of SLE on pregnancy outlined below (e.g., increased rates of preeclampsia, intrauterine growth restriction [IUGR], preterm delivery).

The American Rheumatism Association (now called the American College of Rheumatology) outlined diagnostic criteria in 1982 which were formally revised in 1997 and are outlined in Table 26.1 [8,9]. Patients must fulfill at least four of the 11 criteria at some point in the course of their disease, although not necessarily at the same time. These criteria have been found to be 96% sensitive and 96% specific for the diagnosis of SLE [8]. Women with lupus can develop a number of systemic manifestations including arthralgias, rashes, renal abnormalities, neurologic complications, thromboemboli, myocarditis, and serositis [3].

Lupus is characterized by a variety of autoantibodies with diagnostic and prognostic implications. Antinuclear antibody (ANA) is the most common antibody for screening for autoimmune syndromes. However, 10% of asymptomatic pregnant women without autoimmune disease have ANA antibodies compared to 2% of nonpregnant controls [10]. Because of the high prevalence in the general population, ANA is used mainly as a screening test for lupus. Antibodies to double stranded DNA (dsDNA) and Smith (Sm) are more specific for lupus and anti-dsDNA has been correlated with disease activity (generally renal involvement). Anti-SSA/Ro and anti-SSB/La are more often associated with Sjögren syndrome but are also found in 20–40% of women with SLE and are associated with neonatal lupus syndrome [11,12].

Lupus flares are difficult to characterize, as they represent worsening of a heterogeneous disease process. A variety of scoring systems have been developed to measure SLE disease

Table 26.1 Criteria for diagnosis of SLE.

Criterion	Definition
1 Malar rash	Fixed erythema, flat or raised, over the malar eminences, tending to spare the nasolabial folds
2 Discoid rash	Erythematous raised patches with adherent keratotic scaling and follicular plugging; atrophic scarring may occur in older lesions
3 Photosensitivity	Skin rash as a result of unusual reaction to sunlight, by patient history or physician observation
4 Oral ulcers	Oral or nasopharyngeal ulceration, usually painless, observed by a physician
5 Arthritis	Nonerosive arthritis involving two or more peripheral joints, characterized by tenderness, swelling, or effusion
6 Serositis	(a) Pleuritis—convincing history of pleuritic pain or rub heard by a physician or evidence of pleural effusion *or* (b) Pericarditis—documented by ECG or rub or evidence of pericardial effusion
7 Renal disorder	(a) Persistent proteinuria greater than 0.5 g/day or greater than 3+ proteinuria if quantitation is not performed *or* (b) Cellular casts—may be red cell, hemoglobin, granular, tubular, or mixed
8 Neurologic disorder	(a) Seizures—in the absence of offending drugs or known metabolic derangements (e.g., uremia, ketoacidosis, or electrolyte imbalance) *or* (b) Psychosis—in the absence of offending drugs or known metabolic derangements (e.g., uremia, ketoacidosis, or electrolyte imbalance)
9 Hematologic disorder	(a) Hemolytic anemia—with reticulocytosis *or* (b) Leukopenia—less than 4000/mm^3 on 2 or more occasions *or* (c) Lymphopenia—less than 1500/mm^3 on 2 or more occasions *or* (d) Thrombocytopenia—less than 100,000/mm^3 in the absence of offending drugs

10 Immunologic disorder	(a) Anti-DNA antibody
	or
	(b) Anti-Sm antibody
	or
	(c) Positive findings of antiphospholipid antibodies based on:
	  (i) Abnormal serum level of IgG or IgM anticardiolipin antibodies
	  or
	  (ii) Positive test result for lupus anticoagulant
	  or
	  (iii) False-positive serologic test for syphilis known to be positive for at least 6 months and confirmed by *Treponema pallidum* immobilization or fluorescent treponemal antibody absorption test

11 Antinuclear antibody	An abnormal titer of antinuclear antibody by immunofluorescence or an equivalent assay at any point in time and in the absence of drugs known to be associated with "drug-induced lupus" syndrome

A person is classified as having SLE if any 4 of the 11 criteria are present (serially or simultaneously) during any interval of the evaluation.

From:

Tan EM, *et al*. The 1982 revised criteria for the classification of systemic lupus erythematosus. *Arth Rheum* 1982; **25** (11): 1271–7.

Hochberg MC. Updating the American college of rheumatology revised criteria for the classification of systemic lupus erythematosus (letter). *Arth Rheum* 1997; **40** (9): 1725.

status and to aid the diagnosis of a flare. Symptoms of flares include fatigue, fever, arthralgias/myalgias, weight loss, rash, renal deterioration, serositis, lymphadenopathy, and central nervous system symptoms. The titer of antibodies to Sm, RNP, SSA/Ro, or SSB/La may or may not fluctuate in parallel with disease flares. However, rising titers of antibodies to dsDNA (particularly in the setting of falling complement levels) may suggest an impending flare of disease and thus should trigger closer surveillance of the patient [13].

Differential diagnosis

The main differential diagnosis for SLE is between other rheumatologic and connective tissue disorders. Many of these autoimmune diseases share common diagnostic criteria and it may take time for the varied manifestations of these diseases to appear for ultimate diagnosis. Additionally, because of the varied nature of the criteria for diagnosis, patients presenting with several of the criteria could have other local or systemic disorders.

During pregnancy, differentiation of SLE from normal pregnancy symptoms or preeclampsia can be challenging. Lupus flares often feature inflammatory arthritis, significant leukopenia or thrombocytopenia, inflammatory rashes, pleuritis, and fevers. Many of the manifestations of SLE flare can be similar to preeclampsia (hypertension, proteinuria, activation of the coagulation cascade) although the treatment for each is very different. The treatment for severe preeclampsia often involves delivery, while lupus flares can be treated and the pregnancy can be allowed to continue. A rising anti-dsDNA titer, active urinary sediment, and low complement levels (C3, C4, and CH50) suggest a lupus flare [13–15]. In general, complement levels rise in pregnancy and are unaffected by uncomplicated preeclampsia. Conversely, rising uric acid levels or a greater coagulopathy suggest severe preeclampsia and HELLP (hemolysis, elevated liver enzymes, and low platelet count) syndrome. As the pregnancy approaches term, efforts at discriminating between the two are not likely to be worthwhile: delivery will cure preeclampsia and if the symptoms do not improve, treatment of lupus flare can be initiated.

Morbidity

General morbidity and mortality

Because of the effect of SLE on multiple organ systems, patients with this disease have significantly increased morbidity and mortality. Women with SLE are more prone to cardiovascular disease, thromboembolic phenomena, infection, and renal disease [1]. With better understanding of the disease process and potential complications, survival rates have improved with 5, 10, 15, and 20 year survival rates of 93, 85, 79, and 68%, respectively [16]. Risk factors for mortality include renal damage, thrombocytopenia, lung involvement, high disease activity at diagnosis, and age ≥50 at diagnosis [16]. A summary of the effect of SLE on pregnancy and pregnancy on SLE can be found in Table 26.2.

Table 26.2 Systemic lupus erythematosus (SLE) and pregnancy.

Effect of SLE on Pregnancy	Effect of Pregnancy on SLE
Increased stillbirth rate (25 times baseline)	Worsening of renal status if nephropathy present
Increased preeclampsia rate (20–30%)	Increased flare rates (higher if active at start of pregnancy)
Increased growth restriction rate (12–32%)	
Increased preterm delivery rate (50–60%)	
Increased PPROM rate	
Neonatal lupus (1–2% if α-SSA/SSB present)	

PPROM, preterm premature rupture of membranes.

Effects of pregnancy on SLE

During pregnancy, there is a shift in cytokines from a type 1 helper T response (Th1) to a type 2 helper T response (Th2) pattern with predominance of the anti-inflammatory and pro-B-cell cytokines interleukin-4 (IL-4) and IL-10 [2]. Because SLE is largely a humorally mediated autoimmune syndrome, one might expect that this cytokine shift may worsen the disease process or increase the rate of lupus flares in pregnancy [2].

Because of the heterogeneity of lupus patients and the variety of diagnostic criteria for lupus flares, there have been conflicting data regarding whether SLE exacerbations are more frequent in pregnancy. Some of the contributing factors to this controversy involve the variation in criteria for diagnosing lupus flares and the inherent heterogeneity of patients with lupus with different severity and activity of their lupus [2]. Consequently, the literature data for incidence of lupus flares range from 13% to 74% [17–20]. It is generally believed that the risk for flare in pregnancy is increased if women are not in remission prior to becoming pregnant [2,21]. Approximately 35% of flares occur in the second trimester with another 35% occurring postpartum [18,22]. The majority of flares are minor and do not require immunosuppressive therapy; however, serious manifestations can occur. Ruiz-Irastorza *et al.* [22] found flare rates were higher in pregnancy than nonpregnant controls. When the pregnant women were followed for the year postpartum, they found that the women flared more frequently during pregnancy compared to the year following their deliveries. However, the flares during pregnancy were no more severe than those experienced by the nonpregnant controls or postpartum. Other authors have found equivalent rates of flares in pregnancy compared with nonpregnant controls [21,23].

Lupus nephropathy is the end result of autoimmune-mediated inflammation and renal damage. Pregnancy causes a worsening in renal function in approximately 20% of women with nephropathy but is reversible 95% of the time [24]. The risk of renal deterioration is directly correlated with prepregnant renal status. Additionally, poor renal function is correlated with poor pregnancy outcome, with higher loss rates seen in women with nephrotic proteinuria or baseline creatinine above 1.5 mg/dL. Women with renal disease are also more likely to have pregnancies complicated by gestational hypertension, preeclampsia, growth restriction, and premature birth [25].

Effects of SLE on pregnancy

Pregnancy outcome and risk of stillbirth are related to the baseline disease status prior to pregnancy and do not appear to be affected by the presence or absence of flares in pregnancy [26]. Stillbirth rates in women with SLE have been found to be 150 per 1000 births, 25 times the national average [27]. Much of the effect of SLE on fetal loss rates has been attributed to concomitant antiphospholipid antibody syndrome (APS) [26,28], and approximately 30% of women with SLE have APA [3]. If SLE is diagnosed during pregnancy, complication rates and fetal loss rates are increased. In women with active renal disease, pregnancy loss rates are as high as 30%, and for women with more advanced renal disease fetal loss rates approach 60% [25]. Women with stable lupus nephritis and plasma creatinine values less than 1.5 mg/dL, proteinuria less than 2 g/24 hours, and no hypertension have lower risks of adverse pregnancy outcome [25]. A past history of cyclophosphamide therapy is associated with premature ovarian failure and chronic steroid administration can lead to amenorrhea.

Pregnancy complications are seen more frequently in women with SLE than in controls or in women who later develop SLE [29]. Preeclampsia occurs in 20–30% of women with SLE with higher rates seen in women with underlying hypertension, renal disease, or APS [7,25,27]. IUGR has been reported in 12–32% of lupus pregnancies, which was found to be higher than control populations [19,27,30]. Preterm birth is increased in SLE pregnancies, with rates as high as 50–60% resulting from preeclampsia, IUGR, abnormal fetal testing, and preterm premature rupture of membranes (PPROM) [19,30,31]. Rupture of membranes in women with SLE is more common in preterm and term pregnancies when compared with controls and appears to be unrelated to disease status, treatment, or serology [31].

Neonatal lupus erythematosus (NLE) occurs in 1–2% of women with anti-SSA/Ro or anti-SSB/La antibodies regardless of whether she also has SLE [12]. The pathophysiology is thought to be a result of immune-mediated damage of the fetus by transplacental autoantibodies with resulting inflammation. The syndrome is most commonly characterized by fetal and neonatal congenital heart block (CHB), skin lesions, and occasionally thrombocytopenia, anemia, and hepatitis [12]. While the other manifestations are transient humorally

mediated effects with resolution in the first few months of life, CHB is a permanent condition. The anti-SSA/Ro and anti-SSB/La maternal antibodies cross the placenta and can damage the atrioventricular conducting system, which results in varying degrees of heart block and less often, a myocarditis. Fetal CHB is most commonly diagnosed between 18 and 24 weeks' gestation [32]. These autoantibodies may act via apoptosis [33], or by direct interference with cardiac conduction through calcium channels [34]. The risk of CHB in women with anti-SSA/Ro antibodies and no prior affected infants is 1–2% [11,12,35] but increases to 19% with a prior affected child [35]. Approximately 50% of women whose fetuses or infants have CHB are asymptomatic but more than 85% are anti-SSA/Ro or anti-SSB/La positive [12,35]. Approximately half of these women will develop symptoms of a rheumatic disease, most often these are dry eyes and mouth consistent with Sjögren syndrome. These women should be reassured that they do not have SLE in the absence of other features and they are less than 50% likely to develop SLE in the future. Although third-degree or "complete" CHB is permanent, there is some observational data that first- or second-degree disease can be reversed with antenatal fluorinated steroid therapy, and that progression to more severe forms of heart block may be prevented [36]. Additionally, steroid therapy has shown some reversal of hydropic features in fetuses with CHB and evidence of cardiac failure [36]. At present, there is no evidence supporting the routine use of prophylactic steroid therapy in women with anti-SSA/Ro or anti-SSB-La antibodies to prevent the onset of CHB [33].

Management during pregnancy

Management of SLE during pregnancy begins with preconceptional counseling. At this time, maternal disease status can be assessed and risks of pregnancy discussed. Evaluation for any pre-existing renal disease is performed with a 24-hour urine collection and serum creatinine to measure proteinuria and creatinine clearance. Remission for 6 months prior to pregnancy reduces adverse outcomes.

Early pregnancy assessment should include assessment of maternal disease status including 24-hour urine collection, plasma creatinine, complete blood count, anti-SSA/Ro antibody, anti-SSB/La antibody, anti-dsDNA antibody, lupus anticoagulant, anticardiolipin antibody, C3, and C4 levels. Repeat anti-dsDNA, 24-hour urine, plasma creatinine, C3, and C4 levels to monitor disease status should be performed each trimester. Lupus anticoagulant and anticardiolipin antibodies can be repeated in the second trimester to screen for development of APS. Early genetic risk assessment is important as lupus pregnancies carry increased maternal risk and early diagnosis of genetic abnormalities gives patients the option of termination of a nonviable pregnancy. Because of the

Table 26.3 Systemic lupus erythematosus (SLE) therapeutic agents.

Drug	Safety in Pregnancy	Comments
Glucocorticoids	Safe Pregnancy class C	Association with growth restriction at high dose, need stress-dose steroids at delivery or for medical illnesses if chronic use through pregnancy. Increased risk of preterm rupture of membranes, preterm delivery
Hydroxychloroquine	Generally considered safe Pregnancy class C	Antimalarial. Reduces disease flares
Non-steroidal anti-inflammatory agents	See comments Pregnancy class B	Association with polyhydramnios, and ductus arteriosus closure. Avoid after 28 weeks
Azathioprine (6-mercaptopurine)	See comments Pregnancy class D	Risk of fetal growth restriction and immunosuppression. Use as second-line agent
Cyclophosphamide	Unsafe Pregnancy class D	Alkylating agent. Skeletal and palate defects, also defects in eyes and limbs
Methotrexate	Unsafe Pregnancy class X	Folic acid antagonist. Abortifacient and teratogen

increased risk of premature delivery, establishment of reliable dating is important.

Prepregnant drug regimens, if safe in pregnancy, should be continued in pregnancy to maintain remission. If antiphospholipid syndrome is also present, anticoagulation can reduce the associated complications [1]. Nonsteroidal anti-inflammatory agents (pregnancy class B) are contraindicated after 28 weeks' gestation because of the risk of closure of the fetal ductus arteriosus. Hydroxychloroquine (pregnancy class C), an antimalarial medication helpful in reducing disease flares, is often maintained during pregnancy. Glucocorticoids (pregnancy class C) are also "safe" in pregnancy although if patients are on chronic steroids, stress-dose steroids should be given at delivery. Azathioprine (pregnancy class D) is an immunosuppressive agent that is metabolized to 6-mercaptopurine and is a cytotoxic purine analog. Most investigators have found azathioprine to be "safe" in pregnancy although there is a risk of growth restriction and fetal immunosuppression. Other cytotoxic agents such as cyclophosphamide (pregnancy class D) and methotrexate (pregnancy class X) are contraindicated in pregnancy and are to be avoided. A summary of medications used in the management of SLE is found in Table 26.3.

Making the diagnosis of lupus flare in pregnancy requires excluding the other diagnoses as outlined above. Flares can be managed conservatively with adjustment of medication regimen as outlined above or addition of analgesics such as acetaminophen. Glucocorticoid therapy can be initiated for more severe flares [7]. The exact treatment of the flare will vary with the nature and severity of the flare.

Fetal surveillance includes genetic risk assessment as well as measures of fetal well-being. Fetal growth is assessed in 4-week intervals in the second and third trimester, with more frequent assessment if growth restriction is suspected. Doppler evaluation is reserved for assessment of fetal well-being if estimated fetal weight is less than the 10th percentile. Weekly nonstress testing with assessment of amniotic fluid can begin at 30 weeks.

When women are followed in an intensive multidisciplinary clinic with pregnancies initiated during disease quiescence and treatment of underlying disease, fetal outcomes appear to be improved. Diagnosis and treatment of APS improves fetal loss rates.

Antiphospholipid antibodies

Antiphospholipid antibodies can be present alone or in conjunction with APS. APS has specific diagnostic criteria and results in thrombosis, adverse pregnancy outcome (including growth restriction and third trimester fetal death), or recurrent pregnancy loss (Table 26.4) [37,38]. Prospective evaluation of women with APS without treatment have shown fetal loss rates as high as 50–90% [39]. APA and lupus anticoagulant (LAC) are found in 1–5% of asymptomatic pregnant women but are higher in SLE patients (12–30% and 15–34%, respectively) [5].

APA and LAC bind to β_2-glycoprotein I, other phospholipid associated proteins, or the phospholipids themselves. β_2-glycoprotein I and annexin V are associated with phospholipids in the cell membrane and inhibit platelet and clotting cascade activation. Both molecules are found in high concentrations on the endothelium and syncytiotrophoblast and are thought to provide a protective layer. Anticardiolipin antibody (ACA) and LAC disrupt this protective layer, activating the clotting cascade and allowing complement-mediated injury to the placental vasculature to occur [40].

Table 26.4 Criteria for the classification of antiphospholipid antibody syndrome. Presence of at least one clinical criterion and one laboratory criterion are necessary for the diagnosis of antiphospholipid antibody syndrome. After Wilson *et al.* [37].

Clinical criteria

1 Vascular thrombosis
2 Pregnancy morbidity
   (a) Unexplained IUFD at ≥10 weeks of a morphologically normal fetus
   (b) Severe preeclampsia/eclampsia or severe placental insufficiency before 34 weeks
   (c) Three or more unexplained spontaneous abortions at <10 weeks

Laboratory criteria

1 Anticardiolipin antibody (IgG or IgM) at moderate or high titer,* on two or more occasions at least 6 weeks apart
2 Lupus anticoagulant present on two or more occasions at least 6 weeks apart

Ig, immunoglobulin; IUFD, intrauterine fetal death.
* Test results for anticardiolipin antibody titers according to standards established by Harris [38]: Negative, 0–10 MPL or GPL; Low-positive, >10–20 MPL or GPL; Moderate >20–80 MPL or GPL; High positive, >80 MPL or GPL.

LAC is detected by the prolongation of various clotting assays with failure to normalize with the addition of control plasma (to exclude factor deficiencies) and is reported as present or absent. The presence of LAC is more specific than ACA for APS. ACA are detected by direct β_2-glycoprotein I dependent immunoassays and are reported by antibody class and low or high titer. It appears that the clinically relevant classes are IgG and IgM at high titer [41]. Although LAC and ACA are frequently concordant and sometimes share epitope specificity, they are distinct entities. Other antibodies have been evaluated including anti-β_2-glycoprotein I antibodies, other anticardiolipin antibody classes, and antibodies to other phospholipids, but their clinical significance is unclear and they are not included in the diagnostic criteria. Although β_2-glycoprotein I antibodies are not included in the diagnostic criteria, it appears that there is an association with some of the clinical features of APS.

Treatment goals include improvement of fetal outcomes and reduction in risk for maternal thrombosis. Historic treatment consisted of aspirin (pregnancy class C) or glucocorticoids (pregnancy class C). However, heparin (pregnancy class C) was shown to be as effective as steroids (without the risk for PPROM associated with chronic steroid use), and has become the standard therapy. Either unfractionated or low molecular weight heparin (LMWH) may be used (pregnancy class B). A recent meta-analysis showed that the live birth rate was improved by 54% with heparin and aspirin therapy [42]. One cautionary note is that despite anticoagulation, 20–30% of women with APS have fetal losses. Intravenous immunoglobulin (IVIG) has been shown to be effective, although the cost and side-effects currently limit it to women with severe APS or those who have been refractory to heparin therapy. Aspirin therapy can be initiated at the first positive pregnancy test and heparin therapy can be initiated at 5–7 weeks' gestation. As there is no maternal blood flow through the placenta prior to 5–7 weeks, heparin is not necessary before this point and may potentiate implantation bleeding. Heparin therapy can either be therapeutic (i.e., 1 mg/kg enoxaparin every 12 hours with maintenance of anti-Xa levels between 0.5 and 1.0) or prophylactic (i.e., 40 mg/day enoxaparin). It is not our practice to follow anti-Xa levels in those women receiving prophylactic heparin treatment. A platelet count should be obtained within 2 weeks of initiation of therapy. Because of the 1–2% risk of osteoporosis and fracture with unfractionated heparin anticoagulation in pregnancy [43], we recommend daily calcium, vitamin D supplementation, and daily weight-bearing exercise as tolerated. Recent data suggest that LMWH anticoagulation during pregnancy does not significantly affect bone mineral density [44]. At 36 weeks, aspirin can be discontinued and LMWH switched to unfractionated heparin to facilitate anticoagulation management at delivery. Postpartum anticoagulation (if indicated) can be with either warfarin or LMWH.

Treatment of APS during pregnancy with active fetal surveillance has shown improved outcomes. Nonetheless, antepartum complications remain common with elevated rates of preeclampsia, growth restriction, and premature birth [5].

Case presentation

The patient is a 32-year-old G5P1 at 7 weeks' gestation with a history of a term vaginal delivery 7 years ago to an infant with second-degree heart block. She had three subsequent miscarriages at approximately 10 weeks' gestation. An evaluation revealed the presence of anti-SSA antibodies, ANA positive, dilute Russell viper venum test positive, as well as high titer IgG ACA. She also complains of periodic arthralgias and has had persistent proteinuria. What is her diagnosis and what therapy recommendations and prognosis can be given for her current pregnancy?

The patient can be diagnosed with APS because of her high-titer ACA and recurrent first trimester miscarriages. Additionally, she meets the criteria for SLE (ANA, ACA, arthralgias, renal disease). She has a 19% chance of another child with CHB and a substantial risk of miscarriage given her prior losses. Additionally, she has increased risk for preeclampsia, growth restriction, PPROM, and preterm delivery. She can be offered aspirin and heparin therapy for her APS and close fetal surveillance to monitor for the development of heart block or growth restriction. Therapy for SLE should be reviewed and optimized for her pregnancy. Her renal status should be assessed and a baseline cardiac evaluation including electrocardiography would not be unreasonable.

References

1 Ruiz-Irastorza G, Khamashta MA, Castellino G, Hughes GR. Systemic lupus erythematosus. *Lancet* 2001;**357**:1027–32.

2 Buyon JP. The effects of pregnancy on autoimmune diseases. *J Leukoc Biol* 1998;**63**:281–7.

3 Mills JA. Systemic lupus erythematosus. *N Engl J Med* 1994;**330**:1871–9.

4 Criswell LA, Amos CI. Update on genetic risk factors for systemic lupus erythematosus and rheumatoid arthritis. *Curr Opin Rheumatol* 2000;**12**:85–90.

5 Levine JS, Branch DW, Rauch J. The antiphospholipid syndrome. *N Engl J Med* 2002;**346**:752–63.

6 Hanly JG, Gladman DD, Rose TH, Laskin CA, Urowitz MB. Lupus pregnancy: a prospective study of placental changes. *Arthritis Rheum* 1988;**31**:358–66.

7 Lockshin MD, Sammaritano LR. Lupus pregnancy. *Autoimmunity* 2003;**36**:33–40.

8 Tan EM, Cohen AS, Fries JF, *et al*. The 1982 revised criteria for the classification of systemic lupus erythematosus. *Arthritis Rheum* 1982;**25**:1271–7.

9 Hochberg MC. Updating the American College of Rheumatology revised criteria for the classification of systemic lupus erythematosus. *Arthritis Rheum* 1997;**40**:1725.

10 Farnam J, Lavastida MT, Grant JA, Reddi RC, Daniels JC. Antinuclear antibodies in the serum of normal pregnant women: a prospective study. *J Allergy Clin Immunol* 1984;**73**:596–9.

11 Gladman G, Silverman ED, Yuk L, *et al*. Fetal echocardiographic screening of pregnancies of mothers with anti-Ro and/or anti-La antibodies. *Am J Perinatol* 2002;**19**:73–80.

12 Lee LA. Neonatal lupus erythematosus. *J Invest Dermatol* 1993;**100**:9S–13S.

13 Repke JT. Hypertensive disorders of pregnancy: differentiating preeclampsia from active systemic lupus erythematosus. *J Reprod Med* 1998;**43**:350–4.

14 Buyon JP, Tamerius J, Ordorica S, Young B, Abramson SB. Activation of the alternative complement pathway accompanies disease flares in systemic lupus erythematosus during pregnancy. *Arthritis Rheum* 1992;**35**:55–61.

15 Abramson SB, Buyon JP. Activation of the complement pathway: comparison of normal pregnancy, preeclampsia, and systemic lupus erythematosus during pregnancy. *Am J Reprod Immunol* 1992;**28**:183–7.

16 Abu-Shakra M, Urowitz MB, Gladman DD, Gough J. Mortality studies in systemic lupus erythematosus. Results from a single center. II. Predictor variables for mortality. *J Rheumatol* 1995;**22**:1265–70.

17 Lockshin MD. Pregnancy does not cause systemic lupus erythematosus to worsen. *Arthritis Rheum* 1989;**32**:665–70.

18 Carmona F, Font J, Cervera R, Munoz F, Cararach V, Balasch J. Obstetrical outcome of pregnancy in patients with systemic lupus erythematosus: a study of 60 cases. *Eur J Obstet Gynecol Reprod Biol* 1999;**83**:137–42.

19 Mintz G, Niz J, Gutierrez G, Garcia-Alonso A, Karchmer S. Prospective study of pregnancy in systemic lupus erythematosus: results of a multidisciplinary approach. *J Rheumatol* 1986;**13**:732–9.

20 Nossent HC, Swaak TJ. Systemic lupus erythematosus. VI. Analysis of the interrelationship with pregnancy. *J Rheumatol* 1990;**17**:771–6.

21 Urowitz MB, Gladman DD, Farewell VT, Stewart J, McDonald J. Lupus and pregnancy studies. *Arthritis Rheum* 1993;**36**:1392–7.

22 Ruiz-Irastorza G, Lima F, Alves J, *et al*. Increased rate of lupus flare during pregnancy and the puerperium: a prospective study of 78 pregnancies. *Br J Rheumatol* 1996;**35**:133–8.

23 Lockshin MD, Reinitz E, Druzin ML, Murrman M, Estes D. Lupus pregnancy: case–control prospective study demonstrating absence of lupus exacerbation during or after pregnancy. *Am J Med* 1984;**77**:893–8.

24 Packham DK, Lam SS, Nicholls K, Fairley KF, Kincaid-Smith PS. Lupus nephritis and pregnancy. *Q J Med* 1992;**83**:315–24.

25 Hayslett JP, Lynn RI. Effect of pregnancy in patients with lupus nephropathy. *Kidney Int* 1980;**18**:207–20.

26 Faussett MB, Branch DW. Autoimmunity and pregnancy loss. *Semin Reprod Med* 2000;**18**:379–92.

27 Simpson LL. Maternal medical disease: risk of antepartum fetal death. *Semin Perinatol* 2002;**26**:42–50.

28 Ginsberg JS, Brill-Edwards P, Johnston M, *et al*. Relationship of antiphospholipid antibodies to pregnancy loss in patients with systemic lupus erythematosus: a cross-sectional study. *Blood* 1992;**80**:975–80.

29 Kiss E, Bhattoa HP, Bettembuk P, Balogh A, Szegedi G. Pregnancy in women with systemic lupus erythematosus. *Eur J Obstet Gynecol Reprod Biol* 2002;**101**:129–34.

30 Lima F, Buchanan NM, Khamashta MA, Kerslake S, Hughes GR. Obstetric outcome in systemic lupus erythematosus. *Semin Arthritis Rheum* 1995;**25**:184–92.

31 Johnson MJ, Petri M, Witter FR, Repke JT. Evaluation of preterm delivery in a systemic lupus erythematosus pregnancy clinic. *Obstet Gynecol* 1995;**86**:396–9.

32 Buyon JP, Waltuck J, Kleinman C, Copel J. In utero identification and therapy of congenital heart block. *Lupus* 1995;**4**:116–21.

33 Buyon JP, Clancy RM. Maternal autoantibodies and congenital heart block: mediators, markers, and therapeutic approach. *Semin Arthritis Rheum* 2003;**33**:140–54.

34 Boutjdir M. Molecular and ionic basis of congenital complete heart block. *Trends Cardiovasc Med* 2000;**10**:114–22.

35 Buyon JP, Rupel A, Clancy RM. Neonatal lupus syndromes. *Lupus* 2004;**13**:705–12.

36 Saleeb S, Copel J, Friedman D, Buyon JP. Comparison of treatment with fluorinated glucocorticoids to the natural history of autoantibody-associated congenital heart block: retrospective review of the research registry for neonatal lupus. *Arthritis Rheum* 1999;**42**:2335–45.

37 Wilson WA, Gharavi AE, Koike T, *et al*. International consensus statement on preliminary classification criteria for definite antiphospholipid syndrome: report of an international workshop. *Arthritis Rheum* 1999;**42**:1309–11.

38 Harris EN. Antiphospholipid antibodies. *Br J Haematol* 1990;**74**:1–9.

39 Warren JB, Silver RM. Autoimmune disease in pregnancy: systemic lupus erythematosus and antiphospholipid syndrome. *Obstet Gynecol Clin North Am* 2004;**31**:345–72, vi–vii.

40 Salmon JE, Girardi G, Holers VM. Activation of complement mediates antiphospholipid antibody-induced pregnancy loss. *Lupus* 2003;**12**:535–8.

41 Silver RM, Porter TF, van Leeuween I, Jeng G, Scott JR, Branch DW. Anticardiolipin antibodies: clinical consequences of "low titers". *Obstet Gynecol* 1996;**87**:494–500.

42 Empson M, Lassere M, Craig JC, Scott JR. Recurrent pregnancy loss with antiphospholipid antibody: a systematic review of therapeutic trials. *Obstet Gynecol* 2002;**99**:135–44.

43 Dahlman TC. Osteoporotic fractures and the recurrence of thromboembolism during pregnancy and the puerperium in 184 women undergoing thromboprophylaxis with heparin. *Am J Obstet Gynecol* 1993;**168**:1265–70.

44 Pettila V, Leinonen P, Markkola A, Hiilesmaa V, Kaaja R. Postpartum bone mineral density in women treated for thromboprophylaxis with unfractionated heparin or LMW heparin. *Thromb Haemost* 2002;**87**:182–6.

Perinatal infections

Jeanne S. Sheffield

Perinatal infections, some of which are summarized in the acronym TORCH (toxoplasmosis, rubella, cytomegalovirus, herpes virus), continue to plague pregnancies both in the USA and worldwide. Most perinatal infections are asymptomatic in the mother but may have devastating consequences to the fetus. In the last decade, many advances in maternal and fetal diagnosis as well as treatment have occurred and will be addressed.

Parvovirus B$_{19}$

Parvovirus B$_{19}$, a single-stranded DNA virus, is the only parvovirus causing human disease (erythema infectiosum or Fifth disease). It is an endemic viral infection predominantly seen in preschool and school-age children—by adulthood only 40% of women tested are susceptible [1]. Although often asymptomatic in the mother, parvovirus B$_{19}$ replicates in rapidly proliferating cells such as euthyroid progenitor cells, leading to severe anemia in the fetus, young child, and adults with erythrocyte membrane abnormalities or chronic hemolytic anemias.

Transmission

Transmission of parvovirus B$_{19}$ occurs predominantly through respiratory droplets via person-to-person contact. The virus can also be transmitted parenterally through blood or blood product transfusion, or vertically from mother to fetus. Vertical transmission to the fetus occurs in an estimated one-third of pregnancies when the mother is infected [2].

Parvovirus B$_{19}$ infections occur sporadically or in outbreaks in school systems during late winter and early spring. The incubation period is between 4 and 14 days (as high as 20 days in rare instances) and the secondary attack rate among susceptible household contacts approaches 50%. Patients with erythema infectiosum are infectious before the onset of the rash and remain contagious for only 1–2 days after the rash develops. In contrast, women with transient aplastic crisis are infec-

tious prior to the onset of clinical symptoms through the subsequent week. There is no reactivation phase for parvovirus.

Clinical manifestations

There are a number of clinical manifestations of parvovirus B$_{19}$ infection depending on age and comorbid conditions. *Asymptomatic infection* occurs in 20–30% of adult cases. *Erythema infectiosum* or *Fifth disease*, characterized by mild systemic "flu-like" symptoms, fever, and headache may occur in the initial phase of symptomatic infection. In children, facial erythema or a "slapped cheek" rash then develops followed by a lacy reticular rash on the trunk and extremities. Adults often do not develop the facial rash but develop a rash on the trunk and extremities and frequently acute symmetrical polyarthralgias and arthritis. Myocarditis is rarely seen.

Chronic euthyroid hypoplasia and transient aplastic crisis may occur in women with immunodeficiency or chronic hemolytic anemias. Occasionally, this is accompanied by thrombocytopenia and neutropenia.

Fetal infection has been associated with abortion, fetal death, and nonimmune hydrops [3–6]. Fetal loss rates as high as 15% have been reported although the actual risk is debated. Infection under 20 weeks' gestation is associated with an overall increased risk of death compared to late second and third trimester infection. Parvovirus is the most common infectious etiology of nonimmune hydrops and occurs most commonly in fetuses affected in the first 20 weeks of gestation. Fetal hydrops develops in only 1.1% of infected women overall and frequently resolves within 4–6 weeks without intervention. Intrauterine transfusion for the severely anemic fetus may improve survival (see below).

Diagnosis

A pregnant woman suspected of having parvovirus B$_{19}$ because of symptoms or, more commonly, secondary to exposure to an infected child should have serologic testing performed. A serologic assay for the presence of immuno-globulin G (IgG) and IgM parvovirus specific antibodies by enzyme-linked immunosorbent assay (ELISA) or radioimmu-noassay will determine past and recent infection. IgM develops within days of infection and persists for 2–3 months (up to 6 months in rare cases). IgG develops several days later. The absence of IgM and IgG indicates no prior infection and a susceptible individual. Early infection, prior to antibody formation, may also result in this combination and serology should be repeated 1–2 weeks later. IgG alone indicates prior infection and immunity. IgM alone indicates very recent infection, and IgM and IgG both present indicates recent infection 1 week to 6 months previously (Fig. 27.1).

Fetal parvovirus infection should be considered if nonimmune hydrops is detected on sonography. DNA amplification techniques for parvovirus B_{19} using amniotic fluid or fetal blood samples are now the diagnostic test of choice, as they are more sensitive and specific than fetal serology. Fetal IgM is not recommended for diagnosis—the fetus less than 22 weeks is relatively immuno-incompetent and may not form a detectable IgM response.

Management of parvovirus B_{19} in pregnancy

Figure 27.1 details the evaluation and management of human parvovirus B_{19} infection in pregnancy. The vast majority of

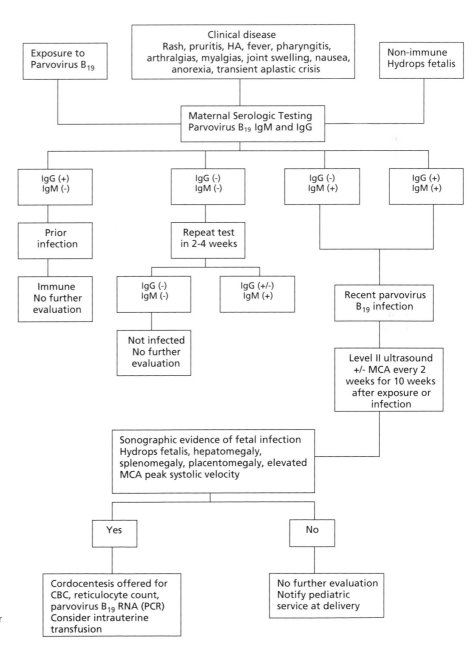

Fig. 27.1 Algorithm for evaluation and management of parvovirus B_{19} infection in pregnancy. MCA, middle cerebral artery Doppler measurements.

fetal parvovirus-associated hydrops occurs in the first 10 weeks after infection—serial sonography every 2 weeks should be performed in women with evidence of recent infection. Middle cerebral artery (MCA) Doppler evaluation may also be used to predict fetal anemia [7,8]. If evidence of fetal infection is noted, a cordocentesis is offered to assess the degree of anemia and confirm infection via DNA or RNA amplification techniques.

At the time of cordocentesis, and depending on gestational age, an intrauterine transfusion may be performed. If a transfusion is performed and the fetus survives, 94% will recover within 6–12 weeks. The overall mortality rate is less than 10% [9–11]. Most fetuses require only one transfusion as fetal hematopoiesis resumes as the parvovirus infection resolves. Long-term neurodevelopmental outcomes of children following intrauterine transfusion for parvovirus infection have recently been reported. No significant delay was noted on standard neurodevelopmental testing, despite severe fetal anemia and intrauterine transfusion [12].

Rubella

Rubella, or German measles, although usually causing a minor maternal illness, is one of the most teratogenic infections known. Fortunately, since the introduction of the rubella vaccine, the incidence of rubella and congenital rubella syndrome has decreased substantially. The number of reported cases in the USA has declined more than 99% over the last three decades, although globally it remains a major issue. Less than 200 cases per year are now seen in the USA.

Pathogenesis and transmission

Rubella is an RNA togavirus with no extrahuman reservoir. Following exposure to the virus via nasopharyngeal secretions, almost 80% of susceptible individuals become infected. Replication occurs in the nasopharynx and regional lymph nodes, with viremia developing 5–7 days after exposure. It is this viremia that results in placental and fetal infection. Adults are infectious during the viremia through 5–7 days of the rash. Subclinical rubella reinfection has been reported during outbreaks, although resultant fetal infection is rare. The peak incidence is in late winter and spring.

Clinical manifestations

After an incubation period of 12–23 days, a prodrome of low-grade fever and malaise, headache, arthralgias, arthritis, pharyngitis, and conjunctivitis develops. A maculopapular rash beginning on the face and spreading to the trunk and extremities occurs in 50–80% of infected women. Posterior cervical, postauricular, and occipital lymphadenopathy is common. Rarely, thrombocytopenia purpura, neuritis, and encephalitis

complicate maternal infection. Up to one-third of women are asymptomatic.

Congenital rubella syndrome is a devastating consequence of maternal infection. The risk of fetal infection varies depending on when in gestation maternal infection occurs. Eighty-five to 90% of pregnant women with rubella in the first trimester have a fetus with congenital infection. As gestation extends beyond 20 weeks, the risk of congenital infection drops markedly. Congenital rubella syndrome may result in abortion and fetal death along with severe infant morbidity. The most common defects are sensorineural deafness, cataracts, heart defects, microcephaly, developmental delay, and mental retardation, although all organs may be affected. Congenitally infected infants shed virus from the throat for 6–12 months following birth and are infectious to susceptible contacts [13].

As many as one-third of asymptomatic neonates at birth will develop late sequelae from fetal infection. Type 1 diabetes, thyroid disease, ocular damage, and progressive panencephalitis may present during the second decade of life [14].

Diagnosis

Although rubella can be isolated from the nasopharynx, urine, and cerebrospinal fluid, the diagnosis of maternal rubella infection usually relies on serologic analysis. Detection of rubella-specific IgM indicates recent infection, although re-exposure to rubella may induce an amnestic response resulting in reappearance of low-titer IgM. Following a primary rubella infection, IgM can be detected within 5–7 days and may persist up to 2 months. Specific IgG develops by 2 weeks and persists for life; re-exposure may increase IgG titers transiently.

As up to 10% of US adults are seronegative and susceptible to infection, rubella immune status should be assessed at initiation of prenatal care. Susceptible women should be counseled regarding prevention strategies and be vaccinated postpartum, as the vaccine is a live attenuated form of the virus.

Women with confirmed maternal rubella in the first 20 weeks of pregnancy should be assessed for fetal infection. Sonography is not a sensitive or specific diagnostic modality. However, cerebral ventriculomegaly, intracranial calcifications, meconium peritonitis, cardiac malformations, hepatosplenomegaly, microcephaly, fetal growth restriction, and microphthalmia have all been found in fetuses subsequently diagnosed with congenital rubella. Diagnosis of fetal rubella using DNA amplification techniques has been reported in a few small series but false-positive and false-negative tests have been noted [15–17].

Management and prevention

There is no treatment for rubella; supportive care should be offered. Droplet precautions are recommended for 7 days after the onset of the rash. Passive immunization using immunoglobulin is not recommended. Primary prevention of rubella relies on comprehensive vaccination programs. The measles-mumps-rubella (MMR) vaccine should be offered to susceptible women of childbearing age. Pregnancy should be avoided for 4 weeks after vaccination as the vaccine is a live attenuated virus with a theoretical malformation risk of 0.5–1.7%. However, if inadvertent vaccination of a pregnant woman does occur, pregnancy termination is no longer recommended as the observed risk to the fetus is minimal. After vaccination, at least 95% of women will seroconvert, developing long-term immunity. Women delivering and who are rubella nonimmune should be offered MMR vaccine prior to discharge. Breastfeeding is safe in those women vaccinated postpartum.

Syphilis

Despite the description of syphilitic infection for more than 500 years and despite the availability of adequate therapy for more than 50 years, syphilis in the adult and neonate remains a nemesis for public health providers. In the USA, in 2004 alone there were 2.7 per 100,000 population new cases of syphilis reported, an increase of 8% from 2003. Although pregnancy itself does not alter the clinical course of syphilis, it is important to diagnose syphilis in pregnancy to ensure prevention of congenital infection and adequate treatment of the mother.

Pathogenesis and transmission

Treponema pallidum, the causative agent of syphilis, is acquired in women primarily by intimate contact with an infected partner. Minute abrasions in the vaginal mucosa provide a portal of entry for the spirochete. The cervical changes associated with pregnancy including eversion or ectropion, hyperemia, and friability increase the risk of spirochete entry. Local replication then occurs and lymphatic dissemination leads to the systemic findings of secondary syphilis. The incubation period averages 3 weeks (3–90 days) depending on inoculum load and host factors [18]. The early stages of syphilis—primary, secondary, and early latent syphilis—are associated with the highest spirochete loads and transmission rates of 30–50% [19–21]. Transmission rates in late-stage disease are much lower.

Fetal acquisition of syphilitic infection may occur by several means. Transplacental passage is the most common. *T. pallidum* has been isolated in the placenta, umbilical cord, and amniotic fluid [22–29]. Transmission may also occur across the membranes or by direct contact with the lesions at delivery. The risk of fetal infection increases as pregnancy advances but infection may occur at any gestational age.

Risk factors associated with maternal syphilis include young age, being black or Hispanic, single, low socioeconomic status, less education, inadequate prenatal care, prostitution, and substance abuse.

Clinical manifestations

Pregnancy has little effect on the clinical course of syphilis. Syphilis, however, has a major impact on pregnancy. Preterm delivery, stillbirth, spontaneous abortion, neonatal demise, and congenital infection are all increased. The fetal risk is directly related to the stage of disease and level of maternal spirochetemia. Maternal syphilis infection is staged according to disease duration and clinical features. Primary syphilis is the initial stage—the chancre is the characteristic lesion. The chancre is usually painless with a smooth base and a red, raised, firm border. The painless nature of the chancre and its location may explain why women often are not diagnosed until later stages. If untreated it will resolve in 3–8 weeks and the woman will progress to the secondary stage.

Secondary syphilis is the time of systemic dissemination which involves many major organ systems. Ninety percent of women with secondary syphilis have dermatologic manifestations. A diffuse macular rash will develop on the trunk and proximal extremities. Plantar and palmar maculopapular target-like lesions are commonly seen. Patchy alopecia may result when hair follicles are involved. Mucosal lesions called mucous patches will develop in 35% of women. These manifest as silver-gray, painless, superficial erosions of the genital, anal, or oral mucosa. They are highly infectious, with very high spirochete loads.

Genital tract involvement will occur in 20% of women at this stage. Condyloma lata (white-gray raised plaques) develop along with generalized lymphadenopathy. Constitutional symptoms are also common in secondary syphilis (70%), with low-grade fever, malaise, anorexia, headache, arthralgias, and myalgias most commonly seen. Finally, 40% of women will have cerebrospinal fluid abnormalities, although only 1–2% will develop aseptic meningitis.

Again, if untreated, the lesions will resolve and the woman will enter the latent stages of syphilis. Early latent syphilis is latent syphilis of less than 12 months' duration. During this stage, 20–25% of women will relapse. Late latent syphilis is diagnosed after being asymptomatic for more than 12 months. The woman is still infectious during latent stages, although the risk decreases with time. Eventually, 20–30% of untreated women will progress to tertiary syphilis.

Tertiary syphilis, involving the integument, cardiovascular, and neurologic systems, is rarely seen in reproductive age women.

Congenital syphilis is rare before 18 weeks' gestation. Common findings of congenital syphilis in the nursery include hepatosplenomegaly, rash, reticuloendothelial abnormalities, osteochondritis, periostitis, rhinitis, and central nervous system (CNS) involvement. Late congenital syphilis, presenting after 2 years of life and often in early adolescence, includes

Hutchinson teeth, interstitial keratitis, and eight nerve deafness (Hutchinson triad) as well as mental retardation, seizures, saddle nose deformity, frontal bossing, saber shins, and cranial nerve palsies. Congenital syphilis is one of the only sexually transmitted diseases infecting a neonate that can be prevented or treated *in utero*.

Diagnosis

Diagnosis of maternal syphilis is commonly performed using a nontreponemal serologic screening test, with a treponemal serologic test used for confirmation. Pregnant women should be screened at the initial visit. A repeat screen may be mandated by state regulation or indicated by maternal risk. The screening tests used are the Rapid Plasma Reagin (RPR) or the Venereal Disease Research Laboratory (VDRL) test. They can be quantitated and usually become negative with adequate therapy, allowing them to be used for follow-up. However, the false-positive rate is approximately 1%, so a positive test must be confirmed using a treponemal test. The treponemal tests used are the fluorescent treponemal antibody absorption (FTA-Abs) test, the microhemagglutination assay for antibodies to *T. pallidum* (MHA-TP), and the *T. pallidum* passive particle agglutination (TP-PA) test.

The diagnosis of congenital syphilis prenatally is difficult. Sonographic findings may include hydrops fetalis, hepatomegaly, placental thickening, and hydramnios, but often the infected fetus will have a normal sonogram. Polymerase chain reaction (PCR) can be performed using infected amniotic fluid. Serologic testing of cord blood at delivery is difficult to interpret. Treponemal tests reflect maternal infection. The nontreponemal tests need cord blood titers to be at least fourfold higher than maternal titers. A non-reactive RPR or VDRL does not exclude infection.

Management

Penicillin remains the drug of choice for the treatment of syphilis in pregnancy. The 2006 Centers for Disease Control (CDC) guidelines recommend 2.4 million units benzathine penicillin G i.m. for primary, secondary, and early latent syphilis (some experts recommend repeating this dose 1 week later). Late latent syphilis or syphilis of unknown duration is treated with 2.4 million units benzathine penicillin G i.m. weekly for three doses. No other antimicrobial agent is recommended in pregnancy. If a woman reports a penicillin allergy, a skin test for major or minor determinant antigens of penicillin should be performed if possible. If reactive, penicillin desensitization should be performed orally (Table 27.1) or intravenously. Up to 50% of women treated for early stage syphilis will have a systemic reaction called the Jarisch–Herxheimer reaction. Although transient with only mild constitutional symptoms, preterm labor and fetal distress may complicate treatment. Treatment after 20 weeks' gestation should be preceded by an

Table 27.1 Oral desensitization protocol for penicillin allergic patients. From Wendel *et al.* [29].

Dose*	Phenoxymethyl Penicillin (units/mL)[†]	Dose (units)	Cumulative dose (units)
1	1000	100	100
2	1000	200	300
3	1000	400	700
4	1000	800	1500
5	1000	1600	3100
6	1000	3200	6300
7	1000	6400	12,700
8	10,000	12,000	24,700
9	10,000	24,000	48,700
10	10,000	48,000	96,700
11	80,000	80,000	176,000
12	80,000	160,000	336,700
13	80,000	320,000	636,700
14	80,000	640,000	1,296,700

Observe for 30 minutes prior to parenteral benzathine penicillin G.
* 15-minute intervals.
[†] 250 mg/5 mL equals 80,000 units/mL.

ultrasound to assess possible fetal infection. If abnormal, antepartum fetal heart rate monitoring should accompany treatment. In fetuses at or near term, delivery with treatment of the mother and infant postpartum may be warranted.

Careful follow-up after treatment should be performed to determine treatment failure (rare) or reinfection. Nontreponemal tests should be performed every month during pregnancy because the consequence of a treatment failure or reinfection in these high-risk women is a congenitally infected infant.

Toxoplasmosis

Toxoplasma gondii, a ubiquitous protozoan transmitted in infected cat feces, undercooked raw meat, and transplacentally, causes an estimated 400–4000 cases of congenital toxoplasmosis in the USA every year [30]. Acute infections, often in asymptomatic pregnant women, can cause severe illness in the fetus or neonate (mental retardation, epilepsy, and blindness). Approximately 15–30% of women in the USA are immune and the incidence of new infection is in the range 0.5–8.1 per 1000 susceptible pregnancies [30–32].

Pathogenesis and transmission

Toxoplasma gondii exists in three forms or stages:
1 *Tachyzoite*: the acute phase in which the organism invades and replicates;
2 *Bradyzoite*: the latent phase when tissue cysts are formed; and

3 *Oocyst sporozoite:* which may survive in the environment for months.

The cat is the definitive host and thus the main reservoir of infection. Infected cats excrete several million oocytes a day—these oocytes then sporulate and become infectious. Ingestion of these sporulated oocytes is the predominant mode of transmission in humans. They may be ingested in raw or undercooked infected meat or in uncooked foods in contact with infected meat or soil, or may be inadvertently ingested from cat litter.

Transplacental passage of toxoplasmosis occurs when a woman becomes infected during pregnancy. The risk of developing congenital toxoplasmosis increases as the gestation advances. The incidence of transmission is 10–25% if infection occurs in the first trimester and highest (60%) in the third trimester. Conversely, however, disease severity is worse if infection occurs during the first trimester. Infection prior to pregnancy confers immunity with little risk of vertical transmission.

Clinical manifestations

Maternal toxoplasmosis is often asymptomatic. If symptoms do occur, fatigue, fever, malaise, and lymphadenopathy (particularly posterior cervical) are usually reported. Photophobia, maculopapular rash, and headache are less common. Most women recover within a few weeks without therapy or sequelae. Women who are immunocompromised, however, may have more severe disease, complicated by encephalitis, pneumonitis, and chorioamnionitis. *T. gondii* infection is one of the AIDS-defining criteria.

Congenital toxoplasmosis has been associated with spontaneous abortion, stillbirth, and intrauterine growth restriction. Although many infected fetuses are born with no evidence of toxoplasmosis, the majority (up to 80%) develop learning and visual disturbances later in life [33,34]. Chorioretinitis is the most common clinical findings among infected newborns. Hydrocephaly, intracerebral calcifications, cataracts, microphthalmia, glaucoma, hepatosplenomegaly, anemia and petechiae, jaundice, and seizures may also manifest in the nursery or over time.

Diagnosis

The parasite is rarely detected in body fluids or tissue; diagnosis is based on serologic evaluation or DNA amplification. A combination of serologic tests is now used to determine recent and past infection. Toxoplasma IgG develops within 1–2 weeks after acquisition, peaks at 1–2 months, and usually persists for life. Avidity testing may help discriminate between recent and past infection. IgM antibodies appear by 10 days after infection and usually become negative within a few months. However, occasionally IgM may be detected in chronic infection and persist for years. The IgM tests available have low specificity and should not be used alone to diagnose acute toxoplasmosis. IgA and IgE antibodies are also used to help diagnose acute infection. IgA persist longer than IgE antibodies. Because of the difficulty in running and interpreting serologic data, the Toxoplasma Serology Laboratory in Palo Alto, California can be consulted. They use a Toxoplasma Serologic Profile and provide to the clinician a detailed interpretation of results [35].

Prenatal diagnosis of toxoplasmosis can now be performed using a number of techniques. DNA amplification by PCR of toxoplasmosis from amniotic fluid or blood is becoming a standard modality with improved sensitivity over standard isolation techniques. Sonographic evidence of hydrocephaly and intracranial calcifications, placental thickening, liver calcifications, hyperechoic bowel, ascites, and growth restriction have all been reported prenatally. *Toxoplasma*-specific IgM and IgA may be found in amniotic fluid or cordocentesis samples but their absence does not indicate lack of infection. When neonatal serology is performed, IgA and IgM may confirm a diagnosis of congenital infection; however, approximately 20% of infected neonates will have nondetectable IgM at birth. The placenta should be evaluated in suspected cases as almost half will have evidence of *T. gondii* cysts.

Management and prevention

Currently, toxoplasma screening is not recommended in the US pregnant population (excepting immunocompromised women). Prevalence rates in the USA are low, and equivocal or false-positive tests high in this setting. Areas where toxoplasmosis is more common (e.g., France and Austria) have screening programs in place and have reported a decline in congenital disease.

Treatment of toxoplasmosis in the infected pregnant women is variable, depending on maternal immune status, gestational age, and presence of fetal infection. Spiramycin can be obtained from the Food and Drug Administration to treat laboratory confirmed acute maternal infection. If fetal infection is documented, a combination of pyrimethamine, folinic acid, and a sulfonamide (usually sulfadiazine) is recommended. Treatment has been shown to decrease the rate of congenital infection and the sequelae of toxoplasmosis in the neonate [35].

Prevention of toxoplasmosis in pregnant women is paramount. Women should be counseled to avoid close contact with cat feces (avoid changing cat litter or wear gloves), cook meat to safe temperatures, wash fruits and vegetables thoroughly prior to eating, wear gloves when gardening, and wash hands after contact with soil and raw meats.

Herpes simplex virus infection

Genital herpes has become the most prevalent sexually transmitted disease with over 1.6 million new herpes simplex virus

(HSV) infections per year in the USA alone [36]. It is estimated that over 50 million adolescents and adults are currently affected. Although the majority of women are unaware of their status, 24.2% of women overall in the USA are seropositive for HSV-2, with higher rates reported in high-risk populations [36,37]. As most cases of HSV are transmitted by persons unaware of their infection or who are asymptomatic, containing this worsening public health problem has become a major concern [38].

Pathogenesis and transmission

There are two serotypes of this DNA virus: HSV-1 and HSV-2. There is a large amount of DNA sequence concordance between the two viruses and prior infection with one type attenuates a new infection with the other type. Transmission occurs secondary to intimate contact with an infected partner or vertically to a fetus or neonate. The incubation period averages 3–6 days.

Following a mucocutaneous infection, the virus travels retrogradely along sensory nerves and remains latent in cranial nerves or dorsal spinal ganglia. The frequency of mucocutaneous recurrences is variable. HSV-1, originally localized to orolabial areas, now causes 5–30% of initial genital herpes. This is probably because of an increase in orogenital sexual practices. HSV-2 occurs almost entirely in the genital region. The majority (over 90%) of recurrent genital herpes is secondary to HSV-2. Recurrences are most frequent in the first years after infection but may recur for many years.

Neonatal infection may occur transplacentally or via ascending infection at any time during pregnancy; however, over 85% of neonatal herpes results by direct contact with the birth canal [39]. It occurs in up to 1 in 3200 live births [38]. Risk factors for neonatal HSV infection include the presence of HSV in the genital tract (often asymptomatic shedding), the type of HSV (HSV-1 more than HSV-2, although usually skin, eye, or mouth disease, not CNS infection), invasive obstetric procedures, mode of delivery and stage of maternal infection. Women acquiring HSV late in the third trimester have the highest likelihood of transmission to the neonate. This is because of high viral loads and the neonate having no protective antibodies acquired transplacentally.

Clinical manifestations

There are four classifications of clinical HSV infection. A *first episode primary infection* occurs when HSV-1 or HSV-2 is isolated from a genital lesion in the absence of any HSV antibodies in serum. Many women with new infections are asymptomatic. However, this group is the one with the highest likelihood of clinical symptoms. Focal painful vesicles may be present or the lesions may appear as painful abraded areas. Inguinal lymphadenopathy, fever, malaise, dysuria, and vulvar pruritus are all more common in this group, although

only noted in approximately one-third of newly acquired infections. Hepatitis, encephalitis, meningitis, or pneumonia are uncommon. Viral shedding and symptomatology usually lasts 1–4 weeks.

First episode non-primary infection is diagnosed when HSV-2 is isolated from the genital tract in the presence of pre-existing HSV-1 serum antibodies. These infections have a shorter clinical course with less severe symptoms and fewer lesions. Transmission risks to a partner, fetus, or neonate is much lower in this group. *Recurrent infection* or *reactivation* occurs when HSV-1 or HSV-2 is isolated from the genital tract in the presence of same serotype antibodies. Reactivation disease has a much shorter course with few lesions and rare systemic symptoms. During pregnancy, 5–10% of women with a history of HSV infection will have a symptomatic recurrence. The risk of vertical transmission is very low.

Finally, *asymptomatic viral shedding* is the presence of HSV on the surface of the skin and mucosa in the absence of signs and symptoms. Most women will shed virus asymptomatically throughout life and the majority of HSV transmission occurs during a period of asymptomatic viral shedding (up to 70%).

Neonatal HSV infection is acquired predominantly intrapartum when the fetus comes in contact with virus shed from the cervix or lower genital tact [40]. Infants born to mothers with a first episode of genital HSV infection near delivery have the highest risk of acquiring HSV. Neonatal infection may manifest as localized infection of the skin, eyes, and mucous membranes. Localized CNS encephalitis may also occur. Disseminated disease with involvement of multiple organs, predominantly liver and lungs, may occur and has the highest reported mortality rate [41].

Diagnosis

History and clinical examination are useful in the diagnosis of HSV infection; however, as genital HSV often has a nonclassic presentation or is asymptomatic, laboratory testing should be performed. Viral culture is the most sensitive test if performed early in an outbreak. The lesion should be unroofed and the fluid cultured. The sensitivity drops markedly as the vesicular lesions ulcerate and then crust over. PCR may be used but is more expensive and not readily available.

Type-specific serology (distinguishing HSV-1 from HSV-2) is now available and proves useful for screening and determining classification of disease for counseling purposes. The best tests available are based on antibodies formed to type-specific G-glycoproteins. Sensitivity approaches 80–90% and specificity ≥96%. If new infection is suspected and antibody testing is negative, repeat the serologic tests in 4–6 weeks.

Management and prevention

Women with symptomatic first episode HSV infection during pregnancy can be treated with systemic acyclovir, valacyclovir, or famciclovir for 7 days. Treatment will attenuate symptoms but not eradicate the latent virus. Severe recurrent disease may also benefit from antiviral therapy, but mild recurrent disease will not. These antiviral medications are pregnancy class B.

Acyclovir or valacyclovir therapy in the latter part of pregnancy (36 weeks' gestation until delivery) has been shown to decrease HSV outbreaks at term, decreasing the need for cesarean delivery. They have also been shown to decrease asymptomatic HSV shedding at delivery. The American College of Obstetricians and Gynecologists (ACOG) states that prophylactic antiviral therapy be considered, especially in the setting of a first episode of HSV infection during the current pregnancy.

Upon presentation for delivery, a woman with a known history of HSV infection should be questioned regarding prodromal symptoms (vulvar itching, burning) and recent HSV lesions. A careful examination of the vulva, vagina, and cervix should be performed for herpetic lesions. Suspicious lesions should be cultured. Women with any evidence of prodromal or active HSV infection should be offered a cesarean delivery. Of note, 10–15% of infants with HSV are born to women undergoing a cesarean delivery—counseling should reflect a decreased risk of HSV transmission with a cesarean delivery but not a negated risk. A nongenital lesion should be covered and vaginal delivery allowed. If a woman presents at term with HSV lesions and ruptured membranes, regardless of rupture duration, a cesarean delivery should be effected. If the infant is preterm, expectant management should be offered as the risk of prematurity outweighs the unknown benefit of delivery. If, at the time of labor, the lesion has resolved, vaginal delivery is allowed.

Women with active HSV infection may breastfeed as long as there is no HSV lesion on the breast. Strict handwashing should be performed before contact with the neonate. Acyclovir may be used in the postpartum period as excretion into breastmilk is low.

Although screening for HSV is not recommended at this time, a women known to be HSV seropositive at her first prenatal visit should be counseled regarding safe sexual practices and counseled to avoid intercourse with a partner known or suspected of having HSV, particularly in the third trimester. Condom use is effective in preventing *most*, but not all, HSV transmission.

Cytomegalovirus

Cytomegalovirus (CMV) remains the most common cause of perinatal infection in the USA, infecting 0.5–2% of all neonates [42,43]. Fifty-five percent of reproductive age women in high socioeconomic classes are seropositive, compared to 85% of women in the lower socioeconomic classes. The risk of seroconversion for a susceptible pregnant woman is 1–4% during the pregnancy—those women acquiring primary CMV infection during pregnancy are at highest risk of transmitting to the neonate.

Pathogenesis and transmission

CMV is a ubiquitous DNA herpesvirus—as with other herpesviruses, it has a latent phase with periodic reactivation despite antibody formation. Transmission occurs with contact from infected nasopharyngeal secretions, urine, saliva, semen, or cervical secretions (sexual contact), blood, or tissue. Children infected with CMV may shed up to 12–16 months [44] and susceptible pregnant women exposed to children are at high risk of acquiring CMV.

Although neonates may acquire infection secondary to passage through the maternal genital tract or from breastfeeding, the majority of neonates are infected transplacentally via hematogenous dissemination. Congenital CMV infection may occur after either primary or recurrent maternal infection. Stagno *et al.* [42,43,45,46], in a series of elegant reports of CMV in pregnancy, defined outcomes of CMV infection depending on the type of maternal infection. These findings are summarized in Fig. 27.2.

Women with primary CMV infection during pregnancy will transmit the virus to the fetus 40% of the time. In contrast, of women with recurrent infection, only 0.15–1% will transmit the virus to the fetus. The risk of clinically apparent disease or sequelae in the neonate is higher in those infants infected during a primary maternal infection. As with many other congenital infections, perinatal transmission is more likely in the third trimester, but outcomes are more severe the earlier in gestation transmission occurs.

Clinical manifestations

The majority of adults infected with CMV are asymptomatic. Fifteen percent of infected pregnant women with primary CMV will develop a mononucleosis-like illness with malaise, headache, fever, lymphadenopathy, pharyngitis, and arthritis. Immunocompromised women may develop more severe complications such as interstitial pneumonitis, myocarditis, hepatitis, retinitis, gastrointestinal disease, and meningoencephalitis, although these are uncommon. Reactivation episodes with CMV are usually asymptomatic, although viral shedding is common.

Congenital CMV infection may present with hepatosplenomegaly, thrombocytopenia, jaundice, and petechiae ("blueberry muffin"). Low birthweight, microcephaly, intracranial calcifications, chorioretinitis, hearing deficits, pneumonitis, microphthalmia, and seizures are also not uncommon. Although the majority of infected infants are asymptomatic at birth, some will develop late-onset sequelae. These commonly include psychomotor retardation, hearing loss, neurologic deficits, chorioretinitis, and learning disabilities.

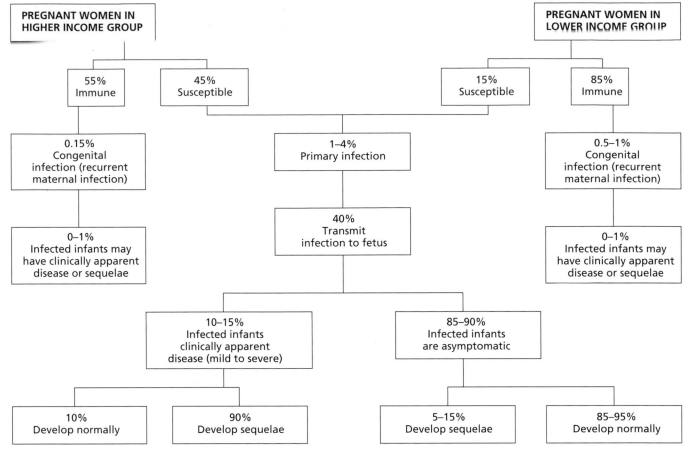

Fig. 27.2 Characteristics of CMV infection in pregnancy. From Stagno and Whitley [45], with permission from the publisher.

Diagnosis

Primary maternal CMV infection, if symptomatic, often presents similarly to Epstein–Barr virus. However, heterophile antibody testing will be negative. CMV IgM is detected within a few days of infection but is only found in 75–90% of women with acute infection [46]. CMV IgM may remain positive for 4–8 months and re-emerge with recurrent infection, making it problematic for diagnosis of acute disease. CMV IgG testing is more reliable—a fourfold rise in paired acute and convalescent sera indicates acute infection. CMV viral culture remains the gold standard for diagnosis although a minimum of 21 days is required for a culture to be reported as negative.

Perinatal infection may be suspected when certain findings on ultrasound are noted. Although nonspecific, fetal hydrops, intrauterine growth restriction, microcephaly, ventriculomegaly, hepatomegaly, cerebral calcifications, hyperechoic bowel, and amniotic fluid abnormalities have all been described. If suspected, amniotic fluid for DNA amplification testing has become the gold standard, although a negative result does not exclude fetal infection [47,48]. Finally, amniotic fluid for CMV culture may be useful but requires a long incubation period.

Management and prevention

The management of an immunocompetent pregnant woman with primary or recurrent CMV infection is controversial. There are no current treatment regimens available for these women beyond symptomatic treatment. If recent primary infection is diagnosed, invasive testing can be offered to identify infected fetuses. Counseling is then carried out regarding the stage of infection and gestational age, understanding that the majority of fetuses develop normally. Pregnancy termination may be an option in rare cases, especially in the face of abnormal ultrasound findings.

Routine serologic screening for CMV infection is not recommended. Preventive measures including handwashing and minimizing exposure to CMV from high-risk areas such as daycare centers and nurseries are the mainstay for preventing primary CMV infection. A CMV vaccine is not available currently for use in pregnancy.

Varicella-zoster virus

Varicella-zoster virus (VZV) is the most contagious viral infection complicating pregnancy—fortunately, more than 95% of adults have serologic evidence of immunity with only 0.1–0.4 cases per 1000 pregnant women occurring each year in the USA. Although uncommon in the pregnant population, if infected, the morbidity for an adult is much greater than that for an infected child.

Pathogenesis and transmission

VZV is a double-stranded DNA herpesvirus that causes clinical infection only in humans. The primary infection, varicella or chicken pox, presents predominantly as a rash with systemic symptoms (see below). The virus then becomes latent with occasional reactivation (herpes zoster or shingles) occurring in certain individuals. Both primary and reactivation diseases are infectious, although viral shedding is less with reactivation. In temperate climates, varicella occurs predominantly in late winter and early spring.

Transmission of VZV occurs primarily by direct contact with an infected individual, although transmission also may occur by inhalation of virus from respiratory droplets or airborne virus particles from skin lesions (predominantly with zoster). The virus usually enters the mucosa of the upper respiratory tract or the conjunctiva. Transplacental passage of the virus may occur, causing congenital varicella in up to 2% of maternal varicella infections prior to 20 weeks' gestation (highest risk 13–20 weeks). Neonatal infection occurs secondary to exposure of the fetus or newborn 5 days prior to delivery to 2 days postpartum before protective maternal antibodies develop.

A susceptible individual has a 60–95% risk of becoming infected after exposure. The incubation period is 10–21 days with a mean of 15 days. An infected person is then contagious from 1 day prior to the onset of the rash until the lesions are crusted over. Once infected, lifelong immunity to reinfection develops in the immunocompetent individual, although subclinical reinfections have been reported. Reactivation disease (shingles) occurs sporadically with an often unknown inciting event.

Clinical manifestations

Varicella or chicken pox often occurs in an adult with a 1–2 day prodrome of fever, malaise, headache, and myalgias. Lesions then appear initially as papules, rapidly progressing to super-ficial clear vesicles surrounded by a halo of erythema. The head and trunk are affected first, spreading then sporadically to the lower abdomen and extremities. The vesicles are intensely pruritic and appear in crops over 3–7 days. The lesions begin to crust during the outbreak. A typical varicella outbreak has at any one time all stages of lesions. Once all the lesions have crusted, the patient is no longer considered infectious.

The risk of varicella pneumonia is increased in adults and may be increased again by pregnancy. In a recently reported series of varicella in pregnancy [49], 5.2% of women with varicella were diagnosed as having pneumonia. Risk factors for developing pneumonia included current smoking and ≥100 skin lesions. The mortality, reportedly as high as 40% in early series, has now decreased to less than 2% with aggressive antiviral use and intensive care facilities. Pneumonia usually develops 2–4 days after the onset of rash, and may present with minimal symptoms (often only a mild cough). A chest X-ray should be performed on all pregnant women presenting with varicella.

Congenital varicella, usually following maternal infection between 12 and 20 weeks, often presents with limb abnormalities such as cutaneous scarring, limb hypoplasia, and muscle atrophy. Microphthalmia, chorioretinitis, microcephaly, seizures, cortical atrophy, and mental retardation may also occur. Neonatal varicella, occurring secondary to exposure near or around delivery, carries a 25–50% attack rate and mortality rate approaching 25%. Clinical manifestations include pneumonia, disseminated mucocutaneous lesions, and visceral infection.

Herpes zoster infection, or shingles, occurs upon reactivation of the VZV virus in 1–3 sensory nerve dermatomes. Pain along the infected dermatome heralds the appearance of papules and then vesicles. These vesicles may coalesce, rupture, and then crust over. Systemic symptoms are uncommon.

Diagnosis

The diagnosis of varicella is usually made clinically. The characteristic rash in susceptible individuals allows for accurate diagnosis in the majority of cases. If the diagnosis is not readily apparent, VZV can be isolated by scraping the base of the vesicles during the acute phase of the infection. Tzanck smear, tissue culture, and direct fluorescent antibody testing are available to test the vesicle specimen. DNA amplification techniques of body fluid or tissue are very sensitive and are rapidly becoming the gold standard. Seroconversion can be documented by antibody assay using acute and convalescent sera. VZV IgM develops rapidly and will remain positive for 4–5 weeks and may be useful in the acute setting. Fetal varicella can be diagnosed using DNA amplification techniques on amniotic fluid specimens.

Management and prevention

The pregnant woman with primary VZV infection should be isolated from other pregnant women and evaluated for evidence of pneumonia. Chest X-ray is useful. Hospitalization and antiviral therapy are reserved for those women with pneumonia or those with systemic symptoms severe enough to require intravenous fluids and symptomatic relief. If antiviral therapy is required, acyclovir is the drug of choice. Acyclovir (500 mg/m² or 10–15 mg/kg every 8 hours) should be started as soon as possible. No fetal side-effects have been reported from acyclovir use in pregnancy. Antiviral use to prevent or treat congenital infection has not been studied.

Prevention is the mainstay of population-based VZV management. The infected individual should be isolated from other susceptible individuals. An exposed pregnant woman should be evaluated as to past disease—if no history of varicella infection, an IgG titer can be rapidly performed. At least 70% of individuals without reported history of VZV actually have VZV IgG. An exposed pregnant woman who is deemed susceptible may be given passive immunity using varicella-zoster immunoglobulin (VZIG). VZIG is a human globulin fraction shown to either prevent or attenuate infection in the majority of susceptible pregnant women [50]. VZIG should be given within 96 hours of exposure to maximize the effect. As VZIG is limited in quantity and is expensive, IgG testing is essential to limit the number of women requiring administration.

The varicella vaccine currently available is a live attenuated vaccine (Varivax). It is not recommended in pregnancy and pregnancy should be avoided within 3 months of administration. To date, there have been no adverse outcomes in women inadvertently receiving the vaccine immediately before or during pregnancy, but the Varicella Vaccine Registry is still accruing data.

Case presentation

The patient is a 30-year-old accountant who presents to your office in January at 26 weeks' gestation. She states that her 6-year-old son was sent home from school that day with a fever and a facial rash with a "slapped cheek" appearance. The pediatrician correctly diagnoses her son with parvovirus B_{19} and is concerned for her fetus. She has never had parvovirus B_{19}, which you confirm with IgG serologic testing.

As she is susceptible, you counsel her on the clinical manifestations in adults including fever, headache, truncal rash, and polyarthralgias. The incubation period is 4–14 days so you repeat the IgM and IgG testing in 3 weeks. Although she is asymptomatic, her parvovirus B_{19} IgM is now positive. A level II ultrasound with MCA Doppler is performed with no evidence of hydrops fetalis or other signs of fetal infection. She undergoes sonographic evaluation every 1–2 weeks for 10–12 weeks after exposure, the fetus develops hepatosplenomegaly, ascites, and an elevated MCA peak systolic velocity consistent with fetal anemia.

She undergoes cordocentesis which reveals a fetal hemoglobin of 6.2 g/dL. Parvovirus B_{19} RNA testing is positive. An intrauterine transfusion is performed at the time of the cordocentesis without complication. Weekly follow-up sonographic evaluation notes a slow resolution of the fetal ascites with normalization of the MCA Doppler findings. No further transfusions are required and she delivers a healthy male infant at term.

References

1 Cohen BJ, Buckley MM. The prevalence of antibody to human parvovirus B_{19} in England and Wales. *Med Microbiol* 1988;**25**:151–3.

2 Public Health Laboratory Service Working Party on Fifth Disease. Prospective study of human parvovirus (B19) infection in pregnancy. *Br Med J* 1990;**300**:1166–70.

3 Harger JH, Adler SP, Koch WC, *et al.* Prospective evaluation of 618 pregnant women exposed to parvovirus B19: risks and symptoms. *Obstet Gynecol* 1998;**91**:413–20.

4 Rodis JF, Quinn DL, Garry GW, *et al.* Management and outcomes of pregnancies complicated by human B19 parvovirus infection: a prospective study. *Am J Obstet Gynecol* 1990;**163**:1168–71.

5 Brown T, Anand A, Ritchie LD. Intrauterine parvovirus infection associated with hydrops fetalis. *Lancet* 1984;**2**:1033–4.

6 Rodis JF, Hovick TJ, Quinn DL, *et al.* Human parvovirus infection in pregnancy. *Obstet Gynecol* 1988;**72**:733–8.

7 Delle Chiaie L, Buck G, Grab D, *et al.* Prediction of fetal anemia with doppler measurement of the middle cerebral artery peak systolic velocity in pregnancies complicated by maternal blood group alloimmunization or parvovirus B_{19} infection. *Ultrasound Obstet Gynecol* 2001;**18**:232–6.

8 Cosmi E, Mari G, Delle Chiaie L, *et al.* Noninvasive diagnosis by doppler ultrasonography of fetal anemia resulting from parvovirus infection. *Am J Obstet Gynecol* 2002;**187**:1290–3.

9 Enders M, Weidner A, Zoellner I, *et al.* Fetal morbidity and mortality after acute human parvovirus B19 infection in pregnancy: prospective evaluation of 1018 cases. *Prenat Diagn* 2004;**24**:513–8.

10 Schild RL, Bald R, Plath H, *et al.* Intrauterine management of fetal parvovirus B19 infection. *Ultrasound Obstet Gynecol* 1999;**13**:161–6.

11 von Kaisenberg CS, Jonat W. Fetal parvovirus B19 infection. *Ultrasound Obstet Gynecol* 2001;**18**:280–8.

12 Dembinski J, Haverkamp F, Hansmann M, *et al.* Neurodevelopmental outcome after intrauterine red cell transfusion for parvovirus B_{19}-induced fetal hydrops. *Br J Obstet Gynaecol* 2002;**109**:1232–4.

13 Zgorniak-Nowosielska I, Zawilinska B, Szostek S. Rubella infection during pregnancy in the 1985–86 epidemic: follow-up after seven years. *Eur J Epidemiol* 1996;**12**:303–8.

14 Webster WS. Teratogen update: congenital rubella. *Teratology* 1998;**58**:13–23.

15 Tanemura M, Suzumori K, Yagami Y, *et al.* Diagnosis of fetal rubella infection with reverse transcription and nested polymerase chain reaction: a study of 34 cases diagnosed in fetuses. *Am J Obstet Gynecol* 1996;**174**:578–82.

16 Tang JW, Aarons E, Hesketh LM, *et al.* Prenatal diagnosis of congenital rubella infection in the second trimester of pregnancy. *Prenat Diagn* 2003;**6**:509–12.

17 Hwa HL, Shyu MK, Lee CN, *et al.* Prenatal diagnosis of congenital rubella infection from maternal rubella in Taiwan. *Obstet Gynecol* 1994;**84**:415–9.

18 Larsen SA, Hunter EF, McGrew BE. Syphilis. In: Wentworth BB, Judson FN, eds. *Laboratory Methods for the Diagnosis of Sexually Transmitted Diseases.* Washington, DC: American Public Health Association, 1984: 1–42.

19 Schober PC, Gabriel G, White P, *et al.* How infectious is syphilis? *Br J Vener Dis* 1983;**59**:217–9.

20 Sanchez PJ, Wendel GD. Syphilis in pregnancy. *Clin Perinatol* 1997;**24**:71–90.

21 Maruti S, Hwany LY, Ross M, *et al.* The epidemiology of early syphilis in Houston, TX, 1994–1995. *Sex Transm Dis* 1997;**24**:475–80.

22 Wendel GE, Sanchez PJ, Peters MT, *et al.* Identification of *Treponema pallidum* in amniotic fluid and fetal blood from pregnancies complicated by congenital syphilis. *Obstet Gynecol* 1991;**78**:890–5.

23 Fojaco RM, Hensely GT, Moskowitz L. Congenital syphilis and necrotizing funisitis. *JAMA* 1989;**12**:1788–90.

24 Qureshi F, Jacques SM, Reyes MP. Placental histopathology in syphilis. *Hum Pathol* 1993;**24**:7779–84.

25 Genest DR, Choi-Hong SR, Tate JE, *et al.* Diagnosis of congenital syphilis from placental examination. *Hum Pathol* 1996;**27**:366–72.

26 Grimprel E, Sanchez PJ, Wendel GD, *et al.* Use of polymerase chain reaction and rabbit infectivity testing to detect *Treponema pallidum* in amniotic fluids, fetal and neonatal sera, and cerebrospinal fluid. *J Clin Microbiol* 1991;**29**:1711–8.

27 Nathan L, Bohman VR, Sanchez PJ, *et al.* In utero infection with *Treponema pallidum* in early pregnancy. *Prenat Diag* 1997;**17**:1119–23.

28 Wendel GD, Maberry MC, Christmas JT, *et al.* Examination of amniotic fluid in diagnosing congenital syphilis with fetal death. *Obstet Gynecol* 1989;**74**:967–70.

29 Wendel GD, Stark BJ, Jamison RB, *et al.* Penicillin allergy and desensitization in serious infections during pregnancy. *N Engl J Med* 1985;**312**:1229–32.

30 Centers for Disease Control and Prevention. CDC recommendations regarding selected conditions affecting women's health. *MMWR* 2000;499RR-2:59–75.

31 Gilbert RE, Peckham CS. Congenital toxoplasmosis in the United Kingdom: to screen or not to screen? *J Med Screen* 2002;**9**:135–6.

32 Jones JL, Kruszon-Moran D, Wilson M. Toxoplasma gondii infection in the United States, 1999–2000. *Emerg Infect Dis* 2003;**9**:1371–4.

33 Carter AO, Frank JW. Congenital toxoplasmosis: epidemiologic features and control. *Can Med Assoc J* 1986;**135**:618–23.

34 Wilson CB, Remington JS, Stagno S, *et al.* Development of adverse sequelae in children born with subclinical congenital *toxoplasma* infection. *Pediatrics* 1980;**66**:767–74.

35 Montoya JG. Laboratory diagnosis of *Toxoplasma gondii* infection and toxoplasmosis. 2002;**185**(Suppl 1):573–82.

36 Armstrong GL, Schillinger J, Markowitz L, *et al.* Incidence of herpes simplex virus type 2 infection in the United States. *Am J Epidemiol* 2001;**153**:912–20.

37 Fleming D, McQuillan G, Johnson R, *et al.* Herpes simplex virus type 2 in the United States, 1976 to 1994. *N Engl J Med* 1997;**337**:1105–11.

38 Brown ZA, Gardella C, Wald A, *et al.* Genital herpes complicating pregnancy. *Obstet Gynecol* 2005;**106**:845–56.

39 Brown ZA, Wald A, Morrow RA, *et al.* Effect of serologic status and cesarean delivery on transmission rates of herpes simplex virus from mother to infant. *JAMA* 2003;**289**:203–9.

40 Kimberlin DW, Rouse DJ. Genital herpes. *N Engl J Med* 2004;**350**:1970–7.

41 Kimberlin DW. Neonatal herpes simplex infection. *Clin Microbiol Rev* 2004;**17**:1–13.

42 Stagno S, Pass RF, Dworsky ME, *et al.* Congenital cytomegalovirus infection. The relative importance of primary and recurrent maternal infection. *N Engl J Med* 1982;**306**:945–9.

43 Stagno S, Cloud G, Pass RF, *et al.* Primary cytomegalovirus infections in pregnancy: incidence, transmission to the fetus and clinical outcome. *JAMA* 1986;**256**:1904–8.

44 Murph JR, Bale JF. The natural history of acquired cytomegalovirus infection among children in group day-care. *Am J Dis Child* 1988;**142**:843–6.

45 Stagno S, Whitley RJ. Herpesvirus infections of pregnancy. Part I: Cytomegalovirus and Epstein–Barr virus infections. *N Engl J Med* 1985;**313**:1270–4.

46 Stagno S, Tinker MK, Irod C, *et al.* Immunoglobulin M antibodies detected by enzyme-linked immunosorbent assay and radioimmunoassay in the diagnosis of cytomegalovirus infections in pregnant women and newborn infants. *J Clin Microbiol* 1985;**21**:930–5.

47 Revello MG, Genna G. Pathogenesis and prenatal diagnosis of human cytomegalovirus infection. *J Clin Virol* 2004;**29**:71–83.

48 Liesnard C, Donner C, Brancart F, *et al.* Prenatal diagnosis of congenital CMV infection: prospective study of 237 pregnancies at risk. *Obstet Gynecol* 2000;**95**:881–8.

49 Harger JH, Ernest JM, Thurnau GR, *et al.* Risk factors and outcome of varicella-zoster virus pneumonia in pregnant women. *J Infect Dis* 2002;**185**:422–7.

50 Centers for Disease Control and Prevention. Varicella-zoster immune globulin for the prevention of chickenpox. *MMWR* 1984;**33**:84.

28

Group B streptococcal infections

Ronald S. Gibbs

In the 1970s, group B streptococci (GBS) dramatically became the leading cause of neonatal infection and important causes of maternal genital tract infection and septicemia [1–4]. Prior to the development of nationally used prevention guidelines in 1996, approximately 6100 early onset cases and 1400 late onset cases occurred annually in the USA [5,6], with a rate of early onset neonatal GBS disease in the range 1.5–2 cases per 1000 live births. Now, with implementation of these guidelines, disease incidence decreased by over 70% [6,7]. In 2002, the rate was 1570 early onset cases (0.4 cases per 1000 live births) and an estimated 110 deaths occurred nationally.

The 1996 guidelines presented culture-based screening and the risk-based approach as equally acceptable alternatives [8]. New guidelines were released in 2002 [9], recommending the single strategy of universal culture-based screening at 35–37 weeks' gestation.

Epidemiology of GBS perinatal infection

An estimated 20–30% of all pregnant women are colonized genitally with GBS. Prenatal screening at 35–37 weeks' gestation is currently recommended in the USA. Early onset neonatal disease occurs within the first week of life; late onset disease occurs after the first week. Meningitis is much more common in late onset disease. Currently, for term infants with GBS sepsis, survival is approximately 98%, but for preterm infants the survival is 90% for cases at 34–36 weeks and 70% for cases at ≤33 weeks [6]. These suboptimal outcomes led to effective prevention strategies. Risk factors for early onset disease include maternal GBS colonization, prolonged rupture of membranes, preterm delivery, GBS bacteriuria during pregnancy, birth of a previous infant with invasive GBS disease, and maternal fever in labor. In pregnant women, GBS can cause urinary tract infection, chorioamnionitis, endometritis, bacteremia, puerperal wound infection, and, most likely, stillbirth.

Isolation of GBS

To optimize recovery of GBS from rectogenital tract specimens, selective media that suppress the growth of competing bacteria should be used. Commercially available selective media include Todd–Hewitt broth (a nutritive broth for Gram-positive organisms) supplemented with either gentamicin plus nalidixic acid or colistin plus nalidixic acid.

Recommended antibiotics for prophylaxis

Resistance to penicillin or ampicillin has not been detected in GBS. Because of its universal activity against GBS and narrow spectrum of activity, penicillin remains the antibiotic of choice for GBS prophylaxis with ampicillin an alternative [4,9].

Resistance to clindamycin and erythromycin increased among GBS isolates in the 1990s. The prevalence of resistance in the USA and Canada was in the range 7–25% for erythromycin and 3–15% for clindamycin from 1998–2001 [10–13]. Resistance to cefoxitin has also been reported [14].

Rising resistance to clindamycin and erythromycin were strongly considered when first- and second-line antibiotics were recommended for GBS chemoprophylaxis in 2002 (Table 28.1). The 2002 guidelines recommend clindamycin or erythromycin only if a patient's GBS isolate has been shown to have *in vitro* susceptibility to both. Vancomycin is recommended for women at high risk of penicillin allergy colonized by clindamycin-resistant or erythromycin-resistant isolates. Vancomycin is recommended even if an isolate shows *in vitro* resistance to either clindamycin *or* erythromycin because of possible inducible resistance.

Table 28.1 Recommended regimens for intrapartum antimicrobial prophylaxis for perinatal group B streptococci GBS disease prevention. From Centers for Disease Control and Prevention [4] with permission.

Recommended	Penicillin G, 5 million units IV initial dose, then 2.5 million units IV every 4 hours until delivery
Alternative	Ampicillin, 2 g IV initial dose, then 1 g IV every 4 hours until delivery
If penicillin allergic† Patients not at high risk for anaphylaxis	Cefazolin, 2 g IV initial dose, then 1 g IV every 8 hours until delivery
Patients at high risk for anaphylaxis‡ GBS susceptible to clindamycin and erythromycin§	Clindamycin, 900 mg IV every 8 hours until delivery *or* Erythromycin, 500 mg IV every 6 hours until delivery
GBS resistant to clindamycin or erythromycin or susceptibility unknown	Vancomycin,¶ 1 g IV every 12 hours until delivery

* Broader-spectrum agents, including an agent active against GBS, may be necessary for treatment of chorioamnionitis.

† History of penicillin allergy should be assessed to determine whether a high risk for anaphylaxis is present. Penicillin-allergic patients at high risk for anaphylaxis are those who have experienced immediate hypersensitivity to penicillin including a history of penicillin-related anaphylaxis; other high-risk patients are those with asthma or other diseases that would make anaphylaxis more dangerous or difficult to treat, such as persons being treated with beta-adrenergic-blocking agents.

‡ If laboratory facilities are adequate, clindamycin and erythromycin susceptibility testing should be performed on prenatal GBS isolates from penicillin-allergic women at high risk for anaphylaxis.

§ Resistance to erythromycin is often but not always associated with clindamycin resistance. If a strain is resistant to erythromycin but appears susceptible to clindamycin, it may still have inducible resistance to clindamycin.

¶ Cefazolin is preferred over vancomycin for women with a history of penicillin allergy other than immediate hypersensitivity reactions, and pharmacologic data suggest it achieves effective intra-amniotic concentrations. Vancomycin should be reserved for penicillin-allergic women at high risk for anaphylaxis.

Prevention of perinatal GBS infection

To date, use of intrapartum antibiotics is the only effective intervention available against perinatal GBS disease. After release of the 2002 guidelines, there was a 34% decline in early onset disease incidence in the following year [15].

Details of 2002 recommendations

For indications for prophylaxis under the 2002 guidelines see Fig. 28.1. In addition, women who had a previous infant with invasive GBS disease or who have any level of GBS bacteriuria during pregnancy should receive intrapartum prophylaxis. Women with unknown culture status at the time of labor should receive intrapartum antibiotic prophylaxis if they present with the risk factors outlined in Fig. 28.1. Figure 28.1 also outlines some common circumstances where intrapartum prophylaxis is not indicated. Women undergoing a planned cesarean delivery in the absence of labor or membrane rupture do not require GBS prophylaxis.

Recommended antibiotics for intrapartum prophylaxis are shown in Table 28.1.

Preterm premature rupture of the membranes

Preterm premature rupture of the membranes (PPROM) places the fetus or newborn at special risk for GBS sepsis. The 2002 Centers for Disease Control (CDC) guidelines provide a sample algorithm (Fig. 28.2), but specifics are individualized, and no single approach is recommended.

Bacteriuria

The 2002 GBS guidelines recommend that all women with GBS bacteriuria, defined as GBS isolated from the urine at any level (even less than 10^5 colony forming units), should receive intrapartum prophylaxis. These women do not require late antenatal screening. Symptomatic or asymptomatic GBS urinary tract infections should be treated according to usual standards.

Case presentation

A 20-year-old primigravida reports a "penicillin allergy" at her first prenatal visit. Details confirm that she had an immediate hypersensitivity reaction including urticaria, hives, and wheezing.

What testing should be performed on the GBS isolate? Because the patient should be given *neither* penicillin nor a cephalosporin, this isolate must be tested for susceptibility to both clindamycin and erythromycin.

What antibiotics should be used for intrapartum prophylaxis? If the isolate is sensitive to both clindamycin *and* erythromycin, *either* may be used for prophylaxis. However, if the isolate is resistant to either (or both) clindamycin or erythromycin, then vancomycin must be used. Isolates reported to have, for example, resistance to erythromycin but susceptibility to clindamycin may actually have inducible resistance to the latter. Thus, vancomycin should be used.

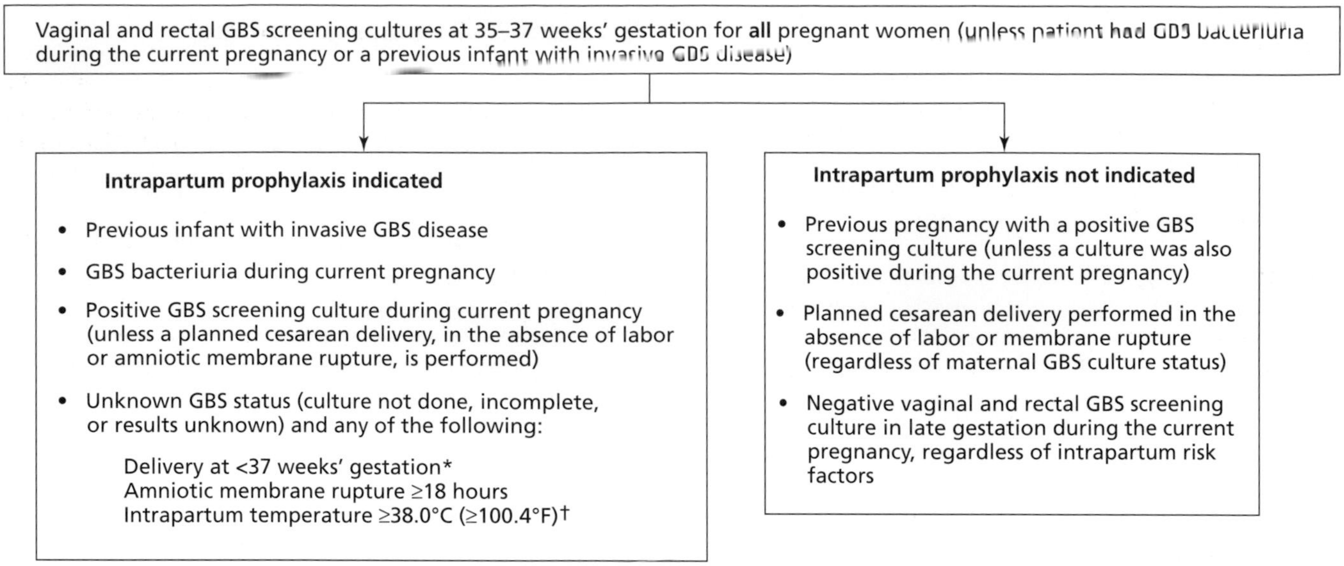

Vaginal and rectal GBS screening cultures at 35–37 weeks' gestation for **all** pregnant women (unless patient had GBS bacteriuria during the current pregnancy or a previous infant with invasive GBS disease)

Intrapartum prophylaxis indicated

- Previous infant with invasive GBS disease

- GBS bacteriuria during current pregnancy

- Positive GBS screening culture during current pregnancy (unless a planned cesarean delivery, in the absence of labor or amniotic membrane rupture, is performed)

- Unknown GBS status (culture not done, incomplete, or results unknown) and any of the following:

  Delivery at <37 weeks' gestation*
  Amniotic membrane rupture ≥18 hours
  Intrapartum temperature ≥38.0°C (≥100.4°F)†

Intrapartum prophylaxis not indicated

- Previous pregnancy with a positive GBS screening culture (unless a culture was also positive during the current pregnancy)

- Planned cesarean delivery performed in the absence of labor or membrane rupture (regardless of maternal GBS culture status)

- Negative vaginal and rectal GBS screening culture in late gestation during the current pregnancy, regardless of intrapartum risk factors

*If onset of labor or rupture of amniotic membranes occurs at <37 weeks' gestation and there is a significant risk for preterm delivery (as assessed by the clinician), a suggested algorithm for GBS prophylaxis managemnt is provide (Figure 3).
†If amnionitis is suspected, broad-spectrum antibiotic therapy that includes an agent known to be active against GBS should replace GBS prophylaxis.

Fig. 28.1 Indications for intrapartum antibiotic prophylaxis to prevent perinatal group B streptococci (GBS) disease under a universal prenatal screening strategy based on combined vaginal and rectal cultures collected at 35–37 weeks' gestation from all pregnant women. From Centers for Disease Control and Prevention [4] with permission.

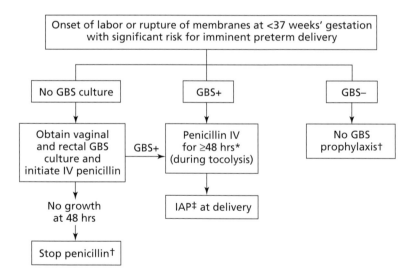

* Penicillin should be continued for a total of at least 48 hours, unless delivery occurs sooner. At the physician's discretion, antibiotic prophylaxis may be continued beyond 48 h in a GBS culture positive woman if delivery has not yet occurred. For women who are GBS culture positive, antibiotic prophylaxis should be reinitiated when labor likely to proceed to delivery occurs or recurs.
† If delivery has not occurred within 4 weeks, a vaginal and rectal GBS screening culture should be repeated and the patient should be managed as described, based on the result of the repeat culture.
‡ IAP, intrapartum antibiotic prophylaxis.

Fig. 28.2 Sample algorithm for group B streptococci (GBS) prophylaxis for women with threatened preterm delivery. This algorithm is not an exclusive course of management. Variations that incorporate individual circumstances or institutional preferences may be appropriate. From Centers for Disease Control and Prevention [4] with permission.

References

1 Gibbs RS, Schrag S, Schuchat A. High risk pregnancy series: an expert's view. Perinatal infections due to group B streptococci. *Obstet Gynecol* 2004;**104**:1062–76.

2 Sweet RL, Gibbs RS. Group B streptococci. In: Sweet RL, Gibbs RS, eds. *Infectious Diseases of the Female Genital Tract*, 4th edn. Philadelphia: Lippincott Williams & Wilkins, 2002: 31–46.

3 Edwards MS, Baker CJ. Group B streptococcal infections. In: Remington JS, Klein JO, eds. *Infectious Diseases of the Fetus and Newborn Infant*, 3rd edn. Philadelphia: W.B. Saunders, 2001: 1091–156.

4 Centers for Disease Control and Prevention. Prevention of perinatal group B streptococcal disease. Revised guidelines from CDC. *MMWR* 2002;**51**(RR-11):1–22.

5 Zangwill KM, Schuchat A, Wenger JD. Group B streptococcal disease in the United States, 1990: report from a multistate active surveillance system. *MMWR* 1992;**41**(SS-6): 25–32.

6 Schrag SJ, Zywicki S, Farley MM, *et al.* Group B streptococcal disease in the era of intrapartum antibiotic prophylaxis. *N Engl J Med* 2000;**342**:15–20.

7 Centers for Disease Control and Prevention. Early-onset group B streptococcal disease, United States, 1998–1999. *MMWR* 2000;**49**:793–6.

8 Centers for Disease Control and Prevention. Prevention of perinatal group B streptococcal disease: a public health perspective. *MMWR* 1996;**45**(RR-7):1–24.

9 Committee on Obstetric Practice, American College of Obstetrics and Gynecology. Prevention of early-onset group B streptococcal disease in newborns. Washington, DC 2002. American College of Obstetrics and Gynecology Committee Opinion Number 279.

10 Fernandez M, Hickman ME, Baker CJ. Antimicrobial susceptibilities of group B streptococci isolated between 1992 and 1996 from patients with bacteremia or meningitis. *Antimicrob Agents Chemother* 1998;**42**:1517–9.

11 Morales WJ, Dickey SS, Bornick P, Lim DV. Change in antibiotic resistance of group B streptococcus: impact on intrapartum management. *Am J Obstet Gynecol* 1999;**181**:310–4.

12 Andrews JI, Diekema DJ, Hunter SK, *et al.* Group B streptococci causing neonatal bloodstream infection: antimicrobial susceptibility and serotyping results from SENTRY centers in the Western hemisphere. *Am J Obstet Gynecol* 2000;**183**:859–62.

13 Bland HL, Vermillion ST, Soper DE, *et al.* Antibiotic resistance patterns of group B streptococci in late third-trimester rectovaginal cultures. *Am J Obstet Gynecol* 2001;**184**:1125–6.

14 Berkowitz K, Regan JA, Greenberg E. Antibiotic resistance patterns of group B streptococci in pregnant women. *J Clin Microbiol* 1990;**28**:5–7.

15 Centers for Disease Control and Prevention. Early-onset neonatal group B streptococcal disease: United States, 2000–2003. *MMWR* 2004;**53**:502–5.

Hepatitis in pregnancy

Patrick Duff

The purpose of this chapter is to review six types of viral hepatitis: A, B, C, D, E, and G; describe the diagnostic tests for each of these infections; define the perinatal complications associated with viral hepatitis; and present the key principles of management of hepatitis in pregnancy (Table 29.1).

Hepatitis A

Hepatitis A is the second most common form of viral hepatitis in the USA. The infection is caused by an RNA virus that is transmitted by fecal–oral contact. The incubation period ranges from 15 to 50 days. Infections in children are usually asymptomatic; infections in adults are usually symptomatic. The disease is most prevalent in areas of poor sanitation and close living [1].

The typical clinical manifestations of hepatitis include low-grade fever, malaise, poor appetite, right upper quadrant pain and tenderness, jaundice, and acholic stools. The diagnosis is best confirmed by detection of immunoglobulin M (IgM) antibody specific for the hepatitis A virus.

Hepatitis A does not cause a chronic carrier state. Perinatal transmission virtually never occurs, and therefore the infection does not pose a major risk to either the mother or the baby unless the mother develops fulminant hepatitis and liver failure. Fortunately, such a situation is extremely rare [1].

Hepatitis A can be prevented by administration of an inactivated vaccine. Two formulations of the vaccine are available: Vaqta and Havrix [2]. Both vaccines require an initial intramuscular injection, followed by a second dose 6–12 months later. The vaccine should be offered to the following individuals:

- International travelers
- Children in endemic areas
- Intravenous drug users
- Individuals who have occupational exposure (e.g., workers in a primate laboratory)
- Residents and staff of chronic care institutions

- Individuals with liver disease
- Homosexual men
- Individuals with clotting factor disorders

Standard immunoglobulin provides reasonably effective passive immunization for hepatitis A if it is given within 2 weeks of exposure. The standard intramuscular dose of immunoglobulin is 0.02 mg/kg.

Hepatitis E

Hepatitis E is caused by an RNA virus. The epidemiology of hepatitis E is similar to that of hepatitis A. The incubation period averages 45 days. The disease is quite rare in the USA but is endemic in developing countries of the world. In these countries, maternal infection with hepatitis E often has an alarmingly high mortality, in the range of 10–20%. This high mortality is probably less the result of the virulence of the microorganism and more related to poor nutrition, poor general health, and lack of access to modern medical care [1].

The clinical presentation of acute hepatitis E is similar to that of hepatitis A. The diagnosis can be established by using electron microscopy to identify viral particles in the stool of infected patients. The most useful diagnostic test, however, is serology.

Hepatitis E does not cause a chronic carrier state. Perinatal transmission can occur but is extremely rare [3].

Hepatitis B

Hepatitis B is caused by a DNA virus that is transmitted parenterally and via sexual contact. The infection also can be transmitted perinatally from an infected mother to her infant.

Acute hepatitis B occurs in approximately 1–2 in 1000 pregnancies in the USA. The chronic carrier state is more frequent, occurring in 6–10 in 1000 pregnancies. Worldwide, over 400 million individuals are chronically infected with hepatitis

Table 29.1 Hepatitis in pregnancy.

Hepatitis Infection	Mechanism of Transmission	Best Diagnostic Test	Carrier State	Perinatal Transmission	Vaccine	Remarks
A	Fecal–oral	Antibody detection	No	No	Yes	Passive immunization with immunoglobulin
E	Fecal–oral	Antibody detection	No	Rare	No	High maternal mortality in developing countries
B	Parenteral/sexual contact	Antigen detection	Yes	Yes	Yes	Passive immunization with hepatitis B immunoglobulin
D	Parenteral/sexual contact	Antibody detection	Yes	Yes	Prevented by hepatitis B vaccine	Virus cannot replicate in absence of hepatitis B infection
C	Parenteral/sexual contact	Antibody detection	Yes	Yes	No	Cesarean delivery for women with detectable serum HCV-RNA
G	Parenteral/sexual contact	Antibody detection	Yes	Yes	No	No clinical significance of infection

B virus. In the USA alone, approximately 1.25 million individuals are chronically infected [1].

Approximately 90% of patients who acquire hepatitis B mount an effective immunologic response to the virus and completely clear their infection. Less than 1% of infected patients develop fulminant hepatitis and die. Approximately 10% of patients develop a chronic carrier state. Some individuals with chronic hepatitis B infection ultimately develop severe chronic liver disease such as chronic active hepatitis, chronic persistent hepatitis, cirrhosis, or hepatocellular carcinoma [1].

The diagnosis of hepatitis B is best confirmed by serologic tests. Patients with acute hepatitis B are positive for the hepatitis B surface antigen and positive for IgM antibody to the core antigen. Patients with chronic hepatitis B are positive for the surface antigen and positive for IgG antibody to the core antigen. Infected patients may or may not be positive for the hepatitis Be antigen. When this latter antigen is present, it denotes active viral replication and a high level of infectivity [4].

In the absence of intervention, approximately 20% of mothers who are seropositive for hepatitis B surface antigen will transmit infection to their neonates. Approximately 90% of mothers who are positive for both the surface antigen and the *e* antigen will transmit infection. Fortunately, there is now excellent immunoprophylaxis for prevention of perinatal transmission of hepatitis B infection. Infants delivered to seropositive mothers should receive hepatitis B immunoglobulin within 12 hours of birth. Prior to their discharge from the hospital, these infants also should begin the hepatitis B vaccination series.

The Centers for Disease Control and Prevention (CDC) now recommend universal vaccination of all infants for hepatitis B. In addition, the vaccine should be offered to all women of reproductive age [4,5].

Hepatitis D (delta virus infection)

Hepatitis D is an RNA virus that depends upon coinfection with hepatitis B for replication. Therefore, the epidemiology of hepatitis D is essentially identical to that of hepatitis B. Patients with hepatitis D may have two types of infection. Some may have acute hepatitis D and hepatitis B (*coinfection*). These individuals typically clear their infection and have a good long-term prognosis. Others may have chronic hepatitis D infection superimposed upon chronic hepatitis B infection (*superinfection*). These women are particularly likely to develop chronic liver disease [1].

The diagnosis of hepatitis D can be established by identifying the delta antigen in liver tissue or serum. However, the most useful diagnostic tests are detection of IgM and/or IgG antibody in serum.

Hepatitis D can cause a chronic carrier state in conjunction with hepatitis B infection. Perinatal transmission of hepatitis D occurs, but it is uncommon. Moreover, the immunoprophylaxis outlined above for hepatitis B is highly effective in preventing transmission of hepatitis D [1].

Hepatitis C

Hepatitis C is caused by an RNA virus. The virus may be transmitted parenterally, via sexual contact, and perinatally. In many patient populations, hepatitis C is actually as common, if not more common, than hepatitis B. Chronic hepatitis C infection now is the number one indication for liver transplantation in the USA [1,6,7].

The disease is usually asymptomatic. The diagnosis is best confirmed by serologic testing. The initial screening test should be an enzyme immunoassay (EIA). The confirmatory test is a recombinant immunoblot assay (RIBA). Seroconversion may not occur for up to 16 weeks following infection. In addition, although these immunologic tests have been available for many years, they still do not distinguish consistently and precisely between IgM and IgG antibody.

In patients who have a low serum concentration of hepatitis C RNA and who do not have coexisting HIV infection, the risk of perinatal transmission of hepatitis C is less than 5%. If the patient's serum concentration of hepatitis C RNA is high and/or she has HIV infection, the perinatal transmission rate may approach 25% [8,9]. Several small, nonrandomized, uncontrolled cohort studies (level II evidence) support the role for an elective cesarean delivery prior to the onset of labor and rupture of membranes in women who have detectable hepatitis C virus RNA. For women who have undetectable serum concentrations of RNA, vaginal delivery appears to be a reasonable plan of management [10–12]. Breastfeeding is acceptable in women who have hepatitis C and does not pose a risk to the neonate [10,12].

Hepatitis G

Hepatitis G is caused by an RNA virus that is related to the hepatitis C virus. Hepatitis G is more prevalent, but less virulent, than hepatitis C. Many patients who have hepatitis G are coinfected with hepatitis A, B, C, and HIV. Interestingly, coinfection with hepatitis G does not adversely affect the prognosis of these other infections [13–16].

Most patients with hepatitis G are asymptomatic. The diagnosis is best established by detection of virus by polymerase chain reaction and by identification of antibody by enzyme-linked immunosorbent assay (ELISA).

Hepatitis G can cause a chronic carrier state, and perinatal transmission has been documented. However, the clinical effects of infection in the mother and baby appear to be minimal. Accordingly, patients should not routinely be screened for this infection, and no special treatment is indicated even if infection is confirmed.

Case presentation

A 32-year-old woman, G3, P1102, at 18 weeks' gestation is seropositive for hepatitis B surface antigen. Additional testing showed that she also was positive for hepatitis C and D and seronegative for HIV infection. There was no evidence of gonorrhea, chlamydia, or syphilis.

What additional testing is indicated in this patient? Patients who are coinfected with hepatitis B, C, and D are particularly likely to develop chronic liver disease such as chronic active hepatitis, chronic persistent hepatitis, and cirrhosis. In some individuals, the liver disease may progress to hepatocellular carcinoma and/or frank hepatic failure. Therefore, this patient should have a battery of liver function tests and a coagulation profile. In addition, she should have a test to determine the serum concentration of hepatitis C virus RNA.

What interventions are appropriate for her sexual partner? The patient's sexual partner should be tested for hepatitis B, C, and D. If he is seronegative for hepatitis B, he should receive an injection of hepatitis B immunoglobulin and begin the hepatitis B vaccine series.

What is the most appropriate method of delivery in this patient? The recommended method of delivery should not be affected by the presence of hepatitis B or D. However, the presence of hepatitis C may influence delivery method. If hepatitis C virus RNA can be detected in the patient's serum, she should be offered an elective cesarean at approximately 38 weeks' gestation prior to rupture of membranes and the onset of labor. Published level II evidence demonstrates that elective cesarean delivery in these highly selected patients results in a decreased risk of perinatal transmission of hepatitis C virus.

What type of immunoprophylaxis is indicated for this patient's neonate? Unfortunately, there is no immunoprophylaxis for hepatitis C. However, effective immunoprophylaxis against hepatitis B and D is available. The infant should receive hepatitis B immunoglobulin within 12 hours of birth. Prior to discharge from the hospital, the infant should receive the first dose of hepatitis B vaccine. A second and third dose should be administered at 1 and 6 months of age.

References

1 Duff P. Hepatitis in pregnancy. *Semin Perinatol* 1998;**22**:277–83.
2 Duff B, Duff P. Hepatitis A vaccine: ready for prime time. *Obstet Gynecol* 1998;**91**:468–71.
3 Khuroo MS, Kamili S, Jameel S. Vertical transmission of hepatitis E virus. *Lancet* 1995;**345**:1025–6.
4 Hepatitis B virus: a comprehensive strategy for eliminating transmission in the United States through universal childhood vaccination. *MMWR* 1991;**40**:1–25.
5 Poland GA, Jacobson RM. Prevention of hepatitis B with the hepatitis B vaccine. *N Engl J Med* 2004;**351**:2832–8.
6 Leikin EL, Reirus JF, Schnell E, *et al*. Epidemiologic predictors of hepatitis C virus infection in pregnant women. *Obstet Gynecol* 1994;**84**:529–34.
7 Bohman VR, Stettler W, Little BB, *et al*. Seroprevalence and risk factors for hepatitis C virus antibody in pregnant women. *Obstet Gynecol* 1992;**80**:609–13.
8 Ohto H, Terazawa S, Sasaki N, *et al*. Transmission of hepatitis C virus from mothers to infants. *N Engl J Med* 1994;**330**:744–50.
9 Steininger C, Kundi M, Jatzko G, *et al*. Increased risk of mother-to-infant transmission of hepatitis C virus by intrapartum infantile exposure to blood. *J Infect Dis* 2003;**187**:345–51.
10 Gibb DM, Goodall RL, Dunn DT, *et al*. Mother-to-child transmission of hepatitis C virus: evidence for preventable peripartum transmission. *Lancet* 2000;**356**:904–7.
11 Zanetti AR, Paccagnini S, Principi N, *et al*. Mother-to-infant transmission of hepatitis C virus. *Lancet* 1995;**345**:289–91.

12 European pediatric hepatitis C virus network. A significant sex— but not elective cesarean section—effect on mother-to-child transmission of hepatitis C virus infection. *J Infect Dis* 2005;**192**: 1872–9.

13 Jarvis LM, Davidson F, Hanley JP, *et al*. Infection with hepatitis G virus among recipients of plasma products. *Lancet* 1996;**348**:1352–5.

14 Kew MC, Kassionides C. HGV: hepatitis G virus or harmless G virus. *Lancet* 1996;**348**(Suppl):10.

15 Alter MJ, Gallagher M, Morris TT, *et al*. Acute non-A-E hepatitis in the United States and the role of hepatitis G infection. *N Engl J Med* 1997;**336**:741–6.

16 Miyakawa Y, Mayuma M. Hepatitis G virus: a true hepatitis virus or an accidental tourist? *N Engl J Med* 1997;**336**:795–6.

30 HIV infection

Howard L. Minkoff

The HIV epidemic is now a quarter of a century old, with a well-defined epidemiology and pathophysiology, and with several effective therapeutic regimens available for use. However, the epidemic is far from contained. In fact, the epicenter is poised to move beyond the bounds of southern Africa; it is projected that India, Nigeria, China, Ethiopia and Russia will have the highest numbers of infected individuals by the end of the decade. Approximately half of these newly infected individuals will be women, the overwhelming majority of whom will be of reproductive age. Thus, obstetricians worldwide will continue to have a central role.

The care of HIV-infected women is more effective than ever and the rates of mother-to-child transmission of HIV are lower than ever in communities with access to therapy. The management of these women and their pregnancies are, not coincidentally, more complex than ever. This chapter is designed to provide guidance to the obstetrician who must identify and treat infected women, and act to reduce rates of HIV transmission and drug toxicity while optimizing pregnant women's health.

Identifying infected patients

Women can only avail themselves of the benefits of effective antiviral therapy if their serostatus is known. Because of the remarkable benefits of antiretroviral therapy, and the reduction in stigma associated with the diagnosis, obstetric and public health organizations have become strong advocates of prenatal HIV screening. However, until recently, the protocols for screening still reflected the social and medical environment that was extant at the time that tests first became available; informed written consents preceded by detailed counseling were required. Those protocols resulted in low testing rates, in part because the process itself contained a stigma, with some providers only screening women they perceived to be at risk. Finally in 1998, the Institute of Medicine proposed, and

the American College of Obstetricians and Gynecologists (ACOG) subsequently endorsed, a process referred to as "opt-out" [1].

In the "opt-out" process, HIV-testing is "routinized." Women are told that testing is part of the standard battery of prenatal tests for all pregnant women and that the test will be performed unless the woman objects. Hence, the "opt-out" policy is also referred to as "informed right of refusal." When "opt-out" is utilized, women are no longer required to sign an informed consent in order to find out their serostatus but they retain the right to refuse the test if they so desire. This approach, in the settings in which it has been adopted, has resulted in improved testing rates. A table detailing the status of the laws in various states can be found at www.ucsf.edu/hivcntr.

The actual laboratory procedure for standard (as distinct from "rapid") testing involves the detection of either antigen from the virus itself, antibodies to portions of the virus, viral nucleic acid, or, less commonly, culture of the virus. The most widely used method (enzyme-linked immunosorbent assay [ELISA] confirmed by Western blot) involves the detection of antibodies to virus in the patient's sera.

In the USA, a disproportionate share of infection occurs among women with no prenatal care [2]. Therefore there is a need to rapidly identify women who are infected and who initially present for care in labor. Several rapid HIV tests have been developed. The OraQuick Advance HIV-1/2 Antibody Test (OraSure Technologies, Inc., Bethlehem, Pennsylvania) with a sensitivity of 99.6% and a specificity of 100%; the Reveal Rapid HIV-1 Antibody Test (MedMira Laboratories, Inc., Halifax, Nova Scotia) with a sensitivity of 99.8% and a specificity of 99.1%; and the Multi-Spot HIV-1/HIV-2 (Biorad) are the only three that have received approval from the Food and Drug Administration (FDA) and are currently available [3]. Rapid HIV testing has been compared with the standard enzyme immunoassay (EIA), which is still utilized extensively by blood transfusion services which perform most of the HIV tests worldwide (although always backed up by a Western blot assay), and they have been found to be comparable.

Post-test counseling of seropositive women

Once an individual's serostatus is determined, there is an emergent need to provide appropriate post-test counseling. This counseling must address psychosocial, as well as medical aspects of the diagnosis. From a patient education standpoint, it is important to draw a clear distinction between HIV infection and AIDS. The patient should be instructed in ways to avoid transmitting the virus to others: safe sex practices, no sharing of razors, and the like. The natural history of HIV disease and long-term follow-up plans should also be incorporated into the counseling. At the current time, advances in the treatment of HIV warrants an air of optimism in these initial conversations, an optimism that may be necessary to dispel the many myths that are still associated with the diagnosis of HIV. Perinatal counseling focuses on the potential consequences of pregnancy on HIV disease (relative rate of disease progression) and the impact of HIV disease status on pregnancy outcome, particularly current estimates of HIV transmission rates. There is no convincing empiric data that pregnancy has an untoward effect on HIV disease [4]. However, pregnancy may have indirect effects—if obstetricians are reticent to utilize the latest pharmacologic interventions then the woman's disease course may indeed be compromised [5].

Perhaps the most important component of counseling relates to the success that obstetricians have had in preventing mother-to-child transmission of HIV with the use of appropriate antiretroviral therapies and cesarean delivery as indicated (see below). Women should be informed of these therapies, as well as risks that may be associated with their use and should be assured that they will have access to these if they so desire.

Although a focus of attention during pregnancy will be on the prevention of mother-to-child transmission of HIV, care begins with a focus on the health of the mother. A baseline CD4 count and viral load provides a reliable picture of the patient's status, the likelihood of progression to clinical illness, and the need for instituting antiviral therapy. If the mother needs medication for her own well-being then therapy should be instituted, albeit modifications of standard regimens may sometimes be necessary. It is also important to screen for infections that may be prevalent in these women, and whose course might be modified by HIV infection (e.g. hepatitis B and C, and syphillis). Appropriate management of co-infections can be achieved by co-management with an infectious disease specialist. Below we discuss, in sequence, care of the mother for her own well-being, and the steps needed to minimize the rates of mother-to-child transmission of HIV.

Care of seropositive women in general

Obtaining a CD4 count and a viral load provides the clinician with a useful snapshot of the patient's status and medication needs when she is first encountered. If her CD4 count is over $350 \, \text{mm}/\text{mL}^3$ and the viral load is under 100,000 copies, then antiviral medications for the woman's health are unnecessary and, were she not pregnant, would be deferred until evidence of immunologic deterioration or viral load increase. However, if the CD4 is below that benchmark or the viral load above 100,000 copies then therapy should be instituted, regardless of pregnancy status. The therapy should be a highly active antiretroviral therapy (HAART) regimen. HAART regimens are medication combinations that are capable of providing sustained reductions in the viral load, and it should be anticipated that the viral load will decrease by more than $1 \log/\text{month}$, and reach an undetectable level within 6 months.

There are several possible regimens that can be used. Most comprise agents from two of the three classes of antiretroviral therapy (nucleoside reverse transcriptase inhibitors [NRTIs], non-nucleoside reverse transcriptase inhibitors [NNRTIs], and protease inhibitors [PIs]) commonly used. Although other classes of drugs are becoming available (e.g., fusion inhibitors and nucleotide reverse transcriptase inhibitors), the experience with these agents in pregnancy is quite limited. The most frequently used regimens comprise two NRTIs and either an NNRTI or a PI (sometimes two PIs are used with one acting as a "booster" of the second). If the chosen regimen fails, the possibility of poor adherence, viral resistance, or both, must be considered. Resistance testing should be performed before the failing regimen is discontinued lest wild-strain virus overgrow resistant strains and mask the identity of the mutated strain. In the latter circumstance, the utility of the resistance test for assisting in the selection of the optimal salvage regimen would be compromised.

Finally, women whose CD4 counts drop below $200 \, \text{mm}/\text{mL}^3$ are at risk of developing opportunistic infection. Therefore, PCP prophylaxis (e.g. Bactrim-DS daily) should be given if the CD4 count drops below $200 \, \text{mm}/\text{mL}^3$, and mycobacterium avium complex prophylaxis (azithromycin, $1200 \, \text{mg}/\text{week}$) should be initiated when the CD4 count equals $50 \, \text{mm}/\text{mL}^3$.

Care of seropositive women in pregnancy

The basic tenets of care are not substantively altered by dint of pregnancy status. The goal remains optimizing the health of the mother. However, during pregnancy that goal is supplemented by the need to minimize the rate of mother-to-child transmission of HIV. Table 30.1 provides a list of antiretroviral drugs and recommendations for use in pregnant HIV-infected women. The virologic and immunologic triggers for therapy,

Table 30.1 Antiretroviral drug use in pregnant HIV-infected women: pharmacokinetic and toxicity data in human pregnancy and recommendations for use in pregnancy (modified from AIDSinfo, a service of the US DHHS).

Antiretroviral Drug	Pharmacokinetics in Pregnancy	Concerns in Pregnancy	Rationale for Recommended Use in Pregnancy
NRTIs/NtRTIs			
Recommended agents			
Zidovudine*	Pharmacokinetics not significantly altered in pregnancy; no change in dose indicated	No evidence of human teratogenicity. Well-tolerated, short-term safety demonstrated for mother and infant	Preferred NRTI for use in combination antiretroviral regimens in pregnancy based on efficacy studies and extensive experience; should be included in regimen unless significant toxicity or stavudine use
Lamivudine*	Pharmacokinetics not significantly altered in pregnancy; no change in dose indicated	No evidence of human teratogenicity. Well-tolerated, short-term safety demonstrated for mother and infant	Because of extensive experience with lamivudine in pregnancy in combination with zidovudine, lamivudine plus zidovudine is the recommended dual NRTI backbone for pregnant women
Alternative agents			
Didanosine	Pharmacokinetics not significantly altered in pregnancy; no change in dose indicated	Cases of lactic acidosis, some fatal, have been reported in pregnant women receiving didanosine and stavudine together	Alternate NRTI for dual nucleoside backbone of combination regimens. Didanosine should be used with stavudine only if no other alternatives are available
Emtricitabine	No studies in human pregnancy	No studies in human pregnancy	Alternate NRTI for dual nucleoside backbone of combination regimens
Stavudine	Pharmacokinetics not significantly altered in pregnancy; no change in dose indicated	No evidence of human teratogenicity. Cases of lactic acidosis, some fatal, have been reported in pregnant women receiving didanosine and stavudine together	Alternate NRTI for dual nucleoside backbone of combination regimens. Stavudine should be used with didanosine only if no other alternatives are available. Do not use with zidovudine due to potential for antagonism
Abacavir*	Phase I/II study in progress	Hypersensitivity reactions occur in ~5–8% of non-pregnant persons; a much smaller percentage are fatal and are usually associated with rechallenge. Rate in pregnancy unknown. Patient should be educated regarding symptoms of hypersensitivity reaction	Alternate NRTI for dual nucleoside backbone of combination regimens. See footnote regarding use in triple NRTI regimen[†]
Insufficient data to recommend use			
Tenofovir	No studies in human pregnancy. Phase I study in late pregnancy in progress	Studies in monkeys show decreased fetal growth and reduction in fetal bone porosity within two months of starting maternal therapy. Clinical studies in humans (particularly children) show bone demineralization with chronic use; clinical significance unknown	Because of lack of data on use in human pregnancy and concern regarding potential fetal bone effects, tenofovir should be used as a component of a maternal combination regimen only after careful consideration of alternatives

Table 30.1 *Continued.*

Antiretroviral Drug	Pharmacokinetics in Pregnancy	Concerns in Pregnancy	Rationale for Recommended Use in Pregnancy
Not recommended Zalcitabine	No studies in human pregnancy	Rodent studies indicate potential for teratogenicity and developmental toxicity	Given lack of data and concerns regarding teratogenicity in animals, not recommended for use in human pregnancy unless alternatives are not available
NNRTIs *Recommended agents* Nevirapine	Pharmacokinetics not significantly altered in pregnancy; no change in dose indicated	No evidence of human teratogenicity. Increased risk of symptomatic, often rash-associated, and potentially fatal liver toxicity among women with CD4$^+$ counts >250/mm^3 when first initiating therapy; unclear if pregnancy increases risk	Nevirapine should be initiated in pregnant women with CD4$^+$ counts >250 cells/mm^3 only if benefit clearly outweighs risk, due to the increased risk of potentially life-threatening hepatotoxicity in women with high CD4$^+$ counts. Women who enter pregnancy on nevirapine regimens and are tolerating them well may continue therapy, regardless of CD4$^+$ count
Not recommended Efavirenz	No studies in human pregnancy	FDA pregnancy class D; significant malformations (anencephaly, anophthalmia, cleft palate) were observed in 3 (15%) of 20 infants born to cynomolgus monkeys receiving efavirenz during the first trimester at a dose giving plasma levels comparable to systemic human therapeutic exposure; there are three case reports of neural tube defects in humans after first trimester exposure; relative risk unclear	Use of efavirenz should be avoided in the first trimester, and women of childbearing potential must be counseled regarding risks and avoidance of pregnancy. Because of the known failure rates of contraception, alternate regimens should be strongly considered in women of child bearing potential. Use after the second trimester of pregnancy can be considered if other alternatives are not available and if adequate contraception can be assured postpartum
Delavirdine	No studies in human pregnancy	Rodent studies indicate potential for carcinogenicity and teratogenicity	Given lack of data and concerns regarding teratogenicity in animals, not recommended for use in human pregnancy unless alternatives are not available

Protease inhibitors

Hyperglycemia, new onset or exacerbation of diabetes mellitus, and diabetic ketoacidosis reported with PI use; unclear if pregnancy increases risk. Conflicting data regarding preterm delivery in women receiving PIs

Recommended agents Nelfinavir	Adequate drug levels are achieved in pregnant women with nelfinavir 1250 mg, given twice daily	No evidence of human teratogenicity. Well-tolerated, short-term safety demonstrated for mother and infant. Nelfinavir dosing at 750 mg three	Given pharmacokinetic data and extensive experience with use in pregnancy compared to other PIs, preferred PI for combination

(Continued)

Table 30.1 *Continued.*

Antiretroviral Drug	Pharmacokinetics in Pregnancy	Concerns in Pregnancy	Rationale for Recommended Use in Pregnancy
		times daily produced variable and generally low levels in pregnant women	regimens in pregnant women, particularly if HAART is being given solely for perinatal prophylaxis. In clinical trials of initial therapy in non-pregnant adults, nelfinavir-based regimens had a lower rate of viral response compared to lopinavir/ritonavir or efavirenz-based regimens, but similar viral response compared with atazanavir or nevirapine-based regimens
Saquinavir-soft gel capsule [SGC] (Fortovase)/ritonavir	Adequate drug levels are achieved in pregnant women with saquinavir-SGC 800 mg boosted with ritonavir 100 mg, given twice daily. Recommended adult dosing of saquinavir-SGC 1000 mg plus ritonavir 100 mg may be used. No pharmacokinetic data on saquinavir-hard gel capsule [HGC]/ritonavir in pregnancy, but better GI tolerance in non-pregnant adults	Well-tolerated, short-term safety demonstrated for mother and infant. Inadequate drug levels observed in pregnant women with saquinavir-SGC given alone at 1200 mg three times daily	Given pharmacokinetic data and moderate experience with use in pregnancy, ritonavir-boosted saquinavir-SGC can be considered a preferred PI for combination regimens in pregnancy
Alternative agents			
Indinavir	Two studies including 18 women receiving indinavir 800 mg three times daily showed markedly lower levels during pregnancy compared to postpartum, although suppression of HIV RNA was seen	Theoretical concern re: increased indirect bilirubin levels, which may exacerbate physiologic hyperbilirubinemia in the neonate, but minimal placental passage. Use of unboosted indinavir during pregnancy is not recommended	Alternate PI to consider if unable to use nelfinavir or saquinavir-SGC/ritonavir, but would need to give indinavir as ritonavir-boosted regimen. Optimal dosing for the combination of indinavir/ritonavir in pregnancy is unknown
Lopinavir/ ritonavir	Phase I/II safety and pharmacokinetic study in progress using twice daily lopinavir 400 mg and ritonavir 100 mg	Limited experience in human pregnancy	Preliminary studies suggest increased dose may be required during pregnancy, though specific dosing recommendations not established. If used during pregnancy, monitor response to therapy closely. If expected virologic result is not observed, consult with a specialist with expertise in HIV in pregnancy
Ritonavir	Phase I/II study in pregnancy showed lower levels during pregnancy compared to postpartum	Minimal experience in human pregnancy	Given low levels in pregnant women when used alone, recommended for use in combination with second PI as low-dose ritonavir "boost" to increase levels of second PI

Table 30.1 *Continued.*

Antiretroviral Drug	Pharmacokinetics in Pregnancy	Concerns in Pregnancy	Rationale for Recommended Use in Pregnancy
Insufficient data to recommend use			
Amprenavir	No studies in human pregnancy	Oral solution contraindicated in pregnant women because of high levels of propylene glycol, which may not be adequately metabolized during pregnancy	Safety and pharmacokinetics in pregnancy data are insufficient to recommend use of capsules during pregnancy
Fosamprenavir	No studies in human pregnancy	No experience in human pregnancy	Safety and pharmacokinetics in pregnancy data are insufficient to recommend use during pregnancy
Atazanavir	No studies in human pregnancy	Theoretical concern re: increased indirect bilirubin levels, which may exacerbate physiologic hyperbilirubinemia in the neonate, although transplacental passage of other PIs has been low	Safety and pharmacokinetics in pregnancy data are insufficient to recommend use during pregnancy
Tipranavir	No studies in human pregnancy	No experience in human pregnancy	Safety and pharmacokinetics in pregnancy data are insufficient to recommend use during pregnancy
Fusion inhibitors			
Insufficient data to recommend use			
Enfuvirtide	No studies in human pregnancy	No experience in human pregnancy	Safety and pharmacokinetics in pregnancy data are insufficient to recommend use during pregnancy

GI, gastrointestinal; HAART, highly active antiretroviral therapy; HGC, hard gel capsule; NNRTI, non-nucleoside reverse transcriptase inhibitor; NRTI, nucleoside reverse transcriptase inhibitor; NtRTI, nucleotide reverse transcriptase inhibitor; PI, protease inhibitor; SGC, soft gel capsule.

* Zidovudine and lamivudine are included as a fixed-dose combination in Combivir; zidovudine, lamivudine, and abacavir are included as a fixed-dose combination in Trizivir.

† Triple NRTI regimens including abacavir have been less potent virologically compared to PI-based HAART regimens. Triple NRTI regimens should be used only when an NNRTI- or PI-based HAART regimen cannot be used (e.g., due to significant drug interactions). A study evaluating use of zidovudine/lamivudine/abacavir among pregnant women with HIV RNA <55,000 copies/mL as a class-sparing regimen is underway.

the timing of initiation, and the choice of components of antiviral therapy may need to be adjusted [6]. For example, if a woman's viral load is 2000 and her CD4 count is 400 mL^3 she would not be a candidate for therapy if she were not pregnant (the usual starting points are CD4 counts <350 mm^3 or a viral load >100,000 copies). However, because of the pregnancy, HAART would be recommended in order to minimize the risk of transmission. In fact, many providers would start HAART in any pregnant woman with detectable virus in order to reduce transmission to the child and to decrease the rate at which resistance develops in the mother. Usually, if HAART were to be used it would be started as soon as criteria for therapy were met. However, if it is being given for the purpose of preventing mother-to-child transmission, therapy would be delayed until the start of the second trimester because there is no immediate threat to the mother's health; unless evidence of demonstrated advantage were known, caution would

dictate that fetal exposure to these agents be delayed until beyond embryogenesis. The three-part zidovudine (ZDV) chemoprophylaxis regimen, initiated after the first trimester, would be recommended, as it is for all pregnant women with HIV-1 infection, regardless of antenatal HIV-1 RNA copy number. The regimen consists of oral administration of 300 mg ZDV b.i.d., initiated at 14–34 weeks' gestation and continued throughout the pregnancy. During labor, intravenous administration of ZDV in a 1-hour initial dose of 2 mg/kg body weight, followed by a continuous infusion of 1 mg/kg body weight/hour until delivery. Finally, oral administration of ZDV is given to the newborn (ZDV syrup at 2 mg/kg body weight/dose every 6 hours) for the first 6 weeks of life, beginning at 8–12 hours after birth.

There are additional pregnancy-specific considerations related to the other agents that might be added to the ZDV. For example, there are several antiretroviral medications that should be avoided in pregnancy. These include efavirenz (Sustiva), which is a class D drug that has been associated with neural tube defects and which should not be used in the first trimester and should only be used thereafter if other alternatives are not available. Another potentially dangerous medication is nevirapine (Viramune), which should be avoided as a component of HAART in pregnant women with CD4 counts ≥250 mm^3 because of the high risk of rapidly progressive and potentially nonreversible liver toxicity (this has not been reported in conjunction with its use in single-dose peripartum regimens) [7]. Additionally, because pregnancy itself can mimic some of the early symptoms of the lactic acidosis or hepatic steatosis syndrome or be associated with other disorders of liver metabolism, physicians caring for HIV-1 infected pregnant women receiving nucleoside analog drugs should be alert for early signs of this syndrome. Pregnant women receiving nucleoside analog drugs should have hepatic enzymes and electrolytes assessed more frequently during the last trimester of pregnancy, and any new symptoms should be evaluated thoroughly. Additionally, because of the reports of several cases of maternal mortality secondary to lactic acidosis with prolonged use of the combination of d4T and ddI by HIV-1 infected pregnant women, clinicians should prescribe this antiretroviral combination during pregnancy with caution and generally only when other nucleoside analog drug combinations have failed or have caused unacceptable toxicity or side-effects.

In addition, the CDC recommends that infected women in the USA refrain from breastfeeding to avoid postnatal transmission of HIV-1 to their infants; women receiving antiretroviral therapy should also follow these recommendations. Women who must temporarily discontinue therapy because of pregnancy-related hyperemesis should not resume therapy until sufficient time has elapsed to ensure that the drugs will be tolerated. To reduce the potential for emergence of resistance, if therapy requires temporary discontinuation for any reason during pregnancy, all drugs should be stopped and reintroduced simultaneously.

HIV-1 infected women receiving antiretroviral therapy whose pregnancy is identified after the first trimester should continue therapy. ZDV should be a component of the antenatal antiretroviral treatment regimen after the first trimester whenever possible, although this may not always be feasible. Women receiving antiretroviral therapy whose pregnancy is recognized during the first trimester should be counseled regarding the benefits and potential risks of antiretroviral administration during this period, and continuation of therapy should be considered. If therapy is discontinued during the first trimester, all drugs should be stopped and reintroduced simultaneously to avoid the development of drug resistance. Regardless of the antepartum antiretroviral regimen, ZDV administration is recommended during the intrapartum period and for the newborn.

Several effective regimens are available for intrapartum therapy for women who have had no prior therapy [6].
• Intrapartum intravenous ZDV followed by 6 weeks of ZDV for the newborn;
• Oral ZDV and 3TC during labor, followed by 1 week of oral ZDV-3TC for the newborn;
• A single dose of nevirapine at the onset of labor, followed by a single dose of nevirapine for the newborn at age 48 hours; and
• The two-dose nevirapine regimen combined with intrapartum intravenous ZDV and 6 weeks of ZDV for the newborn.

If single dose nevirapine is given to the mother, alone or in combination with ZDV, consideration should be given to adding maternal ZDV-3TC starting as soon as possible and continuing for 3–7 days. This may reduce development of nevirapine resistance.

In the immediate postpartum period, the woman should have appropriate assessments (e.g., CD4$^+$ count and HIV-1 RNA copy number) to determine whether antiretroviral therapy is recommended for her own health.

Resistance testing in infected pregnant women should be performed for the same indications as for nonpregnant persons:
• Those with acute infection;
• Those who have virologic failure with persistently detectable HIV-1 RNA levels while receiving antenatal therapy, or suboptimal viral suppression after initiation of antiretroviral therapy;
• Those with a high likelihood of having resistant virus based on community prevalence of resistant virus, known drug resistance in the woman's sex partner, or other source of infection; or
• Those who are about to start therapy.

Several studies performed before viral load testing and combination antiretroviral therapy became a routine part of clinical practice consistently showed that cesarean delivery performed before onset of labor and rupture of membranes (elective or scheduled) was associated with a significant decrease in perinatal HIV-1 transmission compared with other types of delivery, with reductions ranging from 55% to 80%. The ACOG Committee on Obstetric Practice, after reviewing these data, issued a Committee Opinion concerning route of delivery, recommending consideration of scheduled cesarean delivery for HIV-1 infected pregnant women with HIV-1 RNA levels >1000 copies/mL near the time of delivery [8]. More recent observational data from PACTG 367 [9] and the European Collaborative Study [10], evaluating both HIV RNA and maternal antiretroviral therapy along with mode of delivery, do not suggest additional benefit from scheduled cesarean delivery among women on HAART with low HIV RNA, but are conflicting regarding benefit for those on HAART with higher HIV RNA. If cesarean delivery is chosen, the procedure should be scheduled at 38 weeks' gestation, based on the best available clinical information. Amniocentesis for fetal lung maturity should not be performed because, in animal models, contamination of amniotic fluid has been shown to be a vector for fetal infection. For a scheduled cesarean delivery, intravenous ZDV should begin 3 hours before surgery, according to standard dosage recommendations. Other antiretroviral medications taken during pregnancy should not be interrupted near the time of delivery, regardless of route of delivery. Because maternal infectious morbidity is potentially increased, clinicians should consider perioperative antimicrobial prophylaxis.

Ethical and legal considerations

Obstetricians are acutely aware of the fact that in the course of their professional lifetimes, exigencies of law and the less clearly defined issues of ethics will often play a part in how they practice medicine. While the malpractice crisis commands inordinate attention, there are many other highly controversial areas of law and medicine that have involved obstetricians. Included in these are the ethical and legal controversies that swirl around HIV disease. Among the areas that continue to defy consensus are confidentiality, including charting, the appropriateness of "routine" (right of refusal) prenatal HIV testing, and the duty to warn HIV-infected patients' sexual partners of the index patient's seropositive status.

Clinicians should be aware of the relevant statutes within their own jurisdiction. Whatever the law, however, it is important that clinicians attempt to limit knowledge of a patient's serostatus to those with a medical need to know. Discrimination in housing and jobs has waned but has not disappeared.

The clinician also has an obligation to try to persuade the seropositive patient to notify her sex partner(s). The physician will often have the option of contacting exposed partners or utilizing the local health department. A consultation with local health authorities may provide useful information to the provider.

Conclusions

In the 21st century, in the developing world, HIV has become a treatable infection whose transmission from mother to child can be rendered a rare occurrence. However, the remarkable progress in the care of the HIV-infected pregnant woman has been purchased at the price of increasing therapeutic complexity. Obstetricians must be prepared to offer their patients the best prognosis that modern medicine permits by determining women's serostatus as early in pregnancy as possible, assessing their infected patients' immunologic and virologic status, recommending the most efficacious and safest antiretroviral regimens, monitoring their response assiduously, and then choosing the optimum time and method of delivery. By taking those steps, and coordinating their patients' care with experts in the field of HIV, obstetricians can contribute to the diminishing number of HIV-infected children born in this country and to the improved prognosis of their mothers.

Case presentation

The patient is a 27-year-old P0010 at 8 weeks' gestation who underwent routine HIV testing at her first prenatal visit. The ELISA test was repeatedly positive, as was the confirmatory Western blot. When the patient was informed of the results she was unable to recall any specific risk behavior, never having used intravenous drugs, or having a sexual partner known to have HIV, and having had only three lifetime sexual partners. The initial evaluation included a CD4 count that was 380 mm^3 and a viral load of 8000 copies. She was informed that those results would not ordinarily, in a nonpregnant individual, warrant the initiation of antiretroviral therapy but because she was pregnant, consideration should be given to therapy for the purpose of reducing the likelihood of transmission to the child. However, because her condition was good, the initiation of therapy would be deferred until she was beyond the first trimester. When she was 14 weeks pregnant she was started on a HAART regimen of twice-daily Combivir (ZDV + 3TC) and Kaletra (lopinavir + ritonavir). Baseline liver function tests and blood studies were obtained and she was scheduled to return for repeat viral load testing in a month. Within 2 months her viral load was undetectable and her CD4 count had risen to 440/mm^3. At 36 weeks' gestation, when a decision was to be made about mode of delivery, her viral load was still undetectable and a decision was made to allow a trial of labor. When she arrived in labor an intravenous infusion of ZDV was begun and she continued her other medications orally. Immediately after delivery all medications were discontinued. At follow-up, the patient remained well and was referred for ongoing care to a specialist in HIV infection. Her child was uninfected.

References

1 ACOG Committee on Obstetric Practice. ACOG committee opinion number 304, November 2004. Prenatal and perinatal human immunodeficiency virus testing: expanded recommendations. *Obstet Gynecol* 2004;**104**:1119–24.
2 Minkoff HL, O'Sullivan MJ. The case for rapid screening for HIV in labor. *JAMA* 1998;**279**:1743–4.

3 Branson BM. Rapid Tests for HIV Antibody. AIDS Reviews 2, 76-83 (2000). http://www.aidsreviews.com/2000/rev02/art_02.html (Viewed April 2005).

4 Minkoff H, Hershow R, Watts H, *et al*. The relationship of pregnancy to disease progression. *Am J Obstet Gynecol* 2003;**189**:552–9.

5 Minkoff H, Ahdieh L, Watts HD, Greenblatt R, Schmidt J, Schneider M, Stek A. The relationship of pregnancy to the use of highly active antiretroviral therapy. *Am J Obstet Gynecol* 2001;**184**:1221–7.

6 Guidelines for Perinatal care of HIV. AIDSinfo.nih.gov

7 Baylor MS, Johann-Liang R. Hepatotoxicity associated with nevirapine use. *J Acquir Immune Defic Syndr* 2004;**35**:538–9.

8 ACOG committee opinion scheduled cesarean delivery and the prevention of vertical transmission of HIV infection. Number 234, May 2000.

9 Shapiro D, Tuomala R, Pollack H, *et al*. Mother-to-child HIV transmission risk according to antiretroviral therapy, mode of delivery, and viral load in 2895 US women (PACTG 367). Oral presentation at the 11th Conference on Retroviruses and Opportunistic Infections, San Francisco, CA, February, 2004 (Abstract 99).

10 European Collaborative Study. Mother-to-child transmission of HIV infection in the era of highly active antiretroviral therapy. *Clin Infect Dis* 2005;**40**:458–65.

Other recommended reading

Guay LA, Musoke P, Fleming T, *et al*. Intrapartum and neonatal single-dose nevirapine compared with zidovudine for prevention of mother-to-child transmission of HIV-1 in Kampala, Uganda: HIVNET 012 randomized trial. *Lancet* 1999;**354**:795–802.

International Perinatal HIV Group. The mode of delivery and the risk of vertical transmission of human immunodeficiency virus type 1: a meta-analysis of 15 prospective cohort studies. *N Engl J Med* 1999;**340**:977–87.

Mofenson LM; Centers for Disease Control and Prevention. US Public Health Service Task Force. US Public Health Service Task Force recommendations for use of antiretroviral drugs in pregnant HIV-1-infected women for maternal health and interventions to reduce perinatal HIV-1 transmission in the United States. *MMWR Recomm Rep* 2002; **51**(RR-18):1–38.

Sperling RS, Shapiro DE, Coombs RW, *et al*. Maternal viral load, zidovudine treatment and the risk of transmission of human immunodeficiency virus type 1 from mother to infant. *N Engl J Med* 1996;**335**:1621–9.

Tuomala RE, Shapiro D, Mofenson LM, *et al*. Antiretroviral therapy during pregnancy and the risk of an adverse outcome. *N Engl J Med* 2002;**346**:1863–70.

Obstetric Complications

31 Genetic and nongenetic causes of spontaneous abortion

Charles J. Lockwood

Perhaps no area of reproductive medicine, indeed, medicine in general, is more fraught with historical and anecdotal approaches to management and so bereft of evidence-based practices than the work-up and treatment of patients with recurrent miscarriage (aka habitual or recurrent abortion). It is even difficult to obtain a precise estimate of the prevalence of recurrent miscarriage because of definitional and gestational age variations, and the variable requirements for either two vs. three consecutive losses. Some but not all investigators also distinguish between primary recurrent aborters who have no intervening live births and secondary recurrent aborters who do. Further complicating prevalence estimates is the high background rate of pregnancy wastage in the general population which exceeds 50% when losses from conception through discernable fetal development are included [1]. A generally accepted number is that 1% of couples suffer two or more consecutive pregnancy losses prior to the third trimester [2].

Approximately 50–60% of all miscarriages prior to 20 weeks are caused by aneuploidy [1]. The most frequent causes are trisomy (most commonly 16 or 22), followed by polyploidy and monosomy X [1]. As a general rule, the older the mother and the earlier the loss the more likely it is aneuploid. One study suggested that aneuploidy was present in 25% of abortus specimens among women aged 20–29 years and 50% among women over 40 years [3]. Thus, it is not surprising that the risk of pregnancy loss increases in parallel to the risk of fetal Down syndrome. Miscarriage occurs in 9% of pregnancies among women 20–24 years of age but 75% of those occurring in women 44 years and older [4]. While it is difficult to assess the precise rate of aneuploidy in recurrent miscarriage specimens, as initial losses are usually not karyotyped, estimates range from 25% to 57% [4,5]. Data gleaned from preimplantation genetic diagnosis employed at the time of *in vitro* fertilization (IVF) suggests that patients with recurrent miscarriage have far higher rates of abnormal embryos compared with controls (70.7% vs. 45.1%; *P* <0.0001) [6]. They also have far higher rates of embryos with chromosomal abnormalities [6].

Unfortunately, most current "treatments" do not address the general population's high spontaneous wastage rate nor the high aneuploidy risk of attendant recurrent miscarriage. Moreover, proposed treatments must be judged against the high spontaneous remission rate. Indeed, the probability of a live birth after four successive spontaneous abortions is about 40% [7].

Genetic abnormalities

The etiology of recurrent miscarriage resulting from repetitive chromosomal abnormalities is not completely understood. Abnormalities that arise during the oocyte's first meiotic division account for the majority of cases. The clear association of recurrent miscarriage with increasing maternal age has led to a myriad of different theories of causation. For example, because excess oxidative stress leads to premature ovarian failure in animal models, it has been suggested that cumulative oxidative stress in cycling women may impair oocyte quality [8]. Alternatively, it has been posited that because aging is associated with an ever-shrinking oocyte pool, there is a progressive depletion of the number of oocytes available at the requisite stage of maturation for completion of normal meiosis [9]. Supporting this thesis is the observation that women who have lost at least one trisomic fetus have diminished ovarian reserve and enter the menopause at an earlier age than those with no such history [10,11]. Maternal age-related shortening of oocyte telomers has been posited as a cause of accelerated embryo fragmentation and apoptosis [12]. As shortened telomers can also lead to abnormal chiasma formation and nondisjunction, such a phenomenon could also help account for maternal age-associated embryonic aneuploidy [13].

Some have contended that the occurrence of recurrent miscarriage resulting from advanced maternal age-related aneuploidy should be managed through IVF with preimplantation screening for trisomies commonly found in abortus specimens. The argument is that because such losses are stochastic and their frequency increases with increasing age, recruitment of large numbers of embryos with subsequent selection and transfer of those that are putatively euploid will increase the likelihood of a live birth. While such arguments resonate, there is contradictory empiric evidence that live birth rates are improved using IVF with preimplantation screening [14–16].

Low folate levels have been linked to miscarriage when the fetal karyotype is abnormal (odds ratio [OR] 1.95; 95% confidence interval [CI], 1.09–3.48) but not when the fetal karyotype is normal (OR 1.11; 95% CI, 0.55–2.24) [17]. Folate deficiency may also have a role in meiotic nondisjunction. In addition, meta-analysis suggests that fasting hyperhomocysteinemia is modestly associated with recurrent pregnancy loss (<16 weeks) [18]. Thus, given its low toxicity, it would seem prudent to treat patients experiencing recurrent miscarriage with periconceptional folate supplementation (4 mg/day).

Heritable factors that are age-independent may also promote embryonic aneuploidy in up to 10% of affected couples [19]. For example, fragile sites on chromosomes [20,21], mosaicisms and deletions [19], as well as both large pericentric and paracentric chromosomal inversions [22,23] have been associated with recurrent miscarriages. There is a 30-fold increase in the occurrence of balanced translocations among couples with recurrent miscarriage with a prevalence of 3.6% [24]. A recent study observed a 29% rate of miscarriage among clinically recognized pregnancies in couples bearing a balanced translocation with 36% of the abortuses found to have an unbalanced translocation [25]. Thus, high-resolution parental karyotyping should be performed in couples with recurrent miscarriage. It would again be logical to offer affected couples IVF with preimplantation diagnosis but it is not certain that live birth rates will be improved [26].

Skewed inactivation of the X-chromosome appears to be present in 14–20% of women with recurrent miscarriage, about a fourfold increase over the baseline population [27,28]. Affected patients may harbor an X-linked or germline mosaic developmentally lethal mutation on the X chromosome that causes nonrandom X inactivation. Alternatively, such skewing may be associated with a far higher rate of aneuploid conceptuses [29]. Single gene defects may also promote recurrent miscarriage. These may be either X-linked or autosomal recessive. For example, lethal multiple pterygium syndromes are a collection of autosomal recessive and X-linked recessive disorders that are associated with fetal death at 14–20 weeks with variable features including arthrogryposis, hydrocephalus, hydrops and cystic hygromas [30]. Incontinentia pigmenti is an X-linked disorder usually lethal in males [31]. Affected males may also develop hydrops and/or cystic hygromas while affected females have dental anomalies and cutaneous manifestations [31].

Based on the large number of embryonic lethal mutations observed in transgenic mice studies, it is likely that many other developmentally lethal mendelian disorders exist. Unfortunately, until the advent of whole genomic screening there is no simple way to identify such mutations. However, aberrant regulation of trophoblast growth resulting from developmental abnormalities often results in the formation of trophoblast inclusions—abnormal invaginations of the villous surface which on section appear as inverted islands of trophoblasts [32]. Such a phenomenon may also be associated with autism [33]. Thus, careful examination of the placenta may provide valuable clues as to a developmental etiology of recurrent intermittent losses.

Infectious diseases

While acute, severe, bacterial and viral infections can cause an isolated spontaneous abortion, no unequivocal link has been established between chronic genital tract carriage of bacteria and recurrent miscarriage. Ureaplasma urealyticum (serotype 4) is more commonly isolated from women with recurrent miscarriage than controls [34]. Moreover, nonrandomized trials suggest treatment of genital tract mycoplasma with doxycycline may reduce early loss rates [35]. However, there is no evidence from appropriately conducted randomized clinical trials that eradication of mycoplasma species reduces miscarriage rates. There is also no convincing link between either recovery of genital tract Chlamydia trachomatis or the presence of antichlamydial antibodies and recurrent miscarriage [36,37]. The presence of bacterial vaginosis (BV) has been linked to early isolated spontaneous abortion (adjusted OR 2.67; 95% CI, 1.26–5.63) [38]. However, the link between BV and recurrent miscarriage and the benefits of treatment have yet to be firmly established.

Endocrinopathies

While poorly controlled diabetes and thyroid disease are linked to recurrent miscarriage, there is no evidence of such link with either subclinical thyroid disease or diabetes [39,40]. There were initial reports that polycystic ovarian syndrome (PCOS) was associated with recurrent miscarriage. However, recent studies have found no such link [41,42]. In addition, there have been no formal randomized clinical trials of the effect of metformin and other insulin sensitizing agents on the occurrence of spontaneous abortion in PCOS patients, although an anecdotal study suggests metformin improves live birth rates [43].

Progesterone has a crucial role in the maintenance of endometrial hemostasis and architectural integrity [44]. Conversely, the antiprogestin, RU 486 can induce menstruation and early abortion by inhibiting these salutary effects of progesterone [45,46]. These observations provide biological plausibility to the theory that luteal phase defects could promote early pregnancy loss. Indeed, the prevalence of luteal phase defects among recurrent miscarriage patients is reported to be 10–30% [47,48]. Unfortunately, there are no definitive diagnostic criteria because the condition is intermittent [49]. Moreover, meta-analysis of trials of progesterone therapy for recurrent miscarriage do not demonstrate a benefit [50].

It is unclear whether elevated prolactin levels are associated with recurrent pregnancy loss [51], although at least one study has shown that treatment with bromocriptine increases the likelihood of normal pregnancy outcomes [52].

In short, it is unclear whether endocrine disorders including PCOS, luteal phase defects, and hyperprolactinemia are *bona fide* causes of recurrent miscarriage. Equally uncertain is whether their respective treatments (metformin, progesterone supplementation, and bromocriptine) improve live birth rates.

Uterine abnormalities

While müllerian tract anomalies are linked to an increased occurrence of nonvertex presentations and a higher rate of prematurity [53], their association with recurrent miscarriage is generally predicated on descriptive, observational studies replete with ascertainment biases. Salim *et al.* [54] compared women with and without a history of three or more consecutive unexplained pregnancy losses before 14 weeks using three-dimensional ultrasound, and found major congenital anomalies in 23.8% of women with losses compared with 5.3% in controls. However, in both groups the most common anomalies were minor, arcuate and subseptate uteri, which accounted for more than 90% of cases. The former does not appear to be associated with a higher rate of recurrent abortion, and may represent a normal variant [55]. The prevalence of major anomalies was 6.9% in women with recurrent miscarriage compared with 1.7% in controls [55]. Table 31.1 lists the relative distribution of the major anomalies and their associated miscarriage rates (see reference [56] for details).

Various theories have been promulgated to account for the association of uterine anomalies with recurrent miscarriage

Table 31.1 Mullerian duct anomalies and their association with miscarriage.

Mullerian Anomaly	Prevalence Among Patients with Mullerian Anomalies (%)	Risk of Spontaneous Loss (<20 weeks) (%)
Septum	55	65
Unicornuate uterus	20	51
Uterus didelphys	5–7	43
Bicornuate uterus	10	32

including decreased vascularity in the septum, increased inflammation, and a reduction in sensitivity to steroid hormones [56]. However, there is no substantial evidence to favor one putative etiology over another.

There are also no controlled randomized clinical trials of pregnancy outcome following resection of uterine septum, although reductions in recurrent loss have been reported in several large series [57,58]. Traditional open metroplasty is rarely recommended for bicornuate or didelphys uteri because of the attendant risks of infertility and uterine rupture during pregnancy as well as the more favorable associated pregnancy outcomes.

While pregnancy outcomes are generally believed to be relatively unaffected by the presence of myomas [59], submucous myomas that distort the uterine cavity have been posited as causes of recurrent miscarriage and reduced IVF success rates [60]. Hysteroscopic resection may improve fertility, live birth rates, and bleeding patterns [61]. Other uterine defects such as Asherman syndrome and polyps have been posited as causes of recurrent miscarriage, and descriptive series suggest improvements in pregnancy outcomes following hysteroscopic resection [62]. Thus, based on expert opinion, it would seem reasonable to offer patients with recurrent miscarriage screening for uterine defects by sonohysterography. Subsequent magnetic resonance imaging (MRI) or concomitant use of three-dimensional ultrasound can allow differentiation of bicornuate from septate uteri. Operative hysteroscopy can then be employed for the treatment of submucous fibroids, polyps, septae, and synechiae. However, these recommendations are not based upon well-conducted randomized clinical trials.

Inherited thrombophilias

The strength of the association between inherited thrombophilias and recurrent miscarriage appears to be modest at best. Moreover, the risk appears intermittent and restricted to gestational ages greater than 9 weeks. The most robust data are available for the factor V Leiden (FVL) mutation. It represents the most common, significantly thrombogenic, heritable thrombophilia. It is present in about 5% of European-derived populations and 3% of African-Americans but is virtually absent in nonwhite Africans and Asians [63]. It arises from a point mutation in the factor V gene causing the substitution of a glutamine for an arginine at position 506, the site of cleavage by activated protein C, thus conferring activated protein C resistance. A meta-analysis of 31 studies reported a modest link between FVL and first trimester spontaneous abortion with OR 2.01 (95% CI, 1.13–3.58) but a stronger association with late (>19 weeks) nonrecurrent fetal loss (OR 3.26; 95% CI, 1.82–5.83) [64]. A large case–control study of patients with recurrent stillbirths beyond 22 weeks showed an even stronger association with FVL (OR 7.83; 95% CI, 2.83–21.67) [65]. Thus,

Table 31.2 Prevalence and detection of maternal inherited thrombophilias.

Thrombophilia	Prevalence (%)	Detection Methods	References
FVL	5.3	PCR	74, 75
Prothrombin G20201A	2.9	PCR	76, 77
Hyperhomocysteinemia	<5	Fasting assay, ELISA	78
Antithrombin deficiency	0.2	Functional assay with a cut-off of <60%	63, 79
Protein S deficiency	0.2	Measure total free antigen level with a cut-off of <55% in nonpregnant patients and <45% in pregnant patients (repeat to confirm)	80
Protein C deficiency	0.2	Functional assay with a cut-off of <50%	63, 79

ELISA, enzyme-linked immunosorbent assay; PCR, polymerase chain reaction.

the later the fetal loss, the stronger the association with FVL. Indeed, Dudding and Attia [66] conducted a meta-analysis of the link between FVL and adverse pregnancy events and noted no association with first trimester losses but a strong association with two or more second or third trimester fetal losses (OR 10.7; 95% CI, 4.0–28.5).

A similar pattern appears to hold for inherited thrombophilias in general. The European Prospective Cohort on Thrombophilia (EPCOT) consisted of 571 women with thrombophilias followed through 1524 pregnancies compared with 395 controls having 1019 pregnancies [67]. This study found a statistically significant association between inherited thrombophilias in general and stillbirth (OR 3.6; 95% CI, 1.4–9.4) but not between inherited thrombophilias and spontaneous abortion (OR 1.27; 95% CI, 0.94–1.71). Roque et al. [68] assessed a cohort of 491 patients with a history of various adverse pregnancy outcomes and observed that the presence of a maternal thrombophilia was actually protective of recurrent pregnancy loss at less than 10 weeks (OR 0.55; 95% CI, 0.33–0.92). In contrast, maternal thrombophilias were modestly associated with an increased risk of losses at 10 weeks or more (OR 1.76; 95% CI, 1.05–2.94) and more strongly associated with fetal loss after 14 weeks (OR 3.41; 95% CI, 1.90–6.10).

Consistent with this protective effect of FVL and other inherited thrombophilias on early pregnancy is the observation that IVF implantation rates were higher among FVL carriers than among noncarriers (90% vs. 49%; P = 0.02) [69]. Extravillous endovascular trophoblast occlude spiral arteries to minimize uteroplacental blood flow before 10 weeks' gestation. Moreover, intervillous oxygen pressure is substantially lower prior to 10 weeks compared with after 12 weeks (17 ± 6.9 vs. 60.7 ± 8.5 mmHg) [70,71]. Thus, there is no a priori reason why thrombophilias would promote early pregnancy loss. That thrombophilias might be protective of early loss is suggested by the finding of undetectable levels of trophoblast superoxide dismutase, an enzyme responsible for the conversion of the superoxide anions, prior to 10 weeks [72].

In contrast, following restoration of patency in the uteroplacental circulation, subsequent uteroplacental thrombosis would have harmful effects accounting for the link between maternal thrombophilias and later loss. Moreover, anticoagulation therapy may prevent recurrent fetal loss. Gris et al. [73] conducted a randomized clinical trial of the low molecular weight heparin, enoxaparin, versus low dose aspirin in 160 women with one unexplained fetal loss at more than 10 weeks who were heterozygous for FVL, the prothrombin G20210A mutation, or protein S deficiency. They reported that enoxaparin therapy resulted in greater numbers of healthy live births (86.2%) than low dose aspirin (28.8%; P <0.0001) (OR 15.5; 95% CI, 7–34) [73] (see Table 31.2 for list of common inherited thrombophilias, their approximate prevalence in European populations and detection method).

Antiphospholipid antibodies

Antiphospholipid antibody (APA) syndrome is defined by the combination of a prior deep venous or arterial thrombosis, characteristic obstetric complications, or thrombocytopenia associated with APA [81]. Obstetric complications include at least one fetal death at 10 weeks' or more gestation, at least one premature birth before 35 weeks, or at least three consecutive miscarriages before the 10th week. All other causes of pregnancy morbidity must be excluded. The APA have to be present on two or more occasions at least 6 weeks apart.

APA are immunoglobulins against proteins bound to negatively charged (anionic) phospholipids [82]. They can be detected by screening for antibodies binding directly to protein epitopes (e.g., β_2-glycoprotein-1, prothrombin, annexin V) or by indirectly detecting antibodies reacting to proteins present in an anionic phospholipid matrix (e.g., cardiolipin and phosphatidylserine) or by evaluating the "downstream" coagulation effects of these antibodies on in vitro prothrombin activation (i.e., lupus anticoagulants) [83].

Persistently high levels of these antibodies are associated with obstetric complications in about 15–20% of affected patients including fetal loss after 9 weeks' gestation, abruption, severe preeclampsia, and intrauterine growth restriction (IUGR). The most consistent association with fetal loss is seen with lupus anticoagulants with reported odds ratios of 3.0–4.8

while anticardiolipin antibodies display a wider range of reported odds ratios of 0.86–20.0 [82]. While a component of the definition, there is substantial controversy whether APA are also associated with recurrent (three or more) early miscarriage less than 10 weeks in the absence of stillbirth because at least 50% of pregnancy losses in APA patients occur after the 10th week [84]. Moreover, compared with patients having unexplained first trimester losses without APA, those with antibodies more often have documented fetal cardiac activity prior to a loss (86% vs. 43%; P <0.01) [85]. In addition, a meta-analysis of seven studies reported no significant association between APA and either clinical pregnancy (OR 0.99; 95% CI, 0.64–1.53) or live birth rates (OR 1.07; 95% CI, 0.66–1.75) in patients undergoing IVF [86].

Suggested pathogenic mechanism(s) by which APA induce fetal loss include impairment of the anticoagulant effects of placental anionic phospholipid binding proteins β_2-glycoprotein-I and annexin V [87,88], and APA induction of decidual and placental bed complement activation [89]. Treatment includes low molecular weight heparin, low dose aspirin, and hydroxychloroquine, and appears to be associated with an 80% live birth rate.

Immunologic causes

Theoretically, the fetus represents an allograft and maternal immune rejection should result in recurrent pregnancy loss. However, a host of mechanisms exist to prevent such a phenomenon. These include trophoblast expression of non-immunogenic human leukocyte antigen G (HLA-G) and Fas ligand, which can induce programmed cell death in attacking leukocytes. The placenta also produces a myriad of immunosuppressive factors such as human chorionic gonadotropin (hCG), pregnancy-associated plasma protein A (PAPP-A), and progesterone, and facilitates a doubling of free maternal cortisol levels through the production of corticotrophin-releasing hormone.

Two principal theories have been espoused to account for possible maternal immunologically mediated adverse pregnancy outcomes: absence of so-called "blocking" antibodies, and excessive decidual natural killer (NK) cell activity. The nature of the putative blocking antibodies were maternal antipaternal lymphocytotoxic antibodies. The theory was that excessive HLA sharing by prospective parents would lead to the absence of such antibodies. This, in turn, would expose placental antigens to a more cytotoxic maternal immune response. Proponents of this theory advocated treatment of recurrent miscarriage patients lacking such antibodies with infusions of their partner's or third party leukocytes or extracts of placental trophoblast to induce antibody production. However, meta-analyses of such approaches failed to support efficacy [90]. Ober *et al.* [91] conducted a double-blind, placebo-controlled, multicenter, randomized, clinical trial in which 91

recurrent miscarriage patients were assigned to immunization with paternal mononuclear cells, and 92 to sterile saline injections [91]. These investigators noted higher numbers of viable pregnancies in the placebo compared with the treatment group (41/85 [48%] versus 31/86 [36%]; OR 0.60; 95% CI, 0.33–1.12) [91]. Ultimately, the US Food and Drug Administration moved to constrain such treatment.

The link between elevated NK cell activity and recurrent miscarriage has been suggested by several small studies. The underlying theory is that excess decidual NK cell activity may damage the implanting blastocyst or derange early placentation to promote miscarriage. Yamada *et al.* [92] reported that elevated peripheral blood preconception NK cell activity (>46%; relative risk [RR] 3.6; 95% CI, 1.6–8.0) and percentages of circulating NK cells (>16.4%; RR 4.9; 95% CI, 1.7–13.8) predicted subsequent biochemical pregnancy and miscarriage with normal karyotype in the next pregnancy among recurrent aborters. These findings have been supported by other [93,94] but not all investigators [95]. Complicating this issue, we have recently shown that the mRNA repertoire of circulating NK cells is far different from that of decidual NK cells [96]. This calls into question the logic and biologic plausibility of measuring peripheral blood NK cell activity as a proxy for decidual and placental bed NK cell activity. Indeed, decidual NK cell numbers are not increased in spontaneous versus induced abortion specimens [97]. Thus, the scientific underpinning of this innate immune theory of recurrent miscarriage remains suspect.

Morikawa *et al.* [98] evaluated the outcome of intravenous immunoglobulin (IVIG) treatment in 18 pregnancies from 15 women with four or more consecutive miscarriages of unexplained etiology. They noted that 14 treated pregnancies resulted in live births and four resulted in abortions with chromosome abnormalities. Treatment also reduced preinfusion peripheral blood NK cell activity and NK cell number. However, one must exercise extreme caution in interpreting this small, uncontrolled study because IVIG has not been shown to be efficacious when used in unselected women with unexplained recurrent primary miscarriage [90]. Moreover, there is growing evidence that increased decidual NK cell activity is required for normal placentation [99], and that reduced decidual NK cell activity may be associated with preeclampsia and IUGR [100]. Thus, there is very little evidence to support the assessment of peripheral NK cell activity in recurrent miscarriage patients and there is growing evidence against treatment to suppress decidual NK cell activity with IVIG.

Evidence-based evaluation of couples experiencing recurrent miscarriage

A number of social and anthropomorphic factors are modestly associated with the occurrence of isolated and recurrent miscarriage. These include cigarette smoking, heavy caffeine use, and obesity [101,102]. Thus, smoking cessation, reduction in caffeine use, exercise, and diet are all prudent interventions in affected patients.

Based on the most common etiologies and their gestational age association it would appear prudent to classify patients with recurrent loss into those with recurrent early losses (i.e., prior to 10 weeks) and those with later losses (i.e., after 10 weeks). The focus of the evaluation of a patient with recurrent early miscarriages should be on the identification of genetic factors. Thus, parental karyotypes, aggressive karyotyping of abortus specimens, and assessment of the placental pathology for trophoblast inclusions would appear reasonable diagnostic studies. The latter are particularly appropriate when no prior abortus karyotypes were obtained and when there are intermittent euploid losses at around the same gestational ages.

Treatment of patients with recurrent early losses should include nutritional supplementation with folate. Because luteal phase defects may have a role in very early losses, progestational supplementation in the luteal phase (3–14 days after ovulation) and until 10 weeks' gestation appears reasonable. However, the utility of IVF with preimplantational screening for common aneuploidies remains an unproven therapy in patients with recurrent aneuploid losses because of advanced maternal age or parental chromosomal abnormalities.

For losses at or after 10 weeks' gestation, a genetic evaluation should also be performed; evaluation for inherited thrombophilias would also appear prudent (Table 31.2). Treatment of affected patients with low molecular weight heparin may be beneficial in women with recurrent fetal loss and documented thrombophilias other than hyperhomocysteinemia. The latter patient generally can be treated with folate and anticoagulation should be limited to those who fail such therapy and have persistently elevated fasting homocysteine levels.

For patients with either or both early and late miscarriages, a search for uterine anatomic abnormalities should be conducted with sonohysterography and three-dimensional ultrasound. Remediable defects should be corrected prior to attempting a subsequent pregnancy. In addition, a work-up for antiphospholipid antibodies should be performed.

Conclusions

In summary, the evaluation and treatment of patients with recurrent miscarriage should include the following.

1 Parental karyotypes, and assessment of prospective abortus' karyotype. If parental chromosomal abnormalities (e.g., translocation) or abortus' aneuploidy are detected, consider IVF with preimplantation screening.

2 When karyotypes of abortus' specimens are not available and/or the patient's losses are intermittent and generally occur at the same gestation age, analyze the placental specimens of prior losses for trophoblast inclusions. If present, obtain an extended pedigree to rule-out X-linked recessive lethal disorders or autosomal recessive disorders. Consider high-resolution parental karyotyping to rule out subtle chromosomal defects. When mendelian disorders are detected, treatment can consist of further attempts at spontaneous conception or donor gametes. If minor parental chromosomal defects are observed, consider IVF with preimplantation screening.

3 Treat with empiric folate and both luteal phase and gestational progestational supplementation.

4 Consider assessing prolactin levels and ruling out insulin resistant PCOS, treating affected patients with bromocryptine or metformin, respectively.

5 Evaluate uterus with sonohysterography and three-dimensional ultrasonography, and consider hysteroscopic repair of remediable defects prior to conception.

6 Evaluate for APA (lupus anticoagulant, as well as IgM and IgG for anticardiolipin, antiphosphatidylserine, anti-β_2-glycoprotein-I, antiannexin V and antiprothrombin antibodies). Treat with low molecular weight heparin, low dose aspirin, and hydroxychloroquine in subsequent pregnancy.

7 A work-up for inherited thrombophilias if the losses have occurred at or after 10 weeks (Table 31.2). Treat with low molecular weight heparin in next pregnancy.

Further complicating care, patients having miscarriage have high rates of subsequent depression, and repetitive miscarriage may increase risks of post-traumatic stress disorders [103]. As a consequence, they are highly suggestible and more easily accepting of unorthodox treatments. Thus, couples experiencing recurrent miscarriage should be screened for depression and post-traumatic stress disorder, and appropriate psychological support provided. Finally, patients should be reassured of the high spontaneous remission rate.

Case presentation 1

A 39-year-old G5P0050 presents with five consecutive miscarriages in the past 2 years. She has unremarkable past medical, surgical, and gynecological histories, and a 15 pack-year smoking history. Her menses are regular although her cycle has lengthened in the past 18 months from 28 to 34 days. She also notes recent onset of rare hot flushes and night sweats that disturb her sleep. All losses occurred at <9 weeks. Two consisted of chemical pregnancies. Three required curettage. The products of conception of her last loss were karyotyped and revealed trisomy 22.

1 What is the most likely etiology of these losses?

2 What additional diagnostic studies are indicated?

3 What treatment regimen would you recommend?

Case presentation 2

A 28-year-old G5P2032 presents with a history of two term births of healthy unaffected female infants following uncomplicated pregnancies. Her losses all occurred at around 16 weeks' gestation in her initial, middle, and last pregnancies. She has no medical complications, does not smoke or abuse caffeine. Karyotype of her last loss revealed 46 XY. Her placental pathology report revealed no evidence of ischemia, decidual vasculopathy, or infection but made mention of multiple trophoblast inclusions.

1 What is the most likely etiology of these losses?
2 Are there any diagnostic studies indicated?
3 How should she be counseled?

References

1 Rai R, Regan L. Recurrent miscarriage. *Lancet* 2006;**368**:601–11.
2 Regan L. Recurrent miscarriage. *Br Med J* 1991;**302**:543–4.
3 Sullivan AE, Silver RM, LaCoursiere DY, Porter TF, Branch DW. Recurrent fetal aneuploidy and recurrent miscarriage. *Obstet Gynecol* 2004;**104**:784–8.
4 Nybo Andersen AM, Wohlfahrt J, Christens P, Olsen J, Melbye M. Maternal age and fetal loss: population based register linkage study. *Br Med J* 2000;**320**:1708–12.
5 Stern JJ, Dorfmann AD, Gutierrez-Najar AJ, Cerrillo M, Coulam CB. Frequency of abnormal karyotypes among abortuses from women with and without a history of recurrent spontaneous abortion. *Fertil Steril* 1996;**65**:250–3.
6 Rubio C, Simon C, Vidal F, *et al.* Chromosomal abnormalities and embryo development in recurrent miscarriage couples. *Hum Reprod* 2003;**18**:182–8.
7 Stirrat GM. Recurrent miscarriage. *Lancet* 1990;**336**:673–5.
8 Hu X, Roberts JR, Apopa PL, Kan YW, Ma Q. Accelerated ovarian failure induced by 4-vinyl cyclohexene diepoxide in Nrf2 null mice. *Mol Cell Biol* 2006;**26**:940–54.
9 Warburton D. The effect of maternal age on the frequency of trisomy: change in meiosis or *in utero* selection? *Prog Clin Biol Res* 1989;**311**:165–81.
10 Freeman SB, Yang Q, Allran K, Taft LF, Sherman SL. Women with a reduced ovarian complement may have an increased risk for a child with Down syndrome. *Am J Hum Genet* 2000;**66**:1680–3.
11 Kline J, Kinney A, Levin B, Warburton D. Trisomic pregnancy and earlier age at menopause. *Am J Hum Genet* 2000;**67**:395–404.
12 Keefe DL, Franco S, Liu L, *et al.* Telomere length predicts embryo fragmentation after *in vitro* fertilization in women: toward a telomere theory of reproductive aging in women. *Am J Obstet Gynecol* 2005;**192**:1256–60.
13 Liu L, Franco S, Spyropoulos B, Moens PB, Blasco MA, Keefe DL. Irregular telomeres impair meiotic synapsis and recombination in mice. *Proc Natl Acad Sci USA* 2004;**101**:6496–501.
14 Rubio C, Rodrigo L, Perez-Cano I, *et al.* FISH screening of aneuploidies in preimplantation embryos to improve IVF outcome. *Reprod Biomed Online* 2005;**11**:497–506.
15 Rubio C, Pehlivan T, Rodrigo L, Simon C, Remohi J, Pellicer A. Embryo aneuploidy screening for unexplained recurrent miscarriage: a minireview. *Am J Reprod Immunol* 2005;**53**:159–6.
16 Platteau P, Staessen C, Michiels A, Van Steirteghem A, Liebaers I, Devroey P. Preimplantation genetic diagnosis for aneuploidy screening in patients with unexplained recurrent miscarriages. *Fertil Steril* 2005;**83**:393–5.
17 George L, Mills JL, Johansson AL, *et al.* Plasma folate levels and risk of spontaneous abortion. *JAMA* 2002;**288**:1867–73.
18 Nelen WL, Blom HJ, Steegers EA, den Heijer M, Eskes TK. Hyperhomocysteinemia and recurrent early pregnancy loss: a meta-analysis. *Fertil Steril* 2000;**74**:1196–9.
19 Sachs ES, Jahoda MG, Van Hemel JO, Hoogeboom AJ, Sandkuyl LA. Chromosome studies of 500 couples with two or more abortions. *Obstet Gynecol* 1985;**65**:375–8.
20 Toncheva D. Fragile sites and spontaneous abortions. *Genet Couns* 1991;**2**:205–10.
21 Giardino D, Bettio D, Simoni G. 12q13 fragility in a family with recurrent spontaneous abortions: expression of the fragile site under different culture conditions. *Ann Genet* 1990;**33**:88–9.
22 Wolf GC, Mao J, Izquierdo L, Joffe G. Paternal pericentric inversion of chromosome 4 as a cause of recurrent pregnancy loss. *J Med Genet* 1994;**31**:153–5.
23 Turczynowicz S, Sharma P, Smith A, Davidson AA. Paracentric inversion of chromosome 14 plus rare 9p variant in a couple with habitual spontaneous abortion. *Ann Genet* 1992;**35**:58–60.
24 Fryns JP, Van Buggenhout G. Structural chromosome rearrangements in couples with recurrent fetal wastage. *Eur J Obstet Gynecol Reprod Biol* 1998;**81**;171–6.
25 Stephenson MD, Sierra S. Reproductive outcomes in recurrent pregnancy loss associated with a parental carrier of a structural chromosome rearrangement. *Hum Reprod* 2006;**21**:1076–82.
26 Sugiura-Ogasawara M, Suzumori K. Can preimplantation genetic diagnosis improve success rates in recurrent aborters with translocations? *Hum Reprod* 2005;**20**:3267–70.
27 Lanasa MC, Hogge WA, Kubik CJ, *et al.* A novel X chromosome-linked genetic cause of recurrent spontaneous abortion. *Am J Obstet Gynecol* 2001;**185**:563–8.
28 Sangha KK, Stephenson MD, Brown CJ, Robinson WP. Extremely skewed X-chromosome inactivation is increased in women with recurrent spontaneous abortion. *Am J Hum Genet* 1999;**65**: 913–7.
29 Lanasa MC, Hogge WA, Hoffman E. The X chromosome and recurrent spontaneous abortion: the significance of transmanifesting carriers. *Am J Hum Genet* 1999;**64**:934–8.
30 Lockwood C, Irons M, Troiani J, Kawada C, Chaudhury A, Cetrulo C. The prenatal sonographic diagnosis of lethal multiple pterygium syndrome: a heritable cause of recurrent abortion. *Am J Obstet Gynecol* 1988;**159**:474–6.
31 Odent S, Le Marec B, Smahi A, *et al.* Spontaneous abortion of male fetuses with incontinentia pigmenti (apropos of a family). *J Gynecol Obstet Biol Reprod (Paris)* 1997;**26**:633–6.
32 Kliman HJ, Segel L. The placenta may predict the baby. *J Theor Biol* 2003;**225**:143–5.
33 Anderson GM, Jacobs-Stannard A, Chawarska K, Volkmar FR, Kliman HJ. Placental trophoblast inclusions in autism spectrum disorder. *Biol Psychiatry* 2006;Jun 22: [Epub ahead of print].
34 Naessens A, Foulon W, Breynaert J, Lauwers S. Serotypes of *Ureaplasma urealyticum* isolated from normal pregnant women

and patients with pregnancy complications. *J Clin Microbiol* 1988;**26**:319–22.

35 Quinn PA, Shewchuk AD, Shuber J, *et al.* Efficacy of antibiotic therapy in preventing spontaneous pregnancy loss among couples colonized with genital mycoplasmas. *Am J Obstet Gynecol* 1983;**145**:239–44.

36 Sozio J, Ness RB. Chlamydial lower genital tract infection and spontaneous abortion. *Infect Dis Obstet Gynecol* 1998;**6**:8–12.

37 Paukku M, Tulppala M, Puolakkainen M, Anttila T, Paavonen J. Lack of association between serum antibodies to *Chlamydia trachomatis* and a history of recurrent pregnancy loss. *Fertil Steril* 1999;**72**:427–30.

38 Ralph SG, Rutherford AJ, Wilson JD. Influence of bacterial vaginosis on conception and miscarriage in the first trimester: cohort study. *Br Med J* 1999;**319**:220–3.

39 Mills JL, Simpson JL, Driscoll SG, *et al.* Incidence of spontaneous abortion among normal women and insulin-dependent diabetic women whose pregnancies were identified within 21 days of conception. *N Engl J Med* 1988;**319**:1617–23.

40 Rushworth FH, Backos M, Rai R, Chilcott IT, Baxter N, Regan L. Prospective pregnancy outcome in untreated recurrent miscarriers with thyroid autoantibodies. *Hum Reprod* 2000;**15**:1637–9.

41 Rai R, Backos M, Rushworth F, Regan L. Polycystic ovaries and recurrent miscarriage: a reappraisal. *Hum Reprod* 2000;**15**:612–5.

42 Liddell HS, Sowden K, Farquhar CM. Recurrent miscarriage: screening for polycystic ovaries and subsequent pregnancy outcome. *Aust N Z J Obstet Gynaecol* 1997;**37**:402–6.

43 Glueck CJ, Wang P, Goldenberg N, Sieve-Smith L. Pregnancy outcomes among women with polycystic ovary syndrome treated with metformin. *Hum Reprod* 2002;**17**:2858–64.

44 Schatz F, Krikun G, Caze R, Rahman M, Lockwood CJ. Progestin-regulated expression of tissue factor in decidual cells: implications in endometrial hemostasis, menstruation and angiogenesis. *Steroids* 2003;**68**:849–60.

45 Lockwood CJ, Krikun G, Papp C, Aigner S, Nemerson Y, Schatz F. Biological mechanisms underlying RU 486 clinical effects: inhibition of endometrial stromal cell tissue factor content. *J Clin Endocrinol Metab* 1994;**79**:786–9.

46 Lockwood CJ, Krikun G, Hausknecht VA, Papp C, Schatz F. Matrix metalloproteinase and matrix metalloproteinase inhibitor expression in endometrial stromal cells during progestin-initiated decidualization and menstruation-related progestin withdrawal. *Endocrinology* 1998;**139**:4607–13.

47 Lessey BA, Fritz MA. Defective luteal function. In: Fraser JS, Jansen RPS, Lobo RA, Whitehead MI, eds. *Estrogens and Progestogens in Clinical Practice*. Philadelphia: W.B. Saunders; 1998. pp. 437–53.

48 Potdar N, Konje JC. The endocrinological basis of recurrent miscarriages. *Curr Opin Obstet Gynecol* 2005;**17**:424–8.

49 Dawood MY. Corpus luteal insufficiency. *Curr Opin Obstet Gynecol* 1994;**6**:121–7.

50 Oates-Whitehead RM, Haas DM, Carrier JAK. Progestogen for preventing miscarriage (Cochrane Review). In: *The Cochrane Library*, Issue 3, 2004. Oxford: Update Software.

51 Dlugi AM. Hyperprolactinemic recurrent spontaneous pregnancy loss: a true clinical entity or a spurious finding? *Fertil Steril* 1998;**70**:253–5.

52 Hirahara F, Andoh N, Sawai K, Hirabuki T, Uemura T, Minaguchi H. Hyperprolactinemic recurrent miscarriage and results of randomized bromocriptine treatment trials. *Fertil Steril* 1998;**70**:246–52.

53 Stein AL, March CM. Pregnancy outcome in women with mullerian duct anomalies. *J Reprod Med* 1990;**35**:411–4.

54 Salim R, Regan L, Woelfer B, Backos M, Jurkovic D. A comparative study of the morphology of congenital uterine anomalies in women with and without a history of recurrent first trimester miscarriage. *Hum Reprod* 2003;**18**:162–6.

55 Raga F, Bauset C, Remohi J, Bonilla-Musoles F, Simon C, Pellicer A. Reproductive impact of congenital Mullerian anomalies. *Hum Reprod* 1997;**12**:2277–81.

56 Devi Wold AS, Pham N, Arici A. Anatomic factors in recurrent pregnancy loss. *Semin Reprod Med* 2006;**24**:25–32.

57 Daly DC, Maier D, Soto-Albors C. Hysteroscopic metroplasty: six years' experience. *Obstet Gynecol* 1989;**73**:201–5.

58 De Cherney AH, Russell JB, Graebe RA, Polan ML. Resectoscopic management of mullerian fusion defect. *Fertil Steril* 1986;**45**:726–8.

59 Vergani P, Ghidini A, Strobelt N, *et al.* Do uterine leiomyomas influence pregnancy outcome? *Am J Perinatol* 1994;**11**:356–8.

60 Bajeckal N, Li TC. Fibroids, infertility and pregnancy wastage. *Hum Reprod* 2000;**6**:614–20.

61 Fernandez H, Sefrioui O, Virelizier C, Gervaise A, Gomel V, Frydman R. Hysteroscopic resection of submucosal myomas in patients with infertility. *Hum Reprod* 2001;**6**:1489–92.

62 Sanders B. Uterine factors and infertility. *J Reprod Med* 2006;**51**:169–76.

63 Franco RF, Reitsma PH. Genetic risk factors of venous thrombosis. *Hum Genet* 2001;**109**:369–84.

64 Rey E, Kahn SR, David M, Shrier I. Thrombophilic disorders and fetal loss: a meta-analysis. *Lancet* 2003;**361**:901–8.

65 Gris JC, Quere I, Monpeyroux F, *et al.* Case–control study of the frequency of thrombophilic disorders in couples with late foetal loss and no thrombotic antecedent: the Nimes Obstetricians and Haematologists Study5 (NOHA5). *Thromb Haemost* 1999;**81**:891–9.

66 Dudding TE, Attia J. The association between adverse pregnancy outcomes and maternal factor V Leiden genotype: a meta-analysis. *Thromb Haemost* 2004;**91**:700–11.

67 Preston FE, Rosendaal FR, Walker ID, *et al.* Increased fetal loss in women with heritable thrombophilia. *Lancet* 1996;**348**:913–6.

68 Roque H, Paidas MJ, Funai EF, Kuczynski E, Lockwood CJ. Maternal thrombophilias are not associated with early pregnancy loss. *Thromb Haemost* 2004;**91**:290–5.

69 Gopel W, Ludwig M, Junge AK, Kohlmann T, Diedrich K, Moller J. Selection pressure for the factor V Leiden mutation and embryo implantation. *Lancet* 2001;**358**:1238–9.

70 Rodesch F, Simon P, Donner C, Jauniaux E. Oxygen measurements in endometrial and trophoblastic tissues during early pregnancy. *Obstet Gynecol* 1992;**80**:283–5.

71 Jaffe R. Investigation of abnormal first-trimester gestations by color Doppler imaging. *J Clin Ultrasound* 1993;**21**:521–6.

72 Watson AL, Skepper JN, Jauniaux E, Burton GJ. Susceptibility of human placental syncytiotrophoblastic mitochondria to oxygen-mediated damage in relation to gestational age. *J Clin Endocrinol Metab* 1998;**83**:1697–705.

73 Gris JC, Mercier E, Quere I, *et al*. Low-molecular-weight heparin versus low-dose aspirin in women with one fetal loss and a constitutional thrombophilic disorder. *Blood* 2004;**103**:3695–9.

74 Juul K, Tybjaerg-Hansen A, Steffensen R, Kofoed S, Jensen G, Nordestgaard BG. Factor V Leiden: The Copenhagen City Heart Study and 2 meta-analyses. *Blood* 2002;**100**:3–10.

75 Price DT, Ridker PM. Factor V Leiden mutation and the risks for thromboembolic disease: a clinical perspective. *Ann Intern Med* 1997;**127**:895–903.

76 Aznar J, Vaya A, Estelles A, *et al*. Risk of venous thrombosis in carriers of the prothrombin G20210A variant and factor V Leiden and their interaction with oral contraceptives. *Haematologica* 2000;**85**:1271–6.

77 Emmerich J, Rosendaal FR, Cattaneo M, *et al*. Combined effect of factor V Leiden and prothrombin 20210A on the risk of venous thromboembolism: pooled analysis of 8 case–control studies including 2310 cases and 3204 controls. Study Group for Pooled-Analysis in Venous Thromboembolism. *Thromb Haemost* 2001;**86**:809–16.

78 Langman LJ, Ray JG, Evrovski J, Yeo E, Cole DE. Hyperhomocyst(e)inemia and the increased risk of venous thromboembolism: more evidence from a case–control study. *Arch Intern Med* 2000;**160**:961–4.

79 Vossen CY, Conard J, Fontcuberta J, *et al*. Familial thrombophilia and lifetime risk of venous thrombosis. *J Thromb Haemost* 2004;**2**:1526–32.

80 Goodwin AJ, Rosendaal FR, Kottke-Marchant K, Bovill EG. A review of the technical, diagnostic, and epidemiologic considerations for protein S assays. *Arch Pathol Lab Med* 2002;**126**:1349–66.

81 Wilson WA, Gharavi AE, Koike T, *et al*. International consensus statement on preliminary classification criteria for definite antiphospholipid syndrome. *Arthritis Rheum* 1999;**42**:1309–11.

82 Galli M, Barbui T. Antiphospholipid antibodies and thrombosis: strength of association. *Hematol J* 2003;**4**:180–6.

83 Galli M, Luciani D, Bertolini G, Barbui T. Anti-beta 2-glycoprotein I, antiprothrombin antibodies, and the risk of thrombosis in the antiphospholipid syndrome. *Blood* 2003;**102**:2717–23.

84 Branch DW, Silver RM. Criteria for antiphospholipid syndrome: early pregnancy loss, fetal loss or recurrent pregnancy loss? *Lupus* 1996;**5**:409–13.

85 Rai RS, Clifford K, Cohen H, Regan L. High prospective fetal loss rate in untreated pregnancies of women with recurrent miscarriage and antiphospholipid antibodies. *Hum Reprod* 1995;**10**:3301–4.

86 Hornstein M, Davis O, Massey J, Paulson R, Collins J. Antiphospholipid antibodies and *in vitro* fertilization success: a meta-analysis. *Fertil Steril* 2000;**73**:330–3.

87 Field SL, Brighton TA, McNeil HP, Chesterman CN. Recent insights into antiphospholipid antibody-mediated thrombosis. *Baillieres Best Pract Res Clin Haematol* 1999;**12**:407–22.

88 Rand JH, Wu XX, Andree HA, *et al*. Pregnancy loss in the antiphospholipid-antibody syndrome: a possible thrombogenic mechanism. *N Engl J Med* 1997;**337**:154–60.

89 Girardi G, Redecha P, Salmon JE. Heparin prevents antiphospholipid antibody-induced fetal loss by inhibiting complement activation. *Nat Med* 2004;**10**:1222–6.

90 Porter TF, LaCoursiere Y, Scott JR. Immunotherapy for recurrent miscarriage. *Cochrane Database Syst Rev* 2006;**2**:CD000112.

91 Ober C, Karrison T, Odem RR, *et al*. Mononuclear-cell immunisation in prevention of recurrent miscarriages: a randomised trial. *Lancet* 1999;**354**:365–9.

92 Yamada H, Morikawa M, Kato EH, Shimada S, Kobashi G, Minakami H. Pre-conceptional natural killer cell activity and percentage as predictors of biochemical pregnancy and spontaneous abortion with normal chromosome karyotype. *Am J Reprod Immunol* 2003;**50**:351–4.

93 Aoki K, Kajiura S, Matsumoto Y, *et al*. Preconceptional natural-killer-cell activity as a predictor of miscarriage. *Lancet* 1995;**345**:1340.

94 Shakhar K, Ben-Eliyahu S, Loewenthal R, Rosenne E, Carp H. Differences in number and activity of peripheral natural killer cells in primary versus secondary recurrent miscarriage. *Fertil Steril* 2003;**80**:368–75.

95 Shimada S, Iwabuchi K, Kato EH, *et al*. No difference in natural-killer-T cell population, but Th2/Tc2 predominance in peripheral blood of recurrent aborters. *Am J Reprod Immunol* 2003;**50**:334–9.

96 Koopman LA, Kopcow HD, Rybalov B, *et al*. Human decidual natural killer cells are a unique NK cell subset with immunomodulatory potential. *J Exp Med* 2003;**198**:1201–12.

97 Shimada S, Nishida R, Takeda M, *et al*. Natural killer, natural killer T, helper and cytotoxic T cells in the decidua from sporadic miscarriage. *Am J Reprod Immunol* 2006;**56**:193–200.

98 Morikawa M, Yamada H, Kato EH, *et al*. Massive intravenous immunoglobulin treatment in women with four or more recurrent spontaneous abortions of unexplained etiology: down-regulation of NK cell activity and subsets. *Am J Reprod Immunol* 2001;**46**:399–404.

99 Hanna J, Goldman-Wohl D, Hamani Y, *et al*. Decidual NK cells regulate key developmental processes at the human fetal–maternal interface. *Nat Med* 2006;**12**:1065–74.

100 Hiby SE, Walker JJ, O'Shaughnessy KM, *et al*. Combinations of maternal KIR and fetal HLA-C genes influence the risk of preeclampsia and reproductive success. *J Exp Med* 2004;**200**:957–65.

101 George L, Granath F, Johansson AL, Olander B, Cnattingius S. Risks of repeated miscarriage. *Paediatr Perinat Epidemiol* 2006;**20**:119–26.

102 Lashen H, Fear K, Sturdee DW. Obesity is associated with increased risk of first trimester and recurrent miscarriage: matched case–control study. *Hum Reprod* 2004;**19**:1644–6.

103 Neugebauer R, Kline J, Shrout P, *et al*. Major depressive disorder in the 6 months after miscarriage. *JAMA* 1997;**277**:383–8.

Further reading

ACOG Practice Bulletin No 68. Antiphospholipid syndrome. *Obstet Gynecol* 2005;**106**:1113–21.

ACOG Practice Bulletin No 24. Management of recurrent pregnancy loss. February 2001. (Replaces Technical Bulletin Number 212, September 1995). American College of Obstetricians and Gynecologists. *Int J Gynaecol Obstet* 2002;**78**:179–90.

Baart EB, Martini E, van den Berg I, *et al.* Preimplantation genetic screening reveals a high incidence of aneuploidy and mosaicism in embryos from young women undergoing IVF. *Hum Reprod* 2006;**21**:223–33.

Lockwood CJ. Inherited thrombophilias in pregnant patients: detection and treatment paradigm. *Obstet Gynecol* 2002;**99**:333–41.

Oates-Whitehead RM, Haas DM, Carrier JA. Progestogen for preventing miscarriage. *Cochrane Database Syst Rev* 2003: CD003511.

Porter TF, LaCoursiere Y, Scott JR. Immunotherapy for recurrent miscarriage. *Cochrane Database Syst Rev* 2006:CD000112

Rai R, Regan L. Recurrent miscarriage. *Lancet* 2006;**368**:601–11.

32 The incompetent cervix

John Owen

Although the term "cervical incompetence" was first used in the *Lancet* in 1865, the contemporary concept was not widely accepted until the middle of the 20th century after Palmer and Lacomme [1] in 1948 and Lash and Lash [2] in 1950 independently described interval repair of anatomic cervical defects associated with recurrent spontaneous mid-trimester birth. Soon thereafter, Shirodkar [3] in 1955, McDonald [4] in 1957, and later Benson and Durfee [5] in 1965 described the cerclage procedures utilized in contemporary obstetric practice. Nevertheless, the literature on cervical incompetence has been essentially a chronicle of surgical methods to correct often post-traumatic anatomic disruption of the internal os, in women who had experienced recurrent painless dilatation and mid-trimester birth. Evidence-based guidelines for many aspects of the diagnosis and management are still lacking.

Syndrome of spontaneous preterm birth

Spontaneous preterm birth is a syndrome comprised of several anatomic or functional components [6]. These include the uterus and its contractile function (i.e., preterm labor), loss of chorioamnionic integrity (i.e., preterm rupture of membranes), and, finally, diminished cervical competence, either from a primary anatomic defect or from early pathologic cervical ripening (i.e., cervical incompetence). In a particular pregnancy, a single feature may appear to predominate, even though it is more likely that most cases of spontaneous preterm birth result from the interaction of multiple stimuli and functional pathways. Importantly, the relative contribution of each of these components may vary, not only among different women, but also in successive pregnancies of the same woman.

Biologic continuum of cervical competence

As early as 1962, Danforth and Buckingham [7] suggested that cervical competence was not an all-or-nothing phenomenon

as traditionally taught. Rather, it comprised degrees of incompetency, and combinations of factors could cause "cervical failure." In their proposed classification, one group of patients had ostensibly normal cervical tissue, whose integrity as a fibrous ring had been previously damaged as the result of antecedent obstetric trauma. These might even be concealed by a normal-appearing external os and ectocervix. The second group possessed an abnormally low collagen:muscle ratio that would compromise its mechanical function and lead to premature dilatation. The third group comprised women who had no history of antecedent trauma and who also had normal collagen:muscle ratios, but whose obstetric histories mimicked those of groups 1 and 2, presumably from premature triggering of other factors (cervical ripening). These biochemical and ultrastructural findings support the variable, and often unpredictable, clinical course of women with a history of cervical incompetence [8].

Although the traditional paradigm has depicted the cervix as either competent or incompetent, recent evidence, including clinical data [9–12] and interpretative reviews [13–15], suggest that, as with most other biologic processes, cervical competence is rarely an all-or-nothing phenomenon, and it functions along a continuum of reproductive performance. Although some women have tangible anatomic evidence of poor cervical integrity, most women with a clinical diagnosis of cervical incompetence have ostensibly normal cervical anatomy. In a proposed model of cervical competence as a continuum, a poor obstetric history results from a process of premature cervical ripening, induced by infection, inflammation, local or systemic hormonal effects, or even genetic predisposition.

Diagnosis of cervical incompetence

The incidence of cervical incompetence in the general obstetric population is reported to vary between approximately 1 in 100 and 1 in 2000 [16–18]. This wide disparity is likely because of differences among study populations, reporting bias, and the diagnostic criteria used to establish the clinical diagnosis. Most of what is known about cervical incompetence and its treatment indicates that it is a *clinical diagnosis*, characterized by recurrent painless dilatation and spontaneous mid-trimester birth, usually of a living fetus. Associated characteristics, such as uterine contractions, bleeding, overt infection, or premature rupture of membranes, tend to shift the cause of spontaneous preterm birth away from cervical insufficiency and support other components of the preterm birth syndrome. Thus, a history of rapid, relatively painless labor should perhaps better characterize the diagnosis of cervical incompetence. Women with cervical incompetence often have some premonitory symptoms such as increased pelvic pressure, vaginal discharge, and urinary frequency. These symptoms, although neither specific nor uncommon in a normal pregnancy, should not be ignored, particularly in women with risk factors for spontaneous preterm birth.

Because cervical incompetence is part of a broader syndrome, the diagnosis is retrospective and suggested only after poor obstetric outcomes have occurred (or occasionally, are in evolution). Because there are few proven objective criteria, other than a rare, gross cervical malformation, a careful history and review of the past obstetric records are crucial to making an accurate diagnosis. Unfortunately, in many instances, the records are incomplete or unavailable, and many women cannot provide an accurate history. Even with excellent records and history, clinicians might reasonably disagree on the diagnosis in all but the most classic presentation. Confounding factors in the history, medical records, or current physical assessment might be utilized to either support or refute the diagnosis, based on their perceived importance. It is crucial to realize that the physician managing a patient who experiences a spontaneous mid-trimester birth is in the best position to assess and document whether the clinical criteria for cervical incompetence were present.

Because of its unproven efficacy in randomized clinical trials, and the attendant surgical risks, the recommendation for prophylactic cerclage should be limited to women with recurrent spontaneous preterm birth syndrome, after a careful history or physical examination suggest a dominant cervical component. Unless the physical examination confirms a significant cervical anatomic defect, consistent with disruption of its circumferential integrity, the clinician should assess the history for other components of the preterm birth syndrome: cervical incompetence remains a diagnosis of exclusion.

Management

Most of what is known about the management of the incompetent cervix is based on case series that reported surgical correction of the presumed underlying mechanical defect in the cervical stroma. Branch [19] in 1986 and Cousins [20] in 1980

collectively tabulated over 25 case series of cerclage efficacy published between 1959 and 1981. Branch [19] estimated a precerclage survival range of 10–32% versus a perinatal survival range of 75–83% in the same cohorts of women managed with Shirodkar cerclage. Similarly, case series that utilized McDonald cerclage reported a cohort perinatal survival range of 7–50% prior to, and 63–89% after cerclage. Cousins [20] estimated a "mean" survival before Shirodkar cerclage of 22% versus 82% post-therapy, and 27% and 74%, respectively, for investigators who utilized the McDonald technique. In total, over 2000 patients have been reported in these historic cohort comparisons. Interpretation of these series is limited by the following:

1 Diagnostic criteria were not consistent or always reported.
2 Definitions of treatment success were inconsistent (but generally recorded as perinatal survival, as opposed to a gestational age-based endpoint).
3 Treatment approaches were not always detailed and might involve multiple combinations of surgery, medication, bed rest, and other uncontrolled therapies.
4 Cases were not subcategorized according to etiology (i.e., anatomic defects versus a presumed functional cause) [20].

Nevertheless, based on compelling, but potentially biased efficacy data, the surgical management of women with clinically defined cervical incompetence has become standard practice.

Once a patient has been properly evaluated and deemed a suitable candidate for a prophylactic cerclage, a surgical method is chosen. In the presence of normal cervical anatomy and either no prior failed cerclage procedures, or a prior successful McDonald cerclage, a McDonald procedure is the technique of choice, because it is technically easier to perform and appears to be as effective as the Shirodkar technique [21]. Shirodkar cerclage should be reserved for women with anatomic deformities such as an unrepaired cervical laceration or a hypoplastic cervix where a McDonald cerclage is felt to be technically inadvisable. For example, a Shirodkar cerclage should be considered whenever there is less than 1 cm of visible cervix below the vaginal fornix. A patient with a prior failed McDonald cerclage occasionally presents for subsequent obstetric care or preconceptional counseling. If the prior failure is believed to be caused primarily by cervical insufficiency (as opposed to other components of the spontaneous preterm birth syndrome), the patient might be considered a candidate for either a Shirodkar or cervicoisthmic (Benson) procedure. Because few patients are appropriate candidates, and few physicians have surgical experience with the Benson procedure, it would seem prudent to relegate the decision to place a cervicoisthmic cerclage and the procedure itself to a tertiary center.

The chief advantage to prophylactic cerclage is that it can be offered in the early second trimester, after most spontaneous abortions have occurred. It also permits a sonographic evaluation to rule out many fetal anomalies and the potential for first-trimester screening; prenatal diagnosis using chorionic villus sampling can be performed prior to surgery. Many clinicians recommend obtaining cervicovaginal cultures for common pathogens and treating positive cultures prior to placing a cerclage. Active cervicitis should be considered a contraindication to prophylactic cerclage placement, and this must be successfully treated before surgery. Other contraindications to cerclage include ruptured membranes, certain (lethal) fetal anomalies, suspected or confirmed intrauterine infection, vaginal bleeding, and labor.

McDonald cerclage

To place a prophylactic McDonald cerclage, the anesthetized patient is placed in dorsal lithotomy position. At least one assistant is required to provide exposure using right angle or medium-sized Deaver retractors. After an antiseptic vaginal prep, the anterior ectocervix is grasped with a sponge forceps, or similar nontraumatic instrument such as a Babcock clamp, used to provide counter traction. The urinary bladder is generally emptied prior to the procedure, although some recommend leaving some urine in the bladder to better define the position of the bladder as it reflects onto the cervix.

Most surgeons utilize a permanent synthetic material such as No 1 or 2 nylon, Prolene, or Mersilene. Mersilene 5 mm tape has also been proposed, but is more difficult to pull through the stroma and requires more tissue traction and manipulation. For right-handed surgeons, the first tissue bite is taken at the 11–12:00 position on the cervix, exiting at around the 10:00 position. When placing the anterior stitch, the surgeon must avoid the bladder mucosa that can be identified by moving the cervix in and out, and noting where the vaginal mucosa folds in as it reflects off the ectocervix. As the descending branches of the uterine artery are found at 3:00 and 9:00, this area should be avoided when placing the stitches.

The last bite should exit in close proximity to the original entry site. Another variation of the original procedure uses two sutures placed several millimeters apart [22]. This has the theoretic advantage of spreading the suture tension over a larger area and may help prevent the more cephalic stitch from becoming displaced. A second stitch should be considered if the first suture was not optimally placed at the bladder reflection anteriorly or as high as possible in the posterior vaginal fornix. It is necessary to record how many stitches were placed and where the knots were tied to facilitate their later removal.

After the cerclage stitch has been placed, it is important to take up any slack introduced with the multiple tissue bites, utilizing a "laundry bag" technique, whereby traction is applied to each side of the exiting suture while holding counter traction at the exit site with two fingers of the opposite hand. Once this is accomplished, the suture is tied down firmly but should not cause visible blanching of the surrounding tissue. In order to facilitate later identification and removal, a long tag should be left above the knot. After placement, a digital exami-

nation will confirm a closed endocervical canal that is not overly constricted. However, it should not admit a gloved finger.

"Risk factors" for cervical incompetence

While the historic concept of the diagnosis and treatment of cervical incompetence often includes women with past cervical trauma from birth-associated lacerations, forced dilatation, operative injury, or cervical amputation, the prevalence of these antecedent events appears to be decreasing in contemporary US practice. More common in contemporary practice are patients who have undergone prior treatment of cervical dysplasia using cold-knife cone, laser cone, or loop electrosurgical excision procedures (LEEP). These cervical procedures are plausibly risk factors for cervical incompetence. Numerous studies have confirmed that most women with prior LEEP, laser ablation, or cone biopsy do not appear to have a clinically significant rate of second trimester loss or even preterm birth [23–25]. However, women in whom a large cone specimen was removed or destroyed (including cervical amputations), or who have undergone multiple prior procedures, do have an increased risk of spontaneous preterm birth [26,27]. Whether prophylactic cerclage is an effective strategy in these at-risk women remains speculative. The available clinical trial data [28] do not suggest a benefit from prophylactic cerclage in women with these risk factors, and so these women may be followed clinically.

A similar controversy arises over the management of women with *in utero* diethylstilbestrol (DES) exposure. Because many women exposed to DES *in utero* were the products themselves of complicated gestations and were born to women with poor reproductive histories, it is plausible that at least a portion of the presumed DES effect may simply be of genetic origin [29]. Because the use of DES was effectively curtailed in the early 1970s, this congenital risk factor should comprise a steadily diminishing group of patients and will soon be of no clinical concern. Currently, no controlled data support the efficacy of prophylactic cerclage in these patients.

Is cervical incompetence a sonographic diagnosis?

Numerous investigators have asserted that cervical incompetence can be diagnosed by mid-trimester sonographic evaluation of the cervix. Various sonographic findings including shortened cervical length, funneling at the internal os, and dynamic response to provocative maneuvers (e.g., fundal pressure) have been utilized to select women for treatment, generally cerclage. In most of these earlier reports, the sonographic evaluations were not blinded, leading to uncontrolled interventions and difficulty determining their effectiveness.

In many instances, the sonographic criteria for cervical incompetence were only qualitatively described and thus were not reproducible.

Currently, four randomized trials of cerclage for sonographic indications have been published [30–33]. Althuisius *et al.* [30] in the Netherlands enrolled patients believed to have cervical incompetence based on their obstetric history. Of the 19 assigned to cerclage, there was no preterm birth <34 weeks versus a 44% preterm birth rate in the no cerclage–home rest group (*P* = 0.002); none of the women who maintained a cervical length of at least 25 mm experienced a preterm birth. Rust *et al.* [31] enrolled 138 women who had various risk factors for preterm birth (including 12% with multiple gestations) and randomly assigned them to receive McDonald cerclage or no cerclage after their cervical length shortened to <25 mm or they developed funneling >25%. Preterm birth <34 weeks was observed in 35% of the cerclage group versus 36% of the control group.

In a multinational trial comprising 12 hospitals in six countries, To *et al.* [32] screened 47,123 unselected women at 22–24 weeks' gestation with vaginal ultrasound to identify 470 with a shortened cervical length of 15 mm or less. Of these 470, 253 participated in a randomized trial whose primary outcome was the intergroup rates of delivery prior to 33 weeks' gestation. Women assigned to the (Shirodkar) cerclage group (*n* = 127) had a similar rate of preterm birth as the control population (*n* = 126), 22% versus 26% (*P* = 0.44). Berghella *et al.* [33] screened women with various risk factors for spontaneous preterm birth (prior preterm birth, curettage, cone biopsy, DES exposure) with vaginal scans every 2 weeks from 14 to 23 weeks' gestation and randomly assigned 61 with a cervical length <25 mm or funneling >25% to McDonald cerclage or to a no-cerclage control group. Preterm birth <35 weeks was observed in 45% of the cerclage group and 47% of the control group. In none of the four published randomized trials did the authors specifically comment on the proportion of women who were delivered in the mid-trimester after a presentation consistent with clinically defined cervical incompetence.

The findings of Rust *et al.* [31] and Berghella *et al.* [33] seem most applicable to obstetric practice in the USA, and these did not support the use of cerclage for sonographic findings commonly cited as "abnormal" in women with various types of risk factors. The multinational trial by To *et al.* [32] confirmed that shortened cervical length ≤15 mm identified a very high-risk group; however, approximately 100 women in a general obstetric population would have to be screened to find one with this risk factor. None of these three trials demonstrated a benefit from ultrasound-indicated cerclage. The trial by Althuisius *et al.* [30] focused on women whom they believed had a clinical diagnosis of cervical incompetence and who would have likely been candidates for prophylactic cerclage in the USA [34]. Nevertheless, their study does suggest a potential role for cervical ultrasound in women with a clinical diagnosis of cervical incompetence, if the intent is to *avoid* cerclage when the cervical length is maintained at ≥25 mm.

Incompetence in evolution

On occasion, a woman will present with symptoms and physical findings that support an antepartum diagnosis of cervical incompetence. This syndrome, however, comprises a wide spectrum of clinical expression. Women who present with incompetence in evolution, generally defined as a mid-trimester cervical dilatation of at least 2 cm and no other predisposing cause (labor, infection, bleeding, ruptured membranes), are often considered for *emergent* cerclage.

Aarts *et al.* [35] reviewed eight case series published between 1980 and 1992 comprising 249 patients who received an emergent mid-trimester cerclage and estimated a mean neonatal survival rate of 64% (range 22–100%). Smaller, uncontrolled reports of cerclage suggested no benefit [36] or some benefit [37]. Although these reports are not of sufficient scientific quality on which to base firm management recommendations, collectively they demonstrated several important concepts. The earlier the gestational age at presentation and the more advanced the cervical dilatation, the greater the risk of poor neonatal outcome. The finding of membrane prolapse into the vagina is also a significant risk factor for poor outcome [38].

Recently, Althuisius *et al.* [39] reported the results of a randomized clinical trial of emergency cerclage plus bed rest versus bed rest alone in 23 women (singletons and twins) who presented with cervical dilatation and membranes prolapsing to or beyond the external os prior to 27 weeks' gestation. They observed a longer mean interval from presentation to delivery (54 days versus 20 days; *P* = 0.046) in the cerclage group. Neonatal survival was 9/16 with cerclage and 4/14 in the bed rest group. Although the survival differences were not statistically significant, there was significantly lower neonatal composite morbidity (including death) in the cerclage group (10/16 versus 14/14; *P* = 0.02).

Other reports show that women who present with incompetence in evolution have an appreciable (nominal 50%) incidence of bacterial colonization of their amniotic fluid including other markers of subclinical chorioamnionitis [40–42] or proteomic markers of inflammation or bleeding [43]. Women with abnormal amniotic fluid markers have a much shorter presentation-to-delivery interval, regardless of whether they receive cerclage or are managed expectantly with bed rest.

Thus, the optimal management of women who present with incompetence in evolution remains indefinite. Although emergent cerclage may confer some benefit, patient selection remains largely empiric. While not standard care, the evaluation of amniotic fluid makers of infection and inflammation appear to have important prognostic value, although it is still unclear whether and to what extent the results should direct patient management.

Post-cerclage management

There are a number of empiric recommendations regarding physical activity after discharge. A limited interval (24–48 hours) of mandatory bed rest is often advised in the immediate postoperative period. Pelvic rest and sexual abstinence for the remainder of gestation are widely prescribed. Because the use of bed rest in pregnancy as an effective therapy has been seriously questioned [44], it seems reasonable to individualize this recommendation based on a patient's symptoms and physical findings. However, because women with cervical incompetence and cerclage are still at increased risk for preterm birth, physically demanding occupations or prolonged standing should be curtailed.

In the absence of indications for earlier removal, the stitch should be removed around 37 weeks' gestation. Often performed in an outpatient setting, elective removal may be complicated by hemorrhage or appreciable difficulty locating the suture, which may have become embedded in the cervical stroma. Because of its higher placement and use of 5 mm nonabsorbable tape, removal of a Shirodkar cerclage may be particularly troublesome. Difficult removal increases patient discomfort, and, at times, light conscious sedation may be required. Hemorrhage from the suture track may occur, but it can usually be controlled with direct pressure.

Because many women with clinically defined cervical incompetence and cerclage remain at high risk for developing other components of the spontaneous preterm birth syndrome, indications for cerclage removal remote from term may develop. Patients with cerclage should be instructed on the symptoms of preterm labor and be able to present early for evaluation. Women with cerclage and preterm labor can be managed with tocolytic medications and should receive corticosteroids according to published guidelines. Nevertheless, if labor is progressive, the cerclage must be removed. This decision is made by the managing obstetrician based on serial visual and manual examination of the cervix and lower uterine segment.

Preterm premature rupture of membranes (PPROM) complicates 25–30% of pregnancies managed with cerclage [18,42]. Uncontrolled retrospective series have demonstrated that, when the cerclage is removed on admission, perinatal outcomes are indistinguishable from similar cases of PPROM with no antecedent cerclage [45–47]. Other series have addressed the question of whether the cerclage should be left in place or removed immediately after spontaneous membrane rupture [48–50]. While these retrospective series cannot define optimal management, in the absence of clinical trial data confirming a benefit from leaving the cerclage in place after PPROM, the current weight of evidence suggests that the cerclage should be removed.

Cerclage complications

The perceived simplicity and safety of transvaginal cerclage has made this treatment subject to empiric use, in spite of the risk of associated complications [51]. The most commonly reported complications associated with cerclage are membrane rupture and intrauterine infection. Bleeding may occur, but serious hemorrhage is generally limited to the cervicoisthmic procedure. Essentially all transvaginal cerclage procedures are performed under regional anesthesia, which has a low complication rate. Harger [51] tabulated cerclage-associated complications reported in the past 40 years. Chorioamnionitis complicated 0.8–8% of elective cerclage procedures and 9–37% of "urgent" or emergent procedures. Membrane rupture attributed to elective cerclage was observed in 1–18% and was associated with up to 65% of emergent cases. Whether cerclage alone can precipitate overt preterm labor seems doubtful. However, the foreign body might lower the threshold for uterine activity because of local inflammatory effects. Uterine activity often occurs in proximity to cerclage placement and women who have undergone cerclage are more likely to receive tocolytic agents during their gestation [28].

Adjunctive management strategies for the incompetent cervix

Alternative therapies for cervical incompetence can be broadly classified as either providing mechanical support or administering pharmacologic measures to reduce inflammation and infection in order to maintain uterine quiescence. A review of older case series of cerclage indicate that progesterone (usually 17α-hydroxyprogesterone caproate), and, more recently, various tocolytic agents (usually indomethacin) and various prophylactic antibiotic regimens, are widely prescribed adjuncts to cerclage. Whether these agents alone or in combination offer any therapeutic value is unknown, because none has been proved effective in controlled intervention trials. However, of these, progesterone appears to be the most promising [52–54].

Investigators in Europe and the USA have studied vaginal pessaries for the treatment of the incompetent cervix [55]. In 1961, Vitsky [56] proposed the mechanism whereby a lever pessary (Smith, Hodge, or Risser design) might be an effective treatment for the incompetent cervix. A vaginal pessary would displace the cervix posteriorly and shift the gravitational effects of the expanding uterine contents off the internal os and onto the anterior lower uterine segment. Interpretation of the clinical research in this area has been hampered by the frequent use of historic-control study designs, similar to those utilized in most series espousing the efficacy of cerclage. Likewise, the reported success rates of vaginal pessaries closely mirror those observed with cerclage and nominal success rates are in the 80–90% range [55]. Only one randomized trial has been located, and this was a German study published in 1986 by Forster *et al.* [57]. In this trial, 250 women were randomized to cerclage or pessary (the type was not stated). The cerclage group and pessary group had term delivery rates of 69% and 62%, respectively. Another recent retrospective analysis of 36 women with mid-trimester cervical shortening, managed either expectantly or with a Smith–Hodge pessary, showed a significant decrease in the incidence of preterm birth <35 weeks (0% versus 40%; $P=0.03$) [58]. Although further comparative efficacy trials are needed, it would seem reasonable to recommend a trial of vaginal pessary in women with unclear histories or those who demonstrate progressive cervical change on serial mid-trimester evaluations.

Conclusions

Contemporary lines of evidence indicate that cervical incompetence is rarely a distinct and well-defined clinical entity, but only one component of a larger and more complex syndrome of spontaneous preterm birth. The original paradigm of obstetric and gynecologic trauma as a common antecedent of cervical incompetence has been replaced by the recognition of *functional*, as opposed to *anatomic* deficits as the more prevalent etiology. Cervical *competence* functions along a continuum, influenced by both endogenous and exogenous factors that interact through various pathways with other recognized components of the preterm birth syndrome: uterine contractions and decidual activation/membrane rupture. Thus, the convenient term, *cervical incompetence*, may actually represent an oversimplified, incomplete version of the broader pathophysiologic process.

Case presentation

History

A 24-year-old para 0200 presents for preconception counseling. Her obstetric history includes two prior spontaneous preterm births at 21 and 25 weeks' gestation. Hysterosalpingography performed several months after her first loss was normal. Between her first and second birth she underwent a LEEP procedure for dysplasia; review of the path reports shows that the specimen was <10 mm thick. More careful questioning and review of records shows that her first delivery occurred after a relatively short and painless labor. The liveborn infant succumbed quickly to respiratory failure. Review of the placental path report showed chorioamnionitis, although she did not have puerperal fever. In her second pregnancy, she experienced spontaneous membrane rupture at 20 weeks. She was managed expectantly with prophylactic anti-

biotics but at 25 weeks she developed clinical chorioamnionitis. Labor was induced and lasted <4 hours. The infant was liveborn but perished from pulmonary hypoplasia.

Physical examination

Normal cervical anatomy with no palpable defect around the circumference. The cervical length to palpation is 1.5 cm. The external os appears parous but is firmly closed.

Assessment

Cervical incompetence from a nonanatomic functional etiology.

Plan

Discuss risks and benefits of prophylactic cerclage and plan to place a McDonald stitch at 12–14 weeks in her next pregnancy. Adjunctive progesterone (Delalutin) is also recommended beginning at 16 weeks.

Follow-up

In her next pregnancy, following the cerclage, she experiences PPROM at 23 weeks. The cerclage is removed and the patient managed expectantly in the hospital with antibiotics and a course of corticosteroids. At 27 weeks she develops regular contractions, and the cervix is found to be 6 cm dilated. She undergoes a low transverse cesarean for breech presentation. The infant has a protracted neonatal ICU course, but survives with no long-term sequelae.

References

1 Palmer R, Lacomme M. La béance de l'orifice interne, cause d'avortements à répétition? Une observation de déchrure cervico-isthmique répareeé chirurgicalement, avec gestation à terme consécutive. *Gynecol Obstet* 1948;**47**:905–6.
2 Lash AF, Lash SR. Habitual abortion: the incompetent internal os of the cervix. *Am J Obstet Gynecol* 1950;**59**:68–76.
3 Shirodkar VN. A new method of operative treatment for habitual abortions in the second trimester of pregnancy. *Antiseptic* 1955;**52**:299–300.
4 McDonald IA. Suture of the cervix for inevitable miscarriage. *J Obstet Gynecol Br Empire* 1957;**64**:346–53.
5 Benson RC, Durfee RB. Transabdominal cervico-uterine cerclage during pregnancy for the treatment of cervical incompetency. *Obstet Gynecol* 1965;**25**:145–55.
6 Romero R, Mazor M, Munoz H, Gomez R, Galasso M, Sherer DM. The preterm labor syndrome. *Ann N Y Acad Sci* 1994;**734**:414–29.
7 Danforth DN, Buckingham JC. Cervical incompetence: a re-evaluation. *Postgrad Med* 1962;**32**:345–51.

8 Dunn LJ, Dans P. Subsequent obstetrical performance of patients meeting the historical criteria for cervical incompetence. *Bull Sloan Hosp Women* 1962;**7**:43–5.

9 Iams JD, Johnson FF, Sonek J, Sachs L, Gebauer C, Samuels P. Cervical competence as a continuum: a study of ultrasonography cervical length and obstetric performance. *Am J Obstet Gynecol* 1995;**172**:1097–106.

10 Iams JD, Goldenberg RL, Meis PJ, *et al*. The length of the cervix and the risk of spontaneous premature delivery. *N Engl J Med* 1996;**334**:567–72.

11 Buckingham JC, Buethe RA, Danforth DN. Collagen–muscle ratio in clinically normal and clinically incompetent cervixes. *Am J Obstet Gynecol* 1965;**91**:232–7.

12 Ayers JWR, DeGrood RM, Compton AA, Barclay M, Ansbacher R. Sonographic evaluation of cervical length in pregnancy: diagnosis and management of preterm cervical effacement in patients at risk for premature delivery. *Obstet Gynecol* 1988;**71**:939–44.

13 Craigo SD. Cervical incompetence and preterm delivery [Editorial]. *N Engl J Med* 1996;**334**:595–6.

14 Olah KS, Gee H. The prevention of preterm delivery: can we afford to continue to ignore the cervix? *Br J Obstet Gynaecol* 1992;**99**:278–80.

15 Romero R, Gomez R, Sepulveda W. The uterine cervix, ultrasound and prematurity [Editor's comments]. *Ultrasound Obstet Gynecol* 1992;**2**:385–8.

16 Barter RH, Dusbabek JA, Riva HL, Parks J. Surgical closure of the incompetent cervix during pregnancy. *Am J Obstet Gynecol* 1958;**75**:511–24.

17 Jennings CL. Temporary submucosal cerclage for cervical incompetence: report of forty-eight cases. *Am J Obstet Gynecol* 1972;**113**:1097–102.

18 Kuhn R, Pepperell R. Cervical ligation: a review of 242 pregnancies. *Aust N Z J Obstet Gynaecol* 1977;**17**:79–83.

19 Branch DW. Operations for cervical incompetence. *Clin Obstet Gynecol* 1986;**29**:240–54.

20 Cousins JM. Cervical incompetence: 1980. A time for reappraisal. *Clin Obstet Gynecol* 1980;**23**:467–79.

21 Cardwell MS. Cervical cerclage: a ten-year review in a large hospital. *South Med J* 1988;**81**:15.

22 Hofmeister FJ, Schwartz WR, Vondrak BF, Martens W. Suture reinforcement of the incompetent cervix. *Am J Obstet Gynecol* 1968;**101**:58–65.

23 Ferenczy A, Choukroun D, Falcone T, Franco E. The effect of cervical loop electrosurgical excision on subsequent pregnancy outcome: North American experience. *Am J Obstet Gynecol* 1995;**172**:1246–50.

24 Althuisius SM, Shornagel GA, Dekker GA, van Geijn HP, Hummel P. Loop electrosurgical excision procedure of the cervix and time of delivery in subsequent pregnancy. *Int J Gynecol Obstet* 2001;**72**:31–4.

25 Weber T, Obel E. Pregnancy complications following conization of the uterine cervix. *Acta Obstet Gynecol Scand* 1979;**58**:259.

26 Raio L, Ghezzi F, Di Naro E, Gomez R, Luscher K. Duration of pregnancy after carbon dioxide laser conization of the cervix: influence of cone height. *Obstet Gynecol* 1997;**90**:978–82.

27 Sadler L, Saftlas A, Wang W, Exeter M, Whittaker J, McCowan L. Treatment for cervical intraepithelial neoplasia and risk of preterm delivery. *JAMA* 2004;**291**:2100–6.

28 Final report of the Medical Research Council/Royal College of Obstetrics and Gynaecology multicentre randomized trial of cervical cerclage. *Br J Obstet Gynaecol* 1993;**100**:516–23.

29 Mangan CE, Borow L, Burtnett-Rubin MM, Egan V, Giuntoi RL, Mijuta JJ. Pregnancy outcome in 98 women exposed to diethylstibestrol *in utero*, their mothers, and unexposed siblings. *Obstet Gynecol* 1982;**59**:315–9.

30 Althuisius SM, Dekker GA, van Geijn HP, Bekedam DJ, Hummel P. Cervical Incompetence Prevention Randomized Cerclage Trial (CIPRACT): Study design and preliminary results. *Am J Obstet Gynecol* 2000;**183**:823–9.

31 Rust OA, Atlas RO, Reed J, van Gaalen J, Balducci J. Revisiting the short cervix detected by transvaginal ultrasound in the second trimester: why cerclage may not help. *Am J Obstet Gynecol* 2001;**185**:1098–105.

32 To MS, Alfirevic Z, Heath VCF, *et al*. on behalf of the Fetal Medicine Foundation Second Trimester Screening Group. Cervical cerclage for prevention of preterm delivery in women with short cervix: randomised controlled trial. *Lancet* 2004;**363**:1849–53.

33 Berghella V, Odibo AO, Tolosa JE. Cerclage for prevention of preterm birth in women with a short cervix found on transvaginal ultrasound: a randomized trial. *Am J Obstet Gynecol* 2004;**191**:1311–7.

34 American College of Obstetricians and Gynecologists. Cervical insufficiency. *ACOG Pract Bull* No. 48, November 2003.

35 Aarts JM, Jozien T. Brons J, Bruinse HW. Emergency cerclage: a review. *Obstet Gynecol Surv* 1995;**50**:459–69.

36 Novy MJ, Gupta A, Wothe DD, Gupta S, Kennedy KA, Gravett MG. Cervical cerclage in the second trimester of pregnancy: a historical cohort study. *Am J Obstet Gynecol* 2002;**186**: 594–6.

37 Olatunbosun OA, AL-Nuaim L, Turnell RW. Emergency cerclage compared with bed rest for advanced cervical dilatation in pregnancy. *Int Surg* 1995;**80**:170–4.

38 Kokia E, Dor J, Blankenstein J, *et al*. A simple scoring system for treatment of cervical incompetence diagnosed during the second trimester. *Gynecol Obstet Invest* 1991;**31**:12–6.

39 Althuisius SM, Dekker GA, Hummel P, van Geijn HP. Cervical incompetence prevention randomized cerclage trial: emergency cerclage with bed rest versus bed rest alone. *Am J Obstet Gynecol* 2003;**189**:907–10.

40 Romero R, Gonzalez R, Sepulveda W, *et al*. Infection and labor. VIII. Microbial invasion of the amniotic cavity in patients with suspected cervical incompetence: prevalence and clinical significance. *Am J Obstet Gynecol* 1992;**167**:1086–91.

41 Mays JK, Figuerioa R, Shah J, Khakoo H, Kaminsky S, Tejani N. Amniocentesis for selection before rescue cerclage. *Obstet Gynecol* 2000;**95**:652–5.

42 Treadwell MC, Bronsteen RA, Bottoms SF. Prognostic factors and complication rates for cervical cerclage: a review of 482 cases. *Am J Obstet Gynecol* 1991;**165**:555–8.

43 Weiner CP, Lee KY, Buhimschi CS, Christner R, Buhimschi IA. Proteomic biomarkers that predict the clinical success of rescue cerclage. *Am J Obstet Gynecol* 2005;**192**:710–8.

44 Goldenberg RL, Cliver SP, Bronstein J, Cutter GR, Andrews WA, Mennemeyer ST. Bed rest in pregnancy. *Obstet Gynecol* 1994;**84**:131–6.

45 Blickstein I, Katz Z, Lancet M, Molgilner BM. The Outcome of pregnancies complicated by preterm rupture of the membranes with and without cerclage. *Int J Obstet Gynecol* 1989;**28**: 237–42.

46 Yeast JD, Garite TR. The role of cervical cerclage in the management of preterm premature rupture of the membranes. *Am J Obstet Gynecol* 1988;**158**:106–10.

47 McElrath TF, Norwitz ER, Lieberman ES, Heffner LJ. Perinatal outcome after preterm premature rupture of membranes with *in situ* cervical cerclage. *Am J Obstet Gynecol* 2002;**187**:1147–52.

48 Ludmir J, Bader T, Chen L, Lindenbaum C, Wong G. Poor perinatal outcome associated with retained cerclage in patients with premature rupture of membranes. *Obstet Gynecol* 1994;**84**:823–6.

49 Jenkins TM, Berghella V, Shlossman PA, *et al.* Timing of cerclage removal after preterm premature rupture of membranes: maternal and neonatal outcomes. *Am J Obstet Gynecol* 2000;**183**:847–52.

50 McElrath TF, Norwitz ER, Lieberman ES, Heffner LJ. Management of cervical cerclage and preterm premature rupture of the membranes: should the stitch be removed? *Am J Obstet Gynecol* 2000;**183**:840–6.

51 Harger JH. Cerclage and cervical insufficiency: an evidenced-based analysis. *Obstet Gynecol* 2002;**100**:1313–27

52 Sherman AI. Hormonal therapy for control of the incompetent os of pregnancy. *Obstet Gynecol* 1966;**28**:198–205.

53 Keirse MJNC. Progesterone administration in pregnancy may prevent preterm delivery. *Br J Obstet Gynaecol* 1990;**97**:149–54.

54 Meis PJ for the NICHD MFMU Network. Prevention of Recurrent Preterm Delivery by 17 alpha- hydroxyprogesterone caproate prevents recurrent preterm birth. *N Engl J Med* 2003;**348**: 2379–85.

55 Newcomer J. Pessaries for the treatment of incompetent cervix and premature delivery. *Obstet Gynecol Surv* 2000;**55**: 443–8.

56 Vitsky M. Simple treatment of the incompetent cervical os. *Am J Obstet Gynecol* 1961;**81**:1194–7.

57 Forster F, Dunng R, Schwarzlus G. Therapy of cervix insufficiency: cerclage or support pessary? *Zentralbl Gynaekol* 1986;**108**:230–7.

58 Broth R, Pereira L, Slepian J, Berghella V. Role of pessary in management of patients with cervical shortening. *Am J Obstet Gynecol* 2002;**187**:S118 [Abstract 211].

33 Gestational hypertension–preeclampsia and eclampsia

Labib M. Ghulmiyyah and Baha M. Sibai

Hypertension is the most common medical disorder during pregnancy [1]. Approximately 70% of women diagnosed with hypertension during pregnancy will have preeclampsia. The term "preeclampsia" is used to describe a wide spectrum of patients who may have only mild elevation in blood pressure (BP) or severe hypertension with various organ dysfunctions including acute gestational hypertension; preeclampsia; eclampsia; and hemolysis, elevated liver enzymes, low platelet count (HELLP) syndrome.

Gestational hypertension

Gestational hypertension is defined as a systolic BP of at least 140 mmHg and/or a diastolic BP of at least 90 mmHg on at least two occasions at least 6 hours apart after the 20th week of gestation in women known to be normotensive before pregnancy and before 20 weeks' gestation. The BP recordings used to establish the diagnosis should be no more than 7 days apart [2]. Gestational hypertension is considered severe if there is sustained elevations in systolic BP to at least 160 mmHg and/or in diastolic BP to at least 110 mmHg for at least 6 hours [1,3]. Some women with gestational hypertension will subsequently progress to preeclampsia. The rate of progression depends on gestational age at time of diagnosis; the rate reaches 50% when gestational hypertension develops before 30 weeks' gestation [4].

Preeclampsia

Preeclampsia is primarily defined as gestational hypertension plus proteinuria (≥300 mg/24-hour period) [1]. If 24-hour urine collection is not available, then proteinuria is defined as a concentration of at least 30 mg/dL (at least 1+ on dipstick) in at least two random urine samples collected at least 6 hours apart. The urine measurements used to establish proteinuria should be no more than 7 days apart [2]. The concentration of

urinary protein in random urine samples is highly variable. Recent studies have found that urinary dipstick determinations correlate poorly with the amount of proteinuria found in 24-hour urine determinations in women with gestational hypertension [5]. Therefore, the definitive test to diagnose proteinuria should be quantitative protein excretion in a 24-hour period. Severe proteinuria is defined as protein excretion of at least 5 g/24-hour period. Urine dipstick values should not be used to diagnose severe proteinuria [1,6]. In the absence of proteinuria, preeclampsia should be considered when gestational hypertension is associated with persistent cerebral symptoms, epigastric or right upper quadrant pain with nausea or vomiting, thrombocytopenia or abnormal liver enzymes.

Preeclampsia is considered severe if there is severe gestational hypertension in association with abnormal proteinuria or if there is hypertension in association with severe proteinuria (at least 5 g/24-hour period). In addition, preeclampsia is considered severe in the presence of multiorgan involvement such as pulmonary edema, seizures, oliguria (less than 500 mL/24-hour period), thrombocytopenia (platelet count less than 100,000/mm^3), abnormal liver enzymes in association with persistent epigastric or right upper quadrant pain, or persistent severe central nervous system symptoms (altered mental status, headaches, blurred vision, or blindness) [1].

Perinatal outcomes

Gestational hypertension

In general, the majority of cases of mild gestational hypertension develop at or beyond 37 weeks' gestation, and thus pregnancy outcome is similar to that seen in women with normotensive pregnancies. On the other hand, maternal and perinatal morbidities are substantially increased in women with severe gestational hypertension. Indeed, these women have higher morbidities than women with mild preeclampsia.

The rates of abruptio placentae, preterm delivery (at less than 37 and 35 weeks), and small for gestational age (SGA) infants in women with severe gestational hypertension are similar to those seen in women with severe preeclampsia. Therefore, these women should be managed as if they had severe preeclampsia [1].

Preeclampsia

The perinatal death rate and rates of preterm delivery, SGA infants, and abruptio placentae in women with mild preeclampsia are similar to those of normotensive pregnancies. The rate of eclampsia is less than 1%, but the rate of cesarean delivery is increased because of increased rates of induction of labor. In contrast, perinatal mortality and morbidities as well as the rates of abruptio placentae are substantially increased in women with severe preeclampsia. The rate of neonatal complications is markedly increased in those who develop severe preeclampsia in the second trimester, whereas it is minimal in those with severe preeclampsia beyond 35 weeks' gestation.

Severe preeclampsia is also associated with increased risk of maternal mortality (0.2%) and increased rates of maternal morbidities (5%) such as convulsions, pulmonary edema, acute renal or liver failure, liver hemorrhage, disseminated intravascular coagulopathy, and stroke. These complications are usually seen in women who develop preeclampsia before 32 weeks' gestation and in those with preexisting medical conditions [1,7].

Etiology and pathophysiology

The etiology of preeclampsia remains an obstetric enigma. Several etiologies have been proposed but most have not withstood the test of time. Some of these suggested causes include abnormal trophoblast invasion of uterine vessels, immunologic intolerance between fetoplacental and maternal tissues, maladaptation to cardiovascular changes, inflammatory changes of pregnancy, and genetic abnormalities [8]. Some reported pathophysiologic abnormalities of preeclampsia include placental ischemia, generalized vasospasm, abnormal hemostasis with activation of the coagulation system, vascular endothelial dysfunction, abnormal nitric oxide and lipid metabolism, leukocyte activation, and changes in various cytokines and growth factors. Recently, there is substantial evidence suggesting that the pathophysiologic abnormalities of preeclampsia are caused by abnormal angiogenesis, particularly an imbalance in sFlt-1 : PLGF ratio [9].

Management

The objective of management in women with gestational hypertension–preeclampsia must always be safety of the mother and then delivery of a mature newborn who will not require intensive and prolonged neonatal care. This can only be achieved by a plan that takes into consideration one or more of the following: the severity of the disease process, fetal gestational age, maternal and fetal status at time of the initial evaluation, presence of labor, cervical Bishop score, and the wishes of the mother [1].

Mild hypertension or preeclampsia

Once the diagnosis of mild gestational hypertension or mild preeclampsia is made, subsequent therapy will depend on the results of maternal and fetal evaluation. (A suggested algorithm for management of mild preeclampsia is described in Fig. 33.1 [1].)

In general, women with mild disease developing at 37 weeks' gestation or longer have a pregnancy outcome similar to that found in normotensive pregnancy. Thus, those who have a favorable cervix at or near term and patients who are considered noncompliant should undergo induction of labor for delivery [1].

All patients with mild preeclampsia should receive maternal and fetal evaluation at the time of their diagnosis. Maternal evaluation includes measurements of blood pressure, weight, and urine protein, and questioning about symptoms of headache, visual disturbances, and epigastric pain.

Laboratory evaluation includes determinations of hematocrit, platelet counts, liver enzymes levels, and a 24-hour urine collection once a week. This evaluation is important because patients may develop thrombocytopenia and abnormal liver enzyme levels with minimal blood pressure elevation. Fetal evaluation should include ultrasonography to determine fetal growth and amniotic fluid volume every 3 weeks, daily fetal movement count ("kick count"), and nonstress testing at least once weekly. Patients are instructed to receive a regular diet with no salt restriction. Diuretics, antihypertensive drugs, and sedatives are not used. Several studies indicate that these agents do not improve pregnancy outcome, and may increase the incidence of fetal growth restriction [1].

With expectant management, patients are instructed to be on restricted but not complete bed rest, to have BP and urine (dipstick) checked daily and to report symptoms of severe disease.

The women are usually seen twice weekly for evaluation of maternal blood pressure, urine protein and symptoms of impending eclampsia. Maternal and fetal evaluation is performed twice weekly in an ambulatory testing unit. Any evidence of disease progression or development of acute severe hypertension is an indication for prompt hospitalization. Indications for delivery are summarized in Table 33.1.

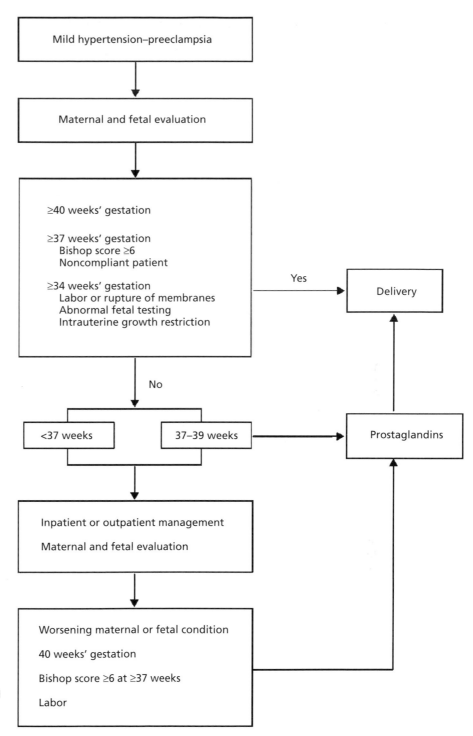

Fig. 33.1 Recommended management of mild gestational hypertension or preeclampsia. From Sibai [1] with permission.

In women with mild gestational hypertension, fetal evaluation should include an nonstress test (NST) and an ultrasound examination of estimated fetal weight and amniotic fluid index. If the results are normal, then there is no need for repeat testing unless there is a change in maternal condition (progression to preeclampsia or severe hypertension) or there is decreased fetal movement or abnormal fundal height growth [1].

Severe preeclampsia

The presence of severe preeclampsia mandates direct admission to labor and delivery. Magnesium sulfate should be administered intravenously to should be given prevent convulsions and antihypertensive medications should be given to lower severe levels of hypertension (systolic pressure greater

Table 33.1 Indication for delivery in mild preeclampsia.

Gestational age >40 weeks

Gestational age ≥37 weeks with:
Bishop score ≥6
Fetal weight <10th percentile
Nonreactive nonstress test pattern

Gestational age ≥34 weeks with:
Labor
Rupture of membranes
Vaginal bleeding
Persistent headaches or visual symptoms
Epigastric pain, nausea, vomiting

Abnormal biophysical profile

Criteria for severe preeclampsia met

than 160 mmHg and/or diastolic pressure of at least 110 mmHg). The aim of the antihypertensive therapy is to keep systolic BP at 140–155 mmHg and diastolic BP at 90–105 mmHg and prevent potential cerebrovascular and cardiovascular complications [1–3]. During the observation period, maternal and fetal conditions are assessed and a plan of management formulated regarding the need for delivery. Betamethasone 12 mg i.m. is administered times two doses 24-hours apart. A suggested algorithm for management of severe preeclampsia is described in Fig. 33.2 [1].

Expectant management of severe preeclampsia

There is disagreement about treatment of patients with severe preeclampsia before 34 weeks' gestation where maternal condition is stable and fetal condition is reassuring. In such patients, some authors consider delivery as the definitive treatment regardless of gestational age, whereas others rec-

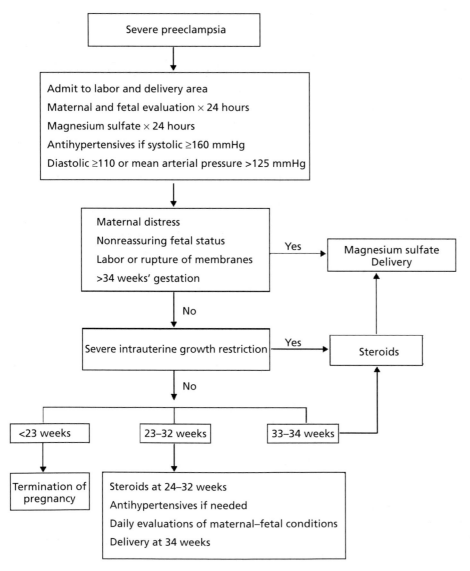

Fig. 33.2 Recommended management of severe preeclampsia. From Sibai [1] with permission.

ommend prolonging pregnancy until development of maternal or fetal indications for delivery, achievement of fetal lung maturity, or at 34 weeks' gestation. Expectant management is safe in properly selected women with severe disease, although maternal and fetal conditions can deteriorate rapidly. Hospitalization and daily monitoring are required. These pregnancies involve higher rates of maternal morbidity and significant risk of neonatal morbidity. For this reason, expectant management should proceed only in a tertiary care center with adequate maternal and neonatal facilities. These patients should be advised of the potential risks and benefits of expectant management, which requires daily monitoring of maternal and fetal conditions. It should be explained that the decision to continue expectant management will be revisited on a daily basis and that the median number of days pregnancy is prolonged in these cases is 7 days (range 2–35 days) [10].

A plan for a vaginal delivery should be attempted for all women with mild disease and for the majority of women with severe disease, particularly those beyond 30 weeks' gestation [2]. Cesarean delivery should be based on fetal gestational age, fetal condition, presence of labor, and cervical Bishop score. The presence of severe preeclampsia is not an indication for cesarean delivery. Elective cesarean section is recommended for women with severe disease below 30 weeks' gestation who are not in labor with a Bishop score of less than 5. Women with severe preeclampsia and fetal growth restriction with unfavorable cervix at less than 32 weeks' gestation are better delivered by cesarean section.

Postpartum management

These women usually receive large amounts of intravenous fluids during labor, as a result of prehydration before the administration of epidural analgesia, and intravenous fluids given during the administration of oxytocin and magnesium sulfate in labor and in the postpartum period. In addition, during the postpartum period there is mobilization of extracellular fluid leading to increased intravascular volume. As a result, women with severe preeclampsia—particularly those with abnormal renal function, those with capillary leaks, and those with early onset—are at increased risk for pulmonary edema and exacerbation of severe hypertension postpartum. These women should receive frequent evaluation of the amount of intravenous fluids, oral intake, blood products, and urine output as well as monitoring by pulse oximetry and pulmonary auscultation.

In general, in most women with gestational hypertension, the BP becomes normotensive during the first week postpartum. In contrast, in women with preeclampsia the hypertension takes a longer time to resolve. In addition, in some women with preeclampsia there is an initial decrease in BP immediately postpartum, followed by development of hypertension again between days 3 and 6. Use of antihypertensive drugs is recommended if the systolic BP is at least 155 mmHg and/or if the diastolic BP is at least 105 mmHg. The drug of choice is oral nifedipine (10 mg every 6 hours) or long-acting nifedipine (10 mg b.i.d.) to keep BP below that level. If BP is well controlled and there are no maternal symptoms, the woman is then discharged home with instructions for daily BP measurements by a home visiting nurse for the first week postpartum or longer as necessary. Antihypertensive medications are discontinued if the pressure remains below the hypertensive levels for at least 48 hours [1].

HELLP syndrome

This term describes preeclamptic patients having hemolysis, elevated liver enzymes, and a low platelet count. The HELLP syndrome has been recognized as a complication of severe preeclampsia–eclampsia for many years [11]. Our criteria for the diagnosis of HELLP syndrome includes laboratory findings summarized in Table 33.2.

Approximately 90% of patients with HELLP syndrome are first seen remote from term, complaining of epigastric or right upper quadrant pain. Approximately half have nausea or vomiting, and others have nonspecific viral syndrome-like symptoms. Hypertension or proteinuria may be absent or mild. Thus, some patients may display various signs and symptoms not diagnostic of severe preeclampsia. Consequently, for all pregnant women having any of these symptoms, it is advisable to obtain a complete blood count, platelet count, and liver enzymes [11].

Some patients may first be seen because of jaundice, gastrointestinal bleeding, hematuria, or bleeding from the gums. As a result, these patients are often misdiagnosed as having viral hepatitis, gallbladder disease, peptic ulcer disease, kidney stones, glomerulonephritis, acute fatty liver of pregnancy, idiopathic or thrombotic thrombocytopenia purpura, or hemolytic uremic syndrome.

Table 33.2 Recommended criteria for HELLP (hemolysis, elevated liver enzymes, and low platelet count) syndrome.

Hemolysis (at least two of these findings)
Peripheral smear (schistocytes, burr cells)
Serum bilirubin (≥1.2 mg/dL)
Low serum haptoglobin
Severe anemia, unrelated to blood loss

Elevated liver enzymes
AST or ALT ≥ twice upper level or normal
LDH ≥ twice upper level of normal

Low platelets (<100,000/mm³)

ALT, alanine aminotransferase; AST, aspartate aminotransferase; LDH, lactic dehydrogenase.

Perinatal outcomes and management

The presence of HELLP syndrome is associated with an increased risk of maternal death (1%) and increased rates of maternal morbidities such as pulmonary edema (8%), acute renal failure (3%), disseminated intravascular coagulopathy (15%), abruptio placentae (9%), liver hemorrhage or failure (1%), adult respiratory distress syndrome, sepsis, and stroke (<1%). Pregnancies complicated by HELLP syndrome are also associated with increased rates of wound hematomas and the need for transfusion of blood and blood products. The development of HELLP syndrome in the postpartum period further increases the risk of renal failure and pulmonary edema [11].

The reported perinatal death rate in recent series is in the range 7.4–20.4%. This high perinatal death rate is mainly experienced at very early gestational age (less than 28 weeks), in association with severe fetal growth restriction or abruptio placentae. Neonatal morbidities are dependent on gestational age at the time of delivery and they are similar to those in preeclamptic pregnancies without the HELLP syndrome. The rate of preterm delivery is approximately 70%, with 15% occurring before 28 weeks' gestation [11].

Patients with the syndrome at less than 37 weeks should be referred to a tertiary care center and managed initially as any patient with severe preeclampsia. The first priority is to assess the mother's condition and stabilize it, particularly if she has coagulation abnormalities. The next step is to investigate fetal well-being with a nonstress test and biophysical profile or Doppler assessment of fetal vessels. Finally, the decision must be made whether or not immediate delivery is indicated. A suggested algorithm for management is summarized in Fig. 33.3 [11]. Delivery may be delayed for 24–48 hours prior to 34 weeks' gestation to administer corticosteroids if the patient is asymptomatic and the fetus has reassuring testing. High-dose steroids have been shown to improve platelet counts transiently in undelivered women with HELLP. However, these studies did not report improvement in clinically important maternal morbidity such as the need for platelet transfusion pulmonary, renal, or hepatic complications [12]. In addition, a recent, double-blind, placebo controlled trial revealed no benefit from high-dose corticosteroids in women with HELLP syndrome [13].

Maternal and fetal conditions are assessed continuously during this time period. In some of these patients, there may be

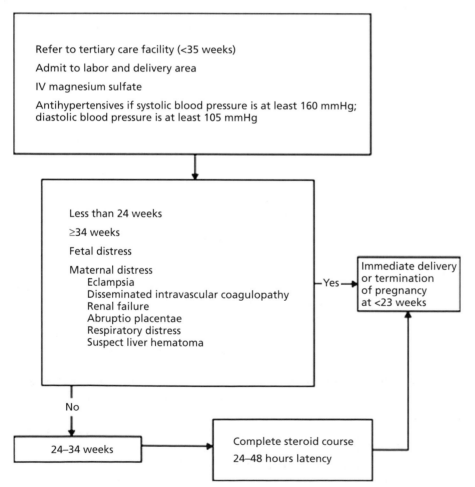

Fig. 33.3 Management of HELLP (hemolysis, elevated liver enzymes, and low platelet count) syndrome. From Sibai [11] with permission.

transient improvement in maternal laboratory tests; however, delivery is still indicated despite such improvement.

HELLP syndrome is not an indication for cesarean delivery, although cesarean delivery may be acceptable prior to 32 weeks' gestation with an unfavorable cervix, because of an anticipated long induction time in a clinically deteriorating gravida. Ripening agents as well as oxytocin can be used to initiate labor with a favorable cervix after 30 weeks. If thrombocytopenia is severe, regional anesthesia and pudendal blocks may be contraindicated. In this situation, intravenous narcotics still can be administered for analgesia during labor.

Maintain platelet counts greater than 20,000/μL for vaginal delivery and 40,000/μL for cesarean delivery. If platelets fall below 40,000/μL prior to cesarean delivery, be prepared to administer platelets just prior to surgery and/or intraoperatively. At the time of skin incision 6–10 units of platelets are usually administered, and an additional 6 units are administered if oozing is noted during surgery. Depending on the platelet count and degree of oozing, leave the bladder flap open and place an intraperitoneal and/or subcutaneous closed suction drain through a separate stab wound in an attempt to prevent wound hematomas. Table 33.3 summarizes the steps taken in cesarean delivery.

After delivery, patients with HELLP syndrome should receive close monitoring of vital signs, fluid intake and output, laboratory values, and pulse oximetry for at least 48 hours. Intravenous magnesium sulfate prophylaxis should be continued for 48 hours.

The clinical and laboratory findings of HELLP syndrome may develop for the first time in the postpartum period. In these patients, the time of onset of the manifestations ranges from a few hours to 7 days, with the majority developing within 48 hours postpartum. Hence, all postpartum women

and health care providers should be educated as to the signs and symptoms of HELLP syndrome. The treatment of patients with postpartum HELLP syndrome should be similar to that in the antepartum period, including the use of magnesium sulfate [11,12].

Eclampsia

Eclampsia is defined as the onset of seizures and/or unexplained coma during pregnancy or postpartum in patients with signs and symptoms of preeclampsia. Although most cases (90%) present in the third trimester or within 48 hours following delivery, rare cases (1.5%) have been reported at or prior to 20 weeks and as late as 23 days postpartum. The diagnosis of eclampsia is straightforward in the presence of hypertension, proteinuria, generalized edema, and convulsions. However, these patients could present with a broad spectrum of signs, ranging from severe hypertension (20–54%), severe proteinuria and generalized edema (48%), to absent or mild hypertension (30–60%), absent proteinuria (14%), and no edema (26%) [14].

Other symptoms may occur before or after the onset of seizures, including persistent frontal or occipital headaches (50–75%), blurred vision (19–32%), photophobia, epigastric/right upper quadrant pain, and altered mental status. All these symptoms in the presence of the above-mentioned risk factors should keep the physician watchful for development of eclampsia [14].

Management

The cardinal steps in the management of eclampsia are as follows.

Do not attempt to arrest the first seizure especially when no intravenous access or skilled personnel for rapid intubation are available. First, support maternal respiratory and cardiovascular functions to prevent hypoxia. Establish airway patency and maternal oxygenation during or immediately after the acute episode. Even if the initial seizure is short, it is important to maintain oxygenation by supplemental oxygen administration via facemask with or without a reservoir at 8–10 L/min because hypoventilation followed by respiratory acidosis often occurs. Pulse oximetry is advisable to monitor oxygenation in these patients. Arterial blood gas analysis is required if the pulse oximetry is abnormal (saturation less than 92%) [14].

Second, prevent maternal injury and aspiration by securing the bed's side rails by elevating them and making sure they are padded. Place patient in lateral decubitus position to minimize aspiration of oral secretions and vomitus in event of emesis.

Third, magnesium sulfate should be started to treat and prevent further seizures. The recommended regimen is to give

Table 33.3 Cesarean delivery in HELLP syndrome.

Epidural anesthesia
   Platelet count >75,000/μL
General anesthesia
Platelet transfusion if necessary
   6–10 units
   Platelet count >40,000/μL
   In operating room at time of surgery
Vesicouterine peritoneum left open
Subfascial drain if oozing at time of surgery and/or platelet count <40,000/μL
Skin closure
   Subcutaneous drain (closed system)
   or
   Secondary closure 3 days later
Perioperative transfusions as needed
Intensive monitoring for 48 hours postpartum

Table 33.4 Magnesium (Mg) toxicity.

Manifestations
Loss of patellar reflex (8–12 mg/dL)
Feeling of warmth, flushing (9–12 mg/dL)
Somnolence (10–12 mg/dL)
Slurred speech (10–12 mg/dL)
Muscular paralysis (15–17 mg/dL)
Respiratory difficulty (15–17 mg/dL)
Cardiac arrest (30–35 mg/dL)

Management
Discontinue magnesium sulfate
Obtain magnesium (serum) level
If magnesium level >15 mg/dL
    Give 1 g calcium gluconate i.v.
    Intubate
    Assist ventilation

Table 33.5 Transitory changes associated with eclamptic convulsions.

Uterine hyperactivity
Increased frequency of contractions
Increased uterine tone
Duration of contraction ≥2–15 minutes

Fetal heart rate changes
Bradycardia
Compensatory tachycardia
Decreased beat–beat variability
Late decelerations

a loading dose of 6 g over 15–20 minutes followed by a continuous infusion of 2 g/hour. Ten percent of patients might have a second convulsion after receiving magnesium sulfate. In this case, another 2 g bolus of magnesium sulfate can be given intravenously over 3–5 minutes. If the patient is still having seizure activity after adequate magnesium sulfate dosing, 250 mg sodium amobarbital may be given intravenously over 3–5 minutes. Be watchful for magnesium toxicity in women with abnormal renal function. Signs and symptoms and management of magnesium toxicity are given in Table 33.4.

Fourth, it is important to reduce and maintain blood pressure in a safe range. The goal is to keep systolic BP at 140–160 mmHg and diastolic BP at 90–110 mmHg. It can be achieved with intravenous bolus doses of 5–10 mg hydralazine or 20–40 mg labetalol every 15 minutes, as needed, or 10–20 mg nifedipine orally every 30 minutes to a maximum dosage of 50 mg in 1 hour. Sodium nitroprusside or nitroglycerine is rarely needed in eclampsia. Diuretics are not used except in setting of pulmonary edema.

Finally, begin induction of labor within 24 hours. It is important to keep in mind that the presence of eclampsia is not an indication for cesarean delivery. The patient should not be rushed to operating room, especially if maternal condition is not stable. It is to the fetus' advantage to be resuscitated *in utero* first. However, if bradycardia or persistent late decelerations occur despite resuscitative measures then a diagnosis of abruptio placentae or nonreassuring fetal status should be considered. The decision to proceed with cesarean delivery after maternal stabilization is based on the fetal gestational age, fetal condition, presence of labor, and cervical Bishop score. Cesarean delivery is recommended for those with eclampsia before 30 weeks, who are not in labor, and have a Bishop score below 5. Patients in labor or with ruptured membranes are allowed to deliver vaginally in the absence of obstetric complications. Labor can be induced with either oxytocin or prostaglandins in all patients after 30 weeks' gestation irrespective of Bishop score.

During the convulsion there is usually a prolonged deceleration and/or bradycardia. Following the convulsion and as a result of maternal hypoxia and hypercarbia, fetal heart rate monitoring might show compensatory tachycardia, decreased beat–beat variability, and transient late decelerations [14]. Additionally, uterine contraction monitors demonstrate both increase in uterine tone and frequency. The duration of the increased uterine activity varies from 2 to 14 minutes (Table 33.5). Because the fetal heart rate pattern usually returns to normal after a convulsion, other conditions should be considered if an abnormal pattern persists. It may take longer for the heart rate pattern to return to baseline in an eclamptic woman whose fetus is preterm with growth restriction. Abruptio placentae may occur after the convulsion and should be considered if uterine hyperactivity remains, if there is repetitive late decelerations, or fetal bradycardia persists.

Magnesium sulfate should be continued for at least 24 hours after delivery and/or after the last convulsion. In the presence of renal insufficiency, rates of both fluid administration and magnesium sulfate should be reduced. After delivery, oral antihypertensive medication can be used to maintain systolic BP below 155 mmHg and diastolic BP below 105 mmHg. Starting 200 mg labetalol every 8 hours (maximum dose 2400 mg/day) or 10 mg nifedipine every 6 hours (maximum dose 120 mg/day) is recommended. Oral nifedipine offers a beneficial diuretic effect in the postpartum period. There are no risks from the combined use of magnesium sulfate and oral nifedipine [14].

Prediction and prevention of preeclampsia

Numerous clinical, biophysical, and biochemical tests have been proposed for the prediction or early detection of preeclampsia. Unfortunately, most of these tests suffer from poor sensitivity, poor positive predictive values, and the majority of them are not suitable for routine use in clinical practice. At present, there is no single screening test that is considered reliable and cost-effective for predicting preeclampsia [8].

During the past two decades, numerous clinical reports and randomized trials described the use of various methods to reduce the rate and/or the severity of preeclampsia. Based on the available data, neither calcium supplementation nor low-dose aspirin should be routinely prescribed for preeclampsia prevention in nulliparous women. In addition, zinc, magnesium, fish oil, and vitamins C and E should not be routinely used for this purpose. Even in studies revealing beneficial effects, the results reveal reductions in a "definition of preeclampsia" without concomitant improvement in perinatal outcome [8].

Case presentation

A 20-year-old white primigravida at 35w 5d of gestation with an uneventful prenatal course was referred to labor and delivery by ambulance with severe preeclampsia. She has been complaining of headache and visual disturbance for the last 2 days. Her past medical/surgical and social history was completely negative. Upon admission, her BP was 180/110 mmHg. She had 2+ protein on urine dipstick. Bedside ultrasound confirmed a singleton intrauterine pregnancy consistent with 35 weeks' gestation. Fetal heart rate tracing was in the 150s and reassuring. Cervical examination revealed a Bishop score of 7.

Intravenous access was secured and laboratory tests were obtained for complete blood count (CBC) including platelet count, liver enzymes, and a metabolic profile. A loading dose of 6 g magnesium sulfate was given over 20 minutes which was followed by a maintenance dose of 2 g/hour. Because of her severe hypertension, an intravenous 10-mg bolus of hydralazine was administered. Blood pressures were monitored every 5–10 minutes; after 30 minutes BP was 150 mmHg systolic and 105 mmHg diastolic. Maternal urine output and reflexes were monitored every hour. The results of the blood tests revealed a platelet count of 110,000/mm^3, a hematocrit of 38%, and normal liver enzymes. Once maternal and fetal conditions were considered stable, intravenous oxytocin was started to initiate labor.

The patient subsequently underwent a spontaneous vaginal delivery of an infant weighing 2650 g with Apgar scores of 6 and 9 at 1 and 5 minutes, respectively. Postpartum magnesium sulfate was continued for 24 hours. In addition, maternal vital signs, intake and urine output as well as patellar reflexes were monitored every hour. She was started on 10 mg oral nifedipine every 6 hours because of elevated blood pressures. Three days postpartum she was discharged home to be seen in 1 week at the outpatient clinic.

Interpreting results

Because this patient was diagnosed with severe preeclampsia at 35w 5d of gestation, she was not a candidate for steroid injections or expectant management. She was started on magnesium sulfate for seizure prophylaxis and antihypertensive medications to stabilize blood pressure and induction of labor was initiated.

References

1 Sibai BM. Diagnosis and management of gestational hypertension and preeclampsia. *Obstet Gynecol* 2003;**102**:181–92.
2 Report of the National High Blood Pressure Education Program. Working group report on high blood pressure in pregnancy. *Am J Obstet Gynecol* 2000;**183**:S1–S22.
3 ACOG Committee on Practice Bulletins: Obstetrics. Diagnosis and management of preeclampsia and eclampsia. *Obstet Gynecol* 2001;**98**:159–67.
4 Barton JR, O'Brien JM, Bergauer NK, Jacques DL, Sibai BM. Mild gestational hypertension remote from term: progression and outcome. *Am J Obstet Gynecol* 2001;**184**:979–83.
5 Knuist M, Bonsel GJ, Zondervan HA, Treffers PE. Intensification of fetal and maternal surveillance in pregnant women with hypertensive disorders. *Int J Gynecol Obstet* 1998;**61**:127.
6 Meyer NL, Mercer BM, Friedman SA, Sibai BM. Urinary dipstick protein: a poor predictor of absent or severe proteinuria. *Am J Obstet Gynecol* 1994;**170**:137–41.
7 Buchbinder A, Sibai BM, Caritis S, Macpherson C, Hauth J, Lindheimer MD. Adverse perinatal outcomes are significantly higher in severe gestational hypertension than in mild preeclampsia. *Am J Obstet Gynecol* 2002;**186**:66–71.
8 Sibai B, Dekker G, Kupferminc M. Preeclampsia. *Lancet* 2005;**365**:785–99.
9 Levine RJ, Thadhani R, Qian C, *et al.* Urinary placental growth factor and risk of preeclampsia. *JAMA* 2005;**293**:77–85.
10 Haddad B. Expectant management of severe preeclampsia remote from term. *Clin Obstet Gynecol* 2005;**48**:430–40.
11 Sibai BM. Diagnosis, controversies, and management of the syndrome of hemolysis, elevated liver enzymes, and low platelet count. *Obstet Gynecol* 2004;**1035**:981–91.
12 Martin JN Jr, Thigpen BD, Rose CH, Cushman J, Moore A, May WL. Maternal benefit of high-dose intravenous corticosteroid therapy for HELLP syndrome. *Am J Obstet Gynecol* 2003;**189**:830–4.
13 Fonseca JE, Mendez F, Catano C, Arias F. Dexamethasone treatment does not improve the outcome of women with HELLP syndrome: a double-blind, placebo-controlled, randomized clinical trial. *Am J Obstet Gynecol* 2005;**193**:1591–8.
14 Sibai BM. Diagnosis, prevention, and management of eclampsia. *Obstet Gynecol* 2005;**105**:402–10.

34 Emergency care in pregnancy

Garrett K. Lam and Michael R. Foley

Incidents requiring emergency care of the gravid patient represent some of the most difficult situations for the practicing clinician. The cause of maternal collapse is varied, with multiple etiologies, and commonly the clinical situation is so dire, there is no time for accurate diagnosis. Attempts to resuscitate the mother are the starting point for intervention; however, as the resuscitation progresses, consideration of the fetus and its well-being must also be taken into account.

It is not the intention of the authors to attempt to cover all the causes of obstetric emergencies in a single chapter. Instead, we focus on amniotic fluid embolism (AFE), and the management of its sequelae: disseminated intravascular coagulopathy (DIC), blood product replacement, and perimortem cesarean delivery. The discussion of these topics and their management should provide guidelines applicable to the treatment of most cases of obstetric emergency.

Amniotic fluid embolism

AFE is one of the most catastrophic causes of maternal collapse. Published literature, including data from a national registry, has estimated the incidence to be between 1 in 8000 and 1 in 80,000 live births worldwide. Illustrative of its severity is its extremely high maternal mortality rate, reported in different sources to be 60–90% [1,2]. In the USA, AFE and pulmonary thromboembolism combine to account for approximately 20% of maternal mortality [3,4].

AFE is a diagnosis of clinical suspicion. Contributing factors include multiparity, precipitous or tumultuous labor, uterine hyperstimulation, rupture of membranes, and use of oxytocin. Episodes usually occur during labor and delivery, or in the immediate postpartum period, although individual cases have occurred around the time of cesarean delivery, D&C for termination of pregnancy, and amniocentesis.

Clinically, the signs of AFE are most notable for the triad of hypoxia, cardiovascular collapse, and coagulopathy. Sudden onset of dyspnea and hypoxia are usually the earliest signs of AFE, with rapid progression to respiratory failure. Indeed, 50% of patients who expire within the first hour of incident have cause of death attributed to profound hypoxemia and bronchospasm [5]. Affected patients may then rapidly develop cardiovascular failure, as manifested through dysrhythmias, pulseless electrical activity, and, ultimately, asystole. Cardiogenic shock is the most malignant expression of AFE, producing an 86% mortality rate in affected patients [1]. DIC is often seen, and has been reported in over 50% of cases. The specific cause of DIC is unclear, but is believed to be related to leakage of thromboplastin-like material into maternal circulation [6]. Symptoms of agitation, nausea, mental status changes, and tonic–clonic seizures have also been reported in AFE patients [1], over and above the major triad of symptoms listed earlier.

In reviewing the symptomatology of AFE, it has been suggested that AFE is really a unique maternal immunologic response to fetal antigens in amniotic fluid that have entered maternal circulation. Studies of patients with AFE have confirmed the presence of elevated serum levels of tryptase, a protein released along with histamine by mast cells in cases of fatal anaphylaxis [7]. Furthermore, a study of registry data revealed that 41% of women with AFE had a history of allergy. Thus, the term "anaphylactoid syndrome of pregnancy" has been suggested in lieu of AFE [1].

No prophylaxis for AFE is known as there are no predisposing factors to serve as forewarning in patients. Thus, the treatment of AFE is unfortunately based solely on supportive care at the time of occurrence. The basic tenets of care, as in any case of maternal collapse, emphasize the need to maintain the patient's ABCs (airway, breathing, circulation). As such, continuous monitoring of oxygen saturation, electrocardiogram (ECG) monitoring, and pulmonary artery catheterization are the quickest ways to monitor respiratory status, intravascular volume, and cardiovascular function accurately. Cardiopulmonary resuscitation with consistent ventilation must be initiated quickly to maintain placental perfusion in women who become unresponsive during an AFE, and continued until the woman is fully resuscitated.

For those patients who weather the initial cardiopulmonary incident, left ventricular failure is seen. In order to ensure organ perfusion, forward flow of circulation must be maintained. Thus, optimizing ventricular preload, even at the potential expense of pulmonary congestion, is imperative. Use of an inotropic medication may also be considered, particularly when hypotension persists, despite aggressive volume expansion. It is at this point where the use of Swan–Ganz catheterization is valuable.

Steroid administration has also been suggested as a treatment based on the anaphylactoid reaction previously described. However, not enough evidence exists to show that steroid administration would have any more significant effect than supportive care.

Disseminated intravascular coagulopathy

DIC is a coagulopathic state caused by the rapid consumption of clotting factors. Although there are two described clinical forms of DIC, this chapter focuses on acute DIC, not chronic DIC from long-term disease (e.g., cancer).

Episodes of DIC are identified by common events. Specifically, the clotting cascade is rapidly activated via exposure of blood to massive amounts of tissue factor, a natural procoagulant. This generates large amounts of thrombin which ultimately cause extensive clot formation that obstructs the microvasculature of tissues and organs. Microscopically, peripheral blood smears will show microangiopathic hemolytic anemia (Fig. 34.1). Initially, affected women exhibit petechiae and ecchymoses (Fig. 34.2). However, as the amount of intravascular thrombi builds, tissue necrosis and ischemia of multiple organ systems occur. An early study by Siegal *et al.* [8] looked at a series of patients with DIC (unrelated to pregnancy), and found that the most commonly affected organ systems were the kidneys, followed by liver, lungs, heart (cardiogenic shock), and then the central nervous system (CNS).

In addition to ischemic sequelae, widespread thrombus formation depletes the patient's intrinsic amounts of clotting factors. A paradoxical state of anticoagulation develops in the patient, which is illustrated clinically by signs such as "oozing" of blood from intravenous sites, catheters, or friable surfaces such as mucosal membranes. In the pregnant patient, vaginal bleeding is one of the most common signs. The inability to clot augments the vicious cycle of organ failure as the loss of blood becomes difficult to stop, intravascular volume and oxygen-carrying capacity drop, exacerbating systemic organ system failure and worsening chances for successful resuscitation. Given the potential severity of the disease, it is not surprising that DIC itself can have a very high mortality rate. In the general literature on DIC, mortality rates are in the range 40–80% [9,10]; however, many of those findings were based on trauma and burn cases, rather than pregnancy-related causes. There does not appear to be any data available directly addressing maternal mortality and DIC specifically.

Treatment of DIC is reviewed partly in the following section on blood product replacement; however, a short discussion on the use of heparin to treat DIC deserves mention. Given that DIC is based on consumption of clotting factors, use of anticoagulants such as heparin to interrupt the clotting cascade is a theoretically sensible treatment option. However, no controlled trials exist that indicate that heparin is beneficial [5].

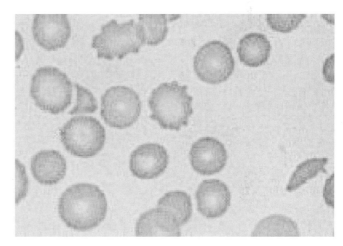

Fig. 34.1 Peripheral smear of patient with disseminated intravascular coagulopathy (DIC). Schistocytes and helmet cells are characteristic of microangiopathic hemolytic anemia. Note the lack of platelets seen in the microscopic field. (From Emedicine with permission.)

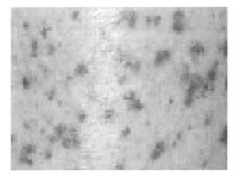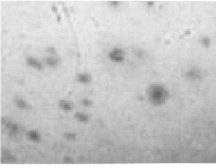

Fig. 34.2 Petechiae and purpura seen in DIC. (From Emedicine with permission.)

Furthermore, there is logical concern that heparinization would exacerbate bleeding, which could create further complications in the patient who is postoperative from delivery. Thus, the mainstay of therapy would appear to be related to replacement therapy with blood products and recombinant factors.

Blood product replacement

In the treatment of DIC from AFE, the cardinal principle is continuing replacement of consumed blood products in order to maintain perfusion and circulation. This is a temporizing measure until the patient has been resuscitated and the bleeding is stabilized. Thus, it is imperative to understand what comprises each type of blood product in order to choose which to use (Table 34.1).

The basic tenets for blood product replacement are to improve oxygen-carrying capacity, maintain intravascular volume, and treat coagulopathy. Transfusion with packed red blood cells (PRBCs) meets the first two purposes. Each unit of packed cells contains approximately 200 mL of red cells in a total volume of 300 mL. In an adult patient without active bleeding, 1 unit should raise the hematocrit by approximately 3%. In nonacute settings, blood that is specifically typed and cross-matched to the patient is used, and a leukopoor option is requested to decrease the risk of febrile transfusion reaction. In an acute setting of bleeding, where blood group and antibody screens are lacking, use of O negative PRBCs is the safest, quickest, temporizing option until properly matched products are available. In most acute care hospitals, typed and screened blood products can be made available within 30 minutes (Transfusion Services, Banner Good Samaritan Regional Medical Center, personal communication, 2005).

Platelet transfusion is considered when thrombocytopenia becomes severe enough that persistent bleeding becomes problematic. It has been our experience that people have individual cut-offs for when platelet transfusion is prescribed; however, a general consensus exists that excessive bleeding from major trauma or surgery follows platelet counts less than $50,000/mm^3$, and spontaneous bleeding occurs with platelet counts below $20,000/mm^3$. Furthermore, dilutional thrombocytopenia requiring platelet transfusion can occur when a patient receives over 1.5–2 times their normal blood volume. Platelets can be collected from single or random donors, but are more commonly available as a group of 10 units from a single donor. One single donor unit should increase the platelet count $7500–10,000/mm^3$ after equilibration, usually occurring within 10 minutes of transfusion [11]. Thus, in the setting of pathologic processes with massive platelet destruction or consumption, such as HELLP (hemolysis, elevated liver enzymes, and low platelet count) or DIC, platelet transfusions have very limited effect, and are often avoided except in a temporizing capacity (e.g., cesarean delivery in an affected patient). Of note, platelet concentrates contain red blood cells (RBCs) in the approximately 50 mL of serum they contain in each unit; thus, Rh negative patients should receive Rh-immune prophylaxis.

The use of plasma products are more germane to the treatment of our AFE patient, as they can replace many of the coagulation products consumed or lost during the course of DIC. Several different preparations of plasma and coagulation products are available.

Fresh frozen plasma (FFP) is separated from freshly drawn blood, and is used to correct any factor deficiency in a patient.

Table 34.1 Table of blood products used for replacement.

Blood Product	Contents	Indications	Volume Added (mL)	Effect
Packed RBCs	Red cells, ~50 mL of plasma, WBCs	Increases red cell mass, oxygen carrying capacity, intravascular volume (secondary)	300	Increases hematocrit on average 3% per unit
Platelets (usually available as 10-pack of single donor platelets)	Platelets, small amount of plasma, RBCs and WBCs	Treats bleeding from thrombocytopenia	50	Increases total platelet count between $7500–10,000/mm^3$
Fresh frozen plasma	Plasma and all clotting factors, fibrinogen	Coagulation disorders, increases intravascular volume (secondary effect)	250	Increases fibrinogen levels 10–15 mg/dL per unit
Cryoprecipitate	Fibrinogen, factors V, VIII, XIII, von Willebrand and fibrinogen	Treats specific bleeding disorders (von Willebrand disease, hemophilia) and any fibrinogen disorders	40	Same as FFP; however, does not add as much intravascular volume

FFP, fresh frozen plasma; RBC, red blood cell; WBC, white blood cell.

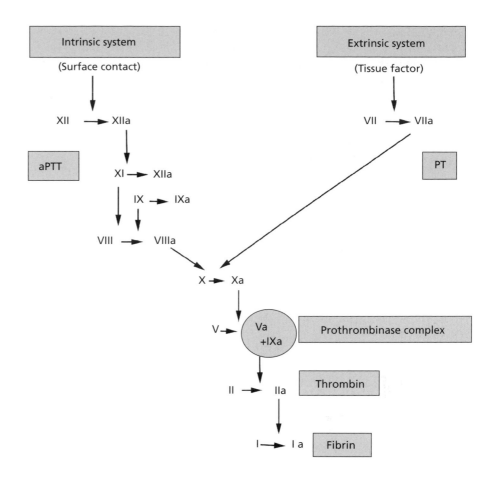

Fig. 34.3 The coagulation cascade. (From Emedicine.com, 2005 with permission.)

It needs to be ABO-compatible with the patient, but does not require antibody cross-matching or Rh typing. A typical unit will provide an extra 250 mL volume, and contains approximately 700 mg fibrinogen, which should raise a patient's fibrinogen level 10–15 mg/dL per unit. Of note, one may notice different recommendations to give FFP based on the number of PRBC units transfused, ranging from 1 unit FFP to every 3–5 units PRBCs. No specific data have shown that prophylactic administration of platelets and FFP based solely upon the amount of transfused PRBCs have been of any benefit [5]. Rather, it is recommended simply to transfuse appropriate products when necessary based on fibrinogen levels and clinical observation.

When specific factors, such as factors VIII, XIII and von Willebrand factor, or fibrinogen is needed, cryoprecipitate is a better choice. Cryoprecipitate is separated from FFP that has been warmed to refrigerator temperatures, given that it is cold-insoluble. It has a similar effect as FFP in raising fibrinogen levels 10–15 mg/dL per unit. Each unit is only 40 mL in volume, making it a logical choice in patients who require fibrinogen but cannot tolerate the larger volumes brought by FFP. Given that it is collected from a single donor unit of FFP, it carries less risk for transmission of hepatitis and HIV.

Recently, recombinant factor VIIa (rVIIa, aka NovoSeven) has been released for treatment of bleeding diathesis, primarily for hemophilias. This synthesized protein, in combination with circulating tissue factor, is given to activate factor X in the common pathway of the coagulation cascade (Fig. 34.3). Thus, it has found novel uses for bleeding disorders from extensive surgery, trauma, thrombocytopenia, liver disease, or qualitative platelet dysfunction [12]. It has been selectively used for individual cases of obstetric hemorrhage [13], and, currently, there is one case report of its successful use for DIC in AFE [14]. Given its novelty, there is no known optimal or minimal dosing regimen for its use in pregnancy. The various case reports have described dosages ranging 20–120 µg/kg for treatment of serious bleeding, and have reported clinically significant hemostasis within 30 minutes of administration. Although there appears to be great potential for the use of rVIIa in obstetric hemorrhage and DIC, reservation of its use for the most severe cases of hemorrhage seems most prudent.

Perimortem cesarean delivery

The final consideration in all cases of obstetric collapse is timing of delivery to salvage the fetus. Unfortunately, there is a lack of depth in the study of this topic for the obvious reason that the opportunity to study this technique is unpredictable, and thus our knowledge is based only on theoretical conclusions drawn from physiologic data and case studies

According to the paper by Katz *et al.* [15], the decision to perform perimortem cesarean delivery must be made quickly and without equivocation. Their paper states that any maternal patient who suffers cardiac arrest in the third trimester should have cesarean delivery initiated within 4 minutes of the time of arrest, and delivery performed within 5 minutes of the seminal event. The recommendation for timing of delivery is based on the physiologic principle that irreversible anoxic damage occurs within 4–6 minutes from cessation of adequate cerebral perfusion. In the pregnant woman, anoxia occurs more quickly given the pre-existing reduction in functional residual capacity caused by the gravid uterus. Furthermore, it is maintained that cardiopulmonary resuscitation likely does not produce adequate blood flow in the pregnant patient. In nonpregnant patients, the thoracic compressions of cardiopulmonary resuscitation produce a stroke volume 30% of normal [15]. This stroke volume is worsened another two-thirds in pregnancy because of caval compression by the gravid uterus, such that chest compressions are likely only producing a cardiac output that is 10% of normal [16]. Therefore, delivery should immediately improve maternal perfusion, and actually improves the chance for successful resuscitation.

The 5-minute rule for delivery of the infant also appears to be supported by physiologic studies and case reports in the literature. Physiologic studies in animals show that a normal fetus has an oxygen reserve of around 2 minutes, but compensatory mechanisms and shunting may preserve oxygenation for vital organs for periods of time longer than 5 minutes. Katz *et al.*'s paper [15] reviewed the available data on fetal survivors from perimortem delivery, and found that most survivors were delivered within 5 minutes of arrest. However, as there are reports of infants who survived past the 5-minute period, and that most term infants have sufficient reserve to recover from hypoxic insult, it has been recommended that any fetus with evidence of a heart rate should be delivered, even if it is past the 5-minute period.

Conclusions

Emergency care in pregnancy is a broad topic encompassing a myriad of causes. It is hoped that the review of the treatment of amniotic fluid embolism and consideration of its attendant comorbidities has provided the reader with guidelines germane to the management of most types of maternal crises. The key principle for treatment of the patient with AFE is devoting full attention towards maintaining her circulation and perfusion, which would benefit both fetus and patient. Awareness of time spent in resuscitation is a critical element in deciding when to perform perimortem cesarean delivery, as the goal for delivery should occur within minutes of complete arrest. Timely delivery may not only salvage a viable infant, but may also improve the mother's chance for successful resuscitation. Finally, with successful resuscitation, attention must be paid to the needs of the patient's associated complications, most notably DIC and blood product replacement. Correct usage of replacement products not only maintains adequate hemostasis and oxygenation, but will also assist in normalization of intravascular volume.

Case presentation

A 29-year-old African-American female, G2P1001 at 38 weeks' gestation, has been on pitocin augmentation for the past 12 hours. Fetal heart rate is consistently in the 140s, with good variability and no signs of hypoxia. At 4 cm dilatation, amniotomy is performed, with light meconium-stained fluid noted. The patient then complains to her labor nurse that she is "feeling strange," with lightheadedness and the inability to "think clearly." She then, oddly, begins counting backwards from 10 spontaneously, and, before she finishes, loses consciousness.

The labor nurse notes that her oxygen saturations are acutely falling, dropping to the 80s.

The resident attempts bedside revival, but no response is obtained. Fetal heart tones become bradycardic to the 80s within minutes from loss of consciousness. She is rushed to the operating room for resuscitation, and has a grand mal seizure on the operating table. The anesthesiologist notes that the patient's rhythm strip shows asystole. The fetal heart monitor verifies a severe bradycardia.

The decision is made to perform a perimortem cesarean delivery of the fetus. Cardiopulmonary resuscitation is performed concurrently. The infant is successfully delivered by low transverse cesarean section, and requires resuscitation in the operating room by the neonatal team.

Full code resuscitation is carried out on the patient throughout the completion of the cesarean delivery. An inordinately small amount of blood loss is noted from the uterine incision. As the patient's skin is being closed, a watery–bloody discharge begins to ooze between the staples. She is also noted to be bleeding from her intravenous sites, and a large pool of blood is noted on the sheets of the operating table between her legs. The code is carried out for a full 50 minutes from the initiation of the cesarean, but the patient never recovers a consistent heart rhythm. Death is pronounced approximately 50 minutes from membrane rupture.

References

1 Clark SL, Hankins GD, Dudley DA, *et al.* Amniotic fluid embolism: analysis of the national registry. *Am J Obstet Gynecol* 1995:**172**:1158–67.

2 Tuffnell DJ. Amniotic fluid embolism. *Curr Opin Obstet Gynecol* 2003;**15**:119–22.

3 Chang J, Elam-Evans LD, Berg CJ, *et al.* Pregnancy-related mortality surveillance, United States, 1991–1999. *MMWR Surveill Summ* 2003;**52**:1–8.

4 Kaunitz AM, Hughes JM, Grimes DA. Causes of maternal mortality in the United States. *Obstet Gynecol* 1985;**65**:605–12.

5 Baldiserri M. Amniotic fluid embolism. UpToDate.com, 2005

6 Davies S. Amniotic fluid embolism and isolated disseminated intravascular coagulation. *Can J Anaesth* 1999;**46**:456–9.

7 Bradley, JM, Collins KM, Harley RA. Ancillary studies in amniotic fluid embolism: a case report and review of the literature. *Am J Forensic Med Pathol* 2005;**26**:92.

8 Siegal T, Seligsohn U, Aghai E, Modan M. Clinical and laboratory aspects of disseminated intravascular coagulation: a study of 118 cases. *Thromb Haemost* 1978;**39**:122–34.

9 Stephan F, Hollande J, Richard O, *et al.* Thrombocytopenia in the surgical ICU. *Chest* 1999;**115**:1363–70.

10 Gando S, Nanzaki S, Kemmotsu O. Disseminated intravascular coagulation and sustained systemic inflammatory response syndrome predict organ dysfunctions after trauma. *Ann Surg* 1999;**229**:121–7.

11 Martin SM, Strong TH. Transfusion of blood components and derivatives in the obstetric intensive care patient. In: Foley MR, Strong TH, Garite TJ, eds. *Obstetric Intensive Care Manual*, 2nd edn. London: McGraw Hill, 2004.

12 Ramanarayanan J, Krishnan G. Factor VII. Emedicine.com, 2005.

13 Bouwmeester FW, Jonkhoff AR, Verheijen RH, van Geijn HP. Successful treatment of life-threatening postpartum hemorrhage with recombinant activated factor VII. *Obstet Gynecol* 2003;**101**:1174–6.

14 Lim Y, Loo CC, Chia V, Fun W. Recombinant factor VIIa after amniotic fluid embolism and disseminated intravascular coagulopathy. *Int J Gynecol Obstet* 2004;**87**:178–9.

15 Katz VL, Dotters DJ, Droegemueller W. Perimortem cesarean delivery. *Obstet Gynecol* 1986;**68**:571–6.

16 Katz VL, Balderston K, DeFreest M. Perimortem cesarean delivery: were our assumptions correct? *Am J Obstet Gynecol* 2005;**192**:1916.

35 Sonographic dating and standard fetal biometry

Alfred Abuhamad and David Nyberg

Pregnancy dating

Accurate pregnancy dating is a critical component of prenatal management. Precise knowledge of gestational age is essential for the management of high-risk pregnancies and in particular fetal growth restriction. Although uterine size, as measured by the fundal height, provides a subjective assessment of the fetal size, ultrasound has a more precise role in confirming gestational age [1].

Overestimation of gestational age based on menstrual dates reflects a preponderance of misdated pregnancies resulting from delayed ovulation in the conception cycle. Overestimation of true gestational age by the menstrual history results in an underestimate of the rate of preterm delivery [2] and an overestimate of the post-dates pregnancies. In a retrospective review of a routinely scan-dated population, Gardosi *et al.* [3] found that 72% of inductions carried out for post-term pregnancy (>294 days) according to menstrual dates were not actually post-term according to ultrasound dating.

Ultrasound has an integral role in confirming gestational age, with a high accuracy when performed in the first or the second trimesters. A study involving *in vitro* fertilization (IVF) pregnancy has shown an ultrasound accuracy for pregnancy dating of 3–4 days when performed between 14 and 22 weeks' gestation [1]. Dating during the third trimester is less predictive because of differences in fetal growth, and should be avoided.

First trimester

Dating by ultrasound in the first half of pregnancy has become a routine part of antenatal care in many institutions around the world. Before 6 weeks, dating can be carried out by measurement and observation of the gestational sac [4]. The gestational sac is visible as early as 4 weeks, and should always be visible by 5 weeks. The size of the gestational sac can be correlated with gestational age [5]. Because the mean sac diameter (MSD) grows at a rate of 1 mm/day, gestational age can be estimated by the formula:

Gestational age (days) = 30 + MSD (mm) [6]

Among all measurements, determination of the maximum embryonic length (crown rump length [CRL]) up to 14 weeks' gestation is the most accurate for determining gestational age. The random error is in the range of 4–8 days at the 95th percentile [7–12].

Second and third trimester

When the CRL is above 60 mm, other biometric parameters are more useful for dating the pregnancy [13]. Standardized measurements include the biparietal diameter (BPD), head circumference (HC), femur length (FL), humeral length (HL), and abdominal circumference (AC). These grow in a predictable way and so can be correlated with gestational age. Virtually any other bone or organ can be measured and compared with gestational age.

In a study that involved pregnancies conceived with IVF, the HC was the most predictive parameter of gestational age between 14 and 22 weeks' gestation as it predicts gestational age by 3.4 days [1]. Other parameters, such as the BPD, AC, and FL have good accuracy. Combining various biometric parameters improves the prediction of gestational age slightly over the HC alone [1].

The AC is a measure of fetal girth. It includes soft tissues of the abdominal wall as well as a measure of internal organs, primarily the liver. Unlike other commonly used fetal measurements, it is not influenced by bone. The importance of the AC is reflected by the fact that, at term, 95% of newborns are found to be within 20% of expected length of 20 cm, whereas the weight may vary by 100% or more. Therefore, differences in weight must be explained primarily by variations in girth.

Not surprisingly then, the AC is among the least predictive measures of fetal age but the most predictive of fetal growth [14–16].

Estimation of fetal weight

The best overall measure of fetal size is obtained by estimating fetal weight. Numerous formulas for estimating fetal weight have been described and utilized [17–19]. Using standard biometry, some formulas use head measurements and AC, others use long bone measurements and AC, and others use all four measurements. The AC is included in all commonly used formulas of estimated fetal weight, and the AC also strongly influences fetal weight estimates [20]. Weight estimates based on AC alone have also been reported [21,22].

Hadlock [17], Dudley [18], Coombs *et al.* [19], Rose and McCallum [23], and Medchill *et al.* [24] estimations of weight formulas, which include BPD, HC, AC, and FL, result in a mean absolute error of approximately 10% [25,26]. Some formulas for estimating fetal weight are volume-based and would be expected to be more accurate in predicting fetal weight; however, these volume-based equations have not been shown to be consistently more accurate and some studies have resulted in large systematic errors [27].

In experienced hands, nearly 80% of estimated weights are within 10% of the actual birth weights and most of the remaining are within 20% of birth weights. However, accuracy decreases with less experienced sonographers [28]. A number of studies have documented that prediction of fetal weight by ultrasound is limited. In one study, Baum *et al.* [28] found that sonographic estimation of fetal weight was no better than clinical or patient estimates at term.

Intrauterine growth restriction

Definition

The term "small for gestational age" (SGA) is commonly used to describe all fetuses that are small. SGA fetuses represent a heterogeneous group of both normal and "growth-restricted" fetuses.

It should be clear that estimated weights and weight percentiles only evaluate fetal size. This approach cannot distinguish growth-restricted compromised fetuses from otherwise healthy fetuses who are simply small for gestational age. Therefore, it is important to correlate estimates of fetal size with other correlates of fetal health including amniotic fluid, Doppler studies, and fetal activity. For this reason, the term intrauterine growth restriction (IUGR) is appropriately applied to fetuses who are SGA and who show other evidence of chronic hypoxemia or malnutrition. Nevertheless, the terms SGA and IUGR are frequently used interchangeably.

Dynamic evaluation of fetal growth with serial ultrasound is more important than a single examination when fetal measurements are below the 10th percentile. This is true irrespective of the methods used, including cross-sectional or longitudinal growth charts, customized growth charts, or predicted fetal growth. The optimal measurement interval in small fetuses that combines acceptable technical error with useful clinical data while minimizing intra- and interobserver variabilities appears to be approximately 10 days [29]. However, longer time intervals will reflect fetal growth in low-risk patients more accurately [30].

Several definitions exist in the literature for the diagnosis of IUGR. The definition that is most commonly used in clinical practice is an estimated fetal weight at less than the 10th percentile for gestational age. At this diagnostic threshold, approximately 70% of "affected" fetuses will be constitutionally small and have no increase in perinatal morbidity or mortality [31]. Using the 5th percentile as a cut-off for the diagnosis of IUGR may be more clinically applicable, given that perinatal morbidity and mortality have been shown to increase beyond this threshold [32]. Of all the ultrasound-derived biometric parameters, the AC is the most sensitive indicator for growth restriction in the fetus. An AC of less than the 2.5th percentile for gestational age carries a sensitivity of greater than 95% for the diagnosis of IUGR [33,34]. The growth profile of the AC should therefore be monitored closely in fetuses at risk for growth abnormalities. Furthermore, when estimating fetal weights by ultrasound, the appropriate growth curves should be used. Curves generated at high altitudes will underestimate IUGR by approximately 50% for sea level population [35].

Symmetric versus asymmetric

"Symmetric" IUGR has been used to describe the growth pattern when all biometric measurements appear affected to the same degree, whereas "asymmetric" IUGR has been used to characterize a smaller AC compared with other growth parameters. Asymmetric IUGR would then show abnormal ratios such as the HC:AC or FL:AC ratio [36].

When first introduced, the term symmetric IUGR was suggested as more likely to reflect underlying fetal condition including aneuploidy, whereas asymmetric IUGR supposedly reflected underlying uterine–placental vascular dysfunction. However, these assumptions have proved to be largely false. Asymmetric IUGR was more likely to be associated with a major fetal anomaly in one study [37], may be seen with aneuploidy (e.g., triploidy), and can initially present as symmetric IUGR [38]. Fetuses with symmetric and asymmetric IUGR also show a similar degree of acid–base impairment [39]. The FL:AC ratio has also been found to be useful for prediction of IUGR [40].

Risk factors

Causes and associations for IUGR are shown in Table 35.1. The most common associations are with maternal hypertension, and/or a history of IUGR in previous pregnancies. Conversely, a history of a prior SGA fetus is a risk factor for preeclampsia [41].

Underlying uterine–placental dysfunction is a commonly evoked cause for otherwise unexplained fetal IUGR. Uterine–placental dysfunction has been correlated with a range of pathologic findings including failure of physiologic transformation of uterine spiral arteries by endovascular trophoblasts, smaller placentas, increase in the thickness of tertiary-stem villi vessel wall, and decrease in lumen circumference of spiral arterioles. Also, confined placental mosaicism has been found to carry a higher risk of IUGR and adverse outcome including fetal death [42]. Uterine–placental dysfunction produces fetal hypoxemia which results in subnormal growth, oligohydramnios, and alterations in blood flow [43].

Various chromosome abnormalities including those confined to the placenta (confined placental mosaicism) may exhibit delayed growth as a prominent feature. Abnormal

Table 35.1 Causes and associations with intrauterine growth restriction (IUGR).

Maternal
Pregnancy induced hypertension/preeclampsia
Severe chronic hypertension
Severe maternal diabetes mellitus
Collagen vascular disease
Heart disease
Smoking
Poor nutrition
Renal disease
Lung disease/hypoxia
Environmental agents
Endocrine disorders
Previous history of IUGR

Uterine–placental
Uterine–placental dysfunction
Placental infarct
Chronic abruption
Multiple gestation/twin transfusion syndrome
Confined placental mosaicism

Fetal
Chromosome abnormalities
Anomalies
Skeletal dysplasias
Multiple anomaly syndromes (see Table 35.2)

Infection

Teratogens

---

growth and development has also been associated with disturbed genomic imprinting (expression of genes depending on whether they are located on the maternal or on the paternal chromosome). This has led to the suggestion that the genomic imprinting has evolved as a mechanism to regulate embryonic and fetal growth [44].

Many fetuses with chromosomal anomalies or other genetic syndromes may exhibit growth delay as a dominant feature (Table 35.2). It may be the primary, or in some cases the only sonographic evidence of underlying fetal anomalies. Early onset IUGR is a common manifestation of major chromosome abnormalities, particularly trisomies 18 and 13, and triploidy [45,46].

Among other variables, smaller fetal size tends to reflect both maternal and paternal birth weights. Magnus *et al.* [47] found the mean maternal birth weight was significantly less among those who had experienced two SGA births compared with those with no SGA births ($3127 \pm 54\,g$ vs. $3424 \pm 22\,g$). Interestingly, the mean paternal birth weight was also lower ($3497 \pm 88\,g$ vs. $3665 \pm 24\,g$) from affected pregnancies with two previous SGA births.

Outcome

When compared with appropriately grown fetuses matched for gestational age, IUGR fetuses have an increased risk of perinatal morbidity and mortality [48]. Long-term follow-up studies have shown an increased incidence of physical handicap and neurodevelopmental delay in growth restricted fetuses [49,50]. The presence of chronic metabolic acidemia *in utero*, rather than actual birth weight appears to be the best predictor of long-term neurodevelopmental delay [51]. In pregnancies with growth restricted fetuses, timing of the delivery is the most critical step in clinical management. Balancing the risk of prematurity with the risk of long-term neurodevelopmental delay is a serious challenge facing physicians involved in the care of these pregnancies. In addition, IUGR fetuses may face long-term adverse adult health outcomes including accelerated atherosclerotic vascular disease, hypertension, and diabetes.

Management

Traditionally, the management of pregnancies with fetal growth restriction relied on cardiotocography for fetal surveillance. During cardiotocography, the physician looks for heart rate variability as a sign of fetal well-being. Heart rate variability is the final result of the rhythmic integrated activity of autonomic neurons generated by organized cardiorespiratory reflexes [52]. In growth restricted fetuses, higher baseline rates, decreased long- and short-term variability, and delayed maturation of reactivity is seen in heart rate tracings [53,54]. These studies have relied on computer generated analyses of fetal heart rate tracings in their evaluation. Unaided visual

Table 35.2 Genetic syndromes that include intrauterine growth restriction (IUGR).

Aarskog syndrome
X-linked. Associated with brachydactyly, shawl scrotum, hypertelorism, vertebral anomalies, and moderate short stature. DNA testing is available

Ataxia-telangiectasia syndrome
Autosomal recessive. Associated with growth deficiency sometimes evident prenatally, ataxia, telangiectasias, and immunodeficiency. DNA testing is available

Bloom syndrome
Autosomal recessive. More common in Ashkenazi Jewish population. Associated with prenatal growth deficiency, butterfly telangiectasia of the face, microcephaly, mild mental retardation in some cases, and occasional syndactyly and/or polydactyly. DNA analysis is available

Cornelia de Lange/Brachman syndrome
Autosomal dominant often *de novo*. Associated with prenatal growth deficiency, micromelia, mental retardation, and synophrys. DNA testing is available

CHARGE syndrome
Characterized by coloboma, heart disease, choanal atresia, retarded growth (typically postnatal onset) or development, CNS abnormalities, genital anomalies, and ear anomalies and/or deafness. DNA testing is available

Coffin–Siris syndrome
Autosomal recessive. Characterized by prenatal growth deficiency, mental retardation, coarse facies, absence of terminal phalanges, and hypoplastic to absent fingernails and toenails. DNA testing is not currently available

Dubowitz syndrome
Autosomal recessive. Characterized by microcephaly, prenatal growth deficiency, mental retardation, dysmorphic facies, 2,3 toe syndactyly, and eczema. DNA testing is not currently available

Fanconi anemia
Autosomal recessive. Characterized by radial ray defects including aplasia of the thumbs or supernumerary thumbs, short stature often of prenatal onset, pancytopenia, renal or other urinary tract abnormalities, cardiac defects, and gastrointestinal abnormalities. DNA testing is available

Johanson–Blizzard syndrome
Autosomal recessive. Rare syndrome associated with prenatal growth deficiency, hypoplastic alae nasi, mental retardation, microcephaly, hydronephrosis, and pancreatic insufficiency. DNA testing is not currently available

Neu–Laxova syndrome
Autosomal recessive. Rare syndrome associated with severe prenatal growth deficiency, microcephaly, exophthalmos, subcutaneous edema,

micrognathia, sloping forehead, syndactyly, contractures, often with pterygia, polyhydramnios, small placenta, and short umbilical cord. Majority of patients are stillborn. DNA testing is not available

Noonan syndrome
Autosomal dominant. Associated with pulmonic stenosis, other congenital heart defects, webbed neck/increased nuchal translucency, short stature typically of postnatal onset, dysmorphic facies, pectus excavatum, and vertebral anomalies. DNA analysis is available

Pena–Shokier phenotype
Autosomal recessive in some families. Characterized by prenatal growth deficiency, arthrogryposis, clubfoot, rocker-bottom feet, micrognathia, pulmonary hypoplasia, polyhydramnios, abnormal placenta, and short umbilical cord. DNA testing is not available

Roberts syndrome/Roberts phocomelia
Autosomal recessive with variable expression. Characterized by thalidomide-type limb reduction defects often more severe in the upper limbs, microcephaly, severe prenatal growth deficiency, mental retardation, cleft lip and/or palate. DNA testing is not available

Seckel syndrome
Autosomal recessive. Characterized by severe prenatal growth deficiency, mental retardation, microcephaly, prominent nose, micrognathia, and missing ribs. DNA analysis is not available

Silver–Russell syndrome
Typically sporadic but has been associated with maternal UPD of chromosome 7 in about 10% of cases. Characterized by prenatal growth deficiency, asymmetry of the limbs, triangular facies, relative microcephaly, and small and/or curved fifth finger. UPD testing is available

Smith–Lemli–Opitz syndrome
Autosomal recessive. Characterized by failure to thrive, microcephaly, 2,3 toe syndactyly, genital abnormalities, polydactyly, and congenital heart defects. Affected fetuses may have low unconjugated estriol MoM on maternal serum screening. Diagnostic testing available

Williams syndrome
Autosomal dominant microdeletion syndrome caused by a deletion of 7p11.23. Characterized by mild prenatal growth deficiency, congenital heart defect particularly supravalvular aortic stenosis, mental retardation, dysmorphic features, contractures, abnormal curvature of the spine, and renal anomalies. Diagnostic testing available by FISH analysis

FISH, fluorescence *in situ* hybridization; MoM, multiples of the median; UPD, uniparental disomy.

analyses of fetal heart rate records have been shown to have limited reliability and reproducibility [55,56]. Furthermore, the presence of overtly abnormal patterns of fetal heart rate tracings represent late signs of fetal deterioration [57,58].

Doppler ultrasound has been shown to improve outcome in high-risk pregnancies [59]. The use of Doppler ultrasound in the management of pregnancies with fetal growth restriction has received significant attention in the literature. Several cross-sectional and longitudinal studies have highlighted the fetal cardiovascular adaptation to hypoxemia and the progressive stages of such adaptation [60–65]. Findings from these studies and the use of Doppler ultrasound in the management of the growth restricted fetus are discussed in the following section.

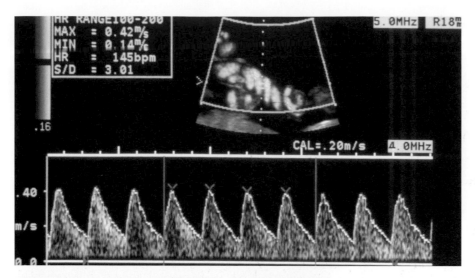

Fig. 35.1 Normal Doppler waveforms obtained from the umbilical artery in the third trimester. In the third trimester of pregnancy, the umbilical circulation is a low impedance circulation. Note the increased amount of flow at end diastole (white arrow). From Abuhamad [92] with permission.

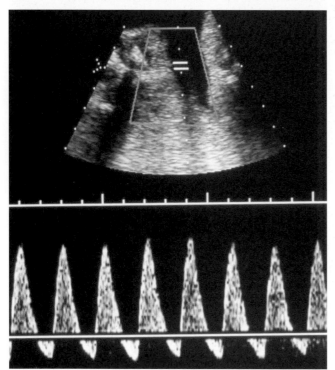

Fig. 35.2 Reversed end-diastolic velocity is noted in the umbilical circulation when downstream impedance is increased. These Doppler waveforms are associated with significant fetal compromise. From Abuhamad [92] with permission.

Fetal arterial Doppler

Umbilical circulation

The umbilical arterial circulation is normally a low impedance circulation, with an increase in the amount of end-diastolic flow with advancing gestation (Fig. 35.1) [66]. Umbilical arterial Doppler waveforms reflect the status of the placental circulation, and the increase in end-diastolic flow that is seen with advancing gestation is a direct result of an increase in the

number of tertiary stem villi with placental maturation [67]. Diseases that obliterate small muscular arteries in placental tertiary stem villi result in a progressive decrease in end-diastolic flow in the umbilical arterial Doppler waveforms until absent and then reverse flow during diastole is noted (Fig. 35.2) [68]. Reversed diastolic flow in the umbilical arterial circulation represents an advanced stage of placental compromise and is associated with obliteration of more than 70% of placental tertiary villi arteries [69,70]. The presence of absent or reversed end-diastolic flow in the umbilical artery is commonly associated with severe IUGR and oligohydramnios [71].

Doppler waveforms of the umbilical arteries can be obtained from any segment along the umbilical cord. Waveforms obtained from the placental end of the cord show more end-diastolic flow than waveforms obtained from the abdominal cord insertion [72]. Differences in Doppler indices of arterial waveforms obtained from different anatomic locations of the same umbilical cord are generally minor and have no significance in clinical practice [66].

Middle cerebral circulation

The cerebral circulation is normally a high impedance circulation with continuous forward flow throughout the cardiac cycle [73]. The middle cerebral artery is the most accessible cerebral vessel to ultrasound imaging in the fetus and it carries more than 80% of cerebral blood flow [74]. In the presence of fetal hypoxemia, central redistribution of blood flow occurs, resulting in an increased blood flow to the brain, heart and adrenals, and a reduction in flow to the peripheral and placental circulations. This blood flow redistribution is known as the brain-sparing reflex and has a major role in fetal adaptation to oxygen deprivation [73,75].

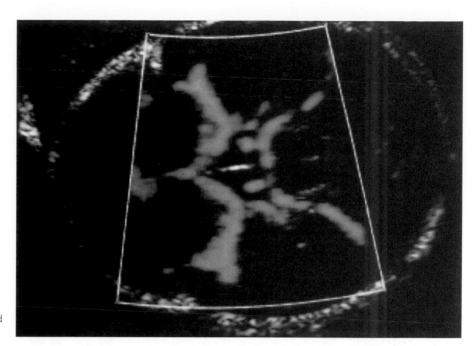

Fig. 35.3 Axial view of the fetal head in the second trimester with color Doppler showing the circulation at the level of the circle of Willis. Note the course of the middle cerebral arteries, almost parallel to the ultrasound beam. From Abuhamad [92] with permission.

The right and left middle cerebral arteries represent major branches of the circle of Willis in the fetal brain. The circle of Willis, which is supplied by the internal carotids and vertebral arteries, can be imaged with color flow Doppler ultrasound in a transverse plane of the fetal head obtained at the base of the skull. In this transverse plane, the proximal and distal middle cerebral arteries are seen in their longitudinal view, with their course almost parallel to the ultrasound beam (Fig. 35.3). Middle cerebral artery Doppler waveforms, obtained from the proximal portion of the vessel, immediately after its origin from the circle of Willis, have shown the best reproducibility [76].

Fetal growth restriction and arterial Doppler

Central redistribution of blood flow to the brain, known as the brain-sparing reflex, represents an early stage in fetal adaptation to hypoxemia [62–65], and follows the lag in fetal growth [77]. At this early stage, the brain-sparing reflex is clinically evident by increased end-diastolic flow in the middle cerebral artery (lower middle cerebral artery pulsatility or resistance index) and decreased end-diastolic flow in the umbilical artery (higher umbilical artery resistance index or S:D ratio). The cerebroplacental ratio, derived by dividing the cerebral resistance index by the umbilical resistance index, defines the brain-sparing reflex and has been shown to predict outcome in IUGR fetuses at less than 34 weeks' gestation [60,78–80].

In the presence of IUGR, Doppler changes in the umbilical artery precede the decrease in cerebroplacental ratio and middle cerebral artery pulsatility or resistance index [62,77]. However, middle cerebral artery Doppler waveforms are of clinical value in differentiating a growth restricted/hypoxemic fetus from a constitutionally small/normoxemic fetus. In the clinical setting of a constitutionally small fetus, the presence of normal middle cerebral artery Doppler waveforms, obtained at less than 32 weeks' gestation, have a 97% negative predictive value for major adverse perinatal outcomes [81].

Several studies have shown that this early stage of arterial redistribution is not associated with the presence of fetal metabolic acidemia [62–65]. It is therefore inferred that infants delivered at this early stage of fetal adaptation are expected to have no adverse long-term neurodevelopmental complications.

Fetal growth restriction and venous Doppler

Chronic fetal hypoxemia results in decreased preload, decreased cardiac compliance, and elevated end-diastolic pressure in the right ventricle [61,82–85]. These changes are evident by an elevated central venous pressure in the chronically hypoxemic fetus, which is manifested by an increased reverse flow in Doppler waveforms of the ductus venosus (Fig. 35.4a,b) and the inferior vena cava (Fig. 35.5a,b) during late diastole. Changes in the fetal central venous circulation are associated with an advanced stage of fetal hypoxemia. At this late stage of fetal adaptation to hypoxemia, cardiac decompensation is often noted with myocardial dysfunction [84]. Furthermore, fetal metabolic acidemia is often present in association with Doppler waveform abnormalities of the inferior vena cava and ductus venosus [57,61,62].

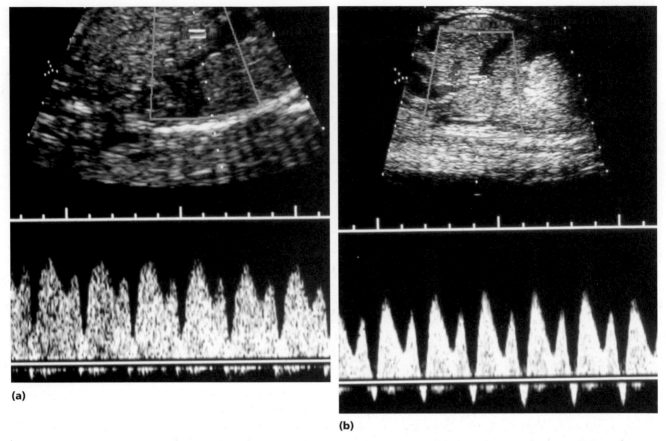

Fig. 35.4 Doppler velocity waveforms of the ductus venosus in a normal fetus (a) and a severely compromised fetus (b) in the third trimester of pregnancy. Note the presence of reverse flow during late diastole in the severely compromised fetus (b). Fig. 35.4b from Abuhamad [92] with permission.

Clinical application

In clinical practice, Doppler ultrasound provides important information on the extent of fetal compromise and thus may aid in the timing of delivery in IUGR fetuses. Arterial Doppler abnormalities, at the level of the umbilical and middle cerebral arteries (brain-sparing reflex), confirm the presence of hypoxemia in the growth restricted fetus, and present early warning signs. Once arterial centralization occurs, however, no clear trend is noted in the observational period and thus arterial redistribution may not be helpful for the timing of the delivery [86–88]. On the other hand, the presence of reversed diastolic flow in the umbilical arteries is a sign of advanced fetal compromise, and strong consideration should be given for delivery except in cases of extreme prematurity. Cesarean delivery following a course of corticosteroids, when appropriate, should be given preference in this setting as labor may cause further fetal compromise.

The current literature is suggestive that venous Doppler abnormalities in the inferior vena cava and ductus venosus and abnormal fetal heart rate monitoring follow arterial Doppler abnormalities and are thus associated with a more advanced stage of fetal compromise [62–65,89]. Furthermore, in the majority of severely growth-restricted fetuses, sequential deterioration of arterial and venous Doppler precedes biophysical profile score deterioration [63]. At least one-third of fetuses will show early signs of circulatory decompensation 1 week before biophysical profile deterioration and, in most cases, Doppler deterioration precedes deterioration of biophysical profile scores by 1 day [63].

The occurrence of such abnormal late stage changes of vascular adaptation by the IUGR fetus appears to be the best predictor of perinatal death, independent of gestational age and weight [65]. In a longitudinal study on Doppler and IUGR fetuses, all intrauterine deaths and all neonatal deaths, with the exception of one case, had late Doppler changes at the time of delivery, whereas only a few of the surviving fetuses showed such changes [65].

This sequential deterioration of the hypoxemic, growth restricted fetus is rarely seen at gestations beyond 34 weeks' [77,90]. Indeed, normal umbilical artery Doppler is common in growth restricted fetuses in late gestation and cerebroplacental ratios have poor correlation with outcome of IUGR

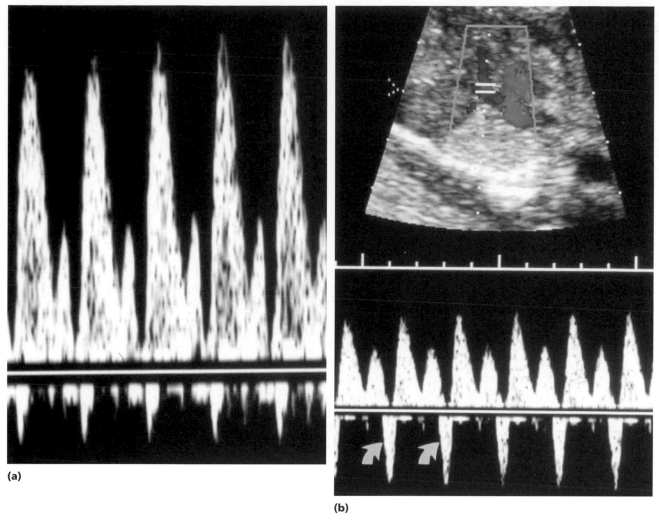

(a)

(b)

Fig. 35.5 Doppler velocity waveforms of the inferior vena cava (IVC) in a normal fetus (a) and a severely compromised fetus (b) in the third trimester of pregnancy. The IVC Doppler waveforms have reverse flow during late diastole (atrial kick) in the normal fetus. Note the increase in reverse flow during late diastole in the severely compromised fetus (b) (white arrowhead). Fig. 35.5(a) from Abuhamad [93] with permission; Fig. 35.5(b) from Abuhamad [92] with permission.

fetuses at more than 34 weeks' gestation [60]. Caution should therefore be exercised when umbilical artery Doppler is used in the clinical management of IUGR fetuses beyond 34 weeks' gestation.

The natural history and pathophysiology of fetal growth restriction have not been fully elucidated as recent studies have highlighted the presence of significant variation in fetal adaptation to hypoxemia. The pattern of incremental deterioration of arterial Doppler abnormalities, followed by venous Doppler abnormalities, then followed by fetal heart tracings and biophysical profile abnormalities is not seen by approximately 20% of preterm fetuses [62]. Furthermore, only 70% of IUGR fetuses showed significant deterioration of all vascular beds by the time they were delivered and approximately 10% showed no significant circulatory change by delivery time [63]. In a recent prospective observational study, more than

50% of IUGR fetuses delivered because of abnormal fetal heart rate tracings did not have venous Doppler abnormalities [65]. In view of these findings, the universal introduction of venous Doppler in the clinical management of the growth restricted fetus should await the results of randomized trials on this subject.

It is currently evident that fetal growth restriction is a complex disorder involving multiple fetal organs and systems [91]. While fetal biometry and arterial Doppler provide information on the early compensatory phase of this disorder, venous Doppler, fetal heart rate analysis, and the biophysical profile provide information on the later stages, commonly associated with fetal cardiovascular collapse. It is hoped that future studies will shed more light on the pathophysiology of this disease and on the various interactions of diagnostic tools in fetal surveillance.

Case presentation

The patient is a 40-year-old G3 P2002 with a pregnancy resulting from assisted reproduction with IVF. She presented to her obstetrician at 29 weeks' gestation for a routine prenatal visit. Prenatal care thus far had been uneventful except for abnormal quad screen with elevated maternal serum alpha-fetoprotein and human chorionic gonadotropin. Detailed ultrasound examination at 19 weeks showed normal fetal anatomy.

Fundal height measured 26 cm and the patient was referred for an obstetric ultrasound examination. The patient reported good fetal movements, and vital signs were within normal limits with no proteinuria. Ultrasound examination revealed the following:

- Cephalic presentation
- Normal amniotic fluid volume
- BPD and HC at the 26th percentile for gestational age
- AC at the 5th percentile for gestational age
- Estimated fetal weight at the 7th percentile for gestational age

When the biometric data were reported to the obstetrician, Doppler studies were ordered. Doppler studies revealed the following:

- Bilateral uterine artery notching (abnormal for gestational age)
- Umbilical artery S : D = 8.0 (abnormal for 29 weeks)
- Middle cerebral artery pulsatility index = 1.50 (abnormal for gestational age)
- Forward flow in the ductus venosus during the entire cardiac cycle (normal)

In view of the presence of IUGR with abnormal arterial Doppler waveforms, the patient was sent to Labor and Delivery where a course of steroids was initiated and a nonstress test (NST) showed reactive fetal heart rate. The patient was discharged home with the following instructions:

- Modified bed rest
- Home nurse visitation in 24 hours to complete the steroid course
- Twice weekly NSTs, including amniotic fluid assessment
- Weekly Doppler studies to include the umbilical artery, the middle cerebral artery, and the ductus venosus
- Follow-up fetal growth in 3 weeks

At 31 weeks' gestation, 3 weeks from diagnosis, absent end-diastolic velocity in the umbilical artery was noted. The patient was admitted to the hospital for daily testing, a second course of steroids, and twice weekly Doppler studies. Fetal biometry showed estimated fetal weight at the 4th percentile with decreased amniotic fluid volume. The patient reported normal fetal activity. Fetal surveillance studies on admission showed the following:

- Absent end-diastolic velocity with intermittent reversed end-diastolic velocity noted in the umbilical artery

- Middle cerebral artery pulsatility index = 1.35
- Absent flow in late diastole in the ductus venosus
- NST with normal reactivity

On the second day of hospitilization, the patient reported decreased fetal movements, NST showed spontaneous decelerations, and Doppler studies showed persistent reversed end-diastolic velocity in the umbilical artery with persistent reversed flow during late diastole (atrial kick) in the ductus venosus. Biophysical profile scored 4/8. The patient was delivered by cesarean of a male infant, weighing 1150 g with Apgar scores of 4 and 7 at 1 and 5 minutes, respectively. Arterial pH was 7.10 with base excess of –11. Both infant and mother did well with no major complications.

References

1 Chervenak FA, Skupski DW, Romero R, *et al*. How accurate is fetal biometry in the assessment of fetal age? *Am J Obstet Gynecol* 1998;**178**:228–37.

2 Goldenberg RL, Davis RO, Cutter GR, *et al*. Prematurity, postdates, and growth retardation: the influence of use of ultrasonography on reported gestational age. *Am J Obstet Gynecol* 1989;**160**:462–70.

3 Gardosi J, Vanner T, Francis A. Gestational age and induction of labour for prolonged pregnancy. *Br J Obstet Gynaecol* 1997;**104**: 792–7.

4 Warren WB, Peisner DB, Raju S, Rosen MG. Dating the early pregnancy by sequential appearance of embryonic structures. *Am J Obstet Gynecol* 1989;**161**:747.

5 Daya S. Accuracy of gestational age estimation by means of fetal crown-rump length measurement. *Am J Obstet Gynecol* 1987;**168**:903–8.

6 Nyberg DA, Mack LA, Laing FC, Patten RM. Distinguishing normal from abnormal gestational sac growth in early pregnancy. *J Ultrasound Med* 1987;**6**:23–7.

7 Robinson HP, Fleming JE. A critical evaluation of sonar "crown-rump length" measurement. *Br J Obstet Gynaecol* 1975;**82**:702–10.

8 Drumm JE, Clinch J, McKenzie G. The ultrasonic measurement of fetal crown rump length as a method of assessing gestational age. *Br J Obstet Gynaecol* 1976;**83**:417–21.

9 Daya S, Woods S, Ward S, Lappainen R, Caco C. Early pregnancy assessment with transvaginal ultrasound scanning. *Can Med Assoc J* 1991;**144**:441–6.

10 Lasser DM, Peisner DB, Wollenbergh J, Timor-Trisch I. First trimester fetal biometry using transvaginal sonography. *Ultrasound Obstet Gynecol* 1993;**3**:104–8.

11 McGregor SN, Tamura RK, Sabbagha RE, Minogue JP, Gibson ME, Hoffman DI. Underestimation of gestational age by conventional crown rump length dating curves. *Am J Obstet Gynecol* 1987;**70**:344–8.

12 Wisser J, Dirscheld P. Estimation of gestational age by transvaginal sonographic measurement of greatest embryonic length in dated human embryos. *Ultrasound Obstet Gynecol* 1994;**4**:457–62.

13 Hadlock FP. Sonographic estimation of fetal age and weight. *Radiol Clin North Am* 1990;**28**:39–50.

14 Kurjak A, Kirkinen P, Latin V. Biometric and dynamic ultrasound assessment of small-for-dates infants: report of 260 cases. *Obstet Gynecol* 1980;**56**:281–4.

15 Landon MB, Mintz MC, Gabbe SG. Sonographic evaluation of fetal abdominal growth: predictor of the large for gestational age infant in pregnancies complicated by diabetes mellitus. *Am J Obstet Gynecol* 1989;**160**:115–21.

16 Basel D, Lederer R, Diamant YZ. Longitudinal ultrasonic biometry of various parameters in fetuses with abnormal growth rate. *Acta Obstet Gynecol Scand* 1987;**66**:143–9.

17 Hadlock FP. Ultrasound evaluation of fetal growth. In: Callen PW, ed. *Ultrasonography in Obstetrics and Gynecology*. Philadelphia: WB Saunders, 1994: 129–43.

18 Dudley NJ. Selection of appropriate ultrasound methods for estimation of fetal weight. *Br J Radiol* 1995;**68**:385–8.

19 Coombs CA, Jaekle RK, Rosenn B, Pope M, Miodovnik M, Siddiqi TA. Sonographic estimation of fetal weight based on a model of fetal volume. *Obstet Gynecol* 1993;**82**:365–70.

20 Hadlock FP, Harrist RB, Carpenter RJ, Deter RL, Park SK. Sonographic estimation of fetal weight. *Radiology* 1984;**150**:535–40.

21 Smith GCS, Smith MFS, McNay MB, Flemming JEE. The relation between fetal abdominal circumference and birthweight: findings in 3512 pregnancies. *Br J Obstet Gynaecol* 1997;**104**: 186–90.

22 Gore D, Williams M, O'Brien W, Gilby J. Fetal abdominal circumference for prediction of intrauterine growth restriction. *Obstet Gynecol* 2000;**95**(Suppl 1):S78–9.

23 Rose BI, McCallum WD. A simplified method for estimating fetal weight using ultrasound measurements. *Obstet Gynecol* 1987;**69**:671–5.

24 Medchill MT, Peterson CM, Garbaciak J. Prediction of estimated fetal weight in extremely low birth weight neonates (500–1000 g). *Obstet Gynecol* 1991;**78**:286–90.

25 Robson SC, Gallivan S, Walkinshaw SA, Vaughan J, Rodeck CH. Ultrasonic estimation of fetal weight: use of targeted formulas in small for gestational age fetuses. *Obstet Gynecol* 1993;**82**:359–64.

26 Sabbagha RE, Minogue J, Tamura RK, Hungerford SA. Estimation of birth weight by use of ultrasonographic formulas targeted to large-, appropriate-, and small-for-gestational-age fetuses. *Am J Obstet Gynecol* 1989;**160**:854–62.

27 Edwards A, Goff J, Baker L. Accuracy and modifying factors of the sonographic estimation of fetal weight 26: *Aust N Z J Obstet Gynaecol* 2001;**41**:187–90.

28 Baum JD, Gussman D, Wirth JC 3rd. Clinical and patient estimation of fetal weight vs. ultrasound estimation. *J Reprod Med* 2002;**47**:194–8.

29 Divon M, Chamberlain P, Sipos L, Manning F, Platt L. Identification of the small for gestational age independent indices of fetal growth. *Am J Obstet Gynecol* 1986;**155**:1197–2003.

30 Owen P, Maharaj S, Khan KS, Howie PW. Interval between fetal measurements in predicting growth restriction. *Obstet Gynecol* 2001;**97**:499–504.

31 Ott WJ. The diagnosis of altered fetal growth. *Obstet Gynecol Clin North Am* 1988;**15**; 237–63.

32 Manning FA. Intrauterine growth restriction. Diagnosis, prognostication, and management based on ultrasound methods. In: Manning FA, ed. *Fetal Medicine: Principles and Practice*. Norwalk, CT: Appleton & Lange; 1995.

33 Hadlock FP, Deter RL, Harrist RB, Roecker E, Park SK. A date-independent predictor of intrauterine growth retardation: femur length/abdominal circumference ration. *Am J Roentgenol* 1993;**141**:979–84.

34 Brown HL, Miller JM Jr, Gabert HA, Kissling G. Ultrasonic recognition of the small-for-gestational-age fetus. *Obstet Gynecol* 1987;**69**:631–5.

35 Creasy RK, Resnick R. Intrauterine growth retardation. In: Creasy RK, Resnick R, eds. *Maternal Fetal Medicine: Principles and Practice*. Philadelphia: Saunders; 1984: 491ff.

36 David C, Gabrielli S, Pilu G, Bovicelli L. The head-to-abdomen circumference ratio: a reappraisal. *Ultrasound Obstet Gynecol* 1995;**5**:256–9.

37 Dashe JS, McIntire DD, Lucas MJ, Leveno KJ. Effects of symmetric and asymmetric fetal growth on pregnancy outcomes. *Obstet Gynecol* 2000;**96**:321–7.

38 Vik T, Vatten L, Jacobsen G, Bakketeig LS. Prenatal growth in symmetric and asymmetric small-for-gestational-age infants. *Early Hum Dev* 1997;**48**:167–76.

39 Blackwell SC, Moldenhauer J, Redman M, Hassan SS, Wolfe HM, Berry SM. Relationship between the sonographic pattern of intrauterine growth restriction and acid–base status at the time of cordocentensis. *Arch Gynecol Obstet* 2001;**264**:191–3.

40 Benson CB, Doubilet PM, Saltzman DH, Jones TB. FL/AC ratio: poor predictor of intrauterine growth retardation. *Invest Radiol* 1985;**20**:727–30.

41 Rasmussen S, Irgens LM, Albrechtsen S, Dalaker K. Predicting preeclampsia in the second pregnancy from low birth weight in the first pregnancy. *Obstet Gynecol* 2000;**96**:696–700.

42 Stipoljev F, Latin V, Kos M, Miskovic B, Kurjak A. Correlation of confined placental mosaicism with fetal intrauterine growth retardation: a case–control study of placentas at delivery. *Fetal Diagn Ther* 2001;**16**:4–9.

43 Mitra SC, Seshan SV, Riachi LE. Placental vessel morphometry in growth retardation and increased resistance of the umbilical artery Doppler flow. *J Matern Fetal Med* 2000;**9**:282–6.

44 Devriendt K. Genetic control of intra-uterine growth. *Eur J Obstet Gynecol Reprod Biol* 2000;**92**:29–34.

45 Snijders RJ, Sherrod C, Gosden CM, Nicolaides KH. Fetal growth retardation: associated malformations and chromosomal abnormalities. *Am J Obstet Gynecol* 1993;**168**:547–55.

46 Dicke JM, Crane JP. Sonographic recognition of major malformations and aberrant fetal growth in trisomic fetuses. *J Ultrasound Med* 1991;**10**:433–8.

47 Magnus P, Bakketeig LS, Hoffman H. Birth weight of relatives by maternal tendency to repeat small-for-gestational-age (SGA) births in successive pregnancies. *Acta Obstet Gynecol Scand Suppl* 1997;**165**:35–8.

48 Bernstein IM, Horbar JD, Badger GJ, Ohlsson A, Golan A. Morbidity and mortality among very-low-birth weight neonates with intrauterine growth restriction. *Am J Obstet Gynecol* 2000;**182**:198–202.

49 Kok JH, den Ouden AL, Verloove-Vanhorick SP, Brand R. Outcome of very preterm small for gestational age infants: the first nine years of life. *Br J Obstet Gynecol* 1998;**105**:162–8.

50 Fattal-Valevski A, Leitner Y, Kutai M, *et al*. Neurodevelopmental outcome in children with intrauterine growth retardation: a 3-year follow-up [Abstract]. *J Child Neurol* 1999;**14**:724–7.

51 Soothill PW, Ajayi RA, Campbell S, *et al*. Relationship between fetal academia at cordocentesis and subsequent neurodevelopment. *Ultrasound Obstet Gynecol* 1992;**2**:80–3.

52 Hanna BD, Nelson MN, White-Traut RC, *et al*. Heart rate variability in preterm brain-injured and very-low-birth-weight infants. *Biol Neonate* 2000;**77**:147–55.

53 Nijhuis IJ, ten Hof J, Mulder EJ, *et al*. Fetal heart rate in relation to its variation in normal and growth retarded fetuses. *Eur J Obstet Gynecol Reprod Biol* 2000;**89**:27–33.

54 Vindla S, James D, Sahota D. Computerised analysis of unstimulated and stimulated behaviour in fetuses with intrauterine growth restriction. *Eur J Obstet Gynecol Reprod Biol* 199;**83**:37–45.

55 Devoe L, Golde S, Kilman Y, Morton D, Shea K, Waller J. A comparison of visual analyses of intrapartum fetal heart rate tracings according to the new National Institute of Child Health and Human Development guidelines with computer analyses by an automated fetal heart rate monitoring system. *Am J Obstet Gynecol* 2000;**183**;361–6.

56 Bracero LA, Roshanfekr D, Byrne DW. Analysis of antepartum fetal heart rate tracing by physician and computer. *J Matern Fetal Med* 2000;**9**:181–5.

57 Hecher K, HackelÖer B. Cardiotocogram compared to Doppler investigation of the fetal circulation in the premature growth-retarded fetus: longitudinal observations. *Ultrasound Obstet Gynecol* 1997;**9**:152–60.

58 Ribbert LS, Visser GH, Mulder EJ, Zonneveld MF, Morssink LP. Changes with time in fetal heart rate variation, movement incidences and haemodynamics in intrauterine growth retarded fetuses: a longitudinal approach to the assessment of fetal well being. *Early Hum Dev* 1993;**31**:195–208.

59 Zarko A, Neilson JP. Doppler ultrasonography in high-risk pregnancies: systematic review with meta-analysis. *Am J Obstet Gynecol* 1995;**172**:1379–87.

60 Bahado-Singh RO, Kovanci E, Jeffres A, *et al*. The Doppler cerebroplacental ratio and perinatal outcome in intrauterine growth restriction. *Am J Obstet Gynecol* 1999;**180**: 750–6.

61 Rizzo G, Capponi A, Talone PE, Arduini D, Romanini C. Doppler indices from inferior vena cava and ductus venosus in predicting pH and oxygen tension in umbilical blood at cordocentesis in growth-retarded fetuses. *Ultrasound Obstet Gynecol* 1996;**7**:401–10.

62 Baschat AA, Gembruch U, Reiss I, Gortner L, Weiner CP, Harman CR. Relationship between arterial and venous Doppler and perinatal outcome in fetal growth restriction. *Ultrasound Obstet Gynecol* 2000;**16**:407–13.

63 Baschat AA, Gembruch U, Harman CR. The sequence of changes in Doppler and biophysical parameters as severe fetal growth restriction worsens. *Ultrasound Obstet Gynecol* 2001;**18**: 571–7.

64 Hecher K, Bilardo CM, Stigter RH, *et al*. Monitoring of fetuses with intrauterine growth restriction: a longitudinal study. *Ultrasound Obstet Gynecol* 2001;**18**:564–70.

65 Ferrazzi E, Bozzo M, Rigano S, *et al*. Temporal sequence of abnormal Doppler changes in the peripheral and central circulatory systems of the severely growth-restricted fetus. *Ultrasound Obstet Gynecol* 2002;**19**:140–6.

66 Fleischer A, Schulman H, Farmakides G, Bracero L, Blattner P, Randolph G. Umbilical artery waveforms and intrauterine growth retardation. *Am J Obstet Gynecol* 1985;**151**:502–5.

67 Giles WB, Trudinger BJ, Baird PJ. Fetal umbilical artery flow velocity waveforms and placental resistance: pathological correlation. *Br J Obstet Gynecol* 1987;**157**:900–2.

68 Trudinger BJ, Stevens D, Connelly A, *et al*. Umbilical artery flow velocity waveforms and placental resistance: the effect of embolizations of the umbilical circulation. *Am J Obstet Gynecol* 1987;**157**:1443–8.

69 Kingdom JC, Burrell SJ, Kaufmann P. Pathology and clinical implications of abnormal umbilical artery Doppler waveforms. *Ultrasound Obstet Gynecol* 1997;**9**:271–86.

70 Morrow RJ, Adamson SL, Bull SB, Ritchie JW. Effect of placental embolization on the umbilical arterial velocity waveform in fetal sheep. *Am J Obstet Gynecol* 1989;**161**:1055–60.

71 Copel JA, Reed KL. *Doppler Ultrasound in Obstetrics and Gynecology*, 1st edn. New York, New York: Raven Press, 1995: 187–98.

72 Trudinger BJ. Doppler ultrasonography and fetal well being. In: Reece EA, Hobbins JC, Mahoney M, Petrie RH, eds. *Medicine of the Fetus and Mother*. Philadelphia: JB Lippincott, 1992.

73 Mari G, Deter RL. Middle cerebral artery flow velocity waveforms in normal and small-for-gestational age fetuses. *Am J Obstet Gynecol* 1992;**166**:1262–70.

74 Veille JC, Hanson R, Tatum K. Longitudinal quantitation of middle cerebral artery blood flow in normal human fetuses. *Am J Obstet Gynecol* 1993;**169**:1393–8.

75 Berman RE, Less MH, Peterson EN, Delannoy CW. Distribution of the circulation in the normal and asphyxiated fetal primate. *Am J Obstet Gynecol* 1970;**108**:956–69.

76 Mari G, Abuhamad AZ, Brumfield J, Ferguson JE III. Doppler ultrasonography of the middle cerebral artery peak systolic velocity in the fetus: reproducibility of measurement. *Am J Obstet Gynecol* 2001;**185**:Abstract 669.

77 Harrington K, Thompson MO, Carpenter RG, *et al*. Doppler fetal circulation in pregnancies complicated by pre-eclampsia or delivery of a small for gestational age baby: 2. Longitudinal analysis. *Br J Obstet Gynaecol* 1999;**106**:453–66.

78 Wladimoroff JW, van den Wijingaard JAGN, Degani S, Noordam MJ, van Eyck J, Tonge HM. Cerebral and umbilical arterial blood flow velocity waveforms in normal and growth retarded pregnancies: a comparative study. *Obstet Gynecol* 1987;**69**:705–9.

79 Gramellini D, Folli MC, Raboni S, Vadora E, Marialdi A. Cerebral–umbilical Doppler ratio as a predictor of adverse perinatal outcome. *Obstet Gynecol* 1992;**74**:416–20.

80 Arduini D, Rizzo G. Prediction of fetal outcome in small for gestational age fetuses: comparison of Doppler measurements obtained from different fetal vessels. *J Perinat Med* 1992;**20**:29–38.

81 Fong KW, Ohlsson A, Hannah ME, *et al*. Prediction of perinatal outcomes in fetuses suspected to have intrauterine growth restriction: Doppler US study of fetal cerebral, renal and umbilical arteries. *Radiology* 1999;**213**:681–9.

82 Rizzo G, Arduini D. Fetal cardiac function in intrauterine growth retardation. *Am J Obstet Gynecol* 1991;**165**:876–82.

83 Chang CH, Chang FM, Yu CH, Liang RI, Ko HC, Chen HY. Systemic assessment of fetal hemodynamics by Doppler ultrasound. *Ultrasound Med Biol* 2000;**26**:777–85.

84 Mäkikallio K, Vuolteenaho O, Jouppila P, Räsänen J. Ultrasonographic and biochemical markers of human fetal cardiac dysfunction in placental insufficiency. *Circulation* 2002;**105**:2058–62.

85 Tsyvian P, Malkin K, Wladimiroff JY. Assessment of mitral a-wave transit time to cardiac outflow tract and isovolumic relaxation time of left ventricle in the appropriate and small-for-gestational-age human fetus. *Ultrasound in Med Biol* 1997;**23**:187–90.

86 Baschat AA, Gembruch U, Gortner L, *et al*. Coronary artery blood flow visualization signifies hemodynamic deterioration in growth restricted fetuses. *Ultrasound Obstet Gynecol* 2000;**16**:425–31.

87 Senat MV, Schwarzler P, Alcais A, *et al*. Longitudinal changes in the ductus venosus, cerebral transverse sinus and cardiotocogram in fetal growth restriction. *Ultrasound Obstet Gynecol* 2000;**16**:19–24.

88 Baschat AA, Gembruch U, Weiner CP, *et al*. Longitudinal changes of arterial and venous Doppler in fetuses with intrauterine growth restriction [Abstract]. *Am J Obstet Gynecol* 2001;**184**:103.

89 Pardi G, Cetin I, Marconi AM, *et al*. Diagnostic value of blood sampling in fetuses with growth retardation. *N Engl J Med* 1993;**328**:692–6.

90 Hecher K, Campbell S, Doyle P, Harrington K, Nicolaides K. Assessment of fetal compromise by Doppler ultrasound investigation of the fetal circulation. Arterial, intracardiac, and venous blood flow velocity studies. *Circulation* 1995;**91**:129–38.

91 Romero R, Kalache KD, Kadar N. Timing the delivery of the preterm severely growth-restricted fetus: venous Doppler, cardiotocography or the biophysical profile? *Ultrasound Obstet Gynecol* 2002;**19**:118–21.

92 Abuhamad A. Uterine size less than dates: a clinical dilemma. In: Bluth EI, Benson CB, Ralls PW, Siegel MJ. *Ultrasound: Practical Approach to Clinical Problems*, 2nd edn. New York: Thieme Medical Publishing, 2006: 56–60.

93 Abuhamad A. Doppler ultrasound in obstetrics. *Ultrasound Clinics* 2006;**6**:293–301.

36 Rh and other blood group alloimmunizations

Kenneth J. Moise, Jr.

The time-honored concept that the placenta is relatively impervious to cell trafficking between the fetus and its mother is no longer accepted. Flow cytometry can detect fetal red cell and red cell precursors in the maternal circulation in virtually all pregnancies [1,2].

In some patients, this exposure to fetal red cell antigens produces an antibody response that can be harmful to future offspring. The process is known as red cell alloimmunization (formerly isoimmunization). Active transplacental transport of these antibodies leads to their attachment to fetal red cells and sequestration in the fetal spleen. The quantity of the maternal antibody (see below), the subclass of immunoglobulin G (IgG), and even the response of the fetal reticuloendothelial system have roles in the development of fetal anemia—a disease state known as hemolytic disease of the fetus and newborn (HDFN). In extreme cases, this severe anemia is associated with the accumulation of extracellular fluid in the form of ascites, pleural effusions, and scalp edema, a condition termed hydrops fetalis.

Prophylaxis

Prevention of maternal alloimmunization is almost uniformly successful in the case of exposure to the RhD or "Rhesus" antigen. Prophylactic immunoglobulin (Rhesus immunoglobulin; RhIg) is now available in the USA in the form of four commercial preparations—two can only be administered intramuscularly while two can be given either intramuscularly or intravenously. RhIg is not effective once the patient has developed endogenous antibodies. Immunoglobulins to prevent sensitization to other red cell antigens are not available.

All pregnant patients should undergo an antibody screen to red cell antigens at the first prenatal visit. In the case of a negative screen in the RhD-negative patient, further testing is unnecessary until 28 weeks' gestation. Unless the patient's partner is documented to be RhD negative, a 300-μg dose of RhIg should be administered. A repeat antibody screen at 28 weeks is recommended by the American Association of Blood Banks, although the American College of Obstetricians and Gynecologists has left this to the discretion of the clinician [3]. Although this has not been studied for cost-effectiveness, a repeat screen will detect the rare patient who becomes RhD sensitized early in pregnancy. If a repeat screen is obtained, the intramuscular RhIg injection can be administered before the patient is sent for venipuncture. The short time interval between procedures will not affect the results of the antibody screen.

At delivery, a cord blood sample should be tested for neonatal RhD typing. If the neonate is determined to be RhD positive, a second dose of 300 μg RhIg should be administered to the mother within 72 hours of delivery. Approximately 0.1% of deliveries will be associated with a fetomaternal hemorrhage (FMH) in excess of 30 mL. More than the standard dose of RhIg will be required in these cases. Because risk factor assessment will only identify 50% of patients who have an excessive FMH at delivery, the routine screening of all postpartum women is now recommended. Typically, this involves a sheep rosette test which is read qualitatively as positive or negative. If negative, one vial of RhIg (300 μg) is given. If positive, the bleed is quantitated with a Kleihauer–Betke stain or fetal cell stain by flow cytometry. Blood bank consultation should then be undertaken to determine the number of doses of RhIg to administer. The mechanism by which RhIg prevents sensitization is not well understood. Biochemical studies have revealed that the standard dose is insufficient to block all of the antigenic sites on the fetal red cells in the maternal circulation [4]. Therefore, if RhIg is inadvertently omitted after delivery, some protection has been proven with administration within 13 days. It should not be withheld as late as 28 days after delivery if the need arises [5].

Additional indications for RhIg are listed in Table 36.1. Although a 50-μg dose of RhIg has been recommended for clinical situations up to 13 weeks' gestation, most hospitals no longer stock this preparation and the cost is comparable to the standard 300-μg dose.

Table 36.1 Indications for administration of Rhesus immunoglobulin. Reproduced with permission from Moise KJ. Red cell alloimmunization. In: Gabbe, Niebyl, Simpson, *et al.* (eds) *Obstetrics: Normal and Abnormal Pregnancies*, 5th edn. Philadelphia, PA: Elsevier, Saunders, (in press).

	Level of Evidence
Spontaneous abortion	A
Elective abortion	A
Threatened abortion	
Ectopic pregnancy	A
Hydatidiform mole	B
Genetic amniocentesis	A
Chorion villus biopsy	A
Fetal blood sampling	A
Placenta previa with bleeding	C
Suspected abruption	C
Intrauterine fetal demise	C
Blunt trauma to the abdomen (includes motor vehicle accidents)	C
At 28 weeks' gestation, unless father of fetus is RhD negative	A
Amniocentesis for fetal lung maturity	A
External cephalic version	C
Within 72 hours of delivery of an RhD-positive infant	A
After administration of RhD-positive blood components	C

Level A evidence (good and consistent scientific evidence) [3].
Level C evidence (consensus and expert opinion) [3].

Methods of surveillance

In recent years, techniques for fetal surveillance in cases of RhD alloimmunization have evolved to a more noninvasive approach. Many of these have led to a reduction in the rate of enhanced maternal immunization as a result of invasive procedures as well as a reduction in the rate of perinatal loss. Consultation with a maternal-fetal specialist should be considered in these cases in an effort to offer the patient the latest advancements in the field.

Antibody titer

In the first affected pregnancy, the maternal antibody titer continues to be used as the first level of surveillance in the USA. Once the maternal antibody screen indicates the presence of an anti-D antibody, a titer should be ordered. A critical titer has been defined as the value for a particular institution that is associated with a risk for fetal hydrops. An anti-D titer of 32 in the first affected pregnancy is often used. However, one must be cautious in the interpretation of antibody titers as they are crude estimates of the amount of circulating antibody. Today titers are performed much the same as they have been

for several decades. Preserved human red cells are used as the indicator for the measurement of a biologic endpoint. These cells have a shelf life of 4 weeks, leading to the likely situation that subsequent titers will be performed using a different batch of indicator cells. In addition, large differences in titer can be seen between laboratories in the same patient, as many commercial facilities use such techniques as enzymatic treatment of the indicator red cells to overestimate the actual value of the titer. Additionally, newer gel technology will often produce titer results that are two or more dilutions higher than expected with older tube technology [6].

Ultrasound

Ultrasound has revolutionized the surveillance of the anemic fetus. An early study is indicated in an affected pregnancy to determine the gestational age accurately. In the past, ultrasound was used to detect fetal hydrops. Unfortunately, this represents an end-stage phase of HDFN with more than two-thirds reduction in the fetal hemoglobin below the norm [7]. The most significant breakthrough in the surveillance of the potentially anemic fetus has been the validation of the peak systolic middle cerebral artery (MCA) Doppler velocity. For many years, alloimmunized women were subjected to repetitive amniocenteses to measure the amount of bilirubin in the amniotic fluid—a surrogate test for the degree of ongoing fetal hemolysis. The test was often referred to as the ΔOD_{450} as it measured the change in optical density at 450 nm for the bilirubin peak using spectrophotometry. Results were plotted on various longitudinal curves named after their authors—the Liley and Queenan curves [8,9]. Recent studies have verified the MCA Doppler to be more sensitive for predicting fetal anemia than the ΔOD_{450} [10]. The MCA can be easily visualized with color flow Doppler. Pulsed Doppler is then used to measure the peak systolic velocity of the MCA just distal to its bifurcation from the internal carotid artery. Enhanced fetal cardiac output and a decrease in blood viscosity contribute to an increased blood flow velocity in fetal anemia. Because the general trend is for the MCA velocity to increase with advancing gestational age, results are reported in multiples of the median (MoM), much like serum alpha fetoprotein. The actual value can be plotted on standard curves (Table 36.2) or entered into a website that will calculate the MoM value (www.perinatology.com). A value greater than 1.5 MoM is suggestive of moderate to severe fetal anemia and requires further investigation through direct ultrasound-guided fetal blood sampling (cordocentesis) [11]. MCA Dopplers can be initiated as early as 18 weeks' gestation and should be repeated every 1–2 weeks as the clinical situation warrants. After 35 weeks' gestation, the false positive rate for the prediction of fetal anemia is increased probably as a result of fetal heart rate accelerations [12]. The advantage of serial MCA measurements is a reduction of over 80% in the

Table 36.2 Peak systolic middle cerebral artery values [11].

Weeks of Gestation	1.29 MoM (mild anemia) (cm/s)	1.50 MoM (moderate–severe anemia) (cm/s)
18	29.9	34.8
20	32.8	38.2
22	36.0	41.9
24	39.5	46.0
26	43.3	50.4
28	47.6	55.4
30	52.2	60.7
32	57.3	66.6
34	62.9	73.1
36	69.0	80.2
38	75.7	88.0
40	83.0	96.6

MoM, multiples of the mean.

need for invasive diagnostic procedures such as amniocentesis and cordocentesis.

Fetal blood typing through DNA analysis

Paternal testing should begin early in the evaluation process of the alloimmunized patient. An RhD-negative result with assurance of paternity requires no further maternal testing after proper documentation of the paternity discussion with the patient in the medical record. Because more than 50% of RhD-positive partners are heterozygous, testing in consultation with the blood bank should be employed to determine the paternal zygosity. This is undertaken by serologic testing for the other paternal Rh antigens (C, c, E, e) and the use of race-specific population tables. Results are reported as a percent chance for an individual to be heterozygous. In the case of a heterozygous paternal phenotype, amniocentesis can be undertaken at 15–17 weeks to obtain fetal DNA from the amniotic fluid to determine the fetal RhD type. Such testing is also available for the majority of the other red cell antigens associated with HDFN. Both paternal and maternal blood samples should be sent to the reference laboratory with the amniotic fluid aliquot in order to exclude gene rearrangements that may invalidate the fetal DNA result. If the patient's partner is not available or if there is a question regarding paternity, paired maternal titers can be tested 8–10 weeks apart. If there is an increase in titer of more than fourfold (i.e., 4–32), an RhD-negative fetal genotype by previous amniocentesis may be erroneous.

An exciting new development in fetal RhD typing involves the isolation of free fetal DNA in maternal serum [13]. In the UK, this technique has virtually replaced amniocentesis for fetal RhD determination in the case of a heterozygous paternal phenotype. It should be available for clinical use in the USA in the near future.

Overall clinical management

First sensitized pregnancy

- Follow maternal titers every 4 weeks up to 20 weeks' gestation; repeat every 2 weeks thereafter.
- Once a critical value (usually 32) is reached in cases of a heterozygous paternal phenotype, perform amniocentesis at 15–17 weeks to determine the fetal RhD status. Send maternal and paternal blood samples (usually in an EDTA tube) with the amniotic fluid.
- If an RhD-negative fetus is found, no further testing is warranted.
- If a homozygous paternal phenotype or RhD-positive fetus by DNA analysis, begin serial MCA Dopplers as early as 24 weeks' gestation. Repeat weekly 3 times and assess trend. If not rising rapidly, consider MCAs every 2 weeks.
- If the MCA Doppler is >1.5 MoM, perform cordocentesis with blood readied for intrauterine transfusion (IUT) for a fetal hematocrit of <30%.
- If repeat MCA velocities remain <1.5 MoM, consider induction by 38 weeks' gestation.
- In the case of an elevated MCA after 35 weeks' gestation, consider repeating the study the following day. If the value remains elevated, perform amniocentesis for fetal lung maturity and ΔOD_{450}. If immature and the ΔOD_{450} value is not in the upper zone 2 of the Liley curve, consider repeat amniocentesis 1 week later to confirm maturity.
- Induce by 38 weeks' gestation.

Previous severely affected fetus or infant
(previous child requiring intrauterine or neonatal transfusion)

- Maternal titers are *not* helpful in predicting the onset of fetal anemia after the first affected gestation.
- In cases of a heterozygous paternal phenotype, perform amniocentesis at 15 weeks' gestation to determine the fetal RhD status. If an RhD-negative fetus is found, no further testing is warranted.
- Begin MCA Doppler assessments at 18 weeks' gestation. Repeat every week.
- When an MCA Doppler >1.5 MoM is noted, perform cordocentesis with blood readied for IUT for fetal hematocrit of <30%.
- If the MCA Doppler value does not become elevated, follow the same protocol after 35 weeks as for the first affected pregnancy (see above).

Intrauterine transfusion

First introduced in 1963 by Sir William Liley, IUT has withstood the test of time as the most successful fetal therapy [14]. Initially the peritoneal cavity was used as the site of transfusion; however, hydropic fetuses were found to exhibit poor absorption of transfused red cells. Today the direct intravascular transfusion (IVT) of donor red cells into the fetal umbilical vein at its placental insertion is the most common method of IUT. Variations in the standard IVT approach include the inclusion of additional transfused cells into the peritoneal cavity at the same setting to prolong the interval between procedures [15]. Additionally, the intrahepatic portion of the umbilical vein is used as the access site for IVT in many centers in Europe [16].

Limited visualization of the umbilical cord insertion precludes successful IVT prior to 18 weeks' gestation. Most centers will not perform an IUT after 35 weeks. After the first IVT, the second procedure is usually planned 7–10 days later with an expected decrement in the fetal hematocrit of approximately 1% per day. Subsequent procedures are repeated at 2–3 week intervals based on fetal response and suppression of fetal erythropoiesis.

After the last procedure, the patient is scheduled for induction of labor at 38–39 weeks' gestation to allow for fetal liver maturity. The addition of oral maternal phenobarbital may further enhance the ability of the fetal liver to conjugate bilirubin, thereby preventing the need for neonatal exchange transfusions [17]. Currently, the typical neonatal course for the fetus treated successfully with serial IUTs includes minimal need for phototherapy and discharge to home with the mother at the end of a routine postpartum stay. Breastfeeding is not contraindicated.

Outcome

In experienced centers, the overall perinatal survival with IUT is 85–90% [18]. Hydropic fetuses fare more poorly, with a 15% decrease in survival over their nonhydropic counterparts [19]. Suppression of fetal erythropoiesis because of serial IUTs can be associated with profound anemia in the first few months of life. Weekly neonatal hematocrit and reticulocyte counts should be followed until there is evidence of renewed production of red cells. Top-up red cell transfusions may be required in as many as 50% of cases [20].

Neurodevelopmental follow-up studies of neonates transfused by IVT are limited in number. Most point to over a 90% chance of intact survival [21]. Hydrops fetalis does not seem to impact this outcome. Sensineural hearing loss may be slightly increased as a result of prolonged exposure of the fetus to high levels of bilirubin. A hearing screen should be performed during the early neonatal course and repeated by 2 years of life.

HDFN caused by non-RhD antibodies

Antibodies to the red cell antigens Lewis, I, and P are often encountered through antibody screening during prenatal care. Because these antibodies are typically of the IgM class, they are not associated with HDFN [22].

Antibodies to more than 50 other red cell antigens have been reported to be associated with HDFN (Table 36.3). However,

Table 36.3 Non-RhD antibodies and associated hemolytic disease of the fetus and newborn (HDFN). Reproduced with permission from Moise KJ. Hemolytic disease of the fetus and newborn. In: Creasy RK, Resnik R, Iams J, (eds). *Maternal-Fetal Medicine*, 5th edition. Philadelphia, PA: W.B. Saunders. 2004.

Antigen System	Specific Antigen	Antigen System	Specific Antigen	Antigen System	Specific Antigen
Frequently associated with severe disease					
Kell	K (K1)				
Rhesus	c				
Infrequently associated with severe disease					
Colton	Co^a	MNS	Mur	Scianna	Sc2
	Co3		M^V		Rd
Diego	ELO		s	Other Ag	Bi
	Di^a		s^D		Good
	Di^b		S		Heibel
	Wr^a		U		HJK
	Wr^b		Vw		Ht^a
Duffy	Fy^a	Rhesus	Be^a		Jones
Kell	Js^b		C		Joslin
	k (K2)		Ce		Kg
	Kp^a		C^w		Kuhn
	Kp^b		ce		Li^a
	K11		E		MAM
	K22		E^w		Niemetz
	Ku		Evans		REIT
	Ul^a		G		Reiter
Kidd	Jk^a		Go^a		Rd
MNS	En^a		Hr		Sharp
	Far		Hr$_o$		Vel
	Hil		JAL		Zd
	Hut		Rh32		
	M		Rh42		
	Mi^a		Rh46		
	Mt^a		STEM		
	MUT		Tar		
Associated with mild disease					
Duffy	Fy^b	Kidd	Jk^b	Rhesus	Riv
	Fy3		Jk3		RH29
Gerbich	Ge2	MNS	Mit	Other	At^a
	Ge3	Rhesus	C^X		JFV
	Ge4		D^w		Jr^a
	Ls^a		e		Lan
Kell	Js^a		HOFM		
			LOCR		

only three of these antibodies cause significant hemolytic disease where treatment with IUT is necessary: anti-RhD, anti-Rhc, and anti-Kell (K1). Most centers use a maternal titer of 32 in cases of non-RhD antibodies to initiate fetal surveillance. Because the Kell antibody affects the fetus both at the level of the bone marrow to suppress erythropoiesis as well as causing the destruction of circulating red cells, a critical titer of 8 is used in the case of Kell antibodies [23].

Case presentation 1

Surveillance of the first affected gestation

A 30-year-old G2 P1001 was noted to have a positive antibody screen for anti-D at her first prenatal visit at 8 weeks' gestation. The patient had not received Rh immunoglobulin after her previous delivery in Mexico 3 years earlier. Her titer was 32 for anti-D. Paternal testing revealed a *CcDe* phenotype consistent with an 85% chance of a heterozygous state. The patient was scheduled for amniocentesis at 16 weeks' gestation. Maternal and paternal blood samples were drawn and forwarded to the reference laboratory with the amniotic fluid sample. Results indicated an RhD-positive fetus. At 24 weeks' gestation the anti-D titer remained stable at 32. Serial MCA Doppler studies were initiated each week. After 3 weeks, these remained at 1.1–1.2 MoM so the testing interval was lengthened to every 2 weeks. The MCA Dopplers remained normal. Induction of labor was undertaken at 38 weeks' gestation. A healthy 3713 g (8 lb 3 oz) female fetus was born vaginally. Cord blood revealed the child to be A, RhD positive, the direct Coombs was 1+, and the total bilirubin was 2.1 mg/dL. The infant required 3 days of bililight therapy with a peak bilirubin of 10 mg/dL. The infant was discharged on the fourth day of life and required no further treatment.

Case presentation 2

Surveillance of a subsequent affected gestation

The patient in case presentation 1 returned 2 years later with her third pregnancy. The current pregnancy had been fathered by the same partner as her previous gestation. At 10 weeks' gestation, the maternal anti-D titer was 128. An amniocentesis at 15 weeks indicated an RhD-positive fetus. Serial MCA Dopplers were initiated each week starting at 18 weeks' gestation. At 25 weeks, the MCA peak systolic velocity was 1.45 MoM. One week later it had risen to 1.7 MoM. The following day, an IUT was scheduled. Initial fetal blood at the time of cordocentesis revealed blood type O, RhD positive, with a 3+ direct Coombs test. The fetal hematocrit was 25% with 15% reticulocytes. An intravascular transfusion of 45 mL raised the fetal hematocrit to 50%. The patient returned for five additional

IUTs, the last one being performed at 35 weeks' gestation. Oral phenobarbital was prescribed to the patient 10 days prior to her planned induction date in an effort to enhance the neonatal capability to conjugate bilirubin. She was induced at 38 weeks' gestation and delivered a healthy 3004 g (6 lb 10 oz) male fetus. Cord blood testing revealed a hematocrit of 45% with a fetal cell stain consisting of 100% adult hemoglobin-containing red cells, indicating suppression of the fetal bone marrow. The infant was discharged on the second day of life and did not require bililight therapy. He was followed with weekly hematocrit and reticulocyte counts by his pediatrician. At 4 weeks of age he was noted to be feeding poorly; the hematocrit had declined to 23%. He was admitted overnight for a "top-up" red cell transfusion. Subsequent testing revealed a rising reticulocyte count. The infant required no further therapy.

References

1 Wataganara T, Chen AY, LeShane ES, *et al.* Cell-free fetal DNA levels in maternal plasma after elective first-trimester termination of pregnancy. *Fertil Steril* 2004;**81**:638–44.

2 Medearis AL, Hensleigh PA, Parks DR, Herzenberg LA. Detection of fetal erythrocytes in maternal blood post partum with the fluorescence-activated cell sorter. *Am J Obstet Gynecol* 1984;**148**:290–5.

3 *Prevention of RhD alloimmunization*. American College of Obstetricians and Gynecologists Practice Bulletin 1999: 4.

4 Kumpel BM. On the mechanism of tolerance to the Rh D antigen mediated by passive anti-D (Rh D prophylaxis). *Immunol Lett* 2002;**82**:67–73.

5 Bowman JM. Controversies in Rh prophylaxis. Who needs Rh immune globulin and when should it be given? *Am J Obstet Gynecol* 1985;**151**:289–94.

6 Novaretti MC, Jens E, Pagliarini T, Bonifacio SL, Dorlhiac-Llacer PE, Chamone DA. Comparison of conventional tube test with diamed gel microcolumn assay for anti-D titration. *Clin Lab Haematol* 2003;**25**:311–5.

7 Nicolaides KH, Warenski JC, Rodeck CH. The relationship of fetal plasma protein concentration and hemoglobin level to the development of hydrops in rhesus isoimmunization. *Am J Obstet Gynecol* 1985;**152**:341–4.

8 Liley AW. Liquor amnii analysis in the management of pregnancy complicated by rhesus sensitization. *Am J Obstet Gynecol* 1961;**82**:1359–70.

9 Queenan JT, Tomai TP, Ural SH, King JC. Deviation in amniotic fluid optical density at a wavelength of 450 nm in Rh-immunized pregnancies from 14 to 40 weeks' gestation: a proposal for clinical management. *Am J Obstet Gynecol* 1993;**168**:1370–6.

10 Opekes D, Seward G, Vandenbussche F, *et al.* Minimally invasive management of Rh alloimmunization: can amniotic fluid delta OD450 be replaced by Doppler studies? A prospective study multicenter trial. *Am J Obstet Gynecol* 2004;**191**:S3.

11 Mari G, for the Collaborative Group for Doppler Assessment of the Blood Velocity in Anemic Fetuses. Noninvasive diagnosis by Doppler ultrasonography of fetal anemia due to maternal red-cell alloimmunization. *N Engl J Med* 2000;**342**:9–14.

12 Zimmerman R, Carpenter RJ Jr, Durig P, Mari G. Longitudinal measurement of peak systolic velocity in the fetal middle cerebral artery for monitoring pregnancies complicated by red cell alloimmunisation: a prospective multicentre trial with intention-to-treat. *Br J Obstet Gynaecol* 2002;**109**:746–52.

13 Finning KM, Martin PG, Soothill PW, Avent ND. Prediction of fetal D status from maternal plasma: introduction of a new noninvasive fetal RHD genotyping service. *Transfusion* 2002;**42**:1079–85.

14 Liley AW. Intrauterine transfusion of foetus in haemolytic disease. *Br Med J* 1963;**2**:1107–9.

15 Moise KJ Jr, Carpenter RJ Jr, Kirshon B, Deter RL, Sala JD, Cano LE. Comparison of four types of intrauterine transfusion: effect on fetal hematocrit. *Fetal Ther* 1989;**4**:126–37.

16 Nicolini U, Nicolaidis P, Fisk NM, Tannirandorn Y, Rodeck CH. Fetal blood sampling from the intrahepatic vein: analysis of safety and clinical experience with 214 procedures. *Obstet Gynecol* 1990;**76**:47–53.

17 Trevett T, Dorman K, Lamvu G, Moise KJ. Does antenatal maternal administration of phenobarbital prevent exchange transfusion in neonates with alloimmune hemolytic disease? *Am J Obstet Gynecol* 2005;**192**:478–82.

18 van Kamp IL, Klumper FJ, Oepkes D, *et al.* Complications of intrauterine intravascular transfusion for fetal anemia due to maternal red-cell alloimmunization. *Am J Obstet Gynecol* 2005;**192**:171–7.

19 van Kamp IL, Klumper FJ, Bakkum RS, *et al.* The severity of immune fetal hydrops is predictive of fetal outcome after intrauterine treatment. *Am J Obstet Gynecol* 2001;**185**:668–73.

20 Saade GR, Moise KJ, Belfort MA, Hesketh DE, Carpenter RJ. Fetal and neonatal hematologic parameters in red cell alloimmunization: predicting the need for late neonatal transfusions. *Fetal Diagn Ther* 1993;**8**:161–4.

21 Hudon L, Moise KJ Jr, Hegemier SE, *et al.* Long-term neurodevelopmental outcome after intrauterine transfusion for the treatment of fetal hemolytic disease. *Am J Obstet Gynecol* 1998;**179**:858–63.

22 Brecher ME. *Technical Manual of the American Association of Blood Banks*. Bethesda, Maryland: American Association of Blood Banks, 2002.

23 Bowman JM, Pollock JM, Manning FA, Harman CR, Menticoglou S. Maternal Kell blood group alloimmunization. *Obstet Gynecol* 1992;**79**:239–44.

37

Multiple pregnancy

Young Mi Lee, Jane Cleary-Goldman, and Mary E. D'Alton

An epidemic of multiple gestations has been noted over the past two decades, attributed largely to an older patient population secondary to delayed childbearing and the rise in assisted reproductive technology (ART) and ovulation induction. According to the National Vital Statistics Report for 2003, the twinning rate was a record high at 31.5 twin births per 1000 total live births, representing a 67% rise since 1980 [1]. More impressive are the numbers of triplets and high-order multiples, which have increased more than 500% since 1980 [1]. Perinatal complications have been strongly impacted by the widespread prevalence of multiple gestations as these pregnancies account for a disproportionate share of adverse outcomes. The most profound implication of this epidemic is the problem of preterm delivery, currently the leading cause of hospitalization among pregnant women and the leading cause of infant death [2]. In addition to prematurity, multiple pregnancy is known to be associated with a greater number of other maternal and fetal problems including gestational hypertension, placental abruption, operative delivery, low birthweight, and adverse neurologic outcomes [3]. The overall increased perinatal risks associated with multiple gestations compared with singleton pregnancies are well documented, in addition to the increasing ways these high-risk pregnancies are affecting medical expenditures and public health [1]. This chapter reviews multiple gestations and the current strategies for managing these complex pregnancies.

Impact of multiple pregnancy on perinatal outcomes

The two most important contributors to increased perinatal morbidity and mortality in multiple gestations appear to be increased rates of prematurity and complications of monochorionicity. In 2002 in the USA, the mean age at delivery was 35.3 weeks for twins, 32.2 weeks for triplets, and 29.9 weeks for quadruplets, compared to 38.8 weeks for singletons [4]. Offspring of multiple pregnancies weigh less than their singleton counterparts. The mean birthweight for singletons is 3332 g compared to 2347 g for twins, 1687 g for triplets, and 1309 g for quadruplets [4]. Neonates from multiple gestations are overrepresented among preterm and low birthweight (LBW) infants. In 2003, multiples accounted for 3% of all live births but more than 25% of very low birthweight (VLBW) infants [1]. In addition, neonates from multiple gestations currently comprise a disproportionate share of neonatal intensive care admissions and recent National Vital Statistics data indicate that nearly 20% of neonatal deaths are from multiple gestations. While the offspring of multiple gestations may be born earlier than singletons, preterm twin and triplet neonates appear to have similar birthweights, morbidities, and mortalities as gestational age-matched controls [5–7]. Therefore, the outcome related to prematurity appears to be similar whether the pregnancy was a singleton or multiple gestation.

Besides prematurity, patients with multiples are at increased risk for adverse perinatal outcomes resulting from complications unique to the twinning process. In particular, monochorionic placentation accounts for 20% of all twin pregnancies and carries a worse prognosis than dichorionicity. Complications from monochorionicity such as twin–twin transfusion syndrome (TTTS) continue to place these offspring at higher risk for long-term adverse outcomes. Cases of single intrauterine fetal death (IUFD) in twins sharing a single placenta can be associated with a coincident insult leading to white matter damage in the surviving co-twin. Other unique but rare problems that occur in monochorionic pregnancies include cord entanglement in monoamniotic twins, conjoined twins, and twin reversed arterial perfusion (TRAP) sequence also known as acardiac twinning.

Multiple gestation is an independent risk factor for long-term neurologic impairment. In various studies, children from a multiple pregnancy have a 4–17 times higher risk of developing cerebral palsy compared to their singleton counterparts [3,8–10]. With more investigators finding this correlation to be true at higher birthweights, this suggests that the risk is not simply related to an increased preterm delivery rate [9,10].

One epidemiologic study reported that the risk of producing one child with cerebral palsy in twin, triplet, and quadruplet gestations was 15 per 1000 twins, 80 per 1000 triplets, and 429 per 1000 quadruplets [10]. While many previous studies regarding this association were not optimally designed, the prevalence of cerebral palsy in multiple pregnancies reported in these studies is similar and ranges 6.7–12.6 per 1000 surviving infants [9]. This consistent conclusion suggests an association between multiple birth and cerebral palsy. While a portion of this risk appears related to the higher rates of prematurity, there are many other risk factors for cerebral palsy seen with higher frequency in multiples including maternal hypertensive disease, bleeding in pregnancy, LBW infants, congenital anomalies, and complications specific to monochorionicity [9,11].

Zygosity and chorionicity

Embryology

Zygosity refers to the genetic constitution of a twin pregnancy, while chorionicity indicates the pregnancy's membrane composition. In dizygotic twins, chorionicity is determined by the mechanism of fertilization, while in monozygotic twins it is determined by the timing of embryonic division. The vast majority of dizygotic twins have separate dichorionic diamniotic placentas (each fetus has its own placental disk with a separate amnion and chorion). This is because dizygotic twins result from the fertilization of two different ova by two separate sperm. The type of placenta that develops in a monozygotic pregnancy is determined by the timing of cleavage of the fertilized ovum. If twinning is accomplished during the first 2–3 days, it precedes the separation of cells that eventually become the chorion. In that case, two chorions and two amnions will be formed. After approximately 3 days, twinning cannot split the chorionic cavity and from that time forward, a monochorionic placenta results. If the split occurs between the third and eighth days, a diamniotic monochorionic placenta develops. Between the 8th and 13th days, the amnion has already formed, and the placenta will therefore be monoamniotic and monochorionic. Embryonic cleavage between the 13th and 15th days results in conjoined twins within a single amnion and chorion; beyond that point, the process of twinning does not occur [12]. Interestingly, rare cases of dizygotic monochorionic twins conceived following ART have been reported [13,14].

Ultrasound diagnosis of chorionicity

The determination of chorionicity is important in the management of multiple gestations as monochorionic twins are at increased risk for poor outcomes. Antenatal knowledge of chorionicity can be critical for determining optimal manage-ment. This is true when deciding whether intrauterine uterine growth restriction (IUGR) in one fetus of a twin gestation is caused by TTTS or uteroplacental insufficiency. Precise knowledge of chorionicity is imperative when contemplating the selective termination (ST) of one abnormal twin or when performing elective first trimester multifetal pregnancy reduction (MPR). If the gestation is monochorionic, a shared placental circulation could result in death or injury to a surviving fetus depending on the technique utilized for the termination procedure.

Chorionicity is most accurately determined in the first trimester. From 6 to 10 weeks, counting the number of gestational sacs with evaluation of the thickness of the dividing membrane is the optimal method. Two separate gestational sacs, each containing a fetus and a thick dividing membrane, suggests a dichorionic diamniotic pregnancy, while one gestational sac with a thin dividing membrane and two fetuses suggests a monochorionic diamniotic pregnancy [15]. The number of yolk sacs can also be used as an indirect method of determining amnionicity [16]. After 9 weeks, the dividing membranes become progressively thinner in monochorionic pregnancies. In dichorionic pregnancies, they remain thick and easy to identify at their attachment to the placenta as a triangular projection (lambda or twin peak sign) [17–19]. Thus, in the late first trimester, sonographic examination of the base of the intertwin membrane for the presence or absence of the lambda sign provides reliable distinction between dichorionic and monochorionic pregnancies [20].

Later in pregnancy, determination of chorionicity and amnionicity becomes less accurate and requires different techniques. The sonographic prediction of chorionicity and amnionicity should be systematically approached by determining the number of placentas visualized and the sex of each fetus and then by assessing the membranes that divide the sacs. If two separate placental disks are seen, the pregnancy is dichorionic. Likewise, if the twins are different genders, the pregnancy is most likely dichorionic. When a single placenta is present and the twins are of the same sex, careful sonographic examination of the dividing membrane will typically result in a correct diagnosis. Evaluation of three features in the intertwin membrane will provide an almost certain diagnosis about the chorionicity of a twin pregnancy:

1 Thickness of the intertwin membrane;
2 Number of layers visualized in the membrane; and
3 Assessment of the junction of the membrane with the placenta for the "twin peak" sign [21].
It should be mentioned that the absence of the twin peak sign does not guarantee that the pregnancy is monochorionic.

In some pregnancies with monochorionic diamniotic placentation, the dividing membranes may not be sonographically visualized because they are very thin. In other cases, they may not be seen because severe oligohydramnios causes them to be closely apposed to the fetus in that sac. This results in a "stuck twin" appearance, where the trapped fetus remains firmly held against the uterine wall despite changes in maternal position. Diagnosis of this condition confirms the presence of a diamniotic gestation, which should be distinguished from a monoamniotic gestation with an absent dividing membrane. In the latter situation, free movement of both twins, and entanglement of their umbilical cords, can be identified [22].

Fetal complications and multiple gestations

The offspring of a multiple gestation are at risk for many complications *in utero* that may lead to long-term adverse outcomes, including growth abnormalities, fetal wastage, and complications unique to the twinning process (Table 37.1).

IUGR and growth discordance

Birthweight is a function of many factors including gestational age, rate of fetal growth, ethnicity, and genetic composition. Two important antenatal markers for growth abnormalities are IUGR and growth discordance. IUGR remains a sonographic and statistical diagnosis consisting of either an estimated fetal weight (EFW) less than the 3rd percentile (2 standard deviations from the mean) for gestational age or an EFW ≤10th percentile for gestational age along with evidence of fetal compromise (usually oligohydramnios or abnormal umbilical artery Doppler velocimetry) [23]. Growth discordance is generally defined as ≥20% difference in EFW between fetuses of the same pregnancy expressed as a percentage of the larger EFW [23]. Both growth abnormalities are seen with increased frequency in multiple gestations.

IUGR has long been known to be associated with adverse perinatal outcomes. Neonatal morbidity (such as meconium aspiration syndrome, hypoglycemia, polycythemia, and pulmonary hemorrhage) may be present in up to 50% of IUGR neonates [23]. Long-term studies show a twofold increased

Table 37.1 Multiple gestation: fetal and neonatal risks.

Fetal wastage
Chromosomal abnormalities
Congenital malformations
Monochorionicity
   TTTS
   Monoamnionicity
   TRAP
Growth discordance/IUGR
Amniotic fluid volume abnormalities
Prematurity
Low birthweight
Perinatal mortality
Cerebral palsy

IUGR, intrauterine growth restriction; TRAP, twin reversed arterial perfusion; TTTS, twin–twin transfusion syndrome.

incidence of cerebral dysfunction (ranging from minor learning disabilities to cerebral palsy) in IUGR infants delivered at term and an even higher incidence if the infant was born preterm [9]. Multiple gestations present a dilemma both in diagnosis and management of IUGR. For example, fetuses suspected to be normally grown may be affected by iatrogenic preterm delivery secondary to interventions for a growth-restricted co-twin. Current management of IUGR is aimed towards early diagnosis and fetal surveillance to aid in timing delivery.

Like IUGR, growth discordance has been associated with an increased risk for adverse perinatal outcomes [24]. Approximately 15% of twins are diagnosed with this condition [24]. Risk factors include monochorionicity, velamentous cord insertion, antenatal bleeding, uteroplacental insufficiency, and gestational hypertensive disease [24]. Growth discordance has different implications depending on chorionicity and is more concerning in monochorionic twinning. Although IUGR can complicate a pregnancy with growth discordance, the second does not necessarily imply the first. While some studies have demonstrated an increased risk for perinatal morbidity in growth discordant twins, others have not. In approximately two-thirds of discordant twin pairs, the smaller twin has a birthweight of less than 10% [25]. In a study of more than 10,000 discordant twins, the neonatal mortality rates were 29 versus 11 per 1000 live births when the smaller twin weighed less than the 10th percentile, compared with those who were above it [25]. Conversely, a recent study suggests that 20% growth discordance may result in an increased risk for some adverse outcomes but not for serious sequelae [26]. After adjusting for chorionicity, antenatal steroids, oligohydramnios, preeclampsia, and gestational age at delivery, discordant twins were at increased risk for low or very low birthweight, neonatal intensive care unit (ICU) admission, neonatal oxygen requirement, and hyperbilirubinemia but did not seem to be at increased risk for serious neonatal morbidity and mortality.

Fetal wastage

The incidence of early pregnancy loss in multiple gestations is higher than previously thought. The routine use of ultrasound has shown that early fetal wastage is common in multiple gestations. In patients with twin gestations scanned in the first trimester, rates of demise ranged from 13% to 78% [27]. This phenomenon has been termed the *vanishing twin*. Explanations for this occurrence include physiologic resorption, artefact, and sonographic error. Although this condition has been associated with first trimester bleeding and spotting, it has not been associated with adverse pregnancy outcomes.

During the second and third trimester, IUFD of one fetus in a multiple gestation is a rare complication affecting approximately 2–5% of twin pregnancies. Death of both fetuses in a twin pregnancy has been reported infrequently. In patients with high-order multiples, however, death of a single fetus may be more common. Studies have indicated single IUFD rates up to 17% in triplet pregnancies [28]. Death of one twin in the second or third trimesters can adversely affect the surviving fetus or fetuses in two ways:

1 Risk for multicystic encephalomalacia and multiorgan damage in monochorionic pregnancies; and
2 Preterm labor and delivery in both dichorionic and monochorionic twins resulting in prematurity.

Two theories explain the pathophysiology of multiorgan damage in surviving monochorionic twins. One theory is based on the premise that the retained dead fetus creates thromboplastic materials which traverse the anastomoses between the placentas causing disseminated intravascular coagulation. This leads to infarctions and cystic changes in myriad organ systems including the kidneys, lungs, spleen, liver, and brain [29].

A more recent and widely accepted theory suggests that blood from the surviving twin may rapidly "back-bleed" into the demised twin through placental anastomosis (a capacitance effect) [30]. Decreased circulatory tone in the dead twin causing blood to flow from the viable to the dead twin, may be the underlying pathophysiology [31]. The dead twin may become congested and the surviving twin anemic. If the hypotension is severe enough, the surviving twin is at risk for ischemic damage to vital organs. Most evidence in the literature suggests that "back-bleeding" is the cause of multiorgan injury in surviving co-twins. As a result, immediate delivery of the co-twin following single IUFD in a monochorionic pregnancy does not improve outcome but rather adds to the additional risk of prematurity. Most cases are managed expectantly with close fetal surveillance. Normal fetal heart rate patterns and biophysical profile scores cannot rule out multicystic encephalomalacia. Normal fetal magnetic resonance imaging, while investigational, may be reassuring [32].

In addition to multiorgan ischemic damage in monochorionic pregnancies, studies have demonstrated that IUFD of one twin can result in preterm delivery. Both dichorionic and monochorionic pregnancies are at risk for preterm delivery. In a study of 17 twin pregnancies complicated by IUFD, 76% of these pregnancies were delivered before 37 weeks. Eighty-six percent of the patients delivering prematurely presented in active labor [33].

When IUFD occurs in a multiple pregnancy, baseline maternal hematologic laboratory investigation is suggested, including prothrombin time (PT), partial thromboplastin time (PTT), fibrinogen level, and platelet count, because of the theoretical risk of maternal consumptive coagulopathy in the setting of a single IUFD. If these values are within normal limits, further surveillance is not indicated. Of note, mothers with IUFD in one twin do not appear to be at increased risk of infection from a retained twin [33]. Dystocia secondary to the dead fetus has been reported infrequently. Cesarean delivery rates appear increased in patients with single IUFD complicating a twin gestation because of higher rates of nonreassuring fetal status in the surviving twin [33].

Discordant anatomic abnormalities

There is general agreement that anomalies occur more frequently in twins than in singletons, but controversy exists regarding the degree of difference [34–37]. The diagnosis of discordance for major genetic disorders or anatomic abnormalities in the second trimester places parents in a difficult position. Management choices include:

1 Expectant management;
2 Termination of the entire pregnancy; and
3 ST of the anomalous fetus.

ST differs from MPR, which is discussed later in this chapter. MPR refers to reduction in the number of fetuses a woman is carrying in order to reduce her risk of preterm delivery. ST, on the other hand, refers to terminating a specific fetus that is known to be abnormal. For dichorionic pregnancies, intracardiac injection with potassium chloride is utilized. In monochorionic pregnancies, various cord occlusive procedures are employed [38].

Several issues should be considered when counseling patients about the management of a multiple pregnancy complicated by a discordant anomaly:

1 Severity of the anomaly;
2 Chorionicity;
3 Effect of the anomalous fetus on the remaining fetus or fetuses; and
4 The parents' personal, moral, and ethical beliefs.

It is important to counsel patients that conservative management can result in adverse outcomes for the healthy twin. Several studies have demonstrated that the normal fetus in a twin pregnancy discordant for major fetal anomalies may be at increased risk for preterm delivery, low birthweight, and perinatal morbidity and mortality [39–41].

Complications unique to monochorionicity

Monoamnionicity

Less than 1% of monozygotic twins are monoamniotic [42]. Monoamniotic twins have been associated with a high rate of perinatal mortality. Previous studies report a fetal mortality rate of greater than 50% but more recent studies indicate a perinatal mortality rate ranging from 10% to 21% [43–45]. Preterm delivery, IUGR, congenital anomalies, cord entanglement, and cord accidents remain common in monoamniotic pregnancies. The management of these pregnancies is controversial, particularly regarding the optimal protocol for antenatal surveillance and the optimal timing for delivery. Because IUFD can occur at any gestational age, some experts suggest early delivery in the late preterm period [46]. Other studies have suggested that early delivery is not prudent secondary to the risks of prematurity [47]. The nonstress test is generally the preferred method of testing over the biophysical profile, as cord compression may be indicated by variable decelerations. While the optimal management and timing of delivery for monoamniotic twins remains uncertain, our current practice includes routine hospitalization beginning at 24–26 weeks, daily nonstress tests, and, if uncomplicated, delivery at 34 weeks is offered after antenatal corticosteroid administration and thorough counseling of the risks and benefits of elective preterm delivery.

Twin–twin transfusion syndrome

Monochorionic twins occur spontaneously in 0.4% of the general population. However, studies have reported that monozygotic twinning may be greater than 10 times higher in pregnancies following fertility treatment [48,49]. The primary concerns from monochorionic placentation include complications such as TTTS characterized by an unequal distribution of the blood flow across the shared placenta of two fetuses. Although all monochorionic twins share a portion of their vasculature, only approximately 15–20% will develop this condition [42,50]. Left untreated, there is up to 60–100% mortality rate for both twins.

Antenatal diagnosis is made sonographically and findings include the presence of a single placenta, same-gender fetuses, weight discordance, and significant amniotic fluid discordance. The recipient twin may have signs of heart failure and hydrops and the donor may demonstrate IUGR and a "stuck" appearance. Umbilical artery Doppler studies can be variable [51]. TTTS may be chronic or acute. A staging system devised by Quintero *et al.* [52] is commonly utilized to categorize disease severity and standardize comparison of different therapies. The net effect of this hemodynamic imbalance is a large, plethoric recipient twin and a small, anemic donor twin. While the exact etiology has not been clearly delineated, the mechanism is likely to involve shunting of arteriovenous anastomoses [53].

Treatment depends on gestational age at diagnosis. Patients with early onset TTTS may opt for selective termination of one twin (usually the donor twin) or voluntary termination of the entire pregnancy. Diagnosis in the middle to late third trimester may be less aggressive depending on disease severity and the proximity to term. Current treatments for severe TTTS require physical intervention and include serial amnioreduction, septostomy, or selective fetoscopic laser coagulation of the communicating vessels. Proponents of laser ablation of the communicating vessels for the treatment of TTTS have argued that amnioreduction and septostomy do not treat the underlying condition. Two nonrandomized studies and one randomized trial comparing both techniques have shown that endoscopic surgery results in lower mortality rates (with the survival of at least one twin in 71–83% of procedures) and

lower rates of neurologic complications than serial amnioreduction [54–56]. The recent randomized trial compared the two therapies in 142 women with severe TTTS identified before 26 weeks' gestation and demonstrated a significant benefit in the laser group, with both improved perinatal survival as well as short-term neurologic outcome [56]. The risk factors for developing TTTS remain elusive and many questions concerning this disease remain unanswered.

Maternal obstetric complications

Antepartum complications develop in over 80% of multiple pregnancies compared to 25% of singleton gestations [23]. Examples of adverse outcomes that may arise include anemia, urinary tract infections, gestational diabetes, abnormal placentation, thromboembolism, preterm premature rupture of membranes, abruption, and postpartum hemorrhage (Table 37.2) [3,57–59]. Pulmonary embolism, the leading cause of maternal death in the USA and around the world, and thromboembolism are about five times more likely during pregnancy or the puerperium than in the nonpregnant state [60]. Women carrying multiples are believed to be at increased risk for both.

Preeclampsia and its related spectrum of diseases occur in approximately 5–8% of singleton pregnancies but the incidence is higher in multiples [61,62]. Hypertensive diseases during pregnancy may manifest as hemolysis, elevated liver enzymes, and low platelet (HELLP) syndrome or eclampsia and can be associated with adverse sequelae including IUGR, placental abruption, disseminated intravascular coagulation, renal failure, and IUFD [61]. Unfortunately, no intervention to date (including aspirin and calcium supplementation) has been shown to prevent or reduce the incidence of preeclampsia in these high-risk pregnancies and delivery remains the only definitive cure [63,64]. Both gestational hypertension

Table 37.2 Multiple gestation: maternal risks.

Hyperemesis
Threatened miscarriage
Anemia
Gestational hypertension
Preterm labor/delivery
Tocolysis complications
Long-term bed rest
Placental abnormalities
Abruption
Abnormal placentation
Urinary tract infection
Gestational diabetes
Postpartum hemorrhage
Operative delivery
Thromboembolism

and preeclampsia are more common in women carrying multiples, with the rates estimated to be 2–2.6 higher in twins compared to singletons [62]. Rates of preeclampsia seem to be the same for both monozygotic and dizygotic twins [65]. When preeclampsia occurs in triplets and higher order multiples, it often occurs earlier, with more severity, and in an atypical presentation [57,66]. Finally, women carrying multifetal pregnancies may also be prone to developing acute fatty liver of pregnancy, one of the most serious maternal obstetric complications [67]. This disease process is characterized by hepatic dysfunction, severe coagulopathy, hypoglycemia, hyperammonemia, and can result in fetal and/or maternal death.

Antepartum management of multiple gestations

The management of multiple pregnancies include adequate nutrition, avoiding strenuous physical activity, and frequent prenatal visits. Patients should be counseled regarding the increased risk of complications associated with multiple gestations. Women with multifetal pregnancies are currently recommended to increase their daily caloric intake approximately 300 kcal more than women with singletons. Iron and folic acid supplementation is also advised. While the optimal weight gain for women with multiples has not been determined, it has been suggested that women with twins gain 15.87–20.41 kg (35–45 lb) [3,68]. Patients with multiples should be followed with serial growth scans because the offspring of these pregnancies are at risk for growth abnormalities.

Multifetal pregnancy reduction

Ovulation induction and ART have greatly contributed to the increasing number of high-order multiples. The purpose of first-trimester MPR is to improve perinatal outcomes by decreasing maternal complications secondary to multiple gestations and by decreasing adverse fetal outcomes associated with preterm delivery. Reducing a high-order multiple gestation to twins lowers the risk of preterm labor and delivery and increases the chances of higher birthweight and gestational age at delivery. In some instances, such as a history of a previous second trimester loss, reduction from twins to a singleton may be indicated.

Nonetheless, MPR is an ethical dilemma. The starting number of fetuses needed to justify the procedure is controversial. There have been conflicting studies regarding whether or not MPR from triplets to twins results in improved perinatal outcomes compared to expectant management [69]. In addition, while most women do not regret their decision, women undergoing multifetal pregnancy reduction may have feelings of loss, guilt, and sadness.

The procedure is most commonly performed transabdominally under ultrasound guidance between 10 and 13 weeks' gestation. Potassium chloride is injected into the fetal heart until asystole is achieved. If chorionic villus sampling is performed prior to the procedure and one fetus is found to have a genetic anomaly, that fetus is targeted. Otherwise, the fetus with a crown rump length smaller than expected for gestational age or the fetus most physically accessible is chosen. The fetus over the cervix is usually avoided. This procedure is reserved for dichorionic pregnancies. In monochorionic pregnancies, selectively reducing one fetus utilizing intracardiac potassium chloride is contraindicated because of the presence of communicating placental anastomoses. Selective reduction in these cases involves more technically challenging procedures.

There are several studies documenting pregnancy loss rates associated with multifetal pregnancy reduction. With extensive experience, the current loss rate is approximately 6% [70]. There is little maternal risk associated with the procedure. The terminated fetus is usually resorbed or becomes a small papyraceous fetus. There have been no reports of coagulation disorders following this procedure [71]. Maternal serum alpha-fetoprotein (MSAFP) is elevated following MPR and ST and therefore cannot be used as a screening tool in these pregnancies.

Prenatal diagnosis

Prenatal diagnosis and genetic counseling are important in the management of patients with a multiple gestation because these pregnancies are at increased risk for both chromosomal and structural anomalies. Dizygotic twinning has been associated with advancing maternal age and many patients who undergo assisted conception, which is associated with an increased risk for multiples, are of advanced maternal age. Prenatal diagnosis has thus become a cornerstone in the management of these patients.

Many known chromosomal anomalies have been reported in twins. Dizygotic twins are usually discordant for these anomalies and monozygotic twins may rarely be as well. In dizygotic pregnancies, the maternal age-related risk for chromosomal abnormalities for each twin is the same as in singleton pregnancies. It has been suggested that the chance of at least one fetus being affected by a chromosomal defect is twice as high as in singletons. In monozygotic twins, the risk for chromosomal abnormalities is the same as in singletons, and in the vast majority of cases both fetuses are affected or both are unaffected [72]. However, there are occasional case reports of monozygotic twins discordant for abnormalities of autosomal or sex chromosomes [73,74].

Genetic consultation should be offered to all patients of advanced maternal age with twins, triplets, and high-order multiples. In patients with singletons and monochorionic twins, "advanced maternal age" is currently defined as age greater than 35 years at expected date of delivery. In the literature, there are a range of maternal ages suggested as being "advanced" when classifying patients with dichorionic twins. Reports suggest that women with twins may be labeled as such between the ages of 31 and 33 because their mid-trimester risk of having one fetus with Down syndrome is similar to that of a 35-year-old woman with a singleton [75,76]. With high-order multiples, this age is thought to be even younger.

Amniocentesis is an appropriate option for women carrying multiples. Chorionic villus sampling of two or more fetuses is also suitable in experienced hands, and there is low risk for cross-contamination [77].

Screening for aneuploidy

In the first trimester, nuchal translucency ultrasound measurements combined with maternal age appears to be a promising method for aneuploidy screening in patients with multiples. Because the nuchal translucency distribution does not differ significantly in singletons compared to twins, the Down syndrome detection rate in multiples using this modality is similar to that of singletons [78]. Increased nuchal translucency appears to be higher in patients with monochoronic pregnancies and it has been suggested that this may reflect an early manifestation of TTTS in a portion of cases [79]. Nuchal translucency can be performed in pregnancies complicated by triplets and high-order multiples with similar accuracy as in singletons.

In singletons, first trimester combined screening—maternal age and nuchal translucency combined with maternal serum free beta human chorionic gonadotropin (β-hCG) and pregnancy-associated plasma protein A (PAPP-A)—has been shown to detect approximately 82% of cases of Down syndrome for a 5% false positive rate [80]. In a recent prospective study, Spencer and Nicolaides reported a 75% detection rate of Down syndrome for a 9% false positive rate using nuchal translucency and first trimester serum markers in 206 twin pregnancies [81]. The combination of nuchal translucency and biochemistry studies in twins may prove to give detection rates similar to singleton pregnancies. Larger prospective studies on first trimester combined screening in twins are needed before definitive conclusions and recommendations for practice can be made.

Second trimester maternal serum screening for Down syndrome is more complex in patients with multiples compared to those with singletons. On average, maternal serum biochemical markers are twice as high in twins as they are in singletons of the same gestational age [82]. In maternal serum screening programs for Down syndrome, these serum markers can be measured in a woman with twins and then divided by the corresponding medians for normal twins ("pseudo-risk" estimation). Nonetheless, experience with maternal serum screening in twins during the second trimester has been limited and interpretation of the analyte data may be difficult. In cases discordant for anomalies, altered serum levels from the affected fetus will be brought closer to the mean by the unaffected twin. Because second trimester maternal serum analytes are difficult to interpret in patients with a twin pregnancy, many medical centers do not offer this screening modality routinely to those individuals.

Screening for neural tube defects in multiples

In singletons, a second trimester MSAFP of greater than 2.5 multiples of the median (MoM) has been used to screen for neural tube defects. Different MSAFP cut-offs are needed for twin pregnancies because the MSAFP level in a twin pregnancy is approximately double that of a singleton pregnancy. A cut-off of 4.5 MoM is often used for twins because it has a detection rate of 50–85% for a 5% false positive rate [83]. If an abnormal MSAFP is found, ultrasound is required for further evaluation. It is important to note that similar to maternal serum screening for aneuploidy, maternal serum screening for neural tube defects in a twin pregnancy will always be limited because it is impossible to confirm which fetus is affected without performing an ultrasound examination. As a result, many centers do not offer this type of serum screening for twin pregnancies.

Screening for anatomic abnormalities

The fetuses of multiple gestations seem to be at increased risk for anatomic abnormalities. Careful sonographic, anatomic evaluation of each fetus should be obtained. No large-scale studies of ultrasound for fetal anatomy in multiples have been performed. Small studies have attempted to determine the predictive value of ultrasound in the detection of fetal anomalies in multiples, and found it effective [84].

Prevention of preterm delivery

Patients with multiples are at increased risk for preterm labor and delivery. No therapy has proven to be efficacious in decreasing the adverse outcomes from prematurity except the administration of corticosteroids and surfactant to improve fetal lung maturity and antibiotics to lengthen the latency period for patients with premature rupture of membranes [85–87]. This therapy does not treat the primary problem of preterm labor. Management strategies aimed at solving this dilemma that have not proven beneficial include prophylactic cervical cerclage, routine bed rest, prophylactic tocolytics, and home uterine monitoring [3].

Prophylactic cervical cerclage in patients with a multiple gestation has not been consistently proven to prevent prematurity. A randomized trial of 128 patients with twins offered elective cerclage at 18–26 weeks did not demonstrate any benefit [88]. Likewise, this intervention has not been shown to significantly improve perinatal outcomes in triplets [89]. A recent meta-analysis of randomized control trials examined individual patient-level data to determine whether cerclage prevented preterm birth in women with a short cervical length [90]. In the subgroup analysis of three trials including 49 twins, cerclage was associated with a significantly higher incidence of preterm birth and perinatal mortality. However, this investigation was limited by small sample size. Until a large prospective randomized trial of cerclage in multiples is performed, it remains difficult to refute a potential benefit from this procedure for a select group of women. Because this surgical procedure carries potential risks for both the mother and her fetuses, cerclage placement for multiple gestations is generally reserved for women with either a strong history or objectively documented cervical incompetence.

The idea that prophylactic bed rest may decrease uterine activity makes common sense to both patients and physicians. However, the literature does not support any significant benefit from routine bed rest or hospitalization in multiples [3,91]. A Cochrane database review of six randomized trials involving over 600 multiples demonstrated a trend toward a decrease in low birthweight infants and a paradoxical increased risk of delivery at less than 34 weeks' gestation with inpatient bed rest [92]. In addition, prophylactic bed rest may be associated with adverse complications such as thromboembolic disease and can be disruptive to families.

Administration of prophylactic tocolytic agents has been attempted but has not been beneficial. Women with multifetal pregnancies appear to be particularly prone to developing pulmonary edema and cardiovascular complications after administration of beta-adrenergic agents because of their higher blood volume and lower colloid osmotic pressure [23,93]. As such, it seems prudent to restrict the use of those agents to women who are confirmed to be in preterm labor.

Ambulatory home monitoring of uterine contractions with a tocodynamometer in an attempt to predict preterm labor has not been shown to be useful. A meta-analysis of six randomized trials was unable to demonstrate a significant benefit of home uterine activity monitoring to reduce the risk of preterm delivery in patients with twins [94]. Furthermore, a prospective trial of 2422 patients (including 844 twins) randomized women to weekly nurse contact, daily nurse contact, or daily nurse contact in addition to home uterine activity monitoring, and demonstrated no difference in preterm delivery prior to 35 weeks' gestation [95].

Specialized twin clinics and transvaginal cervical length surveillance are two current management strategies utilized in attempts to reduce the risk of adverse outcomes associated with multifetal pregnancies. In these clinics, patients have the opportunity to develop rapport with a small group of dedicated caregivers [96]. Heightened awareness can increase compliance with therapeutic directives and mothers are able to provide psychologic support to one another. Another more commonly utilized strategy in managing multiples is cervical length measurements. Premature cervical shortening and cervical funneling detected by transvaginal ultrasound examina-

tion have good predictive capabilities for the development of preterm labor and delivery in women with multiple gestations [97–100]. Studies suggest that a cervical length measurement of ≥35 mm at 24–26 weeks identifies women with twins who are at low risk for delivery prior to 34 weeks' gestation [98]. On the other hand, a cervical length of 25 mm or less with or without funneling at 24 weeks' gestation predicts a high risk for preterm labor and delivery [97]. One study also found that a positive fetal fibronectin test at 28 weeks is a significant predictor of spontaneous preterm labor prior to 32 weeks' gestation [97].

Antenatal surveillance

Although it is prudent to follow fetal growth with serial ultrasound scans, routine antenatal testing in patients with an uncomplicated multiple gestation has not been demonstrated to improve outcomes. Antenatal testing is suggested in all patients with multiple gestations complicated by IUGR, discordant growth, abnormal amniotic fluid volumes, TTTS, monoamnionicity, fetal anomalies, single IUFD, and other medical or obstetric complications (Table 37.3). For women with twins, options for antenatal testing include the nonstress test, the biophysical profile, and Doppler velocimetry assessment if there is suspected IUGR.

When patients with a multiple gestation present for antenatal testing or labor monitoring, each fetal heart rate should be independently identified to ensure precision. Monitoring of triplets and high-order multiples may require frequent sonographic identification of the appropriate fetus.

Routine Doppler studies have not been found to be helpful in the management of women with multiple gestations [101,102]. However, when IUGR or growth discordance is suspected in one or more fetuses, Doppler velocimetry of the umbilical artery is a useful adjunct in assessing and following these pregnancies. Furthermore, in cases of monochorionic twins with IUGR, discordant growth, or amniotic fluid volume abnormalities, Doppler studies of the ductus venosus may be helpful in identifying the possible overlapping pathologies of uteroplacental insufficiency and cardiac dysfunction.

Intrapartum period

A number of factors must be considered when determining the mode of delivery for patients with multiple gestations. These variables include the gestational age and estimated weights of the fetuses, their positions, the availability of real time ultrasound on the labor floor and in the delivery room, the capability of monitoring each twin independently during the entire intrapartum period, and the health care provider experience. When both twins are vertex, vaginal delivery is possible. During the time period between the delivery of the first and second twin, it is important to demonstrate reassuring status of the undelivered twin as evidenced by continuous fetal heart rate monitoring or by ultrasound. If the presenting

Table 37.3 Ultrasound management of patients with twins.

1 Ideally, ultrasound is performed in the first trimester to determine the number of fetuses and amnionicity and chorionicity. Patients are also offered nuchal translucency ultrasound at 10–14 weeks' gestation

2 A detailed ultrasound is scheduled at 18–20 weeks' gestation. This includes standard biometry, assessment of amniotic fluid volume in each sac, and an anatomic survey of each fetus. If the patient did not have a first trimester ultrasound, an attempt is made to determine chorionicity by examining fetal gender, the number of placentas, the thickness as well as number of layers in the membrane separating the sacs, and the presence or absence of the lambda or twin peak sign

3 If the first two scans are suggestive of a dichorionic pregnancy, fetal growth is performed every 3–4 weeks thereafter as long as fetal growth and amniotic fluid volume in each sac remains normal

4 If the initial scan is suggestive of a monochorionic diamniotic pregnancy, subsequent scans are repeated every 2–3 weeks to follow for signs of TTTS. Fetal echocardiography is offered to patients with monochorionic twins because these pregnancies may be at increased risk for congenital heart defects

5 In either dichorionic or monochorionic pregnancies, if there is evidence of IUGR, discordant fetal growth, or discordant fluid volumes, fetal surveillance is intensified and includes frequent nonstress tests along with biophysical profile and Doppler velocimetry studies

6 Daily nonstress testing starting at approximately 24–26 weeks' gestation is suggested for patients with monoamniotic twins because of their risk for sudden IUFD from cord entanglement. Although cord accidents cannot be predicted, daily fetal heart rate monitoring may reveal increasing frequency of variable decelerations. When variable decelerations are identified, continuous monitoring is recommended and may ultimately require delivery for nonreassuring fetal testing

IUFD, intrauterine fetal death; IUGR, intrauterine growth restriction; TTTS, twin–twin transfusion syndrome.

twin is nonvertex, cesarean delivery is suggested. Management of vertex/nonvertex twins is variable. Vaginal delivery of a breech second twin with an estimated fetal weight of 1500–3500 g in a woman with an adequate pelvis is reasonable. Cesarean delivery may be the preferred route of delivery if there is significant growth discordance between the twins or if the provider does not have adequate experience with such deliveries. Some obstetricians have had favorable experiences delivering triplets vaginally. Nonetheless, most providers deliver triplets and higher order multiples by cesarean section because continuous fetal heart rate monitoring of triplets and higher order multiples in labor is challenging [3,68].

Conclusions

Advances in fertility treatment and delayed childbearing have resulted in a substantial increase in the incidence of multiple gestations. The high perinatal morbidity and mortality rates associated with multiple gestations are the result of a variety of factors, some which cannot be altered. Nonetheless, technological advances in recent years have given us new insights

into problems particular to multifetal pregnancies as well as tools with which to detect and treat these problems. Early diagnosis of multiple gestations and serial ultrasound studies are important in the management of these high-risk pregnancies and will hopefully have a beneficial impact on maternal and neonatal outcomes.

Case presentation

A 38-year-old gravida 1 with twins in the moderate preterm gestation presented to a routine prenatal care visit and reported an "upset stomach" the previous weekend. Her prenatal course was significant for a history of polycystic ovarian syndrome and an initial quadruplet pregnancy conceived with ovulation induction and intrauterine insemination. She had elected to have chorionic villus sampling and subsequent MPR to a dichorionic twin gestation. During a routine anatomic ultrasound survey at 20 weeks, the patient was noted to have a short cervix measuring 24 mm. Preterm labor precautions were reviewed, light activity was advised, and serial cervical length measurements were scheduled. At 28 weeks' gestation, the patient was diagnosed with gestational diabetes which subsequently required insulin for glycemic control.

At her office visit at 30w 6d gestation, the patient's blood pressure was 150/92 mmHg and a urine dipstick revealed 2+ proteinuria. She was admitted and corticosteroids administered to assist fetal lung maturation. After 72 hours of hospitalization, a 24-hour urine collection revealed 6 g protein and the patient developed unremitting epigastric pain. Laboratory evaluation revealed a platelet count of 70, liver enzymes of 530 and 478, and a lactic dehydrogenase (LDH) of 990; the findings were consistent with HELLP syndrome. A bedside ultrasound revealed the fetal presentations to be cephalic/breech. The cervix was 3 cm dilated with a Bishop score of 8. However, a 38% twin weight discordancy had been estimated during a routine scan at 30 weeks with a higher estimated fetal weight for twin B.

Immediate delivery was recommended and the risks and benefits of attempted vaginal delivery and cesarean were discussed. The patient underwent an uncomplicated, primary low transverse cesarean delivery. Vigorous male and female infants were born. Although each neonate spent a brief period in the neonatal ICU, they were both discharged home after 2 weeks. There were no postpartum maternal complications and she was discharged home on postoperative day 4.

This case highlights many of the common features of multiple pregnancy including assisted conception, MPR, medical and obstetric complications, and preterm delivery. While the outcome for the majority of multiple gestations is favorable, these high-risk pregnancies can be associated with maternal and neonatal morbidity and mortality and thus warrant increased vigilance.

References

1 Martin JA, Hamilton BE, Sutton PD, Ventura SJ, Menacker F, Munson ML. Births: Final data for 2003. *Natl Vital Stat Rep* 2003;**54**:1–116.

2 Beato CV. *Healthy People 2010 Progress Report: Maternal, Infant, and Child Health*. US Department of Health and Human Services. October 22, 2003.

3 American College of Obstetricians and Gynecologists. Multiple gestation: complicated twin, triplet, and high-order multifetal pregnancy. *ACOG Practice Bulletin No. 56*. October 2004.

4 Martin JA, Hamilton BE, Sutton PD, Ventura SJ, Menacker F, Munson ML. Births: Final Data for 2002. *Natl Vital Stat Rep* 2002;**52**:1–113.

5 Martin JA, Hamilton BE, Ventura SJ, Menacker F, Park MM, Sutton PD. Births: Final Data for 2001. *Natl Vital Stat Rep* 2001;**51**:1–102.

6 Nielson HC, Harvey-Wilkes K, MacKinnon B, Hung S. Neonatal outcome of very premature infants from multiple and singleton gestations. *Am J Obstet Gynecol* 1997;**177**:653–9.

7 Kaufman GE, Malone FD, Harvey-Wilkes KB, Chelmow D, Penzias AS, D'Alton ME. Neonatal morbidity and mortality associated with triplet pregnancy. *Obstet Gynecol* 1998;**91**:342–8.

8 Topp M, Huusom LD, Langhoff-Roos J, *et al.* Multiple birth and cerebral palsy in Europe: a multicenter study. *Acta Obstet Gynecol Scand* 2004;**83**:548–53.

9 Neonatal Encephalopathy and Cerebral Palsy: Defining the Pathogenesis and Pathophysiology. ACOG 2003.

10 Yokoyama Y, Shimizu T, Hayakawa K. Prevalence of cerebral palsy in twins, triplets and quadruplets. *Int J Epidemiol* 1995;**24**:943–8.

11 Russell EM. Cerebral palsied twins. *Arch Dis Child* 1961;**36**:328–36.

12 Benirschke K. The biology of the twinning process: how placentation influences outcome. *Semin Perinatol* 1995;**19**:342–50.

13 Souter VL, Kapur RP, Nyholt DR, *et al.* A report of dizygous monochorionic twins. *N Engl J Med* 2003;**349**:154–8.

14 Miura K, Niikawa NJ. Do monochorionic dizygotic twins increase after pregnancy by assisted reproductive technology? *Hum Genet* 2005;**50**:1–6.

15 Barth RA, Crowe HC. Ultrasound evaluation of multifetal gestations. In: Callen PW, (ed.) *Ultrasonography in Obstetrics and Gynecology*, 4th edn. Philadelphia: W.B. Saunders, 2000: 171.

16 Bromley B, Benacerraf B. Using the number of yolk sacs to determine amnionicity in early first trimester monochorionic twins. *J Ultrasound Med* 1995;**14**:415–9.

17 Bessis R, Papiernik E. Echographic imagery of amniotic membranes in twin pregnancies. In: Gedda L, Parisi P, (eds). *Twin Research 3: Twin Biology and Multiple Pregnancy*. New York: Alan R. Liss, 1981:183.

18 Finberg HJ. The "twin peak" sign: reliable evidence of dichorionic twinning. *J Ultrasound Med* 1992;**11**:571–7.

19 Monteagudo A, Timor-Tritsch IE, Sharma S. Early and simple determination of chorionic and amniotic type in multifetal gestations in the first fourteen weeks by high-frequency transvaginal ultrasonography. *Am J Obstet Gynecol* 1994;**170**:824–9.

20 Sepulveda W, Seibre NJ, Hughes K, *et al.* The lambda sign at 10–14 weeks of gestation as a predictor of chorionicity in twin pregnancies. *Ultrasound Obstet Gynecol* 1996;**7**:421–3.

21 Egan JFX, Borgida AF. Multiple gestations: the importance of ultrasound. *Obstet Gynecol Clin North Am* 2004;**31**:141–58.

22 Nyberg DA, Filly RA, Golbus MS, *et al.* Entangled umbilical cords: a sign of monoamniotic twins. *J Ultrasound Med* 1984;**3**:29–32.

23 Norwitz ER, Valentine E, Park JS. Maternal physiology and complications of multiple pregnancy. *Semin Perinatol* 2005;**29**:338–48.

24 Demissie K, Ananth CV, Martin J, *et al.* Fetal and neonatal mortality among twin gestations in the United States: the role of intrapair birth weight discordance. *Obstet Gynecol* 2002;**100**:474–80.

25 Blickstein I, Keith LG. Neonatal mortality rates among growth-discordant twins, classified according to the birth weight of the smaller twin. *Am J Obstet Gynecol* 2004;**190**:170–4.

26 Amaru RC, Bush MC, Berkowitz RL, Lapinski RH, Gaddipati S. Is discordant growth in twins an independent risk factor for adverse neonatal outcome? *Obstet Gynecol* 2004;**103**:71–6.

27 Landy HJ, Keith L, Keith D. The vanishing twin. *Acta Genet Med Gemellol (Roma)* 1982;**31**:179–94.

28 Cleary-Goldman J, D'Alton M. Management of single fetal demise in a multiple gestation. *Obstet Gynecol Surv* 2004;**59**:285–98.

29 Landry HJ, Weingold AB. Management of a multiple gestation complicated by antepartum fetal demise. *Obstet Gynecol Surv* 1989;**44**:171–6.

30 Okamura K, Murotsuki J, Tanigawara S, Uehara S, Yajima A. Funipuncture for evaluation of hematologic and coagulation indices in the surviving twin following co-twins death. *Obstet Gynecol* 1994;**83**:975–8.

31 Fusi L, McParland P, Fisk N, Wigglesworth J. Acute twin–twin transfusion: a possible mechanism for brain-damaged survivors after intrauterine death of a monochorionic twin. *Obstet Gynecol* 1991;**78**:517–20.

32 Weiss JL, Cleary-Goldman J, Budorick N, Tanji K, D'Alton ME. Multicystic encephalomalacia after first trimester intrauterine fetal demise in monochorionic twins. *Am J Obstet Gynecol* 2004;**190**: 563–5.

33 Carlson N, Towers C. Multiple gestation complicated by the death of one fetus. *Obstet Gynecol* 1989;**73**:685–9.

34 Onyskowova A, Dolezal A, Jedlicka V. The frequency and the character of malformations in multiple birth (a preliminary report). *Teratology* 1971;**4**:496.

35 Hendricks CH. Twinning in relation to birth weight, mortality, and congenital anomalies. *Obstet Gynecol* 1966;**27**:47–53.

36 Kohl SG, Casey G. Twin gestation. *Mt Sinai J Med* 1975;**42**:523–39.

37 Benirschke K, Kim CK. Multiple pregnancy [first of two parts]. *N Engl J Med* 1973;**288**:1276–84.

38 Spadola AC, Simpson LL. Selective termination procedures in monochorionic pregnancies. *Semin Perinatol* 2005;**29**:330–7.

39 Malone FD, Craigo SD, Chelmow D, D'Alton ME. Outcome of twin gestations complicated by a single anomalous fetus. *Obstet Gynecol* 1996;**88**:1–5.

40 Sebire NJ, Sepulveda W, Hughes KS, *et al.* Management of twin pregnancies discordant for anencephaly. *Br J Obstet Gynaecol* 1997;**107**:216–9.

41 Gul A, Cebecia A, Aslan H, *et al*. Perinatal outcomes of twin pregnancies discordant for major fetal anomalies. *Fetal Diagn Ther* 2005;**20**:244–8.

42 D'Alton ME, Simpson LL. Syndromes in twins. *Semin Perinatol* 1995;**19**:375–86.

43 Carr SR, Aronson MP, Coustan DR. Survival rates of monoamniotic twins do not decrease after 30 weeks' gestation. *Am J Obstet Gynecol* 1990;**163**:719–22.

44 Rodis JF, McIlveen PF, Egan JF, *et al*. Monoamniotic twins: improved perinatal survival with accurate prenatal diagnosis and antenatal fetal surveillance. *Am J Obstet Gynecol* 1997;**177**:1046–9.

45 Allen VM, Windrim R, Barrett J, *et al*. Management of monoamniotic twin pregnancies: a case series and systematic review of the literature. *Br J Obstet Gynaecol* 2001;**108**:931–6.

46 Rogue H, Gillen-Goldstein J, Funai E, *et al*. Perinatal outcomes in monoamniotic gestations. *J Mat Fetal Neonatal Med* 2003;**13**:414–21.

47 Tessen JA, Zlatnik FJ. Monoamniotic twins: a retrospective controlled study. *Obstet Gynecol* 1991;**77**:832–4.

48 Blickstein I, Verhoeven HC, Keith LG. Zygotic splitting after assisted reproduction. *N Engl J Med* 1999;**340**:738–9.

49 Blickstein I. Estimation of iatrogenic monozygotic twinning rate following assisted reproduction: pitfalls and caveats. *Am J Obstet Gynecol* 2005;**192**:365–8.

50 Jain V, Fisk NM. The twin–twin transfusion syndrome. *Clin Obstet Gynecol* 2004;**47**:181–202.

51 Malone FD, D'Alton ME. Anomalies peculiar to multiple gestations. *Clin Perinatol* 2000;**27**:1033–46.

52 Quintero RA, Morales WJ, Allen MH, Bornick PW, Johnson PK, Kruger M. Staging of twin–twin transfusion syndrome. *J Perinatol* 1999;**19**:550–5.

53 Bajoria R, Wigglesworth J, Fisk NM. Angioarchitecture of monochorionic placentas in relation to the twin–twin transfusion syndrome. *Am J Obstet Gynecol* 1995;**172**:856–63.

54 Hecher K, Plath H, Bregenzer T, Hansmann M, Hackeloer BJ. Endoscopic laser surgery versus serial amniocenteses in the treatment of severe twin–twin transfusion syndrome. *Am J Obstet Gynecol* 1999;**180**:717–24.

55 Quintero RA, Dickinson JE, Morales WJ, *et al*. Stage-based treatment of twin twin transfusion syndrome. *Am J Obstet Gynecol* 2003;**188**:1333–40.

56 Senat MV, Deprest J, Boulvain M, Paupe A, Winer N, Ville Y. Endoscopic laser surgery versus serial amnioreduction for severe twin-to-twin transfusion syndrome. *N Engl J Med* 2004;**351**:136–44.

57 Devine PC, Malone FD, Athanassiou A, Harvey-Wilkes K, D'Alton ME. Maternal and neonatal outcome of 100 consecutive triplet pregnancies. *Am J Perinatol* 2001;**18**:225–35.

58 Graham G, Simpson LL. Diagnosis and management of obstetrical complications unique to multiple gestations. *Clin Obstet Gynecol* 2004;**47**:163–80.

59 Campbell DM, Templeton A. Maternal complications of twin pregnancy. *Int J Gynaecol Obstet* 2004;**84**:71–3.

60 American College of Obstetricians and Gynecologists. Thromboembolism in pregnancy. *ACOG Practice Bulletin No. 19*. August 2000.

61 American College of Obstetricians and Gynecologists. Diagnosis and management of preeclampsia and eclampsia. *ACOG Practice Bulletin No. 33*. January 2002.

62 Sibai BM, Hauth J, Caritis S, *et al*. Hypertensive disorders in twin versus singleton gestations. National Institute of Child Health and Human Development Network of Maternal-Fetal Medicine Units. *Am J Obstet Gynecol* 2000;**182**:938–42.

63 Caritis S, Sibai B, Hauth J, *et al*. Low-dose aspirin to prevent preeclampsia in women at high risk. National Institute of Child Health and Human Development Network of Maternal-Fetal Medicine Units. *N Engl J Med* 1998;**338**:701–5.

64 Levine RJ, Hauth JC, Curet LB, *et al*. Trial of calcium to prevent preeclampsia. *N Engl J Med* 1997;**337**:69–76.

65 Maxwell CV, Lieberman E, Norton M, Cohen A, Seely EW, Lee-Parritz A. Relationship of twin zygosity and risk of preeclampsia. *Am J Obstet Gynecol* 2001;**185**:819–21.

66 Hardardottir H, Kelly K, Bork MD, Cusick W, Campbell WA, Rodis JF. Atypical presentation of preeclampsia in high-order multifetal gestations. *Obstet Gynecol* 1996;**87**:370–4.

67 Davidson KM, Simpson LL, Knox TA, D'Alton ME. Acute fatty liver of pregnancy in triplet gestation. *Obstet Gynecol* 1998;**91**:806–8.

68 American College of Obstetricians and Gynecologists and the American Academy of Pediatrics. *Guidelines for Perinatal Care*, 5th edn. Washington DC, 2002.

69 Bush MC, Malone FD. Down syndrome screening in twins. *Clin Perinatol* 2005;**32**:373–86.

70 Stone J, Eddleman K, Lynch L, Berkowitz RL. A single center experience with 1000 consecutive cases of multifetal pregnancy reduction. *Am J Obstet Gynecol* 2002;**187**:1163–7.

71 Malone FD, D'Alton ME. Anomalies peculiar to multiple gestations. *Clin Perinatol* 2000;**27**:1033–46.

72 Cleary-Goldman J, D'Alton ME, Berkowitz RL. Prenatal diagnosis and multiple pregnancy. *Semin Perinatol* 2005;**29**:312–20.

73 Rogers JG, Voullaire L, Gold H. Monozygotic twins discordant for trisomy 21. *Am J Med Genet* 1982;**11**:143–6.

74 Dallapiccola B, Stomeo C, Ferranti B, *et al*. Discordant sex in one of three monozygotic triplets. *J Med Genet* 1985;**22**:6–11.

75 Meyers C, Adam R, Dungan J, Prenger V. Aneuploidy in twin gestations: when is maternal age advanced? *Obstet Gynecol* 1997;**89**:248–51.

76 Odibo AO, Elkousy MH, Ural SH, *et al*. Screening for aneuploidy in twin pregnancies: maternal age- and race-specific risk assessment between 9–14 weeks. *Twin Res* 2003;**6**:251–6.

77 Jenkins TM, Wapner RJ. The challenge of prenatal diagnosis in twin pregnancies. *Curr Opin Obstet Gynecol* 2000;**12**:87–92.

78 Odibo AO, Lawrence-Cleary K, Macones GA. Screening for aneuploidy in twins and higher-order multiples: is first-trimester nuchal translucency the solution? *Obstet Gynecol Surv* 2003;**58**:609–14.

79 Sebire NJ, D'Ercole C, Hughes K, Carvalho M, Nicolaides KH. Increased nuchal translucency thickness at 10–14 weeks of gestation as a predictor of severe twin-to-twin transfusion syndrome. *Ultrasound Obstet Gynecol* 1997;**10**:86–9.

80 Malone FD, D'Alton ME, Society for Maternal-Fetal Medicine. First-trimester sonographic screening for Down syndrome. *Obstet Gynecol* 2003;**102**:1066–79.

81 Spencer K, Nicolaides KH. Screening for trisomy 21 in twins using first trimester ultrasound and maternal serum biochemistry in a one stop clinic: a review of three years experience. *Br J Obstet Gynaecol* 2003;**110**:276–80.

82 Graham G, Simpson LL. Diagnosis and management of obstetrical complications unique to multiple gestations. *Clin Obstet Gynecol* 2004;**47**:163–80.

83 Wapner RJ. Genetic diagnosis in multiple pregnancies. *Semin Perinatol* 1995;**19**:351–62.

84 Edwards MS, Ellings JM, Newman RB, *et al*. Predictive value of antepartum ultrasound examination for anomalies in twin gestations. *Ultrasound Obstet Gynecol* 1995;**6**:43–9.

85 National Institutes of Health. National Institutes of Health Consensus Development Conference Statement: Effect of corticosteroids for fetal maturation on perinatal outcomes, February 28–March 2, 1994. *Am J Obstet Gynecol* 1995;**173**:246–52.

86 Mercer BM, Miodovnik M, Thurnau GR, *et al*. Antibiotic therapy for reduction of infant morbidity after preterm premature rupture of the membranes: a randomized controlled trial. *JAMA* 1997;**278**:989–95.

87 Lovett SM, Weiss JD, Diogo MJ, Williams PT, Garite TJ. A prospective double-blind, randomized, controlled clinical trial of ampicillin-sulbactam for preterm premature rupture of membranes in women receiving antenatal corticosteroid therapy. *Am J Obstet Gynecol* 1997;**176**:1030–8.

88 Newman RB, Krombach RS, Myers MC, *et al*. Effect of cerclage on obstetric outcome in twin gestations with a shortened cervical length. *Am J Obstet Gynecol* 2002;**186**:634–40.

89 Elimian A, Figueroa R, Nigam S, *et al*. Perinatal outcome of triplet gestation: does prophylactic cerclage make a difference? *J Maternal Fetal Med* 1999;**8**:119–22.

90 Berghella V, Odibo AO, To MS, Rust OA, Althuisius SM. Cerclage for short cervix on ultrasonography: meta-analysis of trials using individual patient-level data. *Obstet Gynecol* 2005;**106**:181–9.

91 Saunders MC, Dick JS, Brown IM, McPherson K, Chalmers I. The effects of hospital admission for bed rest on the duration of twin pregnancy: a randomized trial. *Lancet* 1985;**2**:793–5.

92 Crowther CA. Hospitalization and bed rest for multiple pregnancy. *Cochrane Database Syst Rev* 2001;**1**:CD000110.

93 Katz M, Robertson PA, Creasy RK. Cardiovascular complications associated with terbutaline treatment for preterm labor. *Am J Obstet Gynecol* 1981;**139**:605–8.

94 Colton T, Kayne HL, Zhang Y, *et al*. A meta-analysis of home uterine activity monitoring. *Am J Obstet Gynecol* 1995;**173**:1499–505.

95 Dyson DC, Danbe KH, Bamber JA, *et al*. Monitoring women at risk for preterm labor. *N Engl J Med* 1998;**338**:15–9.

96 Luke B, Brown MB, Misiunas R, *et al*. Specialized prenatal care and maternal and infant outcomes in twin pregnancy. *Am J Obstet Gynecol* 2003;**189**:934–8.

97 Goldenberg RL, Iams JD, Miodovnik M, *et al*. The preterm prediction study: risk factors in twin gestations. National Institute of Child Health and Human Development Maternal-Fetal Medicine Units Network. *Am J Obstet Gynecol* 1996;**175**:1047–53.

98 Imseis HM, Albert TA, Iams JD. Identifying twin gestations at low risk for preterm birth with a transvaginal ultrasonographic cervical measurement at 24 to 26 weeks' gestation. *Am J Obstet Gynecol* 1997;**177**:1149–55.

99 Ramin KD, Ogburn PL Jr, Mulholland TA, *et al*. Ultrasonographic assessment of cervical length in triplet pregnancies. *Am J Obstet Gynecol* 1999;**180**:1442–5.

100 Gibson JL, Macara LM, Owen P, Young D, Maculey J, Mackenzie F. Prediction of preterm delivery in twin pregnancy: a prospective, observational study of cervical length and fetal fibronectin testing. *Ultrasound Obstet Gynecol* 2004;**23**:561–6.

101 Geipel A, Berg C, Germer U, *et al*. Doppler assessment in the uterine circulation in the second trimester in twin pregnancies: prediction of pre-eclampsia, fetal growth restriction and birth weight discordance. *Ultrasound Obstet Gynecol* 2002;**20**:541–5.

102 Giles W, Bisits A, O'Callahan S, Gill A, DAMP Study Group. The Doppler assessment in multiple pregnancy randomised controlled trial of ultrasound biometry versus umbilical artery Doppler ultrasound and biometry in twin pregnancy. *Br J Obstet Gynaecol* 2003;**110**:593–7.

38 Polyhydramnios and oligohydramnios

Michael G. Ross, Ron Beloosesky, and John T. Queenan

"All that fluid which is contained in the ovum is called by the general name of the waters. The quantity, in proportion to the size of the different parts of the ovum, is greatest by far in early pregnancy. At the time of parturition, in some cases, it amounts to or exceeds four pints. In others, it is scarcely equal to as many ounces. It is usually in the largest quantity when the child has been some time dead, or is born in a weakly state."

T. Denman, 1815

In 1815, Denman [1] recognized the great variation in amniotic fluid (AF) volume and associated polyhydramnios with congenital malformations, fetal death, and fetal disease. Although our current knowledge of the intrauterine environment has expanded manyfold, we have not overturned any of Denman's concepts [1].

Polyhydramnios and oligohydramnios are pathologic conditions representing excess AF and diminished AF, respectively. Numerous serious clinical conditions are associated with polyhydramnios and oligohydramnios. An understanding of the normal AF parameters and the AF turnover is appropriate before embarking into the pathologic considerations.

Normal AF composition and volume

During the first trimester, AF is isotonic with maternal plasma [2] but contains minimal protein. It is thought that the fluid arises either from a transudate of fetal plasma through non-keratinized fetal skin, or maternal plasma across the uterine decidua and/or placenta surface [3]. Thus, fetuses with renal agenesis may demonstrate normal first trimester AF volumes (Table 38.1). With advancing gestation, AF osmolality and sodium concentration decrease, a result of the mixture of dilute fetal urine and isotonic fetal lung liquid production. In comparison with the first half of pregnancy, AF osmolality decreases by 20–30 mOsm/kg with advancing gestation to levels approximately 85–90% of maternal serum osmolality [4] in the human, although there was no osmolality decrease in the AF near term in the rat [5]. AF urea, creatinine, and uric

acid increase during the second half of pregnancy, resulting in AF concentrations of the urinary byproducts two to three times higher than fetal plasma [4].

Throughout the history of medicine, investigators have been intrigued with the concept of quantitating the volume of AF. In 1966, Charles and Jacoby [6] described a technique to measure the volume of AF by *para*-aminohippurate (PAH), a dye dilution technique. In 1972, Queenan *et al.* [7], using this technique, measured the AF volumes in 187 samples from 115 patients with normal pregnancies. The volumes varied widely for the various weeks of gestation. The mean volumes were 239 mL at 25–26 weeks, 984 mL at 33–34 weeks (the peak volume), 836 mL at term, and 544 mL at 41–42 weeks (Fig. 38.1).

Brace and Wolf [8] analyzed AF volumes in 12 published studies including 705 normal pregnancies at 8–43 weeks' gestation. They found that AF volume rises linearly from early gestation until 32 weeks, whereupon it remains constant until term, ranging between 700 and 800 mL. After 40 weeks, AF volume declines at a rate of 8% a week, to an average of 400 mL at 42 weeks. At 30 weeks' gestation, the 95% confidence intervals about the mean (817 mL) covers the range 18–2100 mL. Thus, a volume less than 318 mL is considered oligohydramnios and more than 2100 mL polyhydramnios. The wide biologic variability in the AF volume with advancing gestational age, especially before 32–35 weeks makes an absolute volume criterion for oligohydramnios or polyhydramnios inappropriate. Accordingly, AF volume abnormalities are best defined as a volume below the 5th percentile or above the 95th percentile for gestational age.

Dynamics of AF turnover

AF is produced and resorbed in a dynamic process with large volumes of water circulated between the AF and fetal compartments. During the latter half of gestation, the primary sources of AF include fetal urine excretion and fluid secreted

Table 38.1 Typical increases in amniotic fluid.

Gestation (weeks)	Fluid Volume (mL)
12	50
14	100
16	150
18	200
20	250

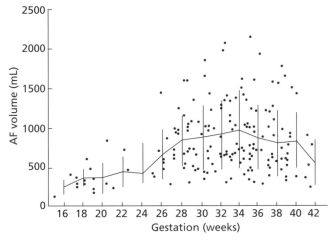

Fig. 38.1 Normal AF (AF) volumes are plotted against weeks of gestation. The mean values 6 ± 1 SD are calculated for each 2-week period. (From Queenan *et al.* [7] with permission.)

by the fetal lung. The primary pathways for water exit from the AF include removal by fetal swallowing and intramembranous absorption across the fetal membranes into fetal blood. If the balance of fluid exchange is disturbed, polyhydramnios or oligohydramnios develops. For instance, if a pathologic condition increased the AF volume by 1 oz or 30 mL/day, 1 L of excess AF would accumulate in a month.

Fetal urine

Since the days of Hippocrates, physicians have believed that the fetus voids *in utero*. Today, fetal micturition is known to be the major source of AF. Chez *et al.* [9] studied fetal urine production with indwelling catheters in rhesus monkeys, and reported the rate to be 5 mL/kg/hour, which correlates with the rate of swallowing in Pritchard's studies [10]. In humans, fetal urine production changes with increasing gestation. The amount of urine produced by the human fetus has been estimated by the use of ultrasound assessment of fetal bladder volume [11], although the accuracy of these measurements has been called into question. Exact human fetal urine production rates across gestation are not established but appear to be in the range of 25% of bodyweight per day or nearly 1000 mL/day near term [11,12]. Biochemical studies also attest to the importance of fetal micturition in determining AF volume. AF

is isotonic in early pregnancy, but by term it becomes hypotonic, a result of the increased contribution of hypotonic urine.

Kurjak *et al.* [13] studied fetal renal function in 255 normal singleton pregnancies and 133 complicated pregnancies between 22 and 41 weeks' gestation. They evaluated the hourly fetal urine production rate (HFUPR), fetal glomerular filtration rate (GFR), fetal tubular water reabsorption (TWR), and the effect of furosemide on fetal micturition by sonography and biochemical tests. In normal pregnancies, the HFUPR increased from 2.2 mL/hour at 22 weeks to 26.3 mL/hour at 40 weeks' gestation. The fetal GFR was 2.66 mL/min at term and the percentage of TWR was 78%. In growth restricted fetuses, the HFUPR was below the 10th centile in 59% and was above normal in only 6%. The diuretic effect of furosemide was the same in growth restricted and in normal fetuses. In diabetic pregnancies, HFUPR values varied considerably and correlated with fetal size. In 90% of pregnancies with polyhydramnios, the HFUPR was normal.

Oligohydramnios is associated with severe malformations of the fetal urinary system (e.g., renal agenesis), which is incompatible with urine production. In a review of 295 fetuses with renal agenesis, Jeffcoate and Scott [14] found sufficient clinical data in 100 to establish a diagnosis of oligohydramnios. From these data, the investigators inferred that conditions affecting fetal urine production would alter the AF volume. On the other hand, they also reported renal agenesis in a fetus with polyhydramnios. Others reported renal agenesis and normal AF volume [15,16].

Fetal lung fluid

As early as 1888, investigators believed that the fetus made respiratory movements near term [17]. Since then, fetal respiratory movements have been documented and are currently one component of a test of fetal well-being, the biophysical profile. It was originally believed that the fetal lungs absorbed fluid, as evidenced by the finding of meconium in the bronchial trees. However, it is now recognized that all mammalian fetuses normally secrete fluid from their lungs. In the human, AF clearly contains phospholipids, such as lecithin and sphingomyelin derived from type II aveolar cells; thus, at least some of the tracheal fluid contributes to the AF volume. Liley [18] described some 800 mothers who had radiologic contrast media injected into the AF and noted that only four had the medium demonstrated in the fetal or neonatal lungs.

The absolute rate of fluid production by the human fetal lungs has not been determined, although animal studies suggest that the respiratory tract has a major role in AF production. Goodlin and Lloyd [19] demonstrated that the fetal lamb produces 50–80 mL/day tracheal fluid. Adamson *et al.* [20] reported that the near term lamb has tracheal secretions of 200–400 mL/day. Tracheal ligation in animals leads to overdistention of the lungs, suggesting a relatively large outflow of fluid from the lungs. This knowledge has been utilized in the development of therapeutic approaches to the treatment of diaphragmatic hernia; tracheal occlusion results in pulmonary distension despite the presence of a thoracic mass. Under physiologic conditions, half of the fluid exiting the lungs enters the AF and half is swallowed [21], therefore an average of approximately 165 mL/day lung liquid enters the AF near term. Fetal lung fluid production is affected by physiologic and endocrine factors, but nearly all stimuli have been demonstrated to reduce fetal lung liquid production, with no evidence of stimulated production and nominal changes in fluid composition. Increased arginine vasopressin [22], catecholamines [23] and cortisol [24] decrease lung fluid production. The marked increase in fetal plasma levels of these hormones during labor results in a cessation of lung fluid production, after which lung liquid is resorbed into pulmonary lymphatics to prepare for newborn respiration.

Fetal swallowing

Swallowing is the major pathway for AF removal. Evidence of fetal swallowing of AF was established many years ago by amniography, a technique used to outline the fetal abdominal cavity for intrauterine transfusions [25]. Studies of near term pregnancies suggest that the human fetus swallows an average of 210–760 mL/day [26], which is considerably less than the volume of urine produced each day. However, fetal swallowing may be reduced beginning a few days before delivery [27], so the rate of human fetal swallowing is probably underestimated. Fetal swallowing is increased during active as compared with quiet sleep states. Furthermore, the near term fetus develops functional ingestive responses such that fetal swallowing may increase in response to thirst or appetite stimulation. Of note, fetal swallowing decreases with acute arterial hypotension [28] or hypoxia [21,29], indicating that oligohydramnios associated with fetal hypoxia is not caused by increased AF resorption via swallowing.

The effect of fetal swallowing can be demonstrated by studying mothers who have delivered babies with tracheoesophageal fistulas. Of 228 such cases, 25 fetuses had complete obstruction between the mouth and the stomach and 19 (76%) of these had polyhydramnios [30]. In a study of 169 cases of polyhydramnios, 54 (32%) of the fetuses were unable to swallow [14].

Anencephaly is also associated with a high incidence of polyhydramnios. Although swallowing has been demonstrated in some of these fetuses, it is reasonable to believe that the swallowing capability is reduced or absent in many. Surprisingly, Abramovich [31] demonstrated in eight anencephalic fetuses and one microcephalic fetus that those with the low AF volumes appeared to have reduced swallowing, whereas three fetuses with polyhydramnios appeared to swallow normal amounts. In light of these findings, he suggested that the presence or absence of swallowing has little effect on the etiology of polyhydramnios in anencephaly.

The exposed meninges in anencephaly have been described as the source of the production of the excess AF [32]. Other authors disagreed [33], noting that the rudimentary and distorted brain is almost always covered with a collagen membrane. They proposed that fetal polyuria may contribute to the polyhydramnios because anencephalic fetuses lack antidiuretic hormone. Naeye et al. [34] also suggested that polyuria of the anencephalic fetus causes polyhydramnios.

How important swallowing is in controlling AF volume remains undefined. An inability to swallow in the setting of esophageal atresia but not in anencephaly appears to result in polyhydramnios in some cases.

Intramembranous flow

The amount of fluid swallowed by the fetus does not equal the amount of fluid produced by both the kidneys and the lungs in either human or ovine gestation. As the volume of AF does not greatly increase during the last half of pregnancy, another route of fluid absorption is needed. The intramembranous (IM) pathway refers to the route of absorption between the fetal circulation and the amniotic cavity directly across the amnion. Although the contribution of the IM pathway to the overall regulation and maintenance of AF volume and composition has yet to be completely understood, results from in vivo and in vitro studies of ovine membrane permeability suggest that the permeability of the fetal chorioamnion is important in determining AF composition and volume [35–37]. This IM flow, recirculating AF water to the fetal compartment, is thought to be driven by the significant osmotic gradient between the hypotonic AF and isotonic fetal plasma [38]. In addition, electrolytes (e.g., Na^+) may diffuse down a concentration gradient from fetal plasma into the AF while - peptides (e.g., arginine vasopressin [39,40]) and other electrolytes (e.g., Cl^-) may be recirculated to the fetal plasma.

Although never directly measured in humans, indirect evidence supports the presence of IM flow. Studies of intra-amniotic ^{51}Cr injection demonstrated appearance of the tracer in the circulation of fetuses with impaired swallowing [41]. Additionally, alterations in IM flow may contribute to AF clinical abnormalities, as membrane ultrastructure changes are noted with polyhydramnios or oligohydramnios [42]. Experimental estimates of the net IM flow averages 200–250 mL/day in fetal sheep and likely balances the flow of urine and lung liquid with fetal swallowing under homeostatic conditions.

AF turnover

The AF is constantly recirculating. When diffusion of water is measured, approximately 500 mL water enters and leaves the amniotic sac each hour, with little effect on the total AF volume. However, estimates of actual bulk flow of water suggest that approximately 1000 mL/day enter and leave the amniotic cavity at term. This results in a turnover of the entire volume of AF each day.

Clinical measurement of AF

A few decades ago, AF volume was estimated in crude ways such as measurement of fundal height, roentgenographic, or direct measurement at the time of delivery. The PAH dye dilution technique provides an accurate measurement but is an invasive technique and therefore limited to research [6].

Ultrasound examination is the only practical clinical means of assessing the AF volume. Several ultrasound methods have been used to estimate the AF volume; each has limitations in the detection of abnormal AF volumes. These methods can better identify true normal AF volumes than abnormal AF volumes (oligohydramnios and polyhydramnios), which they all detect poorly.

The single deepest pocket (SDP) measurement refers to the vertical dimension of the largest pocket of AF not containing umbilical cord or fetal extremities and measured at a right angle to the uterine contour. The horizontal component of this vertical dimension must be at least 1 cm. A normal SDP measurement is 2.1–8 cm, with oligohydramnios defined as less than 2.0 cm and polyhydramnios as more than 8.0 cm. In a comparison of SDP with dye-determined AF volume, SDP poorly identifies patients with oligohydramnios [43,44].

The AF index (AFI) is measured by first dividing the uterus into four quadrants using the linea nigra for the right and left divisions and the umbilicus for the upper and lower quadrants. The maximum vertical AF pocket diameter in each quadrant not containing cord or fetal extremities is measured in centimeters; the sum of these measurements is the AFI. A normal AFI is 5.1–25 cm, with oligohydramnios defined as less than 5.0 cm and polyhydramnios as more than 25 cm (Table 38.2). The accuracy of the AFI has been examined in several studies [43,45–48]. In comparison to dye dilution, the AFI overestimated actual volumes by 89% at low volumes and underestimated actual volumes by 54% at high volumes. Chauhan *et al.* [47] demonstrated the sensitivity, specificity, positive, and negative predictive values of AFI ≤5 for prediction of oligohydramnios were 5%, 98%, 80%, and 49%; these same characteristics for AFI >24 for prediction of polyhydramnios were 30%, 98%, 57%, and 93%, respectively.

Table 38.2 Diagnostic categories of the amniotic fluid index (AFI). (From Moore and Cayle [68] with permission.)

AF Volume	Percent of Patients	AFI Value (cm)
Severe oligohydramnios	2	≤5
Moderate oligohydramnios	20	5.1–8.0
Normal	76	8.1–24.0
Polyhydramnios	2	>24

The two diameter AF pocket is the product of the vertical depth multiplied by the horizontal diameter of the largest pocket of AF not containing umbilical cord or extremities (with the transducer held at a right angle to the uterine contour). A normal two-dimensional measurement is 15.1–50 cm^2, with oligohydramnios defined as less than 15 cm^2 and polyhydramnios as more than 50 cm^2. Two series that compared the two diameter pocket and dye-determined AF volume found that the former identified 81–94% of the dye-determined normal volumes and approximately 60% of pregnancies with low volumes [43,46]. Receiver operator curve analysis showed that for any specific two diameter pocket, the 95% confidence range was so wide that ultrasonographic assessment was not a reasonable reflection of actual AF volume, and thus was not clinically useful [47].

Subjective assessment of AF volume refers to visual interpretation without sonographic measurements [49]. The ultrasonographer scans the uterine contents and subsequently reports the AF volume as oligohydramnios, normal, or polyhydramnios. One study involving 63 pregnancies compared the subjective assessment of AF volume with ultrasound measurement of AFI, the single deepest pocket technique, and the two diameter pocket method in the identification of dye-determined AF volume [49]. The subjective assessment of AF volume by an experienced examiner had a similar sensitivity to the other techniques for identifying dye-determined AF volumes.

All obstetric ultrasound examinations should include an assessment of AF volume. Although the ultrasonographer may elect to use only a subjective assessment, we recommend use of an objective measure (e.g., AFI) if the subjective assessment is abnormal, in patients at increased risk of pregnancy complications, and in all patients examined in the third trimester.

Polyhydramnios

Definition

Historically, polyhydramnios has been characterized by an excessive accumulation of AF, usually more than 2000 mL. However, this definition does not take the normal physiologic changes that occur in the volume of AF as the gestational weeks change. There is a progressive increase in AF volume from a mean of 30 mL at 10 weeks to 190 mL at 16 weeks, peaking at 780 mL at 32–35 weeks' gestation; thereafter, AF volume progressively decreases to approximately 550 mL at 42 weeks [8]. The wide biologic variability in the AF volume with advancing gestational age makes an absolute volume criterion for oligohydramnios or polyhydramnios inappropriate. Accordingly, AF volume abnormalities are best defined as a volume below the 5th percentile or above the 95th percentile for gestational age.

Diagnosis

Polyhydramnios is generally a problem of the late second to early third trimester. The clinician may notice that the uterus is consistently larger than expected for the stage of gestation, or there may be a sudden increase in uterine size. The fetal parts may be difficult to palpate and the fetal heart may be difficult to hear with Doppler ultrasound if the fetus moves about in the large volume of AF.

The diagnosis of polyhydramnios can be confirmed by sonography by quantifying the AF. When one is scanning the pregnant uterus, it is possible to make a qualitative judgment as to the presence or absence of polyhydramnios. At 16 weeks' gestation, when genetic amniocentesis is commonly performed, the fetus and placenta each weigh approximately 100 g and the AF volume is 200 mL. Therefore, at this time the AF volume constitutes approximately 50% of the uterine image (Table 38.3). At 28 weeks, when the fetus weighs 1000 g and the placenta weighs 200 g, the AF volume is approximately 1000 mL, and comprises approximately 45% of the image of the uterus. At term, when the fetus and placenta weigh 3300 and 500 g, respectively, the AF volume is approximately 800 mL and makes up only approximately 17% of the image of the uterus (Table 38.3). Keeping these guidelines in mind will facilitate making a judgment about the normalcy of AF volume versus polyhydramnios or oligohydramnios.

In severe cases, the mere image confirms the diagnosis because the findings are dramatic. Nonetheless, it is useful to have a quantifiable value such as the AFI. The diagnosis of polyhydramnios is established by an AFI ≥25 cm.

Table 38.3 Typical amniotic fluid (AF) volumes.

Gestation (weeks)	Fetus (g)	Placenta (g)	AF Volume (mL)	AF as % of Total
16	100	100	200	50
28	1000	200	1000	45
36	2500	400	900	24
40	3300	500	800	17

Table 38.4 Polyhydramnios: chronic versus acute.

	Chronic	Acute
Week of diagnosis	28–38	20–24
Fundal height by 24 weeks using calipers (cm)	20–26	29–32
Weight gain for 4-week interval at diagnosis (lb)	2–8	10–12
Outcome	Varies according to cause	Perinatal death
Maternal symptoms	Mild to severe	Severe

Polyhydramnios may have both maternal and fetal sequelae. In mild cases, there are minimal maternal symptoms, generally consisting of abdominal discomfort and slight dyspnea. In moderate to severe polyhydramnios (AF volume greater than 4000 mL), there may be marked respiratory distress: dyspnea and orthopnea and usually edema of the lower extremities (Table 38.4).

The increased AF volume and overstretched myometrium place the patient with polyhydramnios at risk of certain complications. Spontaneous labor with intact membranes usually produces contractions that are of poor quality because of the excessive uterine size. There is an increased incidence of abnormal presentations, and therefore there are more operative deliveries. Spontaneous rupture of the membranes causes a sudden decompression of the uterus, which increases the incidence of abruptio placentae and cord prolapse. There is a marked increase in the incidence of postpartum hemorrhage as a result of uterine overdistention resulting in uterine atony. Fetal complications include the myriad of congenital anomalies or abnormalities that result in increased fluid production or reduced fluid resorption.

Associations

Clinically detectable polyhydramnios occurs in 0.4–0.5% of pregnancies. Most cases of mild polyhydramnios (e.g., AFI 25–30 cm) are idiopathic (35–66%), and have a good prognosis, although the risks of preterm labor and fetal malpresentation remain. With increasing degrees of AF volume, the rate of fetal anomalies approaches 50%. It may be associated with diabetes mellitus, structural congenital malformations (usually of the central nervous system or gastrointestinal tract) impairing fetal swallowing, chromosomal abnormalities, multiple pregnancy (especially twin–twin transfusion syndrome or an acardiac twin), or blood group incompatibilities. When associated with fetal hydrops, polyhydramnios may be a result of fetal cardiac abnormalities, anemia or hypoproteinemia. Once polyhydramnios is diagnosed, a systematic maternal work-up is necessary to determine the cause. Management is determined by the underlying cause. The clinician should rule out such conditions as diabetes mellitus, erythroblastosis fetalis, and multiple pregnancy (e.g., twin–twin transfusion) by performing a glucose tolerance test, indirect Coombs test, and sonography, respectively.

In Queenan and Gadow's [50] 1970 series of 358 patients with polyhydramnios, the major associated conditions were diabetes mellitus (25%), congenital malformations (20%), and erythroblastosis fetalis (11%) (Table 38.5). By 1987, the causes had changed considerably, according to Hill *et al.* [51]. The representation of diabetes mellitus was lower, reflecting stricter blood glucose control, and the occurrence of polyhydramnios resulting from Rhesus (Rh) incompatibility was markedly decreased as a result of Rh immunoglobulin prophylaxis. Panting-Kemp *et al.* [52] reported a 66% incidence of idiopathic

Table 38.5 Polyhydramnios: associated conditions.

Cause	1970*	1987†	1999‡
Idiopathic (%)	35	66	65
Diabetes mellitus (%)	25	15	28
Congenital malformations (%)	21	13	4
Rh incompatibility (%)	11	1	
Multiple pregnancy (%)	8	5	3

* Source: Queenan and Gadow [50].
† Source: Hill *et al.* [51].
‡ Source: Panting-Kemp *et al.* [52].

polyhydramnios, with 4% of patients demonstrating fetal congenital malformation and 28% with maternal diabetes mellitus. The reduction in the rate of fetal malformations associated with polyhydramnios may represent a higher detection rate of the malformation by second trimester ultrasound and termination of severe cases before reaching viability.

Management

Treatment of polyhydramnios depends on the etiology and prognosis for effective treatment. Therapeutic amniocentesis is an option for the treatment of twin–twin transfusion syndrome. However, recent studies have indicated that fetoscopic laser ablation of the communicating blood vessels is of greater efficacy in severe cases presenting prior to fetal viability.

Conservative management includes modified bed rest and assessment of uterine activity and fetal well-being. Diuretics are generally contraindicated because they deplete maternal vascular volume with little effect on the total AF volume. If moderate to severe polyhydramnios results in pronounced maternal distress, and sonographic study reveals a normal-appearing fetus, a more aggressive approach becomes necessary. If the fetus is mature, delivery is indicated. If the fetus is too immature for delivery, amniocentesis with drainage to normalize AF volume may be indicated. Complications of rapid removal of AF occur in 2–3% of procedures and include premature separation of the placenta, placental abruption, and premature rupture of membranes [53–55]. Reaccumulation of AF may rapidly occur and the procedure may need to be repeated every 2–3 days. A tocolytic agent should be considered to decrease the occurrence of uterine contractions.

For severe symptomatic polyhydramnios at less than 32 weeks' gestation, we suggest treatment with indomethacin following the amniocentesis to maintain normal AF volume without exposing the fetus to the risks of serial invasive procedures. Prostaglandin synthetase inhibitors may stimulate fetal secretion of arginine vasopressin and facilitate vasopressin-induced renal antidiuretic responses, and reduced renal blood flow, thereby reducing fetal urine flow. These agents may also impair production or enhance reabsorption of lung liquid [56]. Indomethacin is started at 25 mg orally four times daily. If there is no reduction in AF volume, then the dosage is gradually increased to 2–3 mg/kg/day [57]. Maternal side-effects, such as nausea, esophageal reflux, gastritis, and emesis, are seen in approximately 4% of patients treated with indomethacin for preterm labor. The primary fetal concern with use of indomethacin is constriction of the ductus arteriosus and recent information suggests an increased risk of intraventricular hemorrhage. During indomethacin therapy we monitor AF volume two to three times per week. The drug is tapered when there is a reduction in AF volume, and stopped when polyhydramnios is no longer severe. We obtain fetal echocardiographic evaluations at intervals to examine ductal flow. If the fetus is found to have major malformations incompatible with life, delivery may be considered.

Future therapies

Future therapeutic approaches for polyhydramnios include the use of intra-amniotic pharmacologic agents to reduce fetal fluid production. In ovine pregnancy, intra-amniotic administration of either AVP or DDAVP results in rapid fetal plasma absorption and a marked decrease in fetal urine flow [40] although there is no effect on fetal swallowing [58].

Oligohydramnios

Definition

Oligohydramnios is a pathologic condition characterized by a decrease in AF volume. Although it can occur in the first half of pregnancy, it is generally a problem of the second half.

Diagnosis

Oligohydramnios is suspected when the uterus is smaller than the date of gestation would suggest, and the diagnosis is made by sonography. The clinician relies on a quantifying method such as depth of the SDP, or, more commonly, the AFI. An AFI of 5.0–8.0 cm indicates borderline AF, whereas an AFI of 5.0 or less indicates oligohydramnios. The time in pregnancy when it develops has a bearing on the prognosis. When oligohydramnios occurs as early as the second trimester, the prognosis is very poor [59].

Moore *et al.* [60] demonstrated the reliability and the predictive value of a scoring system for oligohydramnios in the second trimester. Sixty-two cases of oligohydramnios were diagnosed sonographically between 13 and 28 weeks' gestation. Three experienced sonographers used a subjective scale to rate the oligohydramnios as mild, moderate, severe, or anhydramniotic. Intraobserver reliability was excellent (intraclass correlation coefficient, 0.81). The overall perinatal mortality was 43% and the incidence of pulmonary hypoplasia was 33%. One-third had lethal congenital anomalies. The frequency of adverse outcomes strongly correlated with the most severe oligohydramnios or anhydramnios; 88% of the fetuses with severe oligohydramnios or anhydramnios had lethal outcomes, compared with 11% in the mild and moderate oligohydramnios group. The presence of an anuric urinary tract anomaly was associated with the most severe grade of oligohydramnios and was uniformly fatal. Pulmonary hypoplasia was diagnosed in 60% of the severe oligohydramnios group versus 6% of the moderate group.

The investigators concluded that subjective grading of oligohydramnios by experienced observers in the second trimester is both reliable and predictive of outcome. The finding of severe oligohydramnios in the second trimester is highly predictive of a poor fetal outcome and should stimulate an extensive search for the etiology and consideration of intervention.

Clinical significance

Oligohydramnios occurring as early as the second trimester is associated with a poor prognosis. Mercer and Brown [61] reported 39 cases of oligohydramnios in the second trimester, diagnosed by sonography. Nine of the pregnancies were associated with fetal malformations: Potter syndrome [7], atrioventricular disassociation [6], congenital absence of the thyroid [1], and multiple anomalies [7]. There were 10 unexplained stillbirths, one death resulting from abruptio placentae, eight with perinatal mortality and morbidity after premature labor or abruptio placentae, and six live-born term infants. Although oligohydramnios in the second trimester is associated with a marked increase in perinatal mortality, it is not uniformly associated with a poor outcome.

Although oligohydramnios can be idiopathic, commonly it is associated with a specific clinical condition. The clinical conditions most commonly associated with oligohydramnios are discussed below.

Premature rupture of membranes

Premature rupture of membranes (PROM) occurs in 2–4% of preterm gestations. The clinical implications for oligohydramnios in the setting of PROM are as follows. If PROM occurs before 24 weeks, there is an 80% chance of labor, infection, or both. The rate of perinatal mortality is 54% and the risk of permanent handicap in survivors is 40% [62]. It is not unusual for a pregnancy complicated by PROM to present initially as oligohydramnios with a normally functioning fetal bladder. Further work-up reveals a slow leak of AF resulting from PROM.

The earlier in pregnancy that PROM occurs, the more likely the risk of fetal pulmonary hypoplasia. If the PROM occurs at 16–24 weeks' gestation, the threat of pulmonary hypoplasia is great.

Oligohydramnios occurring secondary to PROM later in pregnancy creates a risk of umbilical cord compression. If compression occurs during labor, variable decelerations may become very problematic. This can be treated with amnioinfusion to create a cushion to relieve the cord compression (see Chapter 51).

Congenital malformation

When managing oligohydramnios, the clinician should always rule out chromosome abnormalities and structural malformations. Malformations of the urogenital system are the most commonly associated with oligohydramnios. The classic is Potter syndrome, with renal agenesis, low-set ears, and facial pressure deformities. With little or no AF, it is very difficult to image the fetus and adrenal glands may be mistaken for kidneys. Transabdominal amnioinfusion can help in providing fluid contrast for proper imaging (see Chapter 51). Additional urogenital problems can be encountered in the form of obstructive uropathy, such as posterior urethral valve syndrome, ureteropelvic junction syndrome, or ureterocystic junction obstruction. The obstructive uropathies can be detected as early as 14–16 weeks' gestation. Bilateral cystic dysplasia of the fetal kidneys may be detected as early as 12 weeks' gestation. If the problem is unilateral, oligohydramnios is not likely. Cystic kidneys and renal pelvis dilatation are found with trisomy 21 and trisomy 18, so karyotype should be determined.

Intrauterine growth restriction

Between 3% and 7% of all pregnancies are complicated by intrauterine growth restriction (IUGR). These fetuses have a considerably higher incidence of problems including hypoxia, acidosis, meconium aspiration, and polycythemia. After birth, potential complications include hypoglycemia, necrotizing enterocolitis, and impaired growth and development.

Approximately 60% of fetuses with IUGR have decreased AF volume discernible on sonographic examination. This feature may be very useful in differentiating the pathologically growth restricted fetus from the one that is merely constitutionally small. Generally, oligohydramnios in the IUGR fetus is a sign of potential fetal jeopardy and a thorough evaluation of fetal well-being is indicated.

Postdate pregnancy

Approximately 3–7% of pregnancies extend beyond 42 completed weeks of gestation, dated from the first day of the last normal menstrual period. These pregnancies have a higher incidence of perinatal mortality, perinatal morbidity, and macrosomia. Postdate pregnancies are a leading cause of obstetric malpractice litigation, with most of the cases involving neurologically impaired babies [63].

The incidence of oligohydramnios increases in postdate pregnancies, in part a result of normal shifts in the rates of fluid production and resorption (e.g., increased fetal swallowing) as well as a potential response to relative fetal hypoxia or nutrient restriction secondary to placental aging. The significance of oligohydramnios and spontaneous fetal heart rate decelerations during antepartum testing of postdate pregnancies was evaluated by Small *et al.* [64]. The occurrence of oligohydramnios or spontaneous decelerations during testing necessitates consideration of prompt delivery. Fetuses with decreased AF volume are at increased risk for umbilical cord compression, meconium aspiration, and fetal compromise.

Twin pregnancy

Seventy-five percent of twin pregnancies are dichorionic and 25% are monochorionic. The fetal loss rate is much higher in monochorionic pregnancies as a result of twin–twin transfusion syndrome. Monochorionic twin pregnancies may be identified by the telltale "T sign" at the base of the intertwin membrane. The first manifestation of twin–twin transfusion syndrome is an increased nuchal translucency in one or both fetuses at 10–14 weeks' gestation. Subsequently, at 15–17 weeks' gestation there is intertwin disparity of AF volume manifested by folding of the intertwin membrane [65].

In multiple pregnancies where polyhydramnios and oligohydramnios occur in separate sacs, there is a serious danger to the fetus with oligohydramnios. Chescheir and Seeds [66] reported on seven such twins with twin–twin transfusion syndrome resulting in a perinatal mortality rate of 71%. The occurrence of the complication before 26 weeks' gestation resulted in death of all fetuses despite a variety of attempted therapies. In twin–twin transfusion syndrome, the donor twin becomes anemic and, over time, growth restricted, and develops oligohydramnios. When the oligohydramnios is severe, the fetus becomes immobilized, generally against the uterine wall because of pressure from the sac with polyhydramnios. The fetus does not move despite changing of maternal position. This has been called the *trapped twin syndrome*.

Endoscopic laser ablation of the intercommunicating placental vessels [67] is recommended for severe twin–twin transfusion syndrome presenting prior to fetal viability. Following viability, amniodrainage from the twin with polyhydramnios may improve the AF volume of the donor twin with oligohydramnios [65].

Management

Amnioinfusion may be considered in pregnancies complicated by oligohydramnios when the physician feels that augmenting the AF volume will provide diagnostic or therapeutic benefit. Amnioinfusion may be performed therapeutically, prophylactically, or as a diagnostic intervention (see Chapter 51).

Conclusions

Recent clinical and laboratory studies have provided an ever increasing understanding of the dynamics of amniotic fluid volume, the clinical importance of oligo- and polyhydramnios, and the potential use of the amniotic cavity as a route for the administration of therapeutic agents to the fetus. AF is a dynamic body of water which provides essential functions for appropriate fetal growth and development. The extremes of volume—too much or too little—may be associated with an unfavorable prognosis. Appropriate diagnosis and management of polyhydramnios and oligohydramnios is essential to optimize fetal outcome.

Case presentation

A 26-year-old gravida 2, para 1, with a history of one prior term vaginal delivery presented for prenatal care in the first trimester. The patient's fundal height was slightly greater than her dates, and a subsequent ultrasound revealed a twin gestation with a dividing membrane consistent with diamniotic monochorionic placentation. Repeat ultrasounds demonstrated symmetric growth until a 26-week scan revealed a 20% weight discordance. A repeat ultrasound 2 weeks later demonstrated marked oligohydramnios (i.e., stuck twin) in the smaller twin, associated with an absence of bladder filling and polyhydramnios in the larger twin. A diagnosis of twin–twin transfusion syndrome was made. As the gestation was beyond fetal viability, laser ablation of placental anastomoses was not entertained. An amnioreduction procedure was performed with withdrawal of 2 L fluid from the polyhydramnios sac. Subsequent ultrasound confirmed a reduction in amniotic fluid in the polyhydramnios sac, and reaccumulation of fluid in the oligohydramnios sac, although still subjectively reduced. A repeat amnioreduction was performed 1 week later. Shortly thereafter, the patient progressed into spontaneous labor and was operatively delivered at 29 weeks' gestation. Twins demonstrated a 25% discordancy in weight, with evidence of polycythemia and anemia in the larger and smaller twin, repectively.

This case represents an example of twin–twin transfusion syndrome. The donor twin's anemia, reduced intravascular volume, and mild hypoxemia result in relative oliguria. Continued fetal swallowing, despite reduced amniotic fluid (e.g., urine) production contributes to the oligohydramnios. Conversely, the recipient twin develops polycythemia, increased intravascular volume, and elevated plasma atrial natriuretic factor levels. Markedly increased urine production contributes to the polyhydramnios state. Amnioreduction reduces intra-amniotic pressure, potentiating increased maternal to fetal placental water flow, and facilitating intravascular volume repletion and urine output in the donor twin. However, the twin–twin transfusion pathophysiology continues, with continued transfer of plasma and red cells, and polyhydramnios/oligohydramnios recurs.

References

1 Denman T. *An Introduction to the Practice of Midwifery*. London: Bliss and White, 1825.

2 Campbell J, Wathen N, Macintosh M, Cass P, Chard T, Mainwaring BR. Biochemical composition of amniotic fluid and extraembryonic coelomic fluid in the first trimester of pregnancy. *Br J Obstet Gynaecol* 1992;**99**:563–5.

3 Faber JJ, Gault CF, Green TJ, Long LR, Thornburg KL. Chloride and the generation of amniotic fluid in the early embryo. *J Exp Zoolog* 1973;**183**:343–52.

4 Gillibrand PN. Changes in the electrolytes, urea and osmolality of the amniotic fluid with advancing pregnancy. *J Obstet Gynaecol Br Commonw* 1969;**76**:898–905.

5 Desai M, Ladella S, Ross MG. Reversal of pregnancy-mediated plasma hypotonicity in the near-term rat. *J Matern Fetal Neonatal Med* 2003;**13**:197–202.

6 Charles D, Jacoby HE. Preliminary data on the use of sodium aminohippurate to determine amniotic fluid volumes. *Am J Obstet Gynecol* 1966;**95**:266–9.

7 Queenan JT, Thompson W, Whitfield CR, Shah SI. Amniotic fluid volumes in normal pregnancies. *Am J Obstet Gynecol* 1972;**114**:34–8.

8 Brace RA, Wolf EJ. Normal amniotic fluid volume changes throughout pregnancy. *Am J Obstet Gynecol* 1989;**161**:382–8.

9 Chez RA, Smith RG, Hutchinson DL. Renal function in the intrauterine primate fetus. I. Experimental technique; rate of formation and chemical composition of urine. *Am J Obstet Gynecol* 1964;**90**:128–31.

10 Pritchard JA. Deglutition by normal and anencephalic fetuses. *Obstet Gynecol* 1965;**25**:289–97.

11 Rabinowitz R, Peters MT, Vyas S, Campbell S, Nicolaides KH. Measurement of fetal urine production in normal pregnancy by real-time ultrasonography. *Am J Obstet Gynecol* 1989;**161**: 1264–6.

12 Fagerquist M, Fagerquist U, Oden A, Blomberg SG. Fetal urine production and accuracy when estimating fetal urinary bladder volume. *Ultrasound Obstet Gynecol* 2001;**17**:132–9.

13 Kurjak A, Kirkinen P, Latin V, Ivankovic D. Ultrasonic assessment of fetal kidney function in normal and complicated pregnancies. *Am J Obstet Gynecol* 1981;**141**:266–70.

14 Jeffcoate TN, Scott JS. Polyhydramnios and oligohydramnios. *Can Med Assoc J* 1959;**80**:77–86.

15 Shiller W, Toll CM. An inquiry into the cause of oligohydramnios. *Am J Obstet Gynecol* 1927;**12**:689.

16 Sylvester PE, Hughes DR. Congenital absence of both kidneys; a report of four cases. *Br Med J* 1954;**4853**:77–9.

17 Quoting Ahlfeld FL, Farber S, Sweet LK. Amniotic sac contents in the lungs of infants. *Am J Dis Child* 1931;**42**:1372.

18 Liley AW. Disorders of amniotic fluid. In: Assali NS, (ed.) *Pathophysiology of Gestation*. New York: Academic Press; 1972.

19 Goodlin R, Lloyd D. Fetal tracheal excretion of bilirubin. *Biol Neonate* 1968;**12**:1–12.

20 Adamson TM, Brodecky V, Lambert V *et al*. The production and composition of lung liquid in the *in utero* foetal lamb. In: Dawes GS, (ed.) *Foetal and Neonatal Physiology*. Cambridge, UK: Cambridge University Press, 1973.

21 Brace RA, Wlodek ME, Cock ML, Harding R. Swallowing of lung liquid and amniotic fluid by the ovine fetus under normoxic and hypoxic conditions. *Am J Obstet Gynecol* 1994;**171**:764–70.

22 Ross MG, Ervin G, Leake RD, Fu P, Fisher DA. Fetal lung liquid regulation by neuropeptides. *Am J Obstet Gynecol* 1984;**150**:421–5.

23 Lawson EE, Brown ER, Torday JS, Madansky DL, Taeusch HW Jr. The effect of epinephrine on tracheal fluid flow and surfactant efflux in fetal sheep. *Am Rev Respir Dis* 1978;**118**:1023–6.

24 Dodic M, Wintour EM. Effects of prolonged (48 h) infusion of cortisol on blood pressure, renal function and fetal fluids in the immature ovine foetus. *Clin Exp Pharmacol Physiol* 1994;**21**:971–80.

25 Queenan JT, Von Gal HV, Kubarych SF. Amniography for clinical evaluation of erythroblastosis fetalis. *Am J Obstet Gynecol* 1968;**102**:264–74.

26 Pritchard JA. Fetal swallowing and amniotic fluid volume. *Obstet Gynecol* 1966;**28**:606–10.

27 Bradley RM, Mistretta CM. Swallowing in fetal sheep. *Science* 1973;**179**:1016–7.

28 El-Haddad MA, Ismail Y, Guerra C, Day L, Ross MG. Effect of oral sucrose on ingestive behavior in the near-term ovine fetus. *Am J Obstet Gynecol* 2002;**187**:898–901.

29 Sherman DJ, Ross MG, Day L, Humme J, Ervin MG. Fetal swallowing: response to graded maternal hypoxemia. *J Appl Physiol* 1991;**71**:1856–61.

30 Carter CO. Congenital malformation. Ciba Foundation Symposium, 264. 1960.

31 Abramovich DR. Fetal factors influencing the volume and composition of liquor amnii. *J Obstet Gynaecol Br Commonw* 1970;**77**:865–77.

32 Gadd RL. Liquor amnii. In: Phillipp EE, Barnes J, Newton M, (eds). *Scientific Foundations of Obstetrics and Gynaecology*. London: Butterworth Heinemann, 1987:254.

33 Benirschke K, McKay DG. The antidiuretic hormone in fetus and infant; histochemical observations with special reference to amniotic fluid formation. *Obstet Gynecol* 1953;**1**:638–49.

34 Naeye RL, Milic AM, Blanc W. Fetal endocrine and renal disorders: clues to the origin of hydramnios. *Am J Obstet Gynecol* 1970;**108**:1251–6.

35 Lingwood BE, Wintour EM. Amniotic fluid volume and *in vivo* permeability of ovine fetal membranes. *Obstet Gynecol* 1984;**64**:368–72.

36 Gilbert WM, Newman PS, Eby-Wilkens E, Brace RA. Technetium Tc 99m rapidly crosses the ovine placenta and intramembranous pathway. *Am J Obstet Gynecol* 1996;**175**:1557–62.

37 Lingwood BE, Wintour EM. Permeability of ovine amnion and amniochorion to urea and water. *Obstet Gynecol* 1983;**61**:227–32.

38 Gilbert WM, Brace RA. The missing link in amniotic fluid volume regulation: intramembranous absorption. *Obstet Gynecol* 1989;**74**:748–54.

39 Ervin MG, Ross MG, Leake RD, Fisher DA. Fetal recirculation of amniotic fluid arginine vasopressin. *Am J Physiol* 1986;**250**:E253–8.

40 Gilbert WM, Cheung CY, Brace RA. Rapid intramembranous absorption into the fetal circulation of arginine vasopressin injected intraamniotically. *Am J Obstet Gynecol* 1991;**164**:1013–8.

41 Queenan JT, Allen FH Jr, Fuchs F, *et al.* Studies on the method of intrauterine transfusion. I. Question of erythrocyte absorption from amniotic fluid. *Am J Obstet Gynecol* 1965;**92**:1009–13.

42 Hebertson RM, Hammond ME, Bryson MJ. Amniotic epithelial ultrastructure in normal, polyhydramnic, and oligohydramnic pregnancies. *Obstet Gynecol* 1986;**68**:74–9.

43 Magann EF, Nolan TE, Hess LW, Martin RW, Whitworth NS, Morrison JC. Measurement of amniotic fluid volume: accuracy of ultrasonography techniques. *Am J Obstet Gynecol* 1992;**167**:1533–7.

44 Horsager R, Nathan L, Leveno KJ. Correlation of measured amniotic fluid volume and sonographic predictions of oligohydramnios. *Obstet Gynecol* 1994;**83**:955–8.

45 Dildy GA III, Lira N, Moise KJ Jr, Riddle GD, Deter RL. Amniotic fluid volume assessment: comparison of ultrasonographic estimates versus direct measurements with a dye-dilution technique in human pregnancy. *Am J Obstet Gynecol* 1992;**167**:986–94.

46 Magann EF, Morton ML, Nolan TE, Martin JN Jr, Whitworth NS, Morrison JC. Comparative efficacy of two sonographic measurements for the detection of aberrations in the amniotic fluid volume and the effect of amniotic fluid volume on pregnancy outcome. *Obstet Gynecol* 1994;**83**:959–62.

47 Chauhan SP, Magann EF, Morrison JC, Whitworth NS, Hendrix NW, Devoe LD. Ultrasonographic assessment of amniotic fluid does not reflect actual amniotic fluid volume. *Am J Obstet Gynecol* 1997;**177**:291–6.

48 Magann EF, Doherty DA, Chauhan SP, Busch FW, Mecacci F, Morrison JC. How well do the amniotic fluid index and single deepest pocket indices (below the 3rd and 5th and above the 95th and 97th percentiles) predict oligohydramnios and hydramnios? *Am J Obstet Gynecol* 2004;**190**:164–9.

49 Magann EF, Nevils BG, Chauhan SP, Whitworth NS, Klausen JH, Morrison JC. Low amniotic fluid volume is poorly identified in singleton and twin pregnancies using the 2×2 cm pocket technique of the biophysical profile. *South Med J* 1999;**92**:802–5.

50 Queenan JT, Gadow EC. Polyhydramnios: chronic versus acute. *Am J Obstet Gynecol* 1970;**108**:349–55.

51 Hill LM, Breckle R, Thomas ML, Fries JK. Polyhydramnios: ultrasonically detected prevalence and neonatal outcome. *Obstet Gynecol* 1987;**69**:21–5.

52 Panting-Kemp A, Nguyen T, Chang E, Quillen E, Castro L. Idiopathic polyhydramnios and perinatal outcome. *Am J Obstet Gynecol* 1999;**181**:1079–82.

53 Queenan JT. Recurrent acute polyhydramnios. *Am J Obstet Gynecol* 1970;**106**:625–6.

54 Elliott JP, Sawyer AT, Radin TG, Strong RE. Large-volume therapeutic amniocentesis in the treatment of hydramnios. *Obstet Gynecol* 1994;**84**:1025–7.

55 Leung WC, Jouannic JM, Hyett J, Rodeck C, Jauniaux E. Procedure-related complications of rapid amniodrainage in the treatment of polyhydramnios. *Ultrasound Obstet Gynecol* 2004;**23**:154–8.

56 Kramer WB, Van dVI, Kirshon B. Treatment of polyhydramnios with indomethacin. *Clin Perinatol* 1994;**21**:615–30.

57 Cabrol D, Landesman R, Muller J, Uzan M, Sureau C, Saxena BB. Treatment of polyhydramnios with prostaglandin synthetase inhibitor (indomethacin). *Am J Obstet Gynecol* 1987;**157**:422–6.

58 Kullama LK, Nijland MJ, Ervin MG, Ross MG. Intraamniotic deamino(D-Arg8)-vasopressin: prolonged effects on ovine fetal urine flow and swallowing. *Am J Obstet Gynecol* 1996;**174**:78–84.

59 Moore TR. Oligohydramnios. In: Queenan JT, Hobbins JC, (eds). *Protocols in High-Risk Pregnancies*. Cambridge, MA: Blackwell Science, 1996:488.

60 Moore TR, Longo J, Leopold GR, Casola G, Gosink BB. The reliability and predictive value of an amniotic fluid scoring system in severe second-trimester oligohydramnios. *Obstet Gynecol* 1989;**73**:739–42.

61 Mercer LJ, Brown LG. Fetal outcome with oligohydramnios in the second trimester. *Obstet Gynecol* 1986;**67**:840–2.

62 Ghidini A, Romero R. Prelabor rupture of the membranes. In: Queenan JT, Hobbins JC, (eds). *Protocols in High-Risk Pregnancies*. Cambridge, MA: Blackwell Science, 1996: 547.

63 Quilligan EJ. Postdate pregnancies. In: Queenan JT, Hobbins JC, (eds). *Protocols in High-Risk Pregnancies*. Cambridge, MA: Blackwell Science, 1996:633.

64 Small ML, Phelan JP, Smith CV, Paul RH. An active management approach to the postdate fetus with a reactive nonstress test and fetal heart rate decelerations. *Obstet Gynecol* 1987;**70**:636–40.

65 Nicolaides K, Sebire N, d'Ercole C. Prediction, diagnosis and management of twin-to-twin transfusion syndrome. In: Cockburn F, (ed.) *Advances In Perinatal Medicine*. New York: Parthenon Publishing, 1997:200.

66 Chescheir NC, Seeds JW. Polyhydramnios and oligohydramnios in twin gestations. *Obstet Gynecol* 1988;**71**:882–4.

67 Ville Y, Hecher K, Gagnon A, Sebire N, Hyett J, Nicolaides K. Endoscopic laser coagulation in the management of severe twin-to-twin transfusion syndrome. *Br J Obstet Gynaecol* 1998;**105**:446–53.

68 Moore TR, Cayle JE. The AF index in normal human pregnancy. *Am J Obstet Gynecol* 1990;**162**:1168.

39 Prevention of preterm birth

Paul J. Meis

The problem of preterm birth

Preterm birth is defined as a live birth before 37 completed weeks' gestation. Preterm births can be classified by their apparent etiology as spontaneous preterm labor and delivery, constituting approximately 45% of preterm births; births occurring after spontaneous premature preterm rupture of the fetal membranes (PPROM), approximately 35% of preterm births; and preterm births that result from a medical or obstetric complication of the pregnancy, approximately 20% of preterm births [1]. Based on common risk factors for their occurrence, it may be appropriate to consider those births caused by spontaneous preterm labor and PPROM as a single entity and likely to be caused by similar pathogeneses [2].

The rate of preterm birth is high in the USA compared with other developed countries, and the rate has been increasing. In 2004 (the last year for which data are available at the time of writing), 12.5% of all births in the USA were delivered prior to term, representing over half a million births. This rate has shown a steady increase over the past two decades, and represents an increase of more than 30% since the government began tracking preterm births in 1981. Compared with singleton births (one baby), multiple births in the USA were about six times more likely to be preterm in 2002 [3].

Preterm birth demonstrates a marked racial disparity. The rate of preterm birth for black infants is 17.6%, compared to 10.7% for white infants. However, the rate of preterm birth for white infants remains high compared to rates of 6–8% for most European countries [4]. Preterm birth is the most common reason for the death of a newborn infant. Preterm birth is also the leading cause of cerebral palsy in the surviving children and is linked to other long-term developmental problems. In very premature infants, weighing 501–700 g, the mortality rate is approximately 70%, and with neonatal intensive care many of these deaths may occur as late as 100 days of hospitalization. The risk of severe handicap (cerebral palsy, mental retardation, epilepsy, blindness, or deafness) in survivors is approximately 20% [4].

The financial costs of preterm birth are very high. In 2002, prematurity related infant stays resulted in hospital charges of $15,500,000,000. The costs of hospital care for infants born at 25–27 weeks' gestation were more than 28 times those of infants born at term: $280,146 vs. $9803 [5]. Hospital costs in 2005 are likely to be even higher. These figures do not include the financial costs to the families of handicapped children over their lifespan. In addition to the financial costs of preterm birth, the families of very preterm infants are exposed to considerable stress in dealing with this problem and dysfunctional family patterns are common. For these reasons, preterm birth is recognized as a major public health problem and reduction of the rates of preterm birth as the most important goal in contemporary obstetric practice and research.

Preterm birth as a social phenomenon

Many studies have shown that the risk of preterm birth is related to low socioeconomic status. Given this relationship, why does the USA have high rates of preterm birth when it has one of the highest rates of per capita income of all the nations of the world? Several facts may explain this seeming contradiction. Access to health care for individuals in the USA may be limited by the lack of health insurance. From 2001 census data, only 32.7% of the female population was covered through private health insurance or Medicaid. In the USA in 2004, 43.6 million people lacked any kind of health insurance [6]. The increase in the number of people without insurance in 2002 was the largest in a decade.

The racial disparity of insurance coverage is striking. In a study by Families USA, nearly 35% of Hispanics were uninsured, as were 20% of blacks and 12% of whites [7]. While many states have attempted to improve insurance coverage with Medicaid for low-income pregnant women, many gaps in coverage persist, and health problems of the women may not be covered by Medicaid insurance until the time of pregnancy.

Income inequality is greater in the USA than in other major industrialized countries such as Canada, Australia, and European countries. In 2002, a total of 34.6 million Americans, 12.1% of the population, lived in poverty. A monograph by Miller [8] described some of the social support benefits enjoyed by pregnant women in Europe. The countries surveyed were Belgium, Denmark, Germany, France, Ireland, Netherlands, Norway, Spain, Switzerland, and the UK. In all of these countries, prenatal care is available to all without regard to their ability to pay. Many of these countries provide financial incentives to pregnant women for attending prenatal visits. All of these countries provide paid pregnancy leave with job security, and routine home visits by a nurse following the delivery. In the Netherlands, women receive 100% of their salaries during maternity leave, and in Denmark and Sweden 90%. These programs are in contrast to the relative lack of organized social support for pregnant women in the USA.

Tocolytic drugs

Since the 1970s, much of the effort toward preventing preterm birth has been focused on attempts to halt preterm labor through the use of tocolytic drugs. Despite the wide usage of these drugs, the results have been disappointing. Since the time of the introduction of these drugs, no reduction has been observed in the rates of preterm birth in the USA or in other countries. Randomized placebo controlled trials of these drugs have found that the use of these drugs can be effective in delaying preterm delivery for a matter of days, but that ultimate preterm delivery is not prevented [9]. The short-term delay in delivery, however, can be useful in allowing time for the effective use of antenatal steroid therapy to enhance fetal lung maturity. This lack of effectiveness of tocolytic therapy and the lack of other effective methods to reduce rates of preterm birth has led to the opinion by many that no effective and reproducible method of preventing preterm birth has been demonstrated [9].

It would appear that once the labor process has begun, which likely occurs earlier than the clinical onset of labor, attempts to halt this process are futile and that effective prevention for preterm labor must rely on programs or interventions that are introduced early in pregnancy. Current evidence suggests that we may be at the threshold of the discovery of effective and clinically useful methods of preventing preterm birth. However, it may be years before these discoveries impact preterm delivery rates.

Prevention of preterm birth in France

The French experience in preterm birth prevention in the 1970s and 1980s is worthy of attention because it represented a formal program to reduce the rate of preterm births and because France was the only European country to experience a significant decrease in the rate of preterm births. The program was under the direction of Dr. Emile Papiernik. A full description of this program was published by Papiernik and Goffinet [10]. Papiernik first tested this program in a small district of France containing the city of Hagenau in the region of Alsace. The basic features of the program included the availability of early and equal prenatal care for all women without regard for ability to pay; provision of information that would convince the women to change their lifestyles; recognition, during prenatal care, of risk factors and warning signs of preterm birth; and appropriate use of maternity work leave and reduction of physical activity. The program was directed at all pregnant women, not only those at high risk. The success of this program in Hagenau led to its adoption throughout the entire country. In France, the proportion of deliveries at less than 37 weeks decreased from 8.2% in 1972 to 6.8% in 1976, 5.6% in 1982, and 4.9% in 1988. Of even greater significance, births at less than 34 weeks decreased from 2.4% of deliveries in 1972 to 1.7% in 1976, 1.2% in 1981, and 0.9% in 1988 [11]. Analysis of the preterm births revealed that the reduction occurred for spontaneous preterm births, and no decrease occurred for indicated preterm deliveries [11]. The decrease in preterm deliveries occurred mainly for women at low or moderate risk. Women at high risk for preterm delivery, because of a history of a previous preterm delivery or a previous stillbirth, did not experience a decreased rate of preterm delivery.

Since 1988 a trend has been seen in France for a modest increase in preterm births, to 4.43% in 1995 and 6.27% in 1998. The largest increases were identified in the subgroup of indicated preterm births, from 0.51% in 1972 to 2.31% in 1998 [10]. France has experienced an increased number of births to immigrant women who were born outside of continental France. An analysis of births in the Seine–Saint-Denis district in 2000 found that almost half of all births occurred to these women. The only groups who experienced an increased rate of preterm births were women born in the French Caribbean or sub-Saharan Africa, who had rates of preterm birth of 7.9 and 7.2%, respectively [12]. These rates are still low compared with rates of preterm birth in the USA.

Unfortunately, attempts to duplicate the French experience in the USA have not been successful. A multicenter randomized trial of a system of patient education, physician education, and weekly pelvic examination enrolled 2395 women. The results showed no significant reduction in the study group compared to the control group [13]. There are several reasons that can be advanced for this lack of success. The program did not receive the same level of support of popular media as was present in France in helping to promote healthier lifestyles, and no governmental policy was in place that encouraged liberal pregnancy work leave. Perhaps more importantly, the trial was limited to women who were at high risk for preterm birth. In general, this group of women did not show benefit in the French program. The results achieved by the French experience are important, but without changes in health care policy, they may not be translatable to the health delivery system currently present in the USA.

Cervical cerclage

The concept of weakness in the compliance and passive ability of the uterine cervix to retain the fetus in pregnancy was first advanced more than 50 years ago, but has remained controversial up to the present time.

In 1955, Shirodkar [14] proposed surgical cerclage of the cervix as a treatment for women with a history of habitual abortion. The surgical technique that he reported, and other similar procedures, have been frequently used since that time with an estimated current frequency of use between 1 in 200 and 1 in 2000 deliveries [15]. The traditional concept of this entity has been to consider the cervix as being competent or incompetent, with the treatment of cervical incompetence (better referred to as insufficiency) requiring surgical cerclage. Despite the relative popularity of this treatment to prevent preterm delivery, controversies have persisted regarding the best means of diagnosis of cervical insufficiency, appropriate indications for the procedure, and the efficacy of the treatment to prevent preterm birth. The classic indications for the procedure using the patient's historical factors include a history of two or more consecutive second trimester pregnancy losses, a history of painless dilatation of the pregnant cervix to 4–6 cm, and a history of diethylstilbestrol (DES) exposure *in utero* of the pregnant women.

The availability of endovaginal ultrasonography to measure cervical length accurately and identify funneling of the internal os has both focused increased attention on the role of the cervix in preterm delivery and provided a potentially better means of evaluating cervical function.

Cervical length remains relatively stable up to the early third trimester of pregnancy at which time progressive shortening begins. The median cervical length is 35–40 mm at 14–22 weeks and falls to approximately 35 mm at 24–28 weeks, and 30 mm after 32 weeks [16]. The cervical length at 22–32 weeks' gestation displays a normal distribution, with the 50th percentile approximately 35 mm and the 10th and 90th at 25 and 45 mm, respectively [17,18]. The studies reported by Iams and other investigators have shown that the likelihood of preterm delivery is inversely related to the length of the cervix when measured at 24–28 weeks' gestation. While the cervical length can now be measured with accuracy and the associated risk of preterm delivery better assessed, it is less certain that this risk can be altered by surgical cerclage of the shortened cervix.

Perhaps the most common cause of a shortened cervix is inflammation, resulting from local effects of intravaginal and/or intrauterine infection or to decidual hemorrhage with consequent biochemically induced change in the cervix. These inflammatory alterations in the cervix are similar to the changes that occur in preparation to labor at term, and are a prelude to preterm labor and delivery. The cervical appearance in these women is currently indistinguishable from a shortened cervix resulting from intrinsic physical causes, but surgical cerclage in this circumstance would be counterproductive and would likely enhance the inflammatory or hemorrhagic process.

The efficacy of cervical cerclage in preventing preterm delivery has been evaluated by a number of randomized trials. Some of these trials enrolled women on the bases of historical pregnancy factors; other more recent trials enrolled patients on the basis of ultrasound measurement of cervical length. Grant reported a meta-analysis of four earlier trials [19]. Enrollment into these trials was essentially by the subject's past pregnancy history. A total of 1509 women were enrolled. The largest trial was conducted by the Medical Research Council and Royal College of Obstetrics and Gynaecology Working Group (MRC/RCOG) and enrolled 905 subjects [20]. The combined odds ratios (OR) of the trials did not find a statistically significant reduction of delivery at less that 33 weeks' gestation or at less than 37 weeks' gestation. The largest single trial (MRC/RCOG) found OR of delivery at less than 33 weeks of 0.67, which barely met statistical significance (95% confidence intervals [CI], 0.47–0.97). Subgroup analysis of this trial found that the only group of subjects who benefited were women with a history of combination of three or more preterm births or second trimester pregnancy losses [20].

Several randomized trials have reported the results of cervical cerclage for patients with a shortened cervix on ultrasound measurement.

Rush et al. [21] randomly assigned patients with sonographic evidence of cervical shortening (<25 mm) or funneling (>25%) between 16 and 24 weeks' gestation to cerclage ($n=55$) versus no cerclage ($n=58$). There were no significant differences in preterm birth rate (cerclage 35% vs. no cerclage 36%) or other perinatal outcomes between the two groups.

Althuisius et al. [22] recruited 35 women with a history of preterm birth at less than 34 weeks to the Cervical Incompetence Prevention Randomized Cerclage Trial (CIPRACT). Study subjects were followed with endovaginal sonography and randomized to cerclage vs. bed rest if the cervical length fell below 25 mm. Of the 35 women enrolled, 19 were randomly assigned to cerclage with modified bed rest and 16 were assigned to bed rest alone. A preterm birth rate of 44% (7 of the 16 women) occurred in those women treated with bed rest alone, compared with zero in those treated with cerclage and modified bed rest (0 of the 19 women; $P=0.002$).

Berghella et al. [23] randomized 61 women found to have a shortened cervix to either bed rest or bed rest plus cervical cerclage. Some of the women had singleton pregnancies and had risk factors for preterm delivery, some of the women had a twin gestation, and some were at low risk for preterm delivery but were identified on routine screening to have a shortened cervix. Preterm delivery at less than 35 weeks occurred in 45% of the subjects in the cerclage group and 47% of the women in the bed rest group. No difference existed in any obstetric or neonatal outcome.

In 2004, To *et al.* [24] performed the largest randomized multicenter study examining the usefulness of cervical cerclage placement in women with a short cervix. The investigators screened 47,123 women using transvaginal ultrasound at 22–24 weeks' gestation and identified 470 women with a cervical length of 15 mm or less. Two hundred and fifty three patients were randomized to receive either a Shirodkar cervical cerclage (*n*=127) or expectant management (*n*=126). Study subjects in the cerclage arm received a single dose of intravenous intraoperative antibiotics and all participants were administered prophylactic steroids (two doses) for fetal lung maturity at 26–28 weeks' gestation. There were no significant differences in proportion of preterm birth rate before 33 weeks' gestation (cerclage 22% vs. no cerclage 26%; relative risk [RR] 0.84; *P*=0.44) or other differences in perinatal or maternal morbidity or mortality. This study is remarkable for the large number of women screened, the strict definition of shortened cervix (<15 mm), the relatively large number of subjects recruited and randomized, and the careful control of the quality of the surgical procedure used. The researchers concluded that, while transvaginal sonographic measurement of the cervical length at 22–24 weeks identifies a group at high risk of preterm delivery, the insertion of a cerclage suture in such women with short cervices does not substantially reduce the risk of prematurity.

Berghella *et al.* [25] performed a meta-analysis of these four trials, including some additional subjects in the Rust and Althuisius trials. The total number of subjects was 607. The combined OR for these trials did not reach statistical significance for delivery prior to 35 weeks (OR 0.84; 95% CI, 0.67–1.06). Berghella performed subgroup analysis of these data. These analyses found an increased RR for delivery at less than 35 weeks among women with twins having a short cervix who had a cerclage performed, compared with mothers of twins not so treated (RR 2.15; 95% CI, 1.15–4.01). In contrast, subgroup analysis of women with a history of a previous preterm delivery and a shortened cervix had a decreased chance of preterm delivery at less than 35 weeks when cerclage was performed (RR 0.61; 95% CI, 0.40–0.92).

In summary, while the ability to measure the cervix accurately by means of transvaginal ultrasound improves the accuracy of predicting risk for preterm delivery, the use of this method has been disappointing for selecting women who might benefit from cervical cerclage. It seems clear that women with twin gestations who may have a short cervix are poor candidates for a cerclage. Women with a prior preterm delivery and a short cervix may benefit from this procedure and randomized trials of treating this group of women with cerclage are needed.

Infection and preterm birth

Several lines of evidence link the presence of infection and/or inflammation and preterm birth. These include a strong association between histologic chorioamnionitis and preterm birth [26], particularly early preterm birth, an association of bacterial vaginosis with preterm birth [27], and of periodontitis with preterm birth [28]. In addition, a small percentage of women in preterm labor with intact membranes have demonstrated the presence of bacterial invasion of the amniotic space [29].

These associations have stimulated a number of clinical trials of antibiotic therapy for women in preterm labor, and pregnant women with positive vaginal fetal fibronectin, vaginal infections, or periodontal disease [30–34]. Unfortunately, the results of these trials have been disappointing, showing a lack of positive prevention of preterm birth, or, in some cases, an increase in preterm birth in some groups of women treated with antibiotics [31,33,34].

An exception to these disappointing results is the improvement demonstrated by treating women with preterm premature rupture of the fetal membranes with antibiotics such as erythromycin. These results include an increase in latency before labor, and improved neonatal outcome [35,36].

Progesterone prophylactic therapy to prevent preterm birth

The use of progesterone to prevent preterm delivery is not new, and the first randomized trial of progesterone for this purpose was by Papiernik [37]. Several other small trials of progesterone therapy were reported over the next two decades. Recently, interest in this therapy has been reinvigorated as evidenced by the recent publication of five review articles and an American College of Obstetricians and Gynecologists (ACOG) Committee Opinion [38–43]. The origin of this new enthusiasm and interest in progesterone was sparked by the publication in 2003 of two randomized trials; one using progesterone vaginal suppositories and the other 17-alpha hydroxyprogesterone caproate (17P) injections to prevent recurrent preterm delivery [44,45].

The results of the early reported trials of progesterone were evaluated by two meta-analyses. Goldstein *et al.* [46], in 1989, published the results of a meta-analysis of randomized controlled trials involving the use of progesterone or other progestogenic agents for the maintenance of pregnancy. Fifteen trials of variously defined, high-risk subjects were felt to be suitable for analysis. The trials employed six progestational drugs. The pooled OR for these trials showed no statistically significant effect on rates of miscarriage, stillbirth, neonatal death, or preterm birth. The authors concluded that "progestogens should not be used outside of randomized trials at present."

In response to this publication, Keirse [47] presented, in 1990, the results of an analysis of a more focused selection of trials. This meta-analysis was restricted to trials that employed 17P, the most fully studied progestational agent, and included all placebo-controlled trials that used this drug. Pooled OR found no significant effect on rates of miscarriage, perinatal death, or neonatal complications. However, in contrast to Goldstein *et al.*'s review, the OR for preterm birth was significant at 0.5 (95% CI, 0.30–0.85), as was the OR for birthweight less than 2500 g, 0.46 (95% CI, 0.27–0.80). Keirse remarked that the results demonstrated by these trials contrasted markedly with the poor effectiveness of other efforts to reduce the occurrence of preterm birth, but that because no effect was demonstrated to result in lower perinatal mortality or morbidity, "further well-controlled research would be necessary before it is recommended for clinical practice."

A large trial of an oral progestogen was reported by Hobel *et al.* [48] in 1994. As part of a larger preterm birth prevention program, 823 patients were identified as being at risk for preterm birth by a high-risk pregnancy scoring system. The drug used was Provera (medroxyprogesterone acetate), and 411 patients were assigned to take 20 mg/day orally. The control group of 412 patients was given placebo tablets. The allocation to drug or placebo was on the basis of the particular prenatal clinic that the patient attended. The subjects were enrolled prior to 31 weeks' gestation. The outcome of interest was delivery at less than 37 weeks. The rate of preterm delivery in the treatment group was 11.2%, compared with 7.3% in the placebo group. The rate of compliance for the subjects was low, with only 55% of the patients assigned to the Provera group actually taking the drug. This remains the only large trial of an oral progestational agent to prevent preterm birth.

Recently, two large trials have been reported of the use of progestogens to prevent preterm birth. In 2003, da Fonseca *et al.* [44] reported the results of a randomized, placebo controlled trial of vaginal progesterone suppositories in 142 women. The subjects were selected as being at high risk for preterm birth. The risk factor in over 90% of the subjects was that of a previous preterm delivery. The patients were randomly assigned to daily insertion of either a 100-mg progesterone suppository or a placebo suppository. The treatment period was 24–34 weeks' gestation. All patients were monitored for uterine contractions once weekly for 1 hour with an external tocodynamometer. Although 81 progesterone and 76 placebo patients were entered into the study, several patients were excluded from analysis because of PPROM, or were lost to follow-up, leaving 72 progesterone and 70 placebo subjects. The rate of preterm delivery at less than 37 weeks in the progesterone patients was 13.8%, significantly less than the rate in the placebo patients of 28.5%. The rate of preterm delivery at less than 34 weeks' in the treatment group was 2.8% compared to 18.6% in the placebo group. These differences were statistically significant. The rate of uterine contractions measured by the weekly hour-long recording was significantly less at 28–34

weeks in the progesterone patients compared to the placebo patients. Analysis of the results by intent to treat showed smaller differences between the groups but these differences remained statistically significant [49].

Meis *et al.* [45] reported the results of a large multicenter trial of 17P conducted by the Maternal Fetal Medicine Units (MFMU) Network of the National Institute of Child Health and Human Development. The study enrolled women with a documented history of a previous spontaneous preterm delivery, which occurred as a consequence of either spontaneous preterm labor or PPROM. After receiving an ultrasound examination to rule out major fetal anomalies and determine gestational age, the subjects were offered the study and given a test dose of the placebo injection to assess compliance. If they chose to continue, they were randomly assigned, using a 2 : 1 ratio, to weekly injections of 250 mg 17P or a placebo injection. Treatment was begun at 16–20 weeks' gestation and was continued until delivery, or 37 weeks' gestation, whichever came first. The study planned to enroll 500 subjects, a sample size estimated to be sufficient to detect a 37% reduction in the rate of preterm birth. However, enrollment was halted at 463 subjects, 310 in the treatment group and 153 in the placebo group, following a scheduled evaluation by the Data Safety and Monitoring Committee, which found that the evidence of efficacy for the primary outcome was such that further entry of patients was unnecessary. In this study, delivery at less than 37 weeks' was reduced from 54.9% in the placebo group to 36.3% in the treatment group. Similar reductions were seen in delivery at less than 35 weeks', from 30.7% to 20.6%, and in delivery at less than 32 weeks', from 19.6% to 11.4%. All of these differences were statistically significant. Rates of birthweight less than 2500 g were significantly reduced, as were rates of intraventricular hemorrhage, necrotizing enterocolitis, and need for supplemental oxygen and ventilatory support. Rates of neonatal death were reduced from 5.9% in the placebo group to 2.6% in the treatment group, although this difference did not reach statistical significance. The women enrolled in this study had unusually high rates of preterm birth. This could be explained in part by the fact that the mean gestational age of their previous preterm delivery was quite early, at 31 weeks. In addition, one-third of the women had had more than one previous spontaneous preterm delivery. Despite random allocation, more women in the placebo group had had more than one preterm delivery. Adjustment of the analysis controlling for the imbalance found that the treatment effect remained significantly different from that of the placebo. A majority of the women were of African-American ethnicity and the treatment with 17P showed equal efficacy in the African-American women and in the non-African-American subjects.

In 2003, the ACOG Committee on Obstetric Practice published a Committee Opinion about the use of progesterone to reduce preterm birth [38]. The opinion recognized the benefit shown in the two trials for women with a prior spontaneous preterm delivery. The opinion cautioned that progesterone should not be recommended for women with other high-risk conditions (e.g., twin gestation, shortened cervix) outside of randomized trials.

Sanchez-Ramos *et al.* [43], in 2005, published a meta-analysis of trials of progestational agents to prevent preterm births. He included the two recent trials in a total of 10 trials that met the search criteria. The analysis found that "compared with women randomized to the placebo, those who received progestational agents had lower rates of preterm delivery" (26.2% vs. 35.9%; OR 0.45; 95% CI, 0.25–0.80). The comparison of rates of perinatal mortality did not reach a statistically significant difference (OR 0.69; 95% CI, 0.38–1.26). This recommendation was reinforced by the recent report by Caritis *et al.* of the results of a large randomized trial of 17P in women with twin pregnancies [50]. This trial found a lack of efficacy of progesterone treatment to prevent preterm delivery in women with twin gestations and confirmed the earlier report of Hartikainen-Sorri *et al.* [51]. Thus, effective treatments to prevent preterm delivery in multiple gestation pregnancies remain to be discovered.

Petrini *et al.* [42] reported an interesting analysis of the potential impact of 17P treatment of women at risk for recurrent preterm delivery. Their calculations assumed a 33% reduction of preterm births (based on the results of the MFMU Network trial). By their calculations, if all women at risk for recurrent preterm delivery in the USA were treated with 17P, 10,000 spontaneous preterm births would be prevented. However, the overall rate of preterm birth in the USA would be reduced only from 12.1% to 11.8%.

In summary, progesterone treatment has been demonstrated to be an effective reproducible treatment to reduce the rate of preterm delivery in a select group of women (those with a prior spontaneous preterm delivery). Whether this treatment is effective for other groups of high-risk pregnant women must await the results of further randomized trials. It is important to realize that most preterm births in the USA occur to women with no identified risk factors. Large reductions in the rate of preterm birth in the USA will likely depend on policies or treatments that can apply to the broad population of pregnant women.

Case presentation

The patient was a 25-year-old, gravida 2, para 1, whose previous pregnancy was delivered following spontaneous preterm rupture of the fetal membranes at 25 weeks followed by subsequent labor and delivery of a 625-g infant. The child survived but has been diagnosed with spastic quadriplegia form of cerebral palsy. She presented for prenatal care at 12 weeks. Physical examination was unremarkable. At 16 weeks, ultrasonography revealed a 16-week gestation with no obvious fetal anomalies and transvaginal sonography measured the cervix at 3.5 cm.

The patient was started on weekly injections of 250 mg 17P. The prenatal course was unremarkable until 33w 6d when preterm labor contractions began. On admission to labor and delivery, the cervix was fully effaced and 3–4 cm dilatated. Tocolysis with magnesium sulfate was started and the patient was given betamethasone, which was repeated at 24 hours. At 36 hours after admission, uterine contractions recurred despite the tocolytic treatment and the patient was delivered of a 2300-g infant at 34 weeks' gestation. Apgar scores were 8 and 9 at 1 and 5 minutes, respectively. The infant required no ventilatory support in the nursery and mother and infant were discharged home on day 3.

Treatment of this patient with 17P was appropriate as the history of delivery following PPROM is included in the criteria of a prior spontaneous preterm delivery. Tocolysis initially halted labor and allowed time for steroid therapy with betamethasone. However, tocolysis was only effective for a short period, and preterm labor resumed. Treatment with 17P was effective in prolonging the pregnancy compared with the previous delivery, and the birth outcome was excellent. Treatment with 17P is especially effective for women with a history of a very early preterm delivery, but the treatment does not guarantee carrying the pregnancy to term in every case.

References

1 Meis PJ. Indicated preterm births: a review. *Perinat Neonat Med* 1998;**3**:113–5.
2 Klebanoff M. Conceptualizing categories of preterm birth. *Prenat Neonat Med* 1998;**3**:13–5.
3 National Center for Health Statistics, final natality data 2005.
4 Paneth NS. The problem of low birth weight. *Future Child* 1995;**5**:19–34.
5 Agency for Healthcare Research and Quality. Overview of the HCUP National Inpatient Sample 2002.
6 National Centre for Health Statistics Final Natality data. Retrieved 4 Feb 2004 from www.marchofdimes.com/peristats.
7 Families USA. How will association health plans affect minority health. 2005. Accessed at www.familiesusa.org.
8 Miller CA. Maternal Health and infant survival. 1987. National Center for Clinical Infant Programs. Washinton DC.
9 Creasy RK. Preventing preterm birth. *N Engl J Med* 1991;**325**:727–8.
10 Papiernik E, Goffinet F. Prevention of preterm births, the French experience. *Clin Obstet Gynecol* 2004;**47**:755–67.
11 Breart G, Blondel B, Tuppin P, *et al.* Did preterm deliveries continue to decrease in France in the 1980s. *Paediatr Perinat Epidemiol* 1995;**9**:296–356.
12 Zeitlin J, Bucort M, Rivera L, *et al.* Preterm birth and maternal country of birth in a French district with a multiethnic population. *Br J Obstet Gynaecol* 2004;**111**:849–55.
13 Collaborative Group on Preterm Birth Prevention. Multicentered randomized, controlled trial of a preterm birth prevention program. *Am J Obstet Gynecol* 1993;**169**:352–66.
14 Shirodkar VN. A new method of operative treatment for habitual abortion in the second trimester of pregnancy. *Antiseptic* 1955;**52**:299.

15 American College of Obstetricians and Gynecologists Practice Bulletin No. 48. Cervical Insufficiency. *Obstet Gynecol* 2003;**102**:1091–9

16 Iams JD. Abnormal cervical competence. In: Creasy RK, Resnick R, Iams JD (eds) *Maternal-Fetal Medicine: Principles and Practice*, 5th edn. Philadelphia: W.B. Saunders, 2004:603–22.

17 American College of Radiology. ACR Appropriateness Criteria: Expert Panel on Women's Imaging. Premature cervical dilatation. American College of Radiology, Reston Va 1999. Available at http://www.acr.org.

18 American College of Obstetricians and Gynecologists Committee on Quality Assessment. Criteria Set 18, October 1996.

19 Grant A. Cervical cerclage to prolong pregnancy. In: Chalmers I, Enkn M, Keirse M, (eds) *Effective Care in Pregnancy and Childbirth*. Oxford: Oxford University Press, 1989:633–44.

20 MRC/RCOG Working Party on Cervical Cerclage. Interim report of the Medical Research Council/Royal College of Obstetricians and Gynaecologist multicentre randomized trial of cervical cerclage. *Br J Obstet Gynaecol* 1988;**95**:437–55.

21 Rush RW, Isaacs S, McPherson K, *et al.* A randomized controlled trial of cervical cerclage in women at high risk of spontaneous preterm delivery. *Br J Obstet Gynecol* 1984;**91**:724–30.

22 Althuisius SM, Decker GA, Hummel P, *et al.* Final results of the cervical incompetence prevention randomized cerclage trial (CIPRACT): therapeutic cerclage with bed rest versus bed rest alone. *Am J Obstet Gynecol* 2001;**185**:1106–12.

23 Berghella V, Odibo AO, Tolosa JE. Cerclage for prevention of preterm birth in women with a short cervix found on transvaginal ultrasound examination: a randomized trial. *Am J Obstet Gynecol* 2004;**191**:1311–7.

24 To MS, Alfirevic Z, Heath VCF, *et al.* Cervical cerclage for prevention of preterm delivery in women with short cervix: randomized controlled trial. *Lancet* 2004;**363**:1849–53.

25 Berghella V, Odibo AO, To MS, Rust OA, Althuisius SM. Cerclage for short cervix on untrasonography. *Obstet Gynecol* 2005;**106**:181–9.

26 Mueller-Heubach E, Rubinstein DN, Schwarz SS. Histologic chorioamnionitis and preterm delivery in different patient populations. *Obstet Gynecol* 1990;**75**:622–6.

27 Meis PJ, Goldenberg RL, Mercer B, *et al.* The preterm prediction study: significance of vaginal infections. *Am J Obstet Gynecol* 1995;**173**:1231–5.

28 Offenbacher S, Katz V, Fertik G, *et al.* Periodontal infection as a possible risk factor for preterm low birthweight. *J Periodontal* 1996;**67**(Suppl 10):1103–13.

29 Romero R, Sirtori M, Oyarzun E, *et al.* Infection and labor. V. Prevalence, microbiology, and clinical significance of intramniotic infection in women with preterm labor and intact membranes. *Am J Obstet Gynecol* 1989;**161**:817–24.

30 Romero R, Sibai B, Caritis S, *et al.* Antibiotic treatment of preterm labor with intact membranes: a multicenter, randomized, double-blinded, placebo-controlled trial. *Am J Obstet Gynecol* 1993;**169**:764–74.

31 Klebanoff MA, Carey JC, Hauth JC, *et al.* Failure of metronidazole to prevent preterm delivery in women with asymptomatic *Trichomonas vaginalis* infection. *N Engl J Med* 2001;**345**:487–93.

32 Carey JC, Klebanoff MA, Hauth JC, *et al.* Metronidazole to prevent preterm delivery in pregnant women with asymptomatic bacterial vaginosis. *N Engl J Med* 2000;**342**:534–40.

33 Jeffcoat MK, Hauth JC, Geurs NC, *et al.* Periodontal disease and preterm birth. results of a pilot intervention study. *J Periodontol* 2003;**74**:1214–8.

34 Andrews WW, Sibai B, Thom EA, *et al.* Randomized clinical trial of metronidazole plus erythromycin to prevent spontaneous preterm delivery in fetal fibronectin-positive women. *Obstet Gynecol* 2003;**101**:847–55.

35 Mercer BM, Miodovnik M, Thurnau GR, *et al.* Antibiotic therapy for reduction of infant morbidity after preterm premature rupture of the membranes: a randomized controlled trial. National Institute of Child Health and Human Development Maternal-Fetal Medicine Units Network. *JAMA* 1997;**278**:989–95.

36 Kenyon SL, Taylor DJ, Tarnow-Mordi W, *et al.* Broad spectrum antibiotics for preterm, prelabour rupture of fetal membranes: the ORACLE I randomized trial. *Lancet* 2001;**358**:156.

37 Papiernik E. Double blind study of an agent to prevent pre-term delivery among women at increased risk. In: Edition Schering, Serie IV, fiche 3. 1970:65–8.

38 ACOG Committee Opinion No. 291. Use of progesterone to reduce preterm birth. *Obstet Gynecol* 2003;**102**:1115–6.

39 Meis PJ, Connors N. Progesterone treatment to prevent preterm birth. *Clin Obstet Gynecol* 2004;**47**:784–95.

40 Meis PJ, Aleman A. Progesterone treatment to prevent preterm birth. *Drugs* 2004;**64**:2463–74.

41 Meis PJ. For the Society for Maternal Fetal Medicine. 17 Hydroxyprogesterone for the prevention of preterm delivery. *Obstet Gynecol* 2005;**105**:1128–35.

42 Petrini JR, Callaghan WM, Klebanoff M, *et al.* Estimated effect of 17 alpha-hydroxyprogesterone caproate on preterm birth in the United States. *Obstet Gynecol* 2005;**105**:267–72.

43 Sanchez-Ramos L, Kaunitz AM, Delke I. Progestational agents to prevent preterm birth: a meta-analysis of randomized controlled trials. *Obstet Gynecol* 2005;**105**:273–9.

44 da Fonseca EB, Bittar RE, Carvalho MHB, *et al.* Prophylactic administration of progesterone by vaginal suppository to reduce the incidence of spontaneous preterm birth in women at increased risk: a randomized placebo-controlled double-blind study. *Am J Obstet Gynecol* 2003;**188**:419–24.

45 Meis PJ, Klebanoff M, Thom E, *et al.* Prevention of recurrent preterm delivery by 17 alpha-hydroxyprogesterone caproate. *N Engl J Med* 2003;**348**:2379–85.

46 Goldstein P, Berrier J, Rosen S, *et al.* A meta-analysis of randomized control trials of progestational agents in pregnancy. *Br J Obstet Gynecol* 1989;**96**:265–74.

47 Keirse MJNC. Progesterone administration in pregnancy may prevent pre-term delivery. *Br J Obstet Gynecol* 1990;**97**:149–54.

48 Hobel CJ, Ross MG, Bemis RL, *et al.* The West Los Angeles Preterm Birth Prevention Project. I. Program impact on high-risk women. *Am J Obstet Gynecol* 1994;**170**:54–62.

49 da Fonseca EB. Progesterone and preterm birth [Letter reply]. *Am J Obstet Gynecol* 2004;**190**:1803–4.

50 Caritis S, Rouse D. A randomized trial of 17-hydroxyprogesterone caproate (17OHP) for the prevention of preterm birth in twins. *Am J Obstet Gynecol* 2006;**195**:S2.

51 Hartikainen-Sorri A, Kauppila A, Tuimala R. Inefficacy of 17 alpha-Hydroxyprogesterone Caproate in the Prevention of Prematurity in Twin Pregnancy. *Obstet Gynecol* 1980;**56**:692.

40 Pathogenesis and prediction of preterm delivery

Charles J. Lockwood

Preterm delivery (PTD) is defined as a birth before 37 completed weeks' gestation. In 2004, the PTD rate in the USA was 12.5% [1]. This represents an increase of nearly 20% since 1990. Although non-Hispanic white women saw the highest relative increases in their PTD rates, non-Hispanic black women retain a 1.5-fold overall higher PTD rate (11.5% vs. 17.9%, respectively) and a 2.5-fold higher rate of very premature births (<32 weeks) (1.63% vs. 4.04%, respectively). The two principal drivers of the recent increase in PTDs among non-Hispanic white women have been the epidemic of multifetal gestations resulting from the increased availability of assisted reproductive technologies (ART) and those PTDs indicated by deteriorating maternal or fetal health.

Etiology and pathogenesis of spontaneous PTD

Proximate causes of PTD include medically indicated PTDs (18.7–35.2% of cases) and spontaneous PTDs resulting from either preterm labor (PTL) with intact fetal membranes (23.2–64.1%) or preterm premature rupture of membranes (PPROM) (7.1–51.2%) [2]. Ultimately, all spontaneous PTDs utilize a common biochemical pathway of increased genital tract prostaglandin (PG) and protease production coupled with alterations in progesterone receptor (PR) isoform expression in the cervix, decidua, myometrium, and fetal membranes that lead to a functional progesterone withdrawal. This final common pathway is employed by each of four separate pathogenic pathways which have distinctive genetic and/or epidemiologic risk factors and unique biochemical triggers.

Maternal and/or fetal stress: premature activation of the placental–fetal hypothalamic–pituitary–adrenal axis

Periconceptional maternal stress and anxiety are associated with modestly increased rates of spontaneous PTD with odds

ratios (ORs) of 1.16 (95% confidence intervals [CI]: 1.05–1.29) [3]. Depression among women of African descent is associated with an adjusted OR for PTD of 1.96 (95% CI, 1.04–3.72) [4]. Moreover, placental pathologic changes consistent with fetal stress and ischemia are 3–7 times more common in patients with spontaneous PTD compared with term controls [5,6]. Both elevated maternal stress and aberrant placentation are more common with first pregnancies. In addition, there appears to be a genetic predisposition to both maternal mood disorders [7] and impaired placentation [8].

Corticotropin-releasing hormone (CRH), a 41-amino-acid peptide initially discovered in the hypothalamus but also expressed by placental, chorionic, amnionic, and decidual cells, appears to be the mediator of stress-associated PTDs [9]. Maternal plasma free CRH concentrations, which are almost entirely placental-derived, rise during the second half of pregnancy and peak during labor [10]. In contrast to the hypothalamus, where glucocorticoids inhibit CRH release, cortisol enhances placental production of CRH [11]. Both maternal and fetal stress is associated with elevated maternal and/or fetal cortisol levels [12–14]. Lockwood et al. [15] examined paired maternal and fetal hypothalamic–pituitary–adrenal (HPA) axis hormone levels in patients undergoing cordocentesis across the second half of gestation and noted that placental-derived maternal serum CRH values correlated best with fetal cortisol ($r = 0.40$; $P = 0.0002$) but also modestly correlated with maternal cortisol levels ($r = 0.28$; $P = 0.01$). Thus, rising maternal and/or fetal cortisol levels likely establish a positive feedback loop; to wit, placental-derived CRH stimulates the release of fetal pituitary adrenocorticotropin (ACTH) to enhance fetal adrenal cortisol production which further stimulates placental CRH release [15].

The output of prostaglandins $F_{2\alpha}$ and/or E_2 is increased by CRH in cultured amnionic, chorionic, decidual, and placental cells [16,17]. These PGs bind to the uterotonic receptors, FP, EP-1, and EP-3, respectively, in the fundus and corpus of the uterus to mediate calcium flux and increase expression of oxytocin receptor, connexin 43 (gap junctions), and cyclo-oxygenase-2 (COX-2), which triggers effective contractions and generates additional PGs, respectively [18 20]. Prostaglandins also promote premature rupture of the membranes (PROM) and cervical change by enhancing the synthesis of matrix metalloproteinases (MMPs) in the fetal membranes and cervix [19,21]. Moreover, PGs increase cervical expression of interleukin-8 (IL-8), which recruits and activates neutrophils, releasing additional MMPs and elastases which can promote cervical change and PROM [22]. Finally, recent studies suggest that both PGE_2, and $PGF_{2\alpha}$ increase the PR-A isoform and decrease the PR-B isoform in myometrium, cervix, amnion, chorion, and decidua [23–25]. Because PR-A antagonizes the classic PR-mediated genome effects of PR-B, PGs appear to induce a functional progesterone withdrawal. Cortisol released into the amniotic fluid can directly stimulate fetal membrane PG production by increasing amnionic COX-2 expression and inhibiting the chorionic PG metabolizing enzyme, 15-hydroxy-prostaglandin dehydrogenase (PGDH) [26,27].

With the development of the fetal adrenal zone of the fetal adrenal after 28–30 weeks' gestation, stress-associated activation of the placental–fetal HPA axis also mediates PTD by enhancing placental estrogen production. This is because increased fetal adrenal zone production of dehydroepiandrosterone sulfate (DHEAS) accompanies ACTH-induced fetal adrenal cortisol production. In addition, CRH can directly augment fetal adrenal DHEAS production [28]. Placental sulfatases cleave the sulfate conjugates of DHEAS and its 16-hydroxy hepatic derivative allowing their conversion to estradiol (E2) and estrone (E1), as well as estriol (E3), respectively. These estrogens increase expression of contraction-associated proteins (CAPs) such as oxytocin receptor and connexin 43 [29,30]. Because reductions in PR-B expression lead to increased expression of the active form of the estrogen receptor-α (ER-α), rising placental estrogen production would be matched to PG-induced increases in ER-α expression [31].

Decidual-amnion-chorion inflammation

Systemic inflammation resulting from periodontal disease, pneumonia, sepsis, pancreatitis, acute cholecystitis, pyleonephritis, and asymptomatic bacteriuria as well as genital tract inflammatory states such deciduitis, chorioamnionitis, and intra-amniotic infections are all associated with PTD [32–38]. Indeed, genital tract inflammation is the most common antecedent of very early PTDs, accounting for more than half of cases [37,38]. Multiple prospective cohort studies have established a modest association between bacterial vaginosis (BV) and an increased risk of spontaneous PTD (OR 1.4–2.2), with the strongest association noted for BV detected at less than 16 weeks (OR 7.55; 95% CI, 1.80–31.65) [39–41]. The occurrence of BV facilitates overgrowth of upper genital tract facultative bacteria such as mycoplasma species and *Gardnerella vaginalis*, Gram-negative bacteria such as *Escherichia coli*, and

Gram-positive cocci [42,43], as well as urinary tract colonization and infections [44]. In turn, asymptomatic bacteriuria and vaginal *E. coli* colonization are linked to a twofold increase in PTD [45–47].

The link between BV and associated overgrowth of lower and upper genital and urinary tract bacteria with PTD reflects the pivotal role of the innate immune response. Gram-negative bacterial endotoxins bind to cervical and fetal membrane Toll-like receptor 4 (TLR-4) and Gram-positive bacterial exotoxins bind to TLR-2 on decidual cells and leukocytes to elicit production of tumor necrosis factor-α (TNF-α) and IL-1β [48–50]. In turn, TNFα, IL-1β, and/or endotoxins such as lipopolysaccharide (LPS) induce expression of the transcription factor, NFκB, which enhances MMP-1, MMP-3, MMP-9, and COX-2 expression and inhibits PGDH and PR-B gene expression in myometrium, decidua, fetal membranes, and/or cervix while promoting programmed cell death (apoptosis) in amnionic epithelial cells [51–61]. Moreover, TNF-α, IL-1β, and LPS also stimulated IL-6 production in amniochorion and decidua [62,63], which further augments amnionic and decidual PG production [64]. Finally, IL-1β and TNF-α induce IL-8 production in the fetal membranes, decidua, and cervix, effects that are potentiated by IL-6 [63,65]. Given that IL-8 causes recruitment and activation of neutrophils that release additional MMPs and elastases, it further exacerbates the PTD-enhancing effects of genital tract inflammation.

The most common microorganisms identified in the fetal membranes and amniotic fluid of patients with inflammation-associated PTD are *Ureaplasma urealyticum*, *Mycoplasma hominis*, *Gardnerella vaginalis*, and bacteroides species [66,67]. As these organisms are generally of low virulence, it has been posited that a genetically determined exaggerated maternal and/or fetal inflammatory response rather than the presence of microorganisms per se triggers PTD. Indeed, the 15% recurrence risk of PTD coupled with its aggregation in certain families, and concordance in twins are consistent with a genetic link [68–71]. The T2 allele of the TNF-α gene causes increased expression of TNF-α and confers an increased risk of PPROM in African-American women [72]. Moreover, African-American mothers harboring both this polymorphism and BV are at even greater risk of PTD (OR 6.1; 95% CI, 1.9–21.0) [73]. Simhan *et al.* [74] reported the association between the IL-6-174 promoter polymorphism and a decreased risk of PTD among white women [74]. Lorenz *et al.* [75] observed an increased frequency of two (Asp299Gly and Thr399Ile) polymorphisms for TLR-4, the major endotoxin-signaling receptor, in a population of white infants delivering preterm. These findings may help account for disparate ethnic and racial patterns in PTD rates.

Fetal genotypes may also have a role in the genesis of PTD. The presence of a fetal MMP-1 mutation has also been found to increase the risk of PPROM when present in African-American fetuses, suggesting genetic influences on fetal membrane structural integrity contribute to PPROM [76]. Similarly, a 14 CA-repeat allele in the MMP-9 gene enhances transcription and is more common in African-American neonates whose mothers had experienced PPROM [77]. Homozygosity for the IL-1β+3953 allele 1 in African-American fetuses is associated with an increased risk of PTD while Hispanic fetuses carrying the IL-1RN allele 2 have an increased risk for PPROM (OR 6.5; 95% CI, 1.25–37.7) [78]. Finally, gene–environmental interactions may also be important in inflammation-associated PTD. Polymorphisms in drug metabolizing genes, *CYP1A1 Hinc*II RFLP and *GSTT1* shorten gestation among Chinese women exposed to benzene [79] and US women exposed to cigarette smoke [80].

Abruption-associated PTD

Decidual hemorrhage (aka placental abruption) originates in damaged spiral arteries or arterioles and presents clinically as vaginal bleeding or either a retroplacental or retrochorionic hematoma formation noted on ultrasound. When vaginal bleeding occurs in more than one trimester it is associated with a nearly 50% risk of PPROM (OR 7.4; 95% CI, 2.2–25.6) [81]. Decidual hemosiderin deposition and retrochorionic hematoma formation is present in 38% of patients with PTD between 22 and 32 weeks' gestation resulting from PPROM and 36% of patients experiencing PTD after PTL compared with only 0.8% following term delivery ($P < 0.01$) [82]. Uteroplacental vascular lesions associated with abruption include spiral artery vascular thrombosis and failed physiologic transformation of uteroplacental vessels. These vasculopathies may be associated with inherited and acquired thrombophilias [83,84], and hypertension as well as environmental stimuli including heavy cigarette smoking, cocaine, and trauma [85]. Abruption-associated PTDs are more common in older, white, married, parous, college educated patients presenting a demographic profile distinct from that associated with patients with stress-induced PTDs (nulliparous, anxious, or depressed patients) or inflammation-associated PTDs (young, minority, poor) [86]. The association of abruption with increasing maternal age may reflect increase in myometrial artery sclerosis which increases from 11% of spiral arteries at age 17–19 years to 83% after age 39 [87].

The decidua is a rich source of tissue factor, the primary initiator of clotting through thrombin generation [88]. Thus, decidual hemorrhage results in intense local thrombin generation. The expression of MMP-1 and MMP-3 protein and mRNA output by cultured term decidual cells is significantly enhanced by thrombin binding to its receptor, protease-activated receptor type-1 (PAR-1) [89,90]. Lockwood *et al.* [91] recently reported that abruption-associated PPROM is accompanied by dense decidual neutrophil infiltration in the absence of infection. Decidual neutrophils colocalized with areas of thrombin-induced fibrin deposition and thrombin–PAR-1 enhances IL-8 mRNA and protein expression in cultured term decidual cells [91]. Neutrophils are a rich source of elastase

and MMP-9 [92] which contribute to PPROM and cervical effacement. Stephenson *et al.* [93] have shown that thrombin also enhances MMP-9 expression in cultured amniochorion. These studies suggest a mechanism linking abruption-associated PPROM to decidual thrombin–PAR interactions. A link between thrombin and PTL has been described by Phillippe and Chien [94] who reported that thrombin–PAR interactions trigger myometrial contractions.

Mechanical stretching of the uterus resulting from multifetal gestations

There is a decrease in the gestational age at delivery with increasing numbers of fetuses from 35.3 weeks with twins to 29.9 weeks with quadruplets [95], implicating mechanical stretching in the PTD process. Mechanical dilatation of the cervix promotes cervical ripening through the induction of endogenous PG [96] and increased MMP-1 expression [21,97]. Polyhydramnios and multifetal gestation-induced mechanical stretch increases amnion COX-2 expression and related PG production [98,99]. Myometrial stretch induces oxytocin receptor, COX-2, IL-8, and connexin 43 expression [100–103].

Final common pathway of PTD

The generation of PG and proteases reflects the final common pathway of delivery, whether occurring preterm or at term. Levels of PGs increase in reproductive tract tissues, maternal plasma, and amniotic fluid immediately prior to, and during parturition [104–107]. Concomitant with rising PG levels is the upregulation of myometrial PG receptors prior to the onset of labor [108,109]. PGs induce functional progesterone withdrawal, enhance sensitivity to estrogens, and increase MMP and IL-8 expression. Moreover, all the pathways of prematurity described above also directly trigger MMP and IL-8 expression to mediate cervical change and fetal membrane rupture. Prior to 20 weeks' gestation, the myometrium is quiescent because of the high PR-B, low ER-α, low circulating estrogen levels, and inhibition of CAP gene expression. Therefore, inflammation, abruption, and excess stretch occurring prior to 24 weeks presents as "incompetent cervix" with or without subsequent PPROM and not PTL. Figure 40.1 presents a schematic of the discrete pathogenic processes leading to prematurity and their final common biochemical pathway.

Prediction of PTD

The four PTD pathogenic processes outlined above present unique biochemical or biophysical signatures. Efforts to exploit these "signatures" to identify patients at risk from a given pathway have met with modest success. In addition, the

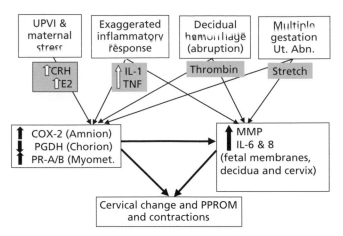

Fig. 40.1 Pathogenesis of preterm delivery (PTD). COX-2, cyclo-oxygenase 2; IL, interleukin; MMP, metalloproteinase; PGDH, 15-hydroxy-prostaglandin dehydrogenase; PR-A/B; PPROM, preterm premature rupture of the membranes; TNF, tumor necrosis factor; UPVI, uteroplacental vascular insufficiency; Ut Abn, uterine abnormality.

final common pathway of cervical and fetal membrane proteolysis can be discerned by assessment of cervicovaginal levels of fetal fibronectin (fFN) derived from the chorion or cervical length determination by ultrasound. The literature examining the efficacy of these various predictors is marked by heterogeneous patient populations with a varying prevalence of PTD, diverse assays and cut-offs, and varying definitions of PTD. Comparison of markers therefore requires conversion of their predictive estimates to positive and negative likelihood ratios (LR). The LR is a measure of the predictive accuracy of a diagnostic test, independent of prevalence. A positive likelihood ratio [LR(+)] is calculated by dividing the sensitivity by the false positive rate. It describes by how much a given positive result raises a priori risk. A negative likelihood ratio [LR(−)] is calculated by dividing the false negative rate by specificity and demonstrates how a given negative test result lowers a priori risks.

Pathway-specific markers

Putative markers of fetal stress include CRH and salivary estriol. Maternal levels of CRH rise in the weeks before labor [10]. However, the largest studies have not found CRH to be predictive of PTD [110,111]. Among those studies finding an association between maternal CRH levels and PTD, the available LRs have been less than robust: 1.8–4.0 for LR(+) and 0.47–0.77 for LR(−) for second trimester maternal CRH levels predicting PTD among asymptomatic patients [112–115]. The test performs no better among symptomatic patients with LR(+) of 3.9 and LR(−) of 0.67 [116]. The detection of salivary estriol levels ≥2.1 ng/mL is predictive of PTD within 72 hours between 32 and 37 weeks but again with only a modest LR(+) of 2.37 and LR(−) of 0.61 [117,118].

Markers of the inflammatory pathway perform modestly better. Lockwood *et al.* [119] conducted a prospective study

cohort among 161 high-risk asymptomatic patients sampled every 3–4 weeks between 24 and 36 weeks and noted a 4.2-fold increase in maximal cervical IL-6 concentrations among patients with subsequent PTDs <37 weeks compared with those with subsequent term deliveries [119]. A single cervical IL-6 value >250 pg/mL identified patients with subsequent PTD compared with those having term deliveries with LR(+) of 3.33 and LR(−) of 0.59. Multiple logistic regression indicated that a cervical IL-6 level >250 pg/mL was an independent predictor of spontaneous PTD with an adjusted OR of 4.8 (95% CI, 1.7–14.3). The Maternal Fetal Medicine (MFM) Network conduced a nested case–control study in an asymptomatic high-risk population and noted that while IL-6 concentrations were significantly higher in cases compared with controls (212 ± 339 vs. 111 ± 186 pg/mL; $P = 0.008$), only 20% of cases had IL-6 values >90th percentile [120]. Moreover, regression analysis suggested that after adjusting for other PTD risk factors, including a positive fFN test result, body mass index <19.8 kg/m², vaginal bleeding in the first or second trimester, previous spontaneous PTD and short cervix, elevated cervical IL-6 levels were not independently associated with spontaneous PTD. Among symptomatic patients, the published LRs for cervical IL-6 for the prediction of PTD were 1.82–3.63 for LR(+) and 0.3–0.8 for LR(−) [65,121–124].

Holst *et al.* [65] found higher cervical IL-8 levels among women who subsequently delivered preterm compared with those delivering at term (median 11.3 ng/mL, range 0.15–98.1 ng/mL vs. 4.9 ng/mL, range 0.15–41.0 ng/mL; $P=0.002$). The presence of cervical IL-8 values ≥7.7 ng/mL predicted PTD ≤7 days with LR(+) of 2.38 and LR(−) of 0.51. Kurkinen-Raty *et al.* [122] observed LR(+) of 1.4 (95% CI, 0.9–2.4) for a cervical IL-8 value >3.74 µg/L among symptomatic patients sampled between 22 and 32 weeks. Rizzo *et al.* [125] observed cervical IL-8 values >450 pg/mL were comparable with that of fFN values >50 ng/mL in predicting PTD and that a cervical IL-8 level >860 pg/mL predicted a positive amniotic fluid culture with LR(+) of 2.4 and LR(−) of 0.28. In contrast, Coleman *et al.* [123] were not able to confirm any PTD predictive value to cervical IL-8 determinations. Other markers of lower genital tract infection including cervical lactoferrin, sialidase, defensins, follistatin-free activin, serum β_2-microglobulin, latex C-reactive protein, intracellular adhesion molecule-1, elevated vaginal pH, and cervical neutrophils do not appear to be predictive of PTD [126–131].

Given the high concentrations of tissue factor in the decidua [88], abruption leads to excess thrombin generation, explaining the consumptive coagulopathy noted in severe cases. Thus, thrombin would appear to be an ideal marker for the detection of abruption-associated PTDs. Rosen *et al.* [132] noted that thrombin–antithrombin complexes (TAT) >3.9 µg/L predict subsequent PPROM in asymptomatic patients with LR(+) of 2.75 and LR(−) of 0.18. Among symptomatic patients TAT complex levels >6.3 µg/L between 24 and 33 weeks predict PTD within 3 weeks with LR(+) of 5.5 and LR(−) of 0.55

[133]. Chaiworapongsa *et al.* [134] observed that TAT complex levels >20 µg/L predict PTD <37 weeks with LR(+) of 2.9 and LR(–) of 0.6.

Markers of the final common pathway

Fibronectins are large extracellular matrix and plasma proteins. A heavily glycosylated form, termed fFN, is present in the amniotic fluid, placental, and fetal membranes [135]. The fFN molecule is produced by extravillous cytotrophoblasts in the anchoring villi and cytotrophoblastic shell as well as the chorion; it is released into cervicovaginal secretions when the extracellular matrix of the chorionic–decidual interface is disrupted prior to labor [136]. It is also produced by amnion epithelium and released into the amniotic fluid where it attains very high concentrations [135]. Thus, fFN is positioned to be deported into the cervicovaginal secretions following occult or overt PPROM [135].

Lockwood *et al.* [135] first described the association between the presence of cervicovaginal fFN (>50 ng/mL) between 22 and 37 weeks' gestation and an increased risk of PTD among symptomatic patients with LR(+) of 4.67 and LR(–) of 0.22. Given evidence that fFN determinations retained their predictive value for only 2–3 weeks, Peaceman *et al.* [137] assessed the value of fFN for predicting PTD within 7–14 days in symptomatic patients and noted LR(+) of 4.9 and 4.9, respectively, and LR(–) of 0.15 and 0.21, respectively. Of note, the corresponding negative predictive values in this population-based study were 99.5 and 99.2%, respectively. Meta-analysis of 14 studies examining the accuracy of fFN reported pooled LRs for the prediction of PTD within 7–14 days in symptomatic patients of 5.43 (95% CI, 4.36–6.74) for LR(+) and 0.25 (95% CI, 0.2–0.31) for the LR(–). The comparable values for predicting PTD prior to 34 weeks were 3.64 (95% CI, 3.32–5.73) and 0.32 (95% CI, 0.16–0.66), respectively, among eight studies [138].

Lockwood *et al.* [139] also assessed the utility of cervicovaginal fFN in the prediction of subsequent PTD amongst high-risk asymptomatic patients sampled every 2–4 weeks between 24 and 37 weeks' gestation. A vaginal fFN value >50 ng/mL predicted PTD with LR(+) of 3.4 and LR(–) of 0.4. Vaginal fFN predicted PTDs resulting from PTL and PPROM with equal efficiency. The MFM Network subsequently assessed the value of cervicovaginal fFN obtained at 22–24 weeks among nearly 3000 asymptomatic women and found LR(+) of 6.3 and LR(–) of 0.84 [140]. A meta-analysis of studies among high-risk asymptomatic patients has demonstrated pooled LRs for the prediction of PTD <34 weeks 4.01 (95% CI, 2.93–5.49) for LR(+) and 0.78 (95% CI, 0.72-0.84) for LR(–) [138].

The fFN test appears equally valid in patients with twins, cervical cerclage, and prior multifetal reduction procedures, and a speculum need not be used to obtain a vaginal specimen [141–144]. While the principal utility of the fFN lies in its very high negative predictive value (>99% for delivery within 2

weeks), most studies suggest a positive predictive value for PTD in general of >50%, suggesting that fFN positive patients beyond 23 completed weeks of gestation should receive corticosteroids.

Between 22 and 30 weeks' gestation, the length of the cervix assumes a Gaussian distribution with the 5th percentile at 20 mm, 10th percentile at 25 mm, 50th percentile at 35 mm, and 90th percentile at 45 mm. The relative risk of PTD increases as the length of the cervix decreases. When women with shorter cervixes at 24 weeks were compared with women with values above the 75th percentile, the relative risks of PTD among the women with shorter cervixes were as follows: 1.98 for cervical lengths ≤40 mm, 2.35 for lengths ≤35 mm, 3.79 for lengths ≤30 mm, 6.19 for lengths ≤26 mm, 9.49 for lengths ≤22 mm, and 13.99 for lengths ≤13 mm [145].

Among symptomatic women who go on to deliver preterm, 80–100% have a cervical length <30 mm when initially evaluated because of contractions. As a rule, a subsequent PTD is highly unlikely in symptomatic women when the cervix is longer than 30 mm, unless abruption is the cause of their contractions. Conversely, PTD is quite likely when a cervix measures <15 mm [146]. In one study of 216 women, in 173 cases the cervical length was ≥15 mm and only one of these women delivered within 7 days, while in the 43 patients with cervical lengths <15 mm, delivery within 7 days occurred in 37% [147]. Vendittelli and Volumenie [148] conducted a meta-analysis of the utility of cervical sonographic length determination for the prediction of PTD among symptomatic patients. Nine articles met their inclusion criteria, the optimal predictive cut-off varied from 18 to 30 mm, and the prevalence of PTD was 37.3%. The authors found that relative risk for the occurrence of PTD when the cervical length was ≤18 mm was 3.9 (95% CI, 1.8–8.5) and that sensitivities for predicting PTD ranged from 68 to 100%, while the specificity ranged from 30 to 78%.

In asymptomatic women with a history of PTD, the gestational age at PTD in the previous pregnancy correlates with the cervical length in the subsequent gestation [149]. Cervical length measurements in the second trimester in asymptomatic women with a history of prior spontaneous PTD predict recurrent spontaneous PTD. The MFM Network examined the value of cervical ultrasound in predicting PTD <35 weeks among high-risk asymptomatic patients [150]. Patients underwent cervical sonography every 2 weeks and lengths <25 mm noted at any time were associated with a relative risk for spontaneous PTD of 4.5 (95% CI, 2.7–7.6) but LR(+) of only 1.5 and LR(–) of 0.39. The efficacy of cervical length in predicting PTD in asymptomatic low-risk women is quite low. In a series of 3694 unselected Finnish women scanned at 18–24 weeks, a 25 mm cut-off yielded insignificant LR(+) and LR(–) [151]. Similar results were found in a large US cohort [152].

The optimal PTD diagnostic accuracy occurs when combining vaginal fFN with cervical length determinations. Hincz *et al.* [153] prospectively evaluated 82 symptomatic patients with cervical sonography and fFN if the cervical length was

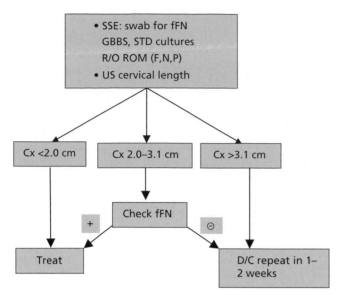

Fig. 40.2 Paradigm for using fetal fibronectin (fFN) and/or cervical ultrasound in symptomatic patients. Cx, cervix; D/C, discharge patient; GBBS, group B β-streptococcus; R/O ROM, rule out rupture of fetal membranes; SSE, sterile speculum exam; STD, sexually transmitted disease; US, ultrasound.

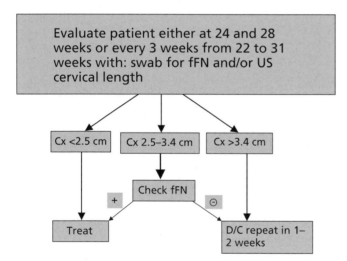

Fig. 40.3 Paradigm for using fFN and/or cervical ultrasound (US) in high-risk asymptomatic patients. Cx, cervix; D/C, discharge patient.

between 2.0 and 3.1 cm. Defining a positive patient as either those with a cervical length <2.1 cm or a positive fFN, they predicted delivery within 28 days with LR(+) of 8.6 and LR(−) of 0.16. The sensitivity of this two-step method was 86%, with a specificity of 90%, positive predictive value of 63%, and negative predictive value of 97%. Interestingly, among patients with a cervical length of 2.0–3.1 mm, 71.4% of those with a positive fFN delivered within 28 days while only 7.4% of those with negative fFN delivered within 28 days. Figure 40.2 describes this algorithm for evaluating symptomatic patients with both fFN and cervical sonography. It represents the most sensitive, specific, and accurate available diagnostic para-

digm. Patients found at risk would qualify for a course of antenatal steroids when ≥24 weeks' gestation, as well as short-term tocolysis, and antibiotic therapy for BV, urinary tract infections, or group B β-streptococcus if present or while cultures are pending.

The MFM Network examined high-risk asymptomatic women between 24 and 28 weeks with fFN and cervical sonography and observed that patients with both a positive fFN and a short cervix on transvaginal ultrasound were at relatively high risk of spontaneous PTD (33.3%) while the absence of either marker places them at very low risk of PTD <34 weeks (1.3%) [154]. Based on expert opinion and these data, we employ the algorithm outlined in Fig. 40.3 for evaluating high-risk asymptomatic patients. Patients are evaluated every 3 weeks from 22 to 32 weeks. Again, patients found at risk can be treated with a course of antenatal corticosteroids and may benefit from decreased work and more intense surveillance.

Conclusions

Substantial strides have been made in our understanding of the pathogenesis of PTD. However, evaluation of the utility of biochemical and biophysical mediators of the major pathogenic markers have not produced efficient predictors of PTD (i.e., markers with high LR(+) and low LR(−) values). Identification of cervicovaginal fFN and cervical shortening on transvaginal sonography are the most accurate and efficient markers of PTD. Both are indicators of the final common pathway of genital tract extracellular matrix breakdown. High-risk asymptomatic patients found with either a short cervix or positive fFN are eligible for antenatal corticosteroids. However, most practitioners rely on the high negative predictive value of a long cervix and/or negative fFN to avoid introduction of costly and potentially dangerous interventions of unproven efficacy. Future methods of risk assessment will likely rely on detection of genetic predispositions to PTD.

Case presentation 1

A 28-year-old primigravida at 28 weeks' gestation returns from her exercise class and notes intermittent abdominal tightening. She contacts her obstetrician who instructs her to decrease activity, increase oral fluids, and call if the pain continues. After several hours the patient notes more frequent pain. She is instructed to come to the hospital. On admission she is noted to have contractions every 6–8 minutes. Intravenous fluids are administered and a vaginal swab is obtained. The attending physician performs a cervical ultrasound. The latter demonstrates a cervical length of 2.8 cm. The vaginal swab is sent for a fFN determination which returns negative. The patient is sent home and instructed to return to the office in 1 week.

Case presentation 2

A 39-year-old G3P2 at 24 weeks notes the onset of heavy vaginal bleeding. Her pregnancy had been complicated by intermittent vaginal bleeding in the first trimester. She is seen by her physician in his office who examines her and notes a long closed posterior cervical exam. An ultrasound reveals a low-lying posterior placenta with a possible retro-chorionic hematoma. The patient is admitted to the hospital with a presumed abruption, given intravenous fluids and a course of corticosteroids. She is discharged in 48 hours and instructed to stop work. The vaginal bleeding continues intermittently for the next 3 weeks. At 27 weeks, she awakens with gross rupture of the membranes and bloody amniotic fluid.

References

1 Martin JA, Hamilton BE, Menacker F, Sutton PD, Mathews TJ. Preliminary births for 2004: Infant and maternal health. Health E-stats. Hyattsville, MD: National Center for Health Statistics. Released November 15, 2005.

2 Moutquin JM. Classification and heterogeneity of preterm birth. *Br J Obstet Gynaecol* 2003;**10**(Suppl 20):30–3.

3 Copper RL, Goldenberg RL, Das A, *et al*. The preterm prediction study: maternal stress is associated with spontaneous preterm birth at less than thirty-five weeks' gestation. National Institute of Child Health and Human Development Maternal-Fetal Medicine Units Network. *Am J Obstet Gynecol* 1996;**175**:1286–92.

4 Orr ST, James SA, Blackmore Prince C. Maternal prenatal depressive symptoms and spontaneous preterm births among African-American women in Baltimore, Maryland. *Am J Epidemiol* 2002;**156**:797–802.

5 Germain AM, Carvajal J, Sanchez M, Valenzuela GJ, Tsunekawa H, Chuaqui B. Preterm labor: placental pathology and clinical correlation. *Obstet Gynecol* 1999;**94**:284–9.

6 Arias F, Rodriquez L, Rayne SC, Kraus FT. Maternal placental vasculopathy and infection: two distinct subgroups among patients with preterm labor and preterm ruptured membranes. *Am J Obstet Gynecol* 1993;**168**:585–91.

7 Craddock N, Forty L. Genetics of affective (mood) disorders. *Eur J Hum Genet* 2006;**14**:660–8.

8 Svensson AC, Pawitan Y, Cnattingius S, Reilly M, Lichtenstein P. Familial aggregation of small-for-gestational-age births: the importance of fetal genetic effects. *Am J Obstet Gynecol* 2006;**194**:475–9.

9 Challis JR, Lye SJ, Gibb W, Whittle W, Patel F, Alfaidy N. Understanding preterm labor. *Ann N Y Acad Sci* 2001;**943**:225–34.

10 McLean M, Bisits A, Davies J, Woods R, Lowry P, Smith R. A placental clock controlling the length of human pregnancy. *Nat Med* 1995;**1**:460–3.

11 Jones SA, Brooks AN, Challis JR. Steroids modulate corticotropin-releasing hormone production in human fetal membranes and placenta. *J Clin Endocrinol Metab* 1989;**68**: 825–30.

12 Sandman CA, Glynn L, Schetter CD, *et al*. Elevated maternal cortisol early in pregnancy predicts third trimester levels of placental corticotropin releasing hormone (CRH): priming the placental clock. *Peptides* 2006;**27**:1457–63.

13 Economides DL, Nicolaides KH, Linton EA, Perry LA, Chard T. Plasma cortisol and adrenocorticotropin in appropriate and small for gestational age fetuses. *Fetal Ther* 1988;**3**:158–64.

14 Amiel-Tison C, Cabrol D, Denver R, Jarreau PH, Papiernik E, Piazza PV. Fetal adaptation to stress. Part I: acceleration of fetal maturation and earlier birth triggered by placental insufficiency in humans. *Early Hum Dev* 2004;**78**:15–27.

15 Lockwood CJ, Radunovic N, Nastic D, Petkovic S, Aigner S, Berkowitz GS. Corticotropin-releasing hormone and related pituitary-adrenal axis hormones in fetal and maternal blood during the second half of pregnancy. *J Perinat Med* 1996;**24**:243–51.

16 Jones SA, Challis JR. Effects of corticotropin-releasing hormone and adrenocorticotropin on prostaglandin output by human placenta and fetal membranes. *Gynecol Obstet Invest* 1990;**29**:165–8.

17 Jones SA, Challis JR. Steroid, corticotrophin-releasing hormone, ACTH and prostaglandin interactions in the amnion and placenta of early pregnancy in man. *J Endocrinol* 1990;**125**:153–9.

18 Myatt L, Lye SJ. Expression, localization and function of prostaglandin receptors in myometrium. *Prostaglandins Leukot Essent Fatty Acids* 2004;**70**:137–48.

19 Olson DM. The role of prostaglandins in the initiation of parturition. *Best Pract Res Clin Obstet Gynaecol* 2003;**17**:717–30.

20 Cook JL, Zaragoza DB, Sung DH, Olson DM. Expression of myometrial activation and stimulation genes in a mouse model of preterm labor: myometrial activation, stimulation, and preterm labor. *Endocrinology* 2000;**141**:1718–28.

21 Yoshida M, Sagawa N, Itoh H, *et al*. Prostaglandin F(2alpha), cytokines and cyclic mechanical stretch augment matrix metalloproteinase-1 secretion from cultured human uterine cervical fibroblast cells. *Mol Hum Reprod* 2002;**8**:681–7.

22 Denison FC, Calder AA, Kelly RW. The action of prostaglandin E2 on the human cervix: stimulation of interleukin 8 and inhibition of secretory leukocyte protease inhibitor. *Am J Obstet Gynecol* 1999;**180**:614–20.

23 Madsen G, Zakar T, Ku CY, Sanborn BM, Smith R, Mesiano S. Prostaglandins differentially modulate progesterone receptor-A and -B expression in human myometrial cells: evidence for prostaglandin-induced functional progesterone withdrawal. *J Clin Endocrinol Metab* 2004;**89**:1010–3.

24 Stjernholm-Vladic Y, Wang H, Stygar D, Ekman G, Sahlin L. Differential regulation of the progesterone receptor A and B in the human uterine cervix at parturition. *Gynecol Endocrinol* 2004;**18**:41–6.

25 Oh SY, Kim CJ, Park I, *et al*. Progesterone receptor isoform (A/B) ratio of human fetal membranes increases during term parturition. *Am J Obstet Gynecol* 2005;**193**:1156–60.

26 Zakar T, Hirst JJ, Mijovic JE, Olson DM. Glucocorticoids stimulate the expression of prostaglandin endoperoxide H synthase-2 in amnion cells. *Endocrinology* 1995;**136**:1610–9.

27 Patel FA, Clifton VL, Chwalisz K, Challis JR. Steroid regulation of prostaglandin dehydrogenase activity and expression in human term placenta and chorio-decidua in relation to labor. *J Clin Endocrinol Metab* 1999;**84**:291–9.

28 Parker CR Jr, Stankovic AM, Goland RS. Corticotropin-releasing hormone stimulates steroidogenesis in cultured human adrenal cells. *Mol Cell Endocrinol* 1999;**155**:19–25.

29 Di WL, Lachelin GC, McGarrigle HH, Thomas NS, Becker DL. Oestriol and oestradiol increase cell to cell communication and connexin43 protein expression in human myometrium. *Mol Hum Reprod* 2001;**7**:671–9.

30 Richter ON, Kubler K, Schmolling J, *et al*. Oxytocin receptor gene expression of estrogen-stimulated human myometrium in extracorporeally perfused non-pregnant uteri. *Mol Hum Reprod* 2004;**10**:339–46.

31 Mesiano S, Chan EC, Fitter JT, Kwek K, Yeo G, Smith R. Progesterone withdrawal and estrogen activation in human parturition are coordinated by progesterone receptor A expression in the myometrium. *J Clin Endocrinol Metab* 2002;**87**:2924–30.

32 Offenbacher S, Boggess KA, Murtha AP, *et al*. Progressive periodontal disease and risk of very preterm delivery. *Obstet Gynecol* 2006;**107**:29–36.

33 Locksmith G, Duff P. Infection, antibiotics, and preterm delivery. *Semin Perinatol* 2001;**25**:295–309.

34 Richey SD, Roberts SW, Ramin KD, Ramin SM, Cunningham FG. Pneumonia complicating pregnancy. *Obstet Gynecol* 1994;**84**:525–8.

35 Ramin KD, Ramin SM, Richey SD, Cunningham FG. Acute pancreatitis in pregnancy. *Am J Obstet Gynecol* 1995;**173**:187–91.

36 Goldenberg RL, Hauth JC, Andrews WW. Intrauterine infection and preterm delivery. *N Engl J Med* 2000;**342**:1500–7.

37 Mueller-Heubach E, Rubinstein DN, Schwarz SS. Histologic chorioamnionitis and preterm delivery in different patient populations. *Obstet Gynecol* 1990;**75**:622–6.

38 Andrews WW, Hauth JC, Goldenberg RL, Gomez R, Romero R, Cassell GH. Amniotic fluid interleukin-6: correlation with upper genital tract microbial colonization and gestational age in women delivered after spontaneous labor versus indicated delivery. *Am J Obstet Gynecol* 1995;**173**:606–12.

39 Meis PJ, Goldenberg RL, Mercer B, *et al*. The preterm prediction study: significance of vaginal infections. National Institute of Child Health and Human Development Maternal-Fetal Medicine Units Network. *Am J Obstet Gynecol* 1995;**173**:1231–5.

40 Hillier SL, Nugent RP, Eschenbach DA, *et al*. Association between bacterial vaginosis and preterm delivery of a low-birth-weight infant. The Vaginal Infections and Prematurity Study Group. *N Engl J Med* 1995;**333**:1737–42.

41 Leitich H, Bodner-Adler B, Brunbauer M, Kaider A, Egarter C, Husslein P. Bacterial vaginosis as a risk factor for preterm delivery: a meta-analysis. *Am J Obstet Gynecol* 2003;**189**:139–47.

42 Hillier SL. The complexity of microbial diversity in bacterial vaginosis. *N Engl J Med* 2005;**353**:1886–7.

43 Meis PJ, Goldenberg RL, Mercer B, *et al*. The preterm prediction study: significance of vaginal infections. National Institute of Child Health and Human Development Maternal-Fetal Medicine Units Network. *Am J Obstet Gynecol* 1995;**173**:1231–5.

44 Hillebrand L, Harmanli OH, Whiteman V, Khandelwal M. Urinary tract infections in pregnant women with bacterial vaginosis. *Am J Obstet Gynecol* 2002;**186**:916–7.

45 Romero R, Oyarzun E, Mazor M, Sirtori M, Hobbins JC, Bracken M. Meta-analysis of the relationship between asymptomatic bacteriuria and preterm delivery/low birth weight. *Obstet Gynecol* 1989;**73**:576–8.

46 Villar J, Gulmezoglu AM, de Onis M. Nutritional and antimicrobial interventions to prevent preterm birth: an overview of randomized controlled trials. *Obstet Gynecol Surv* 1998;**53**:575–85.

47 Krohn MA, Thwin SS, Rabe LK, Brown Z, Hillier SL. Vaginal colonization by *Escherichia coli* as a risk factor for very low birth weight delivery and other perinatal complications. *J Infect Dis* 1997;**175**:606–10.

48 Pioli PA, Amiel E, Schaefer TM, Connolly JE, Wira CR, Guyre PM. Differential expression of Toll-like receptors 2 and 4 in tissues of the human female reproductive tract. *Infect Immun* 2004;**72**:5799–806.

49 Kim YM, Romero R, Chaiworapongsa T, *et al*. Toll-like receptor-2 and -4 in the chorioamniotic membranes in spontaneous labor at term and in preterm parturition that are associated with chorioamnionitis. *Am J Obstet Gynecol* 2004;**191**:1346–5.

50 Holmlund U, Cebers G, Dahlfors AR, *et al*. Expression and regulation of the pattern recognition receptors Toll-like receptor-2 and Toll-like receptor-4 in the human placenta. *Immunology* 2002;**107**:145–51.

51 Belt AR, Baldassare JJ, Molnar M, Romero R, Hertelendy F. The nuclear transcription factor NF-κB mediates interleukin-1β-induced expression of cyclooxygenase-2 in human myometrial cells. *Am J Obstet Gynecol* 1999;**181**:359–66.

52 Yan X, Wu Xiao C, Sun M, Tsang BK, Gibb W. Nuclear factor κB activation and regulation of cyclooxygenase type-2 expression in human amnion mesenchymal cells by interleukin-1β. *Biol Reprod* 2002;**66**:1667–71.

53 Lee Y, Allport V, Sykes A, Lindstrom T, Slater D, Bennett P. The effects of labour and of interleukin 1 beta upon the expression of nuclear factor κB related proteins in human amnion. *Mol Hum Reprod* 2003;**9**:213–8.

54 Arechavaleta-Velasco F, Ogando D, Parry S, Vadillo-Ortega F. Production of matrix metalloproteinase-9 in lipopolysaccharide-stimulated human amnion occurs through an autocrine and paracrine proinflammatory cytokine-dependent system. *Biol Reprod* 2002;**67**:1952–8.

55 Van Meir CA, Sangha RK, Walton JC, Mathews SG, Keirse MJ, Challis JR. Immunoreactive 15-hydroxyprostaglandin dehydrogenase (PGDH) is reduced in fetal membranes from patients at preterm delivery in the presence of infection. *Placenta* 1996;**17**:291–7.

56 McLaren J, Taylor DJ, Bell SC. Prostaglandin E(2)-dependent production of latent matrix metalloproteinase-9 in cultures of human fetal membranes. *Mol Hum Reprod* 2000;**6**:1033–40.

57 Ito A, Nakamura T, Uchiyama T, *et al*. Stimulation of the biosynthesis of interleukin 8 by interleukin 1 and tumor necrosis factor alpha in cultured human chorionic cells. *Biol Pharm Bull* 1994;**17**:1463–7.

58 Arechavaleta-Velasco F, Ogando D, Parry S, Vadillo-Ortega F. Production of matrix metalloproteinase-9 in lipopolysaccharide-stimulated human amnion occurs through an autocrine and paracrine proinflammatory cytokine-dependent system. *Biol Reprod* 2002;**67**:1952–8.

59 So T, Ito A, Sato T, Mori Y, Hirakawa S. Tumor necrosis factor-alpha stimulates the biosynthesis of matrix metalloproteinases

and plasminogen activator in cultured human chorionic cells. *Biol Reprod* 1992;**46**:772–8.

60 Fortunato SJ, Menon R, Lombardi SJ. Role of tumor necrosis factor-alpha in the premature rupture of membranes and preterm labor pathways. *Am J Obstet Gynecol* 2002;**187**: 1159–62.

61 Lei H, Furth EE, Kalluri R, *et al*. A program of cell death and extracellular matrix degradation is activated in the amnion before the onset of labor. *J Clin Invest* 1996;**98**:1971–8.

62 Dudley DJ, Trautman MS, Araneo BA, Edwin SS, Mitchell MD. Decidual cell biosynthesis of interleukin-6: regulation by inflammatory cytokines. *J Clin Endocrinol Metab* 1992;**74**:884–9.

63 Fortunato SJ, Menon RP, Swan KF, Menon R. Inflammatory cytokine (interleukins 1, 6 and 8 and tumor necrosis factor-alpha) release from cultured human fetal membranes in response to endotoxic lipopolysaccharide mirrors amniotic fluid concentrations. *Am J Obstet Gynecol* 1996;**174**:1855–61.

64 Mitchell MD, Dudley DJ, Edwin SS, Schiller SL. Interleukin-6 stimulates prostaglandin production by human amnion and decidual cells. *Eur J Pharmacol* 1991;**192**:189–91.

65 Holst RM, Mattsby-Baltzer I, Wennerholm UB, Hagberg H, Jacobsson B. Interleukin-6 and interleukin-8 in cervical fluid in a population of Swedish women in preterm labor: relationship to microbial invasion of the amniotic fluid, intra-amniotic inflammation, and preterm delivery. *Acta Obstet Gynecol Scand* 2005;**84**:551–7.

66 Hillier SL, Martins J, Krohn M, Kiviat N, Holmes KK, Eschenbach DA. A case–control study of chorioamnionic infection and histologic chorioamnionitis in prematurity. *N Engl J Med* 1988;**319**:972–8.

67 Andrews WW, Goldenberg RL, Hauth JC. Preterm labor: emerging role of genital tract infections. *Infect Agents Dis* 1995;**4**:196–211.

68 Porter TF, Fraser A, Hunter CY, Ward R, Varner MW. The intergenerational predisposition to preterm birth. *Obstet Gynecol* 1997;**90**:63–7.

69 Winkvist A, Mogren I, Hogberg U. Familial patterns in birth characteristics: impact on individual and population risks. *Int J Epidemiol* 1998;**27**:248–54.

70 Treloar SA, Macones GA, Mitchell LE, Martin NG. Genetic influences on premature parturition in an Australian twin sample. *Twin Res* 2000;**3**:80–2.

71 Clausson B, Lichtenstein P, Cnattingius S. Genetic influence on birthweight and gestational length determined by studies in offspring of twins. *Br J Obstet Gynaecol* 2000;**107**:375–81.

72 Roberts AK, Monzon-Bordonaba F, Van Deerlin PG, *et al*. Association of polymorphism within the promoter of the tumor necrosis factor alpha gene with increased risk of preterm premature rupture of the fetal membranes. *Am J Obstet Gynecol* 1999;**180**:1297–302.

73 Macones GA, Parry S, Elkousy M, Clothier B, Ural S, Strauss JF III. A polymorphism in the promoter region of TNF and bacterial vaginosis: preliminary evidence of gene-environment interaction in the etiology of spontaneous preterm birth. *Am J Obstet Gynecol* 2004;**190**:1504–8.

74 Simhan HN, Krohn MA, Roberts JM, Zeevi A, Caritis SN. Interleukin-6 promoter-174 polymorphism and spontaneous preterm birth. *Am J Obstet Gynecol* 2003;**189**:915–8.

75 Lorenz E, Hallman M, Marttila R, Haataha R, Schwartz D. Association between the Asp299Gly polymorphisms in the toll-like receptor 4 and premature births in the Finnish population. *Pediatr Res* 2002;**52**:373–6.

76 Fujimoto T, Parry S, Urbanek M, *et al*. A single nucleotide polymorphism in the matrix metalloproteinase-1 (MMP-1) promoter influences amnion cell MMP-1 expression and risk for preterm premature rupture of the fetal membranes. *J Biol Chem* 2002;**277**:6296–302.

77 Ferrand PE, Parry S, Sammel M, *et al*. A polymorphism in the matrix metalloproteinase-9 promoter is associated with increased risk of preterm premature rupture of membranes in African Americans. *Mol Hum Reprod* 2002;**8**:494–501.

78 Genc MR, Gerber S, Nesin M, Witkin SS. Polymorphism in the interleukin-1 gene complex and spontaneous preterm delivery. *Am J Obstet Gynecol* 2002;**187**:157–63.

79 Wang X, Chen D, Niu T, *et al*. Genetic susceptibility to benzene and shortened gestation: evidence of gene–environment interaction. *Am J Epidemiol* 2000;**152**:693–700.

80 Wang X, Zuckerman B, Pearson C, *et al*. Maternal cigarette smoking, metabolic gene polymorphism, and infant birth weight. *JAMA* 2002;**287**:195–202.

81 Harger JH, Hsing AW, Tuomala RE, *et al*. Risk factors for preterm premature rupture of fetal membranes: a multicenter case–control study. *Am J Obstet Gynecol* 1990;**163**:130–7.

82 Salafia CM, Lopez-Zeno JA, Sherer DM, *et al*. Histologic evidence of old intrauterine bleeding is more frequent in prematurity. *Am J Obstet Gynecol* 1995;**173**:1065–70.

83 Roque H, Paidas MJ, Funai EF, Kuczynski E, Lockwood CJ. Maternal thrombophilias are not associated with early pregnancy loss. *Thromb Haemost* 2004;**91**:290–5.

84 Nurk E, Tell GS, Refsum H, Ueland PM, Vollset SE. Associations between maternal methylenetetrahydrofolate reductase polymorphisms and adverse outcomes of pregnancy: the Hordaland Homocysteine Study. *Am J Med* 2004;**117**:26–31.

85 Misra DP, Ananth CV. Risk factor profiles of placental abruption in first and second pregnancies: heterogeneous etiologies. *J Clin Epidemiol* 1999;**52**:453–61.

86 Strobino B, Pantel-Silverman J. Gestational vaginal bleeding and pregnancy outcome. *Am J Epidemiol* 1989;**129**:806–15.

87 Naeye RL. Maternal age, obstetric complications, and the outcome of pregnancy. *Obstet Gynecol* 1983;**61**:210–6.

88 Lockwood C, Krikun G, Schatz F. The decidua regulates hemostasis in the human endometrium. *Semin Reprod Endocrinol* 1999;**17**:45–51.

89 Mackenzie AP, Schatz F, Krikun G, Funai EF, Kadner S, Lockwood CJ. Mechanisms of abruption-induced premature rupture of the fetal membranes: thrombin enhanced decidual matrix metalloproteinase-3 (stromelysin-1) expression. *Am J Obstet Gynecol* 2004;**191**:1996–2001.

90 Rosen T, Schatz F, Kuczynski E, Lam H, Koo AB, Lockwood CJ. Thrombin-enhanced matrix metalloproteinase-1 expression: a mechanism linking placental abruption with premature rupture of the membranes. *J Matern Fetal Neonatal Med* 2002;**11**:11–7.

91 Lockwood CJ, Toti P, Arcuri F, *et al*. Mechanisms of abruption-induced premature rupture of the fetal membranes: thrombin-enhanced interleukin-8 expression in term decidua. *Am J Pathol* 2005;**167**:1443–9.

92 Lathbury LJ, Salamonsen LA. *In vitro* studies of the potential role of neutrophils in the process of menstruation. *Mol Hum Reprod* 2000;6:899–906.

93 Stephenson CD, Lockwood CJ, Ma Y, Guller S. Thrombin-dependent regulation of matrix metalloproteinase (MMP)-9 levels in human fetal membranes. *J Matern Fetal Neonatal Med* 2005;18:17–22.

94 Phillippe M, Chien EK. Intracellular signaling and phasic myometrial contractions. *J Soc Gynecol Investig* 1998;5:169–77.

95 CDC NCHS Vol 52:1-118 December 17, 2003.

96 Levy R, Kanengiser B, Furman B, Ben Arie A, Brown D, Hagay ZJ. A randomized trial comparing a 30-mL and an 80-mL Foley catheter balloon for preinduction cervical ripening. *Am J Obstet Gynecol* 2004;191:1632–6.

97 Olund A, Jonasson A, Kindahl H, Fianu S, Larsson B. The effect of cervical dilatation by laminaria on the plasma levels of 15-keto-13,14-dihydro-PGF2 alpha. *Contraception* 1984;30:23–7.

98 Leguizamon G, Smith J, Younis H, Nelson DM, Sadovsky Y. Enhancement of amniotic cyclooxygenase type 2 activity in women with preterm delivery associated with twins or polyhydramnios. *Am J Obstet Gynecol* 2001;184:117–22.

99 Terakawa K, Itoh H, Sagawa N, *et al.* Site-specific augmentation of amnion cyclooxygenase-2 and decidua vera phospholipase-A2 expression in labor: possible contribution of mechanical stretch and interleukin-1 to amnion prostaglandin synthesis. *J Soc Gynecol Investig* 2002;9:68–74.

100 Terzidou V, Sooranna SR, Kim LU, Thornton S, Bennett PR, Johnson MR. Mechanical stretch up-regulates the human oxytocin receptor in primary human uterine myocytes. *J Clin Endocrinol Metab* 2005;90:237–46.

101 Sooranna SR, Engineer N, Loudon JA, Terzidou V, Bennett PR, Johnson MR. The mitogen-activated protein kinase dependent expression of prostaglandin H synthase-2 and interleukin-8 messenger ribonucleic acid by myometrial cells: the differential effect of stretch and interleukin-1β. *J Clin Endocrinol Metab* 2005;90:3517–27.

102 Loudon JA, Sooranna SR, Bennett PR, Johnson MR. Mechanical stretch of human uterine smooth muscle cells increases IL-8 mRNA expression and peptide synthesis. *Mol Hum Reprod* 2004;10:895–9.

103 Ou CW, Orsino A, Lye SJ. Expression of connexin-43 and connexin-26 in the rat myometrium during pregnancy and labor is differentially regulated by mechanical and hormonal signals. *Endocrinology* 1997;138:5398–407.

104 Husslein P, Sinzinger H. Concentration of 13,14-dihydro-15-keto-prostaglandin E2 in the maternal peripheral plasma during labour of spontaneous onset. *Br J Obstet Gynaecol* 1984;91:228–31.

105 Sellers SM, Hodgson HT, Mitchell MD, Anderson AB, Turnbull AC. Raised prostaglandin levels in the third stage of labor. *Am J Obstet Gynecol* 1982;144:209–12.

106 Keirse MJNC, Turnbull AC. Prostaglandins in amniotic fluid during late pregnancy and labour. *J Obstet Gynaecol Br Commonw* 1973;80:970–3.

107 Casey ML, MacDonald PC. Biomolecular processes in the initiation of parturition: decidual activation. *Clin Obstet Gynecol* 1988;31:533–52.

108 Matsumoto T, Sagawa N, Yoshida M, *et al.* The prostaglandin E2 and F2 alpha receptor genes are expressed in human myometrium and are down-regulated during pregnancy. *Biochem Biophys Res Commun* 1997;238:838–41.

109 Brodt-Eppley J, Myatt L. Prostaglandin receptors in lower uterine segment myometrium during gestation and labor. *Obstet Gynecol* 1999;93:89–93.

110 Sibai B, Meis PJ, Klebanoff M, *et al.* Maternal Fetal Medicine Units Network of the National Institute of Child Health and Human Development. Plasma CRH measurement at 16 to 20 weeks' gestation does not predict preterm delivery in women at high-risk for preterm delivery. *Am J Obstet Gynecol* 2005;193:1181–6.

111 Berkowitz GS, Lapinski RH, Lockwood CJ, Florio P, Blackmore-Prince C, Petraglia F. Corticotropin-releasing factor and its binding protein: maternal serum levels in term and preterm deliveries. *Am J Obstet Gynecol* 1996;174:1477–83.

112 Holzman C, Jetton J, Siler-Khodr T, Fisher R, Rip T. Second trimester corticotropin-releasing hormone levels in relation to preterm delivery and ethnicity. *Obstet Gynecol* 2001;97:657–63.

113 McLean M, Bisits A, Davies J, *et al.* Predicting risk of preterm delivery by second-trimester measurement of maternal plasma corticotropin-releasing hormone and alpha-fetoprotein concentrations. *Am J Obstet Gynecol* 1999;181:207–15.

114 Leung TN, Chung TK, Madsen G, McLean M, Chang AM, Smith R. Elevated mid-trimester maternal corticotrophin-releasing hormone levels in pregnancies that delivered before 34 weeks. *Br J Obstet Gynaecol* 1999;106:1041–6.

115 Inder WJ, Prickett TC, Ellis MJ, *et al.* The utility of plasma CRH as a predictor of preterm delivery. *J Clin Endocrinol Metab* 2001;86:5706–10.

116 Coleman MA, France JT, Schellenberg JC, *et al.* Corticotropin-releasing hormone, corticotropin-releasing hormone-binding protein, and activin A in maternal serum: prediction of preterm delivery and response to glucocorticoids in women with symptoms of preterm labor. *Am J Obstet Gynecol* 2000;183:643–8.

117 Heine RP, McGregor JA, Goodwin TM, *et al.* Serial salivary estriol to detect an increased risk of preterm birth. *Obstet Gynecol* 2000;96:490–7.

118 McGregor JA, Jackson GM, Lachelin GC, *et al.* Salivary estriol as risk assessment for preterm labor: a prospective trial. *Am J Obstet Gynecol* 1995;173:1337–42.

119 Lockwood CJ, Ghidini A, Wein R, Lapinski R, Casal D, Berkowitz RL. Increased interleukin-6 concentrations in cervical secretions are associated with preterm delivery. *Am J Obstet Gynecol* 1994;171:1097–10.

120 Goepfert AR, Goldenberg RL, Andrews WW, *et al.* National Institute of Child Health and Human Development Maternal-Fetal Medicine Units Network. The Preterm Prediction Study: association between cervical interleukin 6 concentration and spontaneous preterm birth. National Institute of Child Health and Human Development Maternal-Fetal Medicine Units Network. *Am J Obstet Gynecol* 2001;184:483–8.

121 Trebeden H, Goffinet F, Kayem G, *et al.* Strip test for bedside detection of interleukin-6 in cervical secretions is predictive for impending preterm delivery. *Eur Cytokine Netw* 2001;12:359–60.

122 Kurkinen-Raty M, Ruokonen A, Vuopala S, *et al.* Combination of cervical interleukin-6 and -8, phosphorylated insulin-like growth factor-binding protein-1 and transvaginal cervical

ultrasonography in assessment of the risk of preterm birth. *Br J Obstet Gynaecol* 2001;**108**:875–81.

123 Coleman MA, Keelan JA, McCowan LM, Townend KM, Mitchell MD. Predicting preterm delivery: comparison of cervicovaginal interleukin (IL)-1β, IL-6 and IL-8 with fetal fibronectin and cervical dilatation. *Eur J Obstet Gynecol Reprod Biol* 2001;**95**:154–8.

124 Lange M, Chen FK, Wessel J, Buscher U, Dudenhausen JW. Elevation of interleukin-6 levels in cervical secretions as a predictor of preterm delivery. *Acta Obstet Gynecol Scand* 2003;**82**:326–9.

125 Rizzo G, Capponi A, Vlachopoulou A, Angelini E, Grassi C, Romanini C. The diagnostic value of interleukin-8 and fetal fibronectin concentrations in cervical secretions in patients with preterm labor and intact membranes. *J Perinat Med* 1997;**25**:461–8.

126 Goldenberg RL, Andrews WW, Guerrant RL, *et al*. The preterm prediction study: cervical lactoferrin concentration, other markers of lower genital tract infection, and preterm birth. National Institute of Child Health and Human Development Maternal-Fetal Medicine Units Network. *Am J Obstet Gynecol* 2000;**182**:631–5.

127 Andrews WW, Tsao J, Goldenberg RL, *et al*. The preterm prediction study: failure of midtrimester cervical sialidase level elevation to predict subsequent spontaneous preterm birth. *Am J Obstet Gynecol* 1999;**180**:1151–4.

128 Wang EY, Woodruff TK, Moawad A. Follistatin-free activin A is not associated with preterm birth. *Am J Obstet Gynecol* 2002;**186**:464–9.

129 Moawad AH, Goldenberg RL, Mercer B, *et al*. The Preterm Prediction Study: the value of serum alkaline phosphatase, alpha-fetoprotein, plasma corticotropin-releasing hormone, and other serum markers for the prediction of spontaneous preterm birth. *Am J Obstet Gynecol* 2002;**186**:990–6.

130 Simhan HN, Caritis SN, Krohn MA, Hillier SL. Elevated vaginal pH and neutrophils are associated strongly with early spontaneous preterm birth. *Am J Obstet Gynecol* 2003;**189**:1150–4.

131 Simhan HN, Caritis SN, Krohn MA, Hillier SL. The vaginal inflammatory milieu and the risk of early premature preterm rupture of membranes. *Am J Obstet Gynecol* 2005;**192**:213–8.

132 Rosen T, Kuczynski E, O'Neill LM, Funai EF, Lockwood CJ. Plasma levels of thrombin–antithrombin complexes predict preterm premature rupture of the fetal membranes. *J Matern Fetal Med* 2001;**10**:297–300.

133 Elovitz MA, Baron J, Phillippe M. The role of thrombin in preterm parturition. *Am J Obstet Gynecol* 2001;**185**:1059–63.

134 Chaiworapongsa T, Espinoza J, Yoshimatsu J, *et al*. Activation of coagulation system in preterm labor and preterm premature rupture of membranes. *J Matern Fetal Neonatal Med* 2002;**11**:368–73.

135 Lockwood CJ, Senyei AE, Dische MR, *et al*. Fetal fibronectin in cervical and vaginal secretions as a predictor of preterm delivery. *N Engl J Med* 1991;**325**:669–74.

136 Feinberg RF, Kliman HJ, Lockwood CJ. Is oncofetal fibronectin a trophoblast glue for human implantation? *Am J Pathol* 1991;**138**:537–43.

137 Peaceman AM, Andrews WW, Thorp JM, *et al*. Fetal fibronectin as a predictor of preterm birth in patients with symptoms: a multicenter trial. *Am J Obstet Gynecol* 1997;**177**:13–8.

138 Honest H, Bachmann LM, Gupta JK, Kleijnen J, Khan KS. Accuracy of cervicovaginal fetal fibronectin test in predicting risk of spontaneous preterm birth: systematic review. *Br Med J* 2002;**325**:301–4.

139 Lockwood CJ, Wein R, Lapinski R, *et al*. The presence of cervical and vaginal fetal fibronectin predicts preterm delivery in an inner-city obstetric population. *Am J Obstet Gynecol* 1993;**169**:798–804.

140 Goldenberg RL, Mercer BM, Meis PJ, Copper RL, Das A, McNellis D. The preterm prediction study: fetal fibronectin testing and spontaneous preterm birth. NICHD Maternal Fetal Medicine Units Network. *Obstet Gynecol* 1996;**87**:643–8.

141 Goldenberg RL, Iams JD, Miodovnik M, *et al*. The preterm prediction study: risk factors in twin gestations. National Institute of Child Health and Human Development Maternal-Fetal Medicine Units Network. *Am J Obstet Gynecol* 1996;**175**:1047–53.

142 Roman AS, Rebarber A, Sfakianaki AK, *et al*. Vaginal fetal fibronectin as a predictor of spontaneous preterm delivery in the patient with cervical cerclage. *Am J Obstet Gynecol* 2003;**189**:1368–73.

143 Roman AS, Rebarber A, Lipkind H, Mulholland J, Minior V, Roshan D. Vaginal fetal fibronectin as a predictor of spontaneous preterm delivery after multifetal pregnancy reduction. *Am J Obstet Gynecol* 2004;**190**:142–6.

144 Roman AS, Koklanaris N, Paidas MJ, Mulholland J, Levitz M, Rebarber A. "Blind" vaginal fetal fibronectin as a predictor of spontaneous preterm delivery. *Obstet Gynecol* 2005;**105**:285–9.

145 Iams JD, Goldenberg RL, Meis PJ, *et al*. The length of the cervix and the risk of spontaneous premature delivery. National Institute of Child Health and Human Development Maternal Fetal Medicine Unit Network. *N Engl J Med* 1996;**334**:567–72.

146 Iams JD. Prediction and early detection of preterm labor. *Obstet Gynecol* 2003;**10**:402–12.

147 Tsoi E, Akmal S, Rane S, Otigbah C, Nicolaides KH. Ultrasound assessment of cervical length in threatened preterm labor. *Ultrasound Obstet Gynecol* 2003;**21**:552–5.

148 Vendittelli F, Volumenie J. Transvaginal ultrasonography examination of the uterine cervix in hospitalised women undergoing preterm labour. *Eur J Obstet Gynecol Reprod Biol* 2000;**90**:3–11.

149 Iams JD, Johnson FF, Sonek J, Sachs L, Gebauer C, Samuels P. Cervical competence as a continuum: a study of ultrasonographic cervical length and obstetric performance. *Am J Obstet Gynecol* 1995;**172**:1097–103.

150 Owen J, Yost N, Berghella V, *et al*. National Institute of Child Health and Human Development, Maternal-Fetal Medicine Units Network. Mid-trimester endovaginal sonography in women at high risk for spontaneous preterm birth. *JAMA* 2001;**286**:1340–8.

151 Taipale P, Hiilesmaa V. Sonographic measurement of uterine cervix at 18–22 weeks' gestation and the risk of preterm delivery. *Obstet Gynecol* 1998;**92**:902–7.

152 Iams JD, Goldenberg RL, Mercer BM, *et al*. The preterm prediction study: can low-risk women destined for spontaneous preterm birth be identified? *Am J Obstet Gynecol* 2001;**184**:652–5.

153 Hincz P, Wilczynski J, Kozarzewski M, Szaflik K. Two-step test: the combined use of fetal fibronectin and sonographic examination of the uterine cervix for prediction of preterm delivery in symptomatic patients. *Acta Obstet Gynecol Scand* 2002;**81**:58–63.

154 Goldenberg RL, Iams JD, Das A, *et al*. The Preterm Prediction Study: sequential cervical length and fetal fibronectin testing for the prediction of spontaneous preterm birth. National Institute of Child Health and Human Development Maternal-Fetal Medicine Units Network. *Am J Obstet Gynecol* 2000;**182**:636–43.

41 Preterm premature rupture of membranes

Brian M. Mercer

Rupture of fetal membranes before the onset of labor (premature rupture of membranes, PROM) complicates 8–10% of pregnancies, and is responsible for nearly one-third of preterm births [1–3]. PROM, especially preterm PROM (PPROM), has been associated with brief latency from membrane rupture to delivery, an increased risk of chorioamnionitis, and umbilical cord compression. As such PPROM is associated with increased risk of perinatal complications. An understanding of gestational age-dependent risks of delivery, the risks and potential benefits of conservative management, and opportunities to reduce complications of preterm birth will help the clinician improve outcomes after this frequent pregnancy complication.

Mechanisms

Spontaneous membrane rupture at term results from progressive weakening of the membranes because of collagen remodeling and cellular apoptosis, and from increased intrauterine pressure with uterine contractions when membrane rupture occurs subsequent to the onset of labor. While PPROM near term likely results in most cases from these same physiologic processes, PPROM remote from term has been associated with several pathologic processes, especially infection and inflammation. Reported clinical risk factors predisposing to intrauterine infection and/or inflammation, membrane stretch, and local tissue hypoxia have included low socioeconomic status, maternal undernutrition, cigarette smoking, uterine bleeding and work in pregnancy, cervical cerclage *in situ*, prior preterm labor and acute pulmonary disease in the current pregnancy, and bacterial vaginosis in addition to other urogenital infections [1–9]. It has been proposed that there could be a genetic predisposition to PPROM in some women, either through inheritance of non-wild-type polymorphisms for proinflammatory cytokines and metalloproteases [10,11], or through heritable connective tissue disorders of collagen metabolism. Among the strongest risk factors for PPROM is a history of

preterm birth in a previous gestation, particularly one resulting from PPROM (odds ratio [OR] 3.3–6.3) [9].

The role of ascending infection in the pathogenesis of PPROM is particularly plausible as bacterial proteases (collagenases and phospholipases) can cause membrane weakening. Ascending bacterial colonization can also cause a local inflammatory response including production of cytokines, prostaglandins, and metalloproteases which cause membrane degradation and weakening. Preterm contractions can lead to strain hardening of the membranes, while cervical dilatation can result in exposure of the membranes to vaginal microorganisms and reduce underlying tissue support.

Prediction and prevention

Although the above-mentioned clinical risk factors have been associated with PPROM, most women with these characteristics do not develop PPROM and the majority of women with PPROM lack these risk factors. This has led to interest in ancillary testing for prediction of PPROM. Recent study has found both short cervical length on transvaginal ultrasound (less than 25 mm; relative risk [RR] 3.2) and the presence of fetal fibronectin (fFN) in cervicovaginal secretions (RR 2.5) to be associated with an increased risk of preterm birth resulting from PROM [9]. However, like clinical risk factors, these modalities also fail to identify the majority of women destined to have PPROM and thus they are not recommended as routine screening tests for low-risk women.

Identification and treatment of sexually transmitted urogenital infections such as *Chlamydia trachomatis* and *Neisseria gonorrhoea* can reduce the risks of PROM and preterm birth. Treatment of symptomatic bacterial vaginosis and *Trichomonas vaginalis* infection is also likely beneficial, although treatment of women with asymptomatic vaginal infections is controversial and may even be harmful [12,13]. While it is likely that smoking cessation, adequate nutrition before and during pregnancy, and avoidance of unnecessary cervical cerclage could reduce the risk of PPROM, direct benefit has not been demonstrated.

Diagnosis

Diagnosis of membrane rupture is best made by sterile speculum examination of women presenting with a suspicious clinical history or found to have oligohydramnios on ultrasonography. Evident fluid passing through the cervical os is diagnostic. An alkaline vaginal pH (>6.0–6.5) with Nitrazine paper and the presence of a "ferning" pattern on microscopic examination of dried vaginal secretions are supportive when visual inspection is equivocal. These tests are subject to false positive findings because of the presence of cervical mucus, blood, semen, alkaline antiseptics, or bacterial vaginosis, and can be falsely negative with prolonged leakage and oligohydramnios. Repeat speculum examination after prolonged bed rest may provide diagnostic information if initial testing is negative despite a suspicious history. In the absence of fetal growth restriction or urogenital abnormalities, ultrasound evidence of oligohydramnios is suggestive but not diagnostic of membrane rupture. The diagnosis can be confirmed unequivocally by indigo carmine amnioinfusion with observation for passage of dye per vaginum.

Although a variety of substances, including fFN, prolactin, alpha-fetoprotein, human chorionic gonadotropin, insulin-like growth factor binding protein 1 (IGFBP-1), and lacate have been evaluated for their ability to assist in the diagnosis of membrane rupture, these have not generally been studied for their diagnostic ability among women in whom the diagnosis of membrane rupture remains unclear after clinical examination. Further, some of these markers do not require membrane rupture to be present in cervicovaginal secretions. For these reasons, routine testing with these markers is not recommended until their clinical value is clarified.

Clinical course

Brief latency from membrane rupture to delivery, increased risk of intrauterine and neonatal infection, and oligohydramnios have been considered hallmarks of PPROM. Each can impact pregnancy outcomes, and each has implications regarding clinical management of women with PPROM.

While it is true that mean and median latency from membrane rupture to delivery increase with decreasing gestational age at membrane rupture, the clinical importance of this finding is overstated. The likelihood of delivery within 1 week, during conservative management of PROM at 24–32 weeks, is approximately half of those remaining pregnant at any given time, up to 34 weeks [14,15]. Approximately one-quarter of those with membrane rupture near the limit of viability will remain pregnant for 1 month or more. Those with PROM at or near term are rarely given the opportunity to remain pregnant

for an extended time. Benefits of conservative management include additional time for induction of fetal pulmonary maturity and prevention of intraventricular hemorrhage through administration of antenatal corticosteroids (24–48 hours latency required), and reduction of gestational age-dependent morbidity through extended latency (more than approximately 1 week latency required).

Chorioamnionitis complicates 13–60% of pregnancies with PROM, and is increasingly common with decreasing gestational age at membrane rupture [16]. Abruptio placentae, amnionitis, and endometritis complicate 4–12%, 13–60%, and 2–13% of pregnancies, respectively, when membrane rupture occurs remote from term [16–18]. Amniotic fluid cultures from amniocentesis specimens are positive in 25–35% of asymptomatic women after PPROM [19]. Maternal sepsis is uncommon (approximately 1%) but is a serious complication of PROM remote from term. Conservative management of PROM at any gestational age increases the risk of chorioamnionitis. Fetal demise after PPROM is believed to result in most cases from umbilical cord compression. Fetal infection, placental abruption, and umbilical cord prolapse can also lead to fetal death. Overall, fetal death complicates approximately 1% of pregnancies conservatively managed after PPROM. This risk increases in the face of chorioamnionitis, and when PROM occurs near the limit of potential viability. Abruptio placentae (approximately 4–12%) may occur before or after membrane rupture [20,21].

Therefore, expeditious delivery should be considered if the fetus is considered to be at low risk for gestational age-dependent morbidity, if antenatal corticosteroids are not going to be administered when only brief pregnancy prolongation is anticipated, or if continued attempts to extend latency more than approximately 1 week is not planned after antenatal corticosteroid treatment has been completed.

Evaluation

In general, women with PROM at term do not require additional specific evaluations unless additional complications occur. Initial evaluation of the woman presenting with PPROM includes (Table 41.1):

1 Maternal uterine activity and fetal heart rate monitoring for labor, umbilical cord compression, and for fetal well-being if the limit of potential viability has been reached;
2 Clinical assessment for chorioamnionitis (fever ≥38.0°C [100.4°F] with uterine tenderness, maternal or fetal tachycardia, vaginal discharge); and
3 Ultrasound to confirm gestational age and to identify fetal malformations associated with PROM and oligohydramnios if not previously performed, to determine fetal presentation, and to estimate fetal weight and amniotic fluid volume.

Digital cervical examination should be avoided if possible until the diagnosis of PROM has been excluded or a decision to

Table 41.1 Considerations for initial evaluation of the woman with preterm premature rupture of membranes (PPROM).

Maternal uterine activity monitoring for labor

Fetal heart rate monitoring for umbilical cord compression (and fetal well-being if the limit of viability has been reached)

Clinical assessment for chorioamnionitis

Ultrasound to confirm gestational age, estimate fetal growth, and amniotic fluid volume, identify fetal malformations associated with PROM/oligohydramnios if not previously carried out, and to determine fetal presentation

Visual inspection of cervical dilatation and effacement if not in active labor

Cervical cultures for *Neisseria gonorrhoeae* and *Chlamydia trachomatis* if not recently performed

Anovaginal culture for group B streptococcus if not recently performed

Urinalysis with urine culture if not recently performed

Baseline maternal blood white blood cell

Vaginal pool or ultrasound guided amniocentesis sampling for fetal pulmonary maturity at 32–33 weeks' gestation

PROM, premature rupture of membranes.

Table 41.2 Adjuncts to the evaluation of the woman with equivocal findings of intra-amniotic infection.

Maternal blood white blood cell count
Rising values and a value above 16,000/mm^3 are supportive of the diagnosis if antenatal corticosteroids not administered within 5–7 days

Ultrasound guided amniocentesis
Positive culture considered abnormal

Positive Gram stain supportive but may be falsely positive as a result of contamination

White blood cell count ≥30 cells/µL considered abnormal

Glucose concentration <16–20 mg/dL considered abnormal

deliver has been made. Digital examination in this setting shortens latency and increases the risk of chorioamnionitis while adding little information over that obtained by visual examination [22]. Cervical cultures for *Neisseria gonorrhoeae* and *Chlamydia trachomatis*, anovaginal culture for group B streptococci (GBS), and urinalysis with urine culture should be considered if not recently performed. Positive cultures should lead to appropriate therapy. Intrapartum prophylaxis should be administered to those with positive GBS cultures, regardless of intervening antibiotic treatments [23].

If the diagnosis of chorioamnionitis is suspected but not clear, maternal blood white blood cell (WBC) count and ultrasound guided amniocentesis can sometimes be helpful. A maternal WBC count above 16,000/mm^3 is supportive of suspicious clinical findings. It is helpful to obtain a baseline WBC count on presentation after PPROM to be used during initial assessment and for subsequent comparison if needed during conservative management. It is important to remember that there is significant variation in WBC count between patients,

and that the WBC count is elevated in pregnancy and for 5–7 days after administration of antenatal corticosteroids. As such, this test should not be used in isolation. Amniotic fluid Gram stain, WBC count (≥30 cells/µL considered abnormal), and glucose concentration (less than 16–20 mg/dL considered abnormal) can also provide rapid supportive information regarding the presence of intra-amniotic infection [24–26]. Elevated amniotic fluid, blood, and vaginal fluid cytokine levels have also been associated with intrauterine infection after PPROM; however, tests for these markers are not generally available for clinical use. Culture for aerobic and anaerobic bacteria and for mycoplasma can be helpful, but results are generally not available before a management decision is needed.

Management

Delivery after PPROM is mandated by the presence of clinical chorioamnionitis, nonreassuring fetal testing, significant vaginal bleeding, and advanced labor. In the absence of these conditions, conservative management may be appropriate. If conservative management of the patient with PPROM is being considered, initial extended monitoring followed by intermittent monitoring at least daily is appropriate. Biophysical profile testing can be helpful if fetal heart rate testing is nonreactive. A nonreactive fetal heart rate or a nonreassuring biophysical profile score can be a sign of intrauterine infection, particularly if testing had previously been reassuring [26,27]. In the stable patient, gestational age is important in determining whether conservative management or expeditious delivery should be pursued [19].

Preterm PROM near term (34–36w 6d)

Infants born after PROM near term (34–36w 6d) have a relatively low risk of serious morbidity and antenatal corticosteroids are not generally recommended for fetal maturation at this gestation. Although there are risks of neonatal morbidity at this gestation, these risks are not likely to be reduced with the relatively brief latency anticipated at this gestation, and the risks related to intrauterine infection and umbilical cord compression outweigh the potential benefits of conservative management [28,29]. Because of these factors, women with PPROM at 34–36w 6d are best treated by expeditious delivery. Intrapartum GBS prophylaxis should be given in the absence of a recent (less than 6 weeks) negative anovaginal GBS culture.

PROM near term (32–33w 6d)

When PROM occurs at 32–33w 6d gestation, fetal pulmonary maturity should be assessed from amniotic fluid collected from the vaginal pool or by amniocentesis if feasible. From

Table 41.3 Options for management of the woman with preterm premature rupture of membranes (PROM) according to gestational age at membrane rupture.

PROM near term (34–36w 6d)[a]

Expeditious delivery, by labor induction or cesarean delivery as indicated

Intrapartum GBS prophylaxis in the absence of a recent negative anovaginal culture

Broad-spectrum intrapartum antibiotics for suspected chorioamnionitis

*PROM near term (32–33w 6d)**

Expeditious delivery, by labor induction or cesarean delivery as indicated, if fetal pulmonary maturity evident on sampling from the vaginal pool or by amniocentesis

Antenatal corticosteroids for fetal maturation if amniotic fluid testing reveals an immature profile or if fluid unavailable, followed by;

• Delivery 24–48 hours after antenatal corticosteroids if ≥33 weeks' gestation

or

• Delivery 24–48 hours after antenatal corticosteroids if or at 34 weeks if <33 weeks' gestation (if conservatively managed, treat as described for PROM at 23–31w 6d)

Intrapartum GBS prophylaxis in the absence of a recent negative culture

Broad-spectrum intrapartum antibiotics for suspected chorioamnionitis

*PROM remote from term (23–31w 6d)**

Conservative inpatient management

Transfer to a tertiary care facility if adequate facilities for neonatal care not available

At least daily assessment for labor, amnionitis, placental abruption, and fetal well-being

Leg exercises, antiembolic stockings, and/or prophylactic heparin

Fetal growth assessment by ultrasound every 3–4 weeks

Antenatal corticosteroids for fetal maturation if not previously administered

Broad-spectrum antibiotics to prolong pregnancy and reduce neonatal morbidity

Tocolytic therapy for labor can be given but should not be administered if there is suspicion of intrauterine infection, fetal compromise, or placental abruption

Consider elective delivery at 34 weeks' gestation if remains pregnant to this time

Intrapartum GBS prophylaxis in the absence of a recent negative culture

Broad-spectrum intrapartum antibiotics for suspected chorioamnionitis

Previable PROM (<23 weeks)

Counsel regarding:

• Potential for previable, periviable, and preterm birth

• Impact of oligohydramnios on pulmonary development and risk of lethal pulmonary hypoplasia and restriction deformities

• Risks of adverse fetal, neonatal, and long-term infant outcomes with early preterm birth

• Risks of maternal morbidities with conservative management

Deliver by labor induction or dilatation and evacuation according to individual circumstances

or

Manage conservatively with:

• Initial evaluation for intrauterine infection, labor, fetal death, or placental abruption

• Strict pelvic rest and modified bed/couch rest

• Serial ultrasound for fetal weight and pulmonary growth, and amniotic fluid volume

• Broad-spectrum antibiotics to prolong pregnancy and reduce neonatal morbidity may be helpful but no specific data are available for this gestational age

• Treat as for PROM at 23–31w 6d once the limit of viability has been reached

GBS, group B streptococcus.

* Delivery is mandated by the presence of chorioamnionitis, nonreassuring fetal testing/fetal death, significant vaginal bleeding, and for advanced labor.

---

either site, a foam stability index ≥47, phosphatidyl glycerol positive, lecithin:sphingomyelin (L:S) ratio ≥2/1 or TDx-FLMassay ≥55 can be considered indicative of fetal pulmonary maturity [30–33]. The L:S ratio and FLM results may be falsely immature in the presence of blood or meconium contamination, although the presence of either should lead to consideration of delivery [34–36]. If a mature fetal pulmonary profile is obtained, expeditious delivery should be considered in accordance with the recommendations for PROM at 34–36w

6d as these infants are at low risk for complications of prematurity and conservative management increases the risk of infectious morbidity [29]. If testing reveals an immature pulmonary profile or if fluid cannot be obtained, induction of fetal pulmonary maturation with antenatal corticosteroids followed by delivery at 24–48 hours or at 34 weeks' gestation is recommended. If after antenatal corticosteroid administration the patient is ≥33 weeks' gestation, it is unlikely that further delay of delivery to 34 weeks will result in substantial reduction in infant morbidities. Delivery is recommended before complications ensue. If conservative management is pursued, evaluation and treatment should be as described below for PROM at 23–31w 6d.

PROM remote from term (23–31w 6d)

Delivery at 23–31w 6d gestation is associated with significant risks of neonatal morbidity and mortality resulting from prematurity. These women are generally best served by conservative inpatient management after PROM to prolong pregnancy and reduce gestational age-dependent morbidity in the absence of chorioamnionitis, placental abruption, advanced labor, or nonreassuring fetal testing. Because the latency is frequently brief and clinical findings can change over a short period of time, transfer to a tertiary care facility before acute complications occur should be considered if adequate facilities are not available at the initial institution. During conservative management, patients should have at least daily assessment for evidence of labor, chorioamnionitis, placental abruption, and fetal well-being. Leg exercises, antiembolic stockings, and/or prophylactic doses of subcutaneous heparin may be of value in preventing thromboembolic complications [37]. Fetal growth should be assessed with ultrasound every 3–4 weeks. Although initial severe oligohydramnios has been associated with brief latency, this finding is an inaccurate predictor of latency or neonatal outcomes and should not be used to determine clinical management other than as an adjunct to confirm resealing of the membranes with restoration of a normal amniotic fluid index. The patient who remains stable is generally delivered at 34 weeks' gestation because of the ongoing but low risk of fetal loss with conservative management and the high likelihood of survival without long-term complications after delivery at this gestational age.

Several adjunctive therapies have been proposed during conservative management of PROM remote from term. A single course of antenatal corticosteroids for fetal maturation is recommended to reduce the risks of neonatal respiratory distress and intraventricular hemorrhage (without increasing the risk of neonatal infection) [38,39]. Either 12 mg betamethasone i.m. every 24 hours for two doses, or 6 mg dexamethasone i.m. every 12 hours for four doses is appropriate. Broad-spectrum antibiotic therapy should be administered to treat or prevent ascending subclinical decidual infection in order to prolong pregnancy, and to reduce neonatal infectious and gestational age-dependent morbidity [40,41]. Intravenous therapy (48 hours) with ampicillin (2 g i.v. every 6 h) and erythromycin (250 mg i.v. every 6 h) followed by limited duration oral therapy (5 days) with amoxicillin (250 mg p.o. every 8 h) and enteric-coated erythromycin base (333 mg p.o. every 8 h) has been recommended by the National Institute of Child Health and Human Development and the Maternal Fetal Medicine Units (NICHD-MFMU) Network. Therapy for shorter periods has not been studied with adequate numbers,

has not been shown to offer equivalent neonatal benefits [42,43], and is not recommended. Recent shortages have led to the need for substitution of alternative antibiotic agents. Oral ampicillin, erythromycin, and azithromycin are likely appropriate substitutions for the above agents, as needed. The optimal broad-spectrum therapy for women who are penicillin allergic has not been determined. The Oracle trial [44] has suggested that single-agent erythromycin may be appropriate, and has also raised concern that broad-spectrum antibiotic therapy might increase the risk of necrotizing enterocolitis. This latter finding is not consistent with the NICHD-MFMU trial in which broad-spectrum antibiotic therapy in a higher risk population reduced the risk of stage 2–3 necrotizing enterocolitis [40]. Management of GBS carriers after the initial 7 days of antibiotic therapy has not been well studied. Options include:

1 Subsequent intrapartum prophylaxis only;

2 Continued narrow-spectrum GBS prophylaxis from completion of the initial 7-day course through delivery;

3 Follow-up anovaginal culture after completion of the 7-day course, with continued narrow spectrum therapy against GBS until delivery for those with persistently positive cultures; or

4 Follow-up anovaginal culture of those having extended latency after initial antibiotic treatment, with repeat treatment of women with subsequently positive cultures.

Regardless of antepartum antibiotic treatments, intrapartum prophylaxis should be given to all known GBS carriers. Tocolytic therapy for women with PPROM has been shown to reduce the likelihood of delivery at 24–48 hours in some studies [45–48]. However, such treatment has not been shown to improve neonatal outcomes. Tocolytic therapy should not be administered after PPROM if there is suspicion of intrauterine infection, fetal compromise, or placental abruption. Further study is needed regarding tocolytic therapy after PPROM.

Previable PROM (less than 23 weeks)

PPROM before the limit of viability (currently 23 weeks' gestation) is particularly grave as it can lead to previable delivery with no potential for survival, delivery near the limit of viability where the majority of survivors are at risk for acute and long-term complications, or to delivery after extended latency with pulmonary hypoplasia and restriction deformities resulting from severe oligohydramnios at the time of critical pulmonary development and/or prolonged severe oligohydramnios. Alternatively, some conservatively managed patients will have extended latency with survival of a healthy infant and some may have spontaneous resealing of the membranes with reaccumulation of amniotic fluid. Gestational age should be estimated based on the earliest available ultrasound and menstrual history. These patients should be counseled realistically regarding potential fetal and neonatal outcomes after early preterm birth [19]. The risk of stillbirth during conservative management and delivery is approximately 15%.

Most of these pregnancies will deliver before or near the limit of viability, where neonatal death is either assured or common. The risk of long-term sequelae will depend on the gestational age at delivery. Persistent oligohydramnios is a prognostic indicator of poor outcomes after PROM before 20 weeks, with a high risk of lethal pulmonary hypoplasia regardless of extended latency. Conservative management is also associated with a frequent chorioamnionitis (39%), endometritis (14%), retained placenta/postpartum hemorrhage necessitating curettage (12%), and placental abruption (3%).

Should the patient desire delivery after counseling, options for labor induction include high-dose intravenous oxytocin, intravaginal prostaglandin E_2, and oral or intravaginal prostaglandin E_1 (misoprostol) according to clinical circumstances. Dilatation and evacuation can be an option for caregivers with experience in this technique. Placement of intracervical laminaria before labor induction or dilatation and evacuation may be helpful. Women undergoing conservative management should be initially evaluated for evidence of intrauterine infection, labor, or placental abruption. Although supportive data are lacking, it is prudent to advise the patient to pursue strict pelvic rest to reduce the potential for ascending infection and it may be helpful to pursue modified bed or couch rest to enhance the potential for membrane resealing. In the absence of data supporting either approach, inpatient or outpatient monitoring may be considered appropriate with consideration given to individual clinical circumstances. Serial ultrasound can be helpful to evaluate for fetal growth and persistent oligohydramnios, and estimate fetal pulmonary growth (thoracic/abdominal circumference ratio or chest circumference) [49–51]. Information from such testing is useful in counseling and ongoing care of the patient with PROM before the limit of viability. Women with PROM before the limit of viability have been included in some studies of broad-spectrum antibiotic therapy after PROM. However, the numbers of these women are too small to know if treatment of this subgroup is effective, and most studies do not present data separately for these women. A number of small studies have evaluated the potential to reseal the fetal membranes after previable PROM. Some techniques have included transabdominal/transcervical amnioinfusion, and Gelfoam or fibrin-platelet-cryoprecipitate instillation [52–54]. Data regarding efficacy and safety of these techniques are too limited at this time to warrant their incorporation into clinical practice. Once the limit of viability has been reached, many clinicians will admit the patient for ongoing bed rest in order to allow early diagnosis and intervention for infection, abruption, labor, and nonreassuring fetal heart rate patterns (see management of PROM at 23–31w 6d above). Administration of antenatal corticosteroids for fetal maturation is appropriate at this time. It is not known if administration of broad-spectrum antibiotics for pregnancy prolongation will assist women with PPROM who have already had prolonged latency before admission with no evident infection.

Special circumstances

Cerclage

Cerclage is a well-described risk factor for PROM [55,56]. When the cerclage is removed after PROM occurs, the risk of perinatal complications is as those with PROM who had no cerclage [56,57]. Although no individual study has achieved statistical significance, reviews of studies comparing cerclage retention or removal after PPROM suggest a trend towards increased maternal infection with retained cerclage [58–60]. Perhaps more important is that no study has found cerclage retention after PPROM to significantly reduce infant morbidity, and one study has found increased infection-related neonatal death with cerclage retention. As such, cerclage should generally be removed when PROM occurs. If the cerclage is retained concurrent to antenatal corticosteroid treatment for fetal maturation, broad-spectrum antibiotic administration should be given to reduce the risk of infection and the cerclage should be removed after steroid benefit has been achieved (24–48 hours).

Herpes simplex virus

Typically, women with active primary or secondary herpes simplex virus (HSV) infection should be delivered expeditiously by caesarean section when PROM occurs at or near term. Alternatively, when PROM complicates HSV infection near the limit of fetal viability and the mother shows no evidence of systemic infection, conservative management may be appropriate [61]. During conservative management, treatment with acyclovir (200 mg p.o. five times a day or 500 mg i.v. every 6 hours) would be appropriate to reduce viral shedding and the likelihood of recurrences before delivery.

Human immunodeficiency virus

Given the poor prognosis of perinatally acquired HIV infection and increasing risk of vertical transmission with increasing duration of membrane rupture, expeditious cesarean delivery is recommended when PROM occurs after the limit of fetal viability is recommended. Vaginal delivery may be appropriate for selected women with a low viral titer. If conservative management is undertaken, multiagent antiretroviral therapy with serial monitoring of maternal viral load and CD4 counts should be initiated.

Resealing of the membranes

A small number of women will have cessation of leakage with resealing of the membranes, particularly those with PROM after amniocentesis [14,62,63]. In the absence of data in this regard, we empirically continue inpatient observation for approximately 1 week after cessation of leakage and normalization of the amniotic fluid index to encourage healing of the membrane rupture site. These women are subsequently discharged with instructions for modified bed rest, pelvic rest, and are advised to return should labor, vaginal bleeding, abdominal tenderness or fever, or recurrent membrane rupture ensue.

Case presentation

A 23-year-old, G2P0101, with singleton gestation presented at 28 weeks with perineal wetness for approximately 2 hours. She denied contractions, abdominal pain, vaginal bleeding, fever, or chills. She had a prior 32-week preterm birth resulting from preterm labor, but no other pregnancy complications. Past medical and allergy histories were negative. Specific clinical findings included: temperature 37.2°C, pulse 92 beats/min, RR 18, symphysis-fundal height (SFH) 32 cm, with no fundal tenderness. A catheterized urine specimen revealed no leukocytes and culture was subsequently negative. Sterile speculum examination revealed moist vaginal side walls but no fluid pool in the posterior fornix. A sterile swab of the vaginal sidewalls revealed a complex arborized ferning pattern and Nitrazine paper applied to this site turned blue, confirming membrane rupture. Visual inspection suggested a cervix 2 cm dilatated and approximately 1.5 cm long. Endocervical swabs for *Neisseria gonorrhoeae* and *Chlamydia trachomatis*, and distal vagina/anal swabs for GBS were obtained. Ultrasound revealed appropriate fetal growth, a longitudinal cephalic lie, and oligohydramnios (amniotic fluid index 36 mm). The fetal bladder was normal in size and position. There was no evident hydronephrosis. Monitoring revealed a fetal heart rate of 140–150 beats/min with intermittent accelerations and no decelerations or contractions. Maternal WBC count was 12,000/mm³.

After counseling regarding the risks of preterm birth at 28 weeks and of conservative management, the potential benefits of conservative management, antibiotics (NICHD-MFMU protocol) and corticosteroid treatment (12 mg betamethasone i.m. every 24 h for two doses) were initiated, and neonatology consultation was obtained. The patient was transferred to the antepartum unit after 6 hours of reassuring continuous fetal/contraction monitoring, for continued bed rest with bathroom privileges. Daily assessments revealed no clinically evident chorioamnionitis, abruption, or contractions. Fetal testing remained reassuring. Cultures were negative. On hospital day 23, at 31 weeks' gestation, the patient reported mild lower abdominal cramping. External monitoring revealed irregular brief contractions with moderate variable-type decelerations. Speculum examination revealed umbilical cord at the external os. With the patient in knee–chest position and a vaginal hand elevating the presenting part, the patient was taken for immediate cesarean delivery resulting in a liveborn infant with Apgar scores of 4 and 7 at 1 and 5 minutes, respectively. Newborn resuscitation and intubation were performed before transfer to the neonatal ICU. Cord blood pH was within normal limits and placental evaluation revealed no chorioamnionitis. The mother was discharged home on postoperative day 3 for outpatient postoperative evaluation and for counseling regarding her risk of recurrent preterm birth. The infant suffered mild respiratory distress syndrome and hyperbilirubinemia requiring phototherapy, but no sepsis or intraventricular hemorrhage, and is gaining weight at 2 weeks of life.

References

1 Meis PJ, Ernest JM, Moore ML. Causes of low birth weight births in public and private patients. *Am J Obstet Gynecol* 1987;**156**:1165–8.

2 Tucker JM, Goldenberg RL, Davis RO, Copper RL, Winkler CL, Hauth JC. Etiologies of preterm birth in an indigent population: is prevention a logical expectation? *Obstet Gynecol* 1991;**77**:343–7.

3 Martin JA, Hamilton BE, Sutton PD, Ventura SJ, Menacker F, Munson ML. Births: final data for 2002. *Natl Vital Stat Rep* 2003;**52**:1–116.

4 Skinner SJM, Campos GA, Liggins GC. Collagen content of human amniotic membranes: effect of gestation length and premature rupture. *Obstet Gynecol* 1981;**57**:487–9.

5 Lavery JP, Miller CE, Knight RD. The effect of labor on the rheologic response of chorioamniotic membranes. *Obstet Gynecol* 1982;**60**:87–92.

6 Taylor J, Garite T. Premature rupture of the membranes before fetal viability. *Obstet Gynecol* 1984;**64**:615–20.

7 Naeye RL. Factors that predispose to premature rupture of the fetal membranes. *Obstet Gynecol* 1992;**60**:93.

8 Harger JH, Hsing AW, Tuomala RE, *et al.* Risk factors for preterm premature rupture of fetal membranes: a multicenter case–control study. *Am J Obstet Gynecol* 1990;**163**:130.

9 Mercer BM, Goldenberg RL, Meis PJ, *et al.* and the NICHD-MFMU Network. The preterm prediction study: prediction of preterm premature rupture of the membranes using clinical findings and ancillary testing. *Am J Obstet Gynecol* 2000;**183**:738–45.

10 Roberts AK, Monzon-Bordonaba F, Van Deerlin PG, *et al.* Association of polymorphism within the promoter of the tumor necrosis factor alpha gene with increased risk of preterm premature rupture of the fetal membranes. *Am J Obstet Gynecol* 1999;**180**:1297–302.

11 Ferrand PE, Parry S, Sammel M, *et al.* A polymorphism in the matrix metalloproteinase-9 promoter is associated with increased risk of preterm premature rupture of membranes in African Americans. *Mol Hum Reprod* 2002;**8**:494–501.

12 Klebanoff MA, Carey JC, Hauth JC, *et al.* for the NICHD-MFMU Network. Failure of metronidazole to prevent preterm delivery among pregnant women with asymptomatic *Trichomonas vaginalis* infection. *N Engl J Med* 2001;**345**:487–93.

13 Carey JC, Klebanoff MA, Hauth JC, *et al.* for the NICHD-MFMU Network. Metronidazole to prevent preterm delivery in pregnant women with asymptomatic bacterial vaginosis. *N Engl J Med* 2000;**342**:534–40.

14 Mercer B, Arheart K. Antimicrobial therapy in expectant management of preterm premature rupture of the membranes. *Lancet* 1995;**346**:1271–9.

15 Mercer BM, Goldenberg RL, Das AF, *et al.* for the NICHD-MFMU Network. What we have learned regarding antibiotic therapy for the reduction of infant morbidity? *Semin Perinatol* 2003;**27**:217–30.

16 Hillier SL, Martius J, Krohn M, Kiviat N, Holmes KK, Eschenbach DA. A case–control study of chorioamnionic infection and histologic chorioamnionitis in prematurity. *N Engl J Med* 1988;**319**:972–8.

17 Gunn GC, Mishell DR, Morton DG. Premature rupture of the fetal membranes: a review. *Am J Obstet Gynecol* 1970;**106**:469–82.

18 Garite TJ, Freeman RK. Chorioamnionitis in the preterm gestation. *Obstet Gynecol* 1982;**59**:539–45.

19 Mercer BM. Preterm premature rupture of the membranes. *Obstet Gynecol* 2003;**101**:178–93.

20 Vintzileos AM, Campbell WA, Nochimson DJ, Weinbaum PJ. Preterm premature rupture of the membranes: a risk factor for the development of abruptio placentae. *Am J Obstet Gynecol* 1987;**156**:1235–8.

21 Mercer BM, Moretti ML, Prevost RR, Sibai BM. Erythromycin therapy in preterm premature rupture of the membranes: a prospective, randomized trial of 220 patients. *Am J Obstet Gynecol* 1992;**166**:794–802.

22 Alexander JM, Mercer BM, Miodovnik M, *et al.* The impact of digital cervical examination on expectantly managed preterm rupture of membranes. *Am J Obstet Gynecol* 2000;**183**:1003–7.

23 American College of Obstetricians and Gynecologists. ACOG Committee Opinion: number 279, December 2002. Prevention of early-onset group B streptococcal disease in newborns. *Obstet Gynecol* 2002;**100**:1405–12.

24 Broekhuizen FF, Gilman M, Hamilton PR. Amniocentesis for gram stain and culture in preterm premature rupture of the membranes. *Obstet Gynecol* 1985;**66**:316–21.

25 Romero R, Yoon BH, Mazor M, *et al.* A comparative study of the diagnostic performance of amniotic fluid glucose, white blood cell count, interleukin-6, and Gram stain in the detection of microbial invasion in patients with preterm premature rupture of membranes. *Am J Obstet Gynecol* 1993;**169**:839–51.

26 Vintzileos AM, Campbell WA, Nochimson DJ, Weinbaum PJ. Fetal breathing as a predictor of infection in premature rupture of the membranes. *Obstet Gynecol* 1986;**67**:813–7.

27 Vintzileos AM, Campbell WA, Nochimson DJ, Connolly ME, Fuenfer MM, Hoehn GJ. The fetal biophysical profile in patients with premature rupture of the membranes: an early predictor of fetal infection. *Am J Obstet Gynecol* 19851;**152**:510–6.

28 Naef RW 3rd, Allbert JR, Ross EL, Weber BM, Martin RW, Morrison JC. Premature rupture of membranes at 34 to 37 weeks' gestation: aggressive versus conservative management. *Am J Obstet Gynecol* 1998;**178**:126–30.

29 Mercer BM, Crocker L, Boe N, Sibai B. Induction versus expectant management in PROM with mature amniotic fluid at 32–36 weeks: a randomized trial. *Am J Obstet Gynecol* 1993;**82**:775–82.

30 Shaver DC, Spinnato JA, Whybrew D, Williams WK, Anderson GD. Comparison of phospholipids in vaginal and amniocentesis specimens of patients with premature rupture of membranes. *Am J Obstet Gynecol* 1987;**156**:454.

31 Estol PC, Poseiro JJ, Schwarcz R. Phosphatidylglycerol determination in the amniotic fluid from a PAD placed over the vulva: a method for diagnosis of fetal lung maturity in cases of premature ruptured membranes. *J Perinatol Med* 1992;**20**:65.

32 Edwards RK, Duff P, Ross KC. Amniotic fluid indices of fetal pulmonary maturity with preterm premature rupture of membranes. *Obstet Gynecol* 2000;**96**:102.

33 Russell JC, Cooper CM, Ketchum CH, *et al.* Multicenter evaluation of TDx test for assessing fetal lung maturity. *Clin Chem* 1989;**35**:1005.

34 Cotton DB, Spillman T, Bretaudiere JP. Effect of blood contamination on lecithin to sphingomyelin ratio in amniotic fluid by different detection methods. *Clin Chim Acta* 1984;**137**:299.

35 Carlan SJ, Gearity D, O'Brien WF. The effect of maternal blood contamination on the TDx-FLM II assay. *Am J Perinatol* 1997;**14**:491.

36 Tabsh KM, Brinkman CR 3rd, Bashore R. Effect of meconium contamination on amniotic fluid lecithin : sphingomyelin ratio. *Obstet Gynecol* 1981;**58**:605.

37 Kovacevich GJ, Gaich SA, Lavin JP, *et al.* The prevalence of thromboembolic events among women with extended bed rest prescribed as part of the treatment for premature labor or preterm premature rupture of membranes. *Am J Obstet Gynecol* 2000;**182**:1089–92.

38 Harding JE, Pang J, Knight DB, Liggins GC. Do antenatal corticosteroids help in the setting of preterm rupture of membranes? *Am J Obstet Gynecol* 2001;**184**:131–9.

39 American College of Obstetricians and Gynecologists. Committee Opinion. Antenatal corticosteroid therapy for fetal maturation. *Obstet Gynecol* 2002;**99**:871–3.

40 Mercer B, Miodovnik M, Thurnau G, *et al.* and the NICHD-MFMU Network. Antibiotic therapy for reduction of infant morbidity after preterm premature rupture of the membranes: a randomized controlled trial. *JAMA* 1997;**278**:989–95.

41 Kenyon S, Boulvain M, Neilson J. Antibiotics for preterm rupture of the membranes: a systematic review. *Obstet Gynecol* 2004;**104**:1051–7.

42 Lewis DF, Adair CD, Robichaux AG, *et al.* Antibiotic therapy in preterm premature rupture of membranes: are seven days necessary? A preliminary, randomized clinical trial. *Am J Obstet Gynecol* 2003;**188**:1413–6; discussion 1416–7.

43 Segel SY, Miles AM, Clothier B, Parry S, Macones GA. Duration of antibiotic therapy after preterm premature rupture of fetal membranes. *Am J Obstet Gynecol* 2003;**189**:799–802.

44 Kenyon SL, Taylor DJ, Tarnow-Mordi W. Oracle Collaborative Group. Broad spectrum antibiotics for preterm, prelabor rupture of fetal membranes: the Oracle I randomized trial. *Lancet* 2001;**357**:979–88.

45 Christensen KK, Ingemarsson I, Leideman T, Solum T, Svenningsen N. Effect of Ritodrine on labor after premature rupture of the membranes. *Obstet Gynecol* 1980;**55**:187–90.

46 Weiner CP, Renk K, Klugman M. The therapeutic efficacy and cost-effectiveness of aggressive tocolysis for premature labor associated with premature rupture of the membranes. *Am J Obstet Gynecol* 1988;**159**:216–22.

47 Garite TJ, Keegan KA, Freeman RK, Nageotte MP. A randomized trial of Ritodrine tocolysis versus expectant management in patients with premature rupture of membranes at 25 to 30 weeks of gestation. *Am J Obstet Gynecol* 1987;**157**:388–93.

48 How HY, Cook CR, Cook VD, Miles DE, Spinnato JA. Preterm premature rupture of membranes: aggressive tocolysis versus expectant management. *J Matern Fetal Med* 1998;**7**:8–12.

49 Lauria MR, Gonik B, Romero R. Pulmonary hypoplasia: pathogenesis, diagnosis, and antenatal prediction. *Obstet Gynecol* 1995;**86**:466–75.

50 D'Alton M, Mercer B, Riddick E, Dudley D. Serial thoracic versus abdominal circumference ratios for the prediction of pulmonary hypoplasia in premature rupture of the membranes remote from term. *Am J Obstet Gynecol* 1992;**166**:658–63.

51 Vintzileos AM, Campbell WA, Rodis JF, Nochimson DJ, Pinette MG, Petrikovsky BM. Comparison of six different ultrasonographic methods for predicting lethal fetal pulmonary hypoplasia. *Am J Obstet Gynecol* 1989;**161**:606–12.

52 Sciscione AC, Manley JS, Pollock M, *et al*. Intracervical fibrin sealants: a potential treatment for early preterm premature rupture of the membranes. *Am J Obstet Gynecol* 2001;**184**:368–73.

53 Quintero RA, Morales WJ, Bornick PW, Allen M, Garabelis N. Surgical treatment of spontaneous rupture of membranes: the amniograft—first experience. *Am J Obstet Gynecol* 2002;**186**:155–7.

54 O'Brien JM, Barton JR, Milligan DA. An aggressive interventional protocol for early midtrimester premature rupture of the membranes using gelatin sponge for cervical plugging. *Am J Obstet Gynecol* 2002;**187**:1143–6.

55 Treadwell MC, Bronsteen RA, Bottoms SF. Prognostic factors and complication rates for cervical cerclage: a review of 482 cases. *Am J Obstet Gynecol* 1991;**165**:555–8.

56 Blickstein I, Katz Z, Lancet M, Molgilner BM. The outcome of pregnancies complicated by preterm rupture of the membranes with and without cerclage. *Int J Gynaecol Obstet* 1989;**28**: 237–42.

57 Yeast JD, Garite TR. The role of cervical cerclage in the management of preterm premature rupture of the membranes. *Am J Obstet Gynecol* 1988;**158**:106–10.

58 Ludmir J, Bader T, Chen L, Lindenbaum C, Wong G. Poor perinatal outcome associated with retained cerclage in patients with premature rupture of membranes. *Obstet Gynecol* 1994;**84**:823–6.

59 Jenkins TM, Berghella V, Shlossman PA, *et al*. Timing of cerclage removal after preterm premature rupture of membranes: maternal and neonatal outcomes. *Am J Obstet Gynecol* 2000;**183**:847–52.

60 McElrath TF, Norwitz ER, Lieberman ES, Heffner LJ. Perinatal outcome after preterm premature rupture of membranes with *in situ* cervical cerclage. *Am J Obstet Gynecol* 2002;**187**:1147–52.

61 Major CA, Towers CV, Lewis DF, Garite TJ. Expectant management of preterm premature rupture of membranes complicated by active recurrent genital herpes. *Am J Obstet Gynecol* 2003;**188**:1551–4.

62 Johnson JWC, Egerman RS, Moorhead J. Cases with ruptured membranes that "reseal." *Am J Obstet Gynecol* 1990;**163**: 1024–32.

63 Gold RB, Goyer GL, Schwartz, Evans MI, Seabolt LA. Conservative management of second trimester post-amniocentesis fluid leakage. *Obstet Gynecol* 1989;**74**:745–7.

42 Management of preterm labor

Vincenzo Berghella

Major advances with prematurity will come only from a better understanding of the pathophysiology leading to preterm birth (PTB). Prevention efforts in asymptomatic women are more beneficial than treatment of symptomatic women. Despite massive research efforts in primary or secondary prevention, millions of women in the USA present with symptoms of preterm labor (PTL) every year. Given the dire consequences of PTB, especially very early PTB, all should be done to avoid PTB even when it is most difficult (i.e., the woman has manifest symptoms of PTL).

Management of the woman with symptoms of PTL starts with initial assessment of history, physical exam, and specific laboratory and other screening tests to establish diagnosis and prognosis, so as to obtain an accurate initial assessment and decide the correct interventions.

Evaluation: history, physical exam, and screening tests

The history should include at least a review of specific symptoms, such as cramps, abdominal "tightenings," low backache, pelvic pressure, increased vaginal discharge, or spotting. It is paramount to obtain the exact determination of gestational age. To assess prognosis, specific risk factors for PTB should be reviewed. Such risks are listed in Table 42.1.

The physical exam should include an assessment of vital signs, fetal heart monitoring, an abdominal exam for uterine tenderness and contractions, cervical exam by speculum for Nitrazine, pooling, ferning, visual examination of cervix (especially if preterm premature rupture of membranes [PPROM]), collection for fetal fibronectin (fFN) and group B streptococci (GBS), and *Chlamydia* and gonorrhea DNA tests. If there is no PPROM diagnosis, a manual cervical exam can be performed for dilatation, cervical length and/or effacement, station, and presentation.

Laboratory tests that should be considered include Rapid Plasma Reagin (RPR) or Venereal Disease Research Labora-

tory (VDRL) to rule out syphilis in high-risk women, rapid HIV (if status unknown), cervicovaginal fFN, vaginorectal GBS, urinary drug screen (UDS), urinalysis, and urine culture. In women without specific symptoms of these infections, there is no evidence that screening for BV, *Trichomonas*, *Mycoplasma* or *Ureaplasma* is beneficial.

In addition, there are other important screening tests that are suggested. An ultrasound should assess for fetal demise, major anomaly, compromise, polyhydramnios, placenta previa, placental abruption, fetal presentation, and estimated fetal weight. A transvaginal ultrasound (TVU) can be performed for cervical length (CL) evaluation. Amniocentesis may be considered to check for intra-amniotic infection (IAI) (incidence approximately 5–15%) if equivocal signs of chorioamnionitis are present, and fetal lung maturity (FLM) (especially between 33 and 37 weeks). If the diagnosis of IAI is made (≥2 of uterine tenderness, maternal fever ≥38°C (≥100.4°F), maternal tachycardia, fetal tachycardia—in the absence of other infection), delivery is recommended even without amniocentesis. The rates of IAI (documented by amniotic fluid culture) by pregnancy status at <37 weeks are approximately: 5–15% for PTL (intact membranes), 20–30% for PPROM (no labor), 30–40% for PPROM (labor), and 50% if cervix ≥2 cm/80% in second trimester. The rates of infection are indirectly proportional to gestational age. There is insuffient evidence to recommend amniocentesis in all cases of PTL.

Initial assessment

Diagnosis of PTL

The vast majority of the women who present with symptoms of PTL do not deliver preterm even without intervention. Therefore, it is important to establish the diagnosis of PTL before any treatment is ever considered. One of the most commonly used PTL diagnoses is the presence of uterine contractions (≥4/20 minutes or ≥8/hour) *and* documented cervical

Table 42.1 Risk factors for preterm birth (PTB).

Obstetric gynecologic history: prior spontaneous PTB; prior STL; prior ≥2 D&Es; prior cone biopsy; uterine anomalies; DES exposure; myomata; extremes of interpregnancy intervals; ART

Maternal lifestyle (e.g., smoking, drug abuse, STD)

Maternal prepregnancy weight <50 kg (<120 lb); poor nutritional status

Maternal age extremes (<19; >35 years)

Race (especially African-American)

Education (<12 grade)

Certain medical conditions (e.g., DM, HTN)

Low socioeconomic status

Limited prenatal care

Family history of spontaneous PTB (poorly studied)

Vaginal bleeding (especially during second trimester)

Stress (mostly related to above risks)

Anemia

Periodontal disease

ART, assisted reproductive technologies; D&E, dilatation and evacuation; DES, diethylstilbestrol; DM, diabetes mellitus; HTN, hypertension; STD, sexually transmitted disease; STL, second trimester loss.

change with intact membranes at 20–36w 6d. In fact, 70–80% of women even with this diagnosis of PTL do not deliver preterm. Women without cervical change do not have PTL and should not receive tocolysis.

Fetal fibronectin and cervical length

Because so many women with a diagnosis of PTL do not deliver preterm, two predictive tests, fFN and TVU CL, can aid in the initial assessment of the true chance of delivering preterm. These tests have been studied extensively for over 10 years, and are now becoming more common in the assessment of PTL, as they are the best predictive screening tests available. Because no trial has yet demonstrated their benefit, these tests cannot yet be considered standard of care. Women with PTL but negative fFN and TVU CL ≥30 mm have a less than 1% chance of delivering within 1 week, and a more than 95% chance of delivering ≥35 weeks without therapy [1], and should therefore not receive any treatment. Women with positive fFN, or with TVU CL less than 20 mm, are at highest risk of PTB, and should receive treatment interventions.

Interventions

The main interventions for the woman with PTL at high risk for delivering preterm are aimed at increasing fetal maturation and stopping uterine contractions to avoid PTB. In addition, it is important to consider referral to a tertiary care center if the neonatal intensive care unit (ICU) is not adequate for the gestational age of the potential neonate. The woman and her family members should be counseled regarding morbidity

and mortality for the possible preterm infant, using the most up-to-date data. Current (2007) survival is 0% at 21 weeks, 75% at 25 weeks, and more than 95% at 29 weeks, while intact survival at 18 months is over 50% after 25 weeks. Disabilities in mental and psychomotor development, neuromotor function (including cerebral palsy), or sensory and communication function are present in at least 50% of fetuses born ≤25 weeks' gestation [2]. A neonatology consult at 22–34 weeks should always be obtained to discuss neonatal prognosis and management. Obstetric counseling should review the principles and progress of management of PTL. Specific interventions should aim to treat any positive tests or infections, such as urinary tract infections, sexually transmitted diseases (STDs), GBS, and HIV.

Women with multiple gestations should not be treated differently from those with singletons, except for caution in that their risk of pulmonary edema is greater when exposed to betamimetics or magnesium sulfate [3]. There is insufficient evidence to justify the use of steroids for FLM and tocolysis before 23 weeks and after 33w 6d.

Prophylaxis to prevent neonatal morbidity/mortality from PTB (fetal maturation)

Betamethasone and dexamethasone are the only two corticosteroids that cross the placenta reliably and have been shown to benefit the fetus. The regimen for one course of betamethasone is 12 mg IM every 24 hours for 2 doses and for dexamethasone is 6 mg IM every 6 hours for 4 doses. Betamethasone, if available, is preferred to dexamethasone [4]. Corticosteroids given prior to PTB (either spontaneous or indicated) are effective in preventing respiratory distress syndrome (RDS), intraventricular hemorrhage (IVH), and neonatal mortality [5]. Antenatal administration of 24 mg of betamethasone or of dexamethasone to women expected to give birth preterm is associated with a 40% reduction in neonatal mortality, 47% reduction in RDS, and 52% reduction in IVH in preterm infants. There is a trend for a 41% reduction in necrotizing enterocolitis (NEC). These benefits apply to at least 24–33w 6d, and are not limited by gender or race. The effects are significant mostly at 48 hours to 7 days from the first dose, but treatment should not be withheld even if delivery appears imminent, and effects even for babies delivered more than 7 days later have been reported. Such steroids should therefore be administered to any woman at these gestational ages at significant PTB risk upon identification of that risk. The results are mostly from singleton gestations, with insufficient data on multiple gestations.

There is not enough evidence to evaluate the use of repeated doses of corticosteroids in women who remain undelivered more than 7 days after the first course, but who are at continued risk of PTB [5]. Fewer infants (36% less) in the repeat dose(s) of corticosteroids group had severe lung disease compared with infants in the placebo group [6]. No statistically significant differences have been reported for any of the other primary outcomes which included other measures of respiratory morbidity, small for gestational age at birth, perinatal death, IVH, periventricular leukomalacia, and maternal infectious morbidity. Fewer infants in the repeat dose(s) of corticosteroids group needed surfactant compared with infants in the placebo group [7].

There are no contraindications. When used for only one course, no significant side-effects have been reported. If four courses or more are used, there is a possible association with birthweight <10th percentile and small neonatal head circumference (<10th percentile), with evidence of some later "catch-up" growth. No adverse consequences of prophylactic corticosteroids for PTB in either the mothers or, most importantly, the infants, even at 10+years follow-up, have been identified. There is no increase in maternal or fetal/neonatal infection.

Thyrotropin-releasing hormone, phenobarbital, and vitamin K have not been shown to be beneficial for fetal maturation and PTL management.

Nontocolytic interventions

Bed rest, hydration, and sedation have not been shown to be beneficial in the management of PTL. Bed rest has never been tested in singleton gestations complicated by PTL or PPROM. In twin pregnancies with cervical dilatation, bed rest in the hospital has not been shown to decrease PTB [8].

Hydration

Intravenous hydration does not seem to be beneficial, even during the period of evaluation soon after admission, in the management of women with PTL. Compared with bed rest alone, hydration is associated with similar incidence of PTB at <37, <34, or <32 weeks [9]. Admission to neonatal ICU occurs with similar frequency in both groups. Cost of treatment is obviously higher in the hydration group. No studies evaluated oral hydration in women with evidence of dehydration [9].

Antibiotics

There is no clear overall benefit or detriment from prophylactic antibiotic treatment for women with PTL with intact membranes on neonatal outcomes, and there are concerns about a trend for increased neonatal mortality for those who received antibiotics (relative risk [RR] 1.52; 95% confidence interval [CI], 0.99–2.34) [10]. Rates of PTB at less than 36–37 weeks are similar in antibiotics and placebo groups, as is perinatal mortality. There is a 26% reduction in maternal infection with the use of prophylactic antibiotics. Of the different antibiotics or combinations studied so far (macrolide antibiotics, beta-lactam antibiotics, a combination of beta-lactam and macrolide

antibiotics, and antibiotics active against anaerobes), antibiotics active against anaerobes, which included three trials [11–13] and a total of 294 women, show a statistically significant increase (about 10 days) in the interval from randomization to delivery, a 38% reduction in the number of women giving birth within 7 days of enrollment, and fewer (by 37%) admissions to neonatal ICU (one trial). Further research is needed to determine if there is a subgroup of women who could experience benefit from antibiotic treatment for PTL, and to identify which antibiotic or combination of antibiotics is most effective [10].

GBS prophylaxis

Until GBS maternal status is known, penicillin (or ampicillin if not available) should be given to women with a diagnosis of PTL receiving steroids to prevent GBS neonatal infections, unless allergic [14].

Tocolysis

The principles of tocolytic therapy are listed in Table 42.2, and contraindications are listed in Table 42.3.

Primary tocolysis—single agent

Betamimetics
Ritodrine and terbutaline have been the more commonly studied agents.

Table 42.2 Principles of tocolytic therapy.

At 24–33w 6d, steroids for fetal maturation should always be given if tocolysis is initiated. Tocolytics should not be used without concomitant use of steroids for fetal maturation

Tocolysis is typically used for 48 hours to allow steroid effect. Given side-effects, consider stopping tocolytic therapy at 48 hours after steroids given if PTL under control

No tocolytic agent has been shown to improve perinatal mortality

There is no tocolytic agent that is more safe and efficacious. COX inhibitors are the only class of primary tocolytics shown to decrease PTB <37 weeks compared with placebo, while COX inhibitors, betamimetics and ORA have been shown to significantly prolong pregnancy at 48 hours and 7 days compared with placebo. COX inhibitors, CCB, and ORA, properly used, have significantly less side-effects than betamimetics

There is no *maintenance* tocolytic agent that prevents PTB or perinatal morbidity/mortality. There is insufficient evidence to evaluate multiple tocolytic agents for primary tocolysis, refractory (primary agent is failing, so another is started) tocolysis, or repeated tocolysis (after successful primary tocolysis)

CCB, calcium-channel blocker; COX, cyclo-oxygenase; ORA, oxytocin receptor antagonist; PTB, preterm birth; PTL, preterm labor.

Table 42.3 Contraindications to tocolytic therapy.

Maternal
Chorioamnionitis
Severe vaginal bleeding/abruption
Preeclampsia
Medical contraindications to specific tocolytic agent (see text)
Other maternal medical condition that makes continuing the pregnancy
  inadvisable

Fetal
IUFD
Major (especially if lethal) fetal anomaly or chromosome abnormality
Other fetal conditions in which prolongation of pregnancy is inadvisable
Documented fetal maturity

IUFD, intrauterine fetal death.

Dose. Ritodrine: 50–100 μg/min i.v. initial dose, increase 50 μg/min every 10 min (max 350 μg/min) (p.o. 1–20 mg every 2–4 hours).

Terbutaline: 25 mg s.q. every 20 min at first, then 2–3 hours; or 5–10 μg/min i.v., max 80 μg/min; or 2.5–5 mg p.o. every 2–4 hours (hold if maternal heart rate over 120/min).

Mechanism of action. Stimulate B_2 receptor through cyclic adenosine monophosphate, so no free calcium for myometrial contraction.

Evidence for effectiveness. Betamimetics decrease by 37% the number of women in PTL giving birth within 48 hours compared with placebo, and decrease by 22% the number of births within 7 days [15]. There is a trend for reduction of PTB at less than 37 weeks' gestation (RR 0.95; 95% CI, 0.88–1.03). No benefit is demonstrated for betamimetics on RDS or perinatal death. A few trials reported the following outcomes, with no difference detected in cerebral palsy, infant death, and NEC. Ritodrine has been the agent studied usually, with insufficient evidence to evaluate effectiveness of other betamimetics [15].

Comparison with other tocolytics. See below.

Specific contraindications. Cardiac arrhythmia or other significant cardiac disease; diabetes mellitus (DM); poorly controlled thyroid disease (for ritodrine).

Side-effects. MATERNAL: Hyperglycemia (140–200 mg/dL glucose in 20–50%. Mechanism: decreased peripheral insulin sensitivity and increased endogenous glucose production); hyperinsulinemia; hypokalemia (K <3 mEq/L in 50%); tremors, nervousness, dyspnea (10%), chest pain (5–10%), tachycardia/palpitations, arrhythmia (3%); ECG changes (2–3%); hypotension (2–3%); pulmonary edema (<1–5%; mechanism: reduced sodium excretion, leading to sodium and therefore fluid retention); headaches; nausea/vomiting; and

nasal stuffiness. Ritodrine specific: altered thyroid function, antidiuresis.

FETAL/NEONATAL: Ritodrine: tachycardia, hypoglycemia, hypocalcemia, hyperbilirubinemia, hypotension, IVH. Terbutaline: tachycardia, hyperinsulinemia, hyperglycemia, myocardial and septal hypertrophy, myocardial ischemia.

Calcium-channel blockers
Nifedipine (most commonly) and nicardipine have been the calcium-channel blocker (CCB) agents studied.

Dose. Nifedipine 20–30 mg for one dose, then 10–20 mg every 4–8 hours (max. 90 mg/day) (nicardipine dose similar).

Mechanism of action. Impair calcium channels, so inhibit influx of calcium into cell, and therefore myometrial contraction.

Evidence for effectiveness. There are no studies of CCB compared with placebo for PTB prevention. When compared with any other tocolytic agent (mainly betamimetics), CCB reduce the number of women giving birth within 7 days of receiving treatment by 24% and PTB at less than 34 weeks' gestation by 17% [16]. CCB show a trend to reduce PTB within 48 hours of initiation of treatment (RR 0.80; 95% CI, 0.61–1.05), and PTB at less than 37 weeks' gestation (RR 0.95; 95% CI, 0.83–1.09). CCB also reduces the frequency of neonatal RDS by 37%, NEC by 79%, IVH by 41%, and neonatal jaundice by 27%. CCB also reduce the requirement for women to have treatment ceased for adverse drug reaction by an impressive 86%. There are insufficient data regarding the effects of different dosage regimens and formulations of CCB on maternal and neonatal outcomes; the most studied is nifedipine, at the dosage shown above. CCB should therefore be preferred to betamimetics for tocolysis [16].

Specific contraindications. Cardiac disease; hypotension (<90/50 mmHg); concominant use of magnesium; caution in renal disease.

Side-effects. MATERNAL: Flushing, headache, dizziness, nausea, transient hypotension. Caution in women with hypotension and renal disease, as well as women on magnesium (cardiovascular collapse).
FETAL/NEONATAL: None.

Cyclo-oxygenase inhibitors
Non-selective cyclo-oxygenase (COX) inhibitor: indomethacin (Indocin). Selective COX-inhibitors (preferential COX-2 inhibitors): sulindac (Clinoril); rofecoxib (Vioxx); celecoxib (Celebrex); ketorolac (Toradol); nimesulide.

Dose. Indomethacin: 50–100 mg loading dose (rectal or vaginal route preferred, oral otherwise), then 25–50 mg every 6 hours for 48 hours max, and always <32 weeks. Sulindac: 200 mg p.o.

every 12 hours for 48 hours. Ketorolac: 60 mg i.m., then 30 mg i.m. every 6 hours for 48 hours.

Mechanism of action. COX inhibitors, so inhibit prostaglandin synthesis, therefore inhibit myometrial contraction.

Evidence for effectiveness. The nonselective COX inhibitor, indomethacin, was used in 10/13 trials.

When compared with placebo, COX inhibition (indomethacin only studied) results in a 79% reduction in PTB at less than 37 weeks, an increase in gestational age of 3.5 weeks, and an increase in birthweight of approximately 700 g in two small trials [17–19]. There is a trend towards a reduction in delivery within 48 hours of initiation of treatment (RR 0.20; 95% CI, 0.03–1.28) and within 7 days (RR 0.41; 95% CI, 0.10–1.66) [17]. No differences are detected in any other reported outcomes including perinatal mortality and RDS.

Used for 48 hours only, the intravaginal route (100 mg every 12 hours) decreases delivery at 48 hours (3/23 vs. 8/23) and at less than 7 days (5/23 vs. 13/23) compared with rectal/oral (100 mg rectally, followed by 25 mg p.o. every 6 hours), with some improvement in neonatal morbidities [20].

Compared with betamimetics, COX inhibitors significantly reduce by 63% the number of women delivering within 48 hours of initiation of treatment. Compared with magnesium sulfate, COX inhibitors have a trend for a lower number of women delivering within 48 hours of initiation of treatment (RR 0.75; 95% CI, 0.40–1.40) and lower PTB at less than 37 weeks (RR 0.55; 95% CI, 0.17–1.73).

A comparison of nonselective (indomethacin and sulindac) versus selective (rofecoxib and nimesulide) COX-2 inhibitor [21,22] does not demonstrate any differences in maternal or neonatal outcomes. Because of the small numbers, all estimates of effect are imprecise and need to be interpreted with caution.

Specific contraindications. Renal or hepatic disease, active peptic ulcer disease, poorly controlled hypertension (HTN), nonsteroidal anti-inflammatory drug (NSAID) sensitive asthma, coagulation disorders/thrombocytopenia.

Side-effects. When used for only 48 hours, no serious maternal or fetal/neonatal side-effects occur, and fetal surveillance is not indicated. Usually COX inhibitors are better tolerated by the mother than other tocolytics such as magnesium and betamimetics.

MATERNAL: As with any NSAID, mild gastrointestinal upset—nausea, heartburn (take with some food/milk) (COX-1). Gastrointestinal bleeding (COX-1), coagulation and platelet abnormalities (COX-1), asthma if aspirin-sensitive. NSAIDs may obscure elevation in temperature. Longterm rofecoxib (Vioxx) use in adults has been associated with stroke, so this drug is now not available in many countries.

FETAL/NEONATAL: In randomized controlled trials (RCTs) 403 women received short term tocolysis (up to 48 hours) with COX inhibitors (mainly indomethacin) and there was only one case of antenatal closure of the ductus arteriosus (incidence <0.3%). There was no increase in the incidence of patent ductus arteriosus postnatally [17]. No difference in incidences of IVH, bronchopulmonary dysplasia, patent ductus arteriosus, NEC, or perinatal mortality was noted in a review of RCTs aimed at evaluating safety [23]. Use for more than 48 hours, especially ≥32 weeks, is associated with significant fetal effects such as constriction of the ductus arteriosus, which can lead to hydrops, pulmonary hypertension, and death, and renal insufficiency, manifested *in utero* by oligohydramnios. Other effects with prolonged use such as hyperbilirubinemia, NEC, and IVH have not been shown with less than 72-hour use. Selective COX-2 inhibitors have not been shown consistently to be any safer for the fetus/neonate than nonselective COX inhibitors such as indomethacin. Therefore, continuous use of COX inhibitors for more than 48 hours and ≥32 weeks is contraindicated.

Magnesium sulfate (MgSO₄)

Dose. 40 g $MgSO_4$ in 1 L d51/2NS. Initial: 4–6 g/30 min, then 2–4 g/hour. A dose of 5 g/hour has not been shown to be beneficial in perinatal outcome compared with a dose of 2 g/hour, and is associated with significant side-effects [24]. Weaning $MgSO_4$ tocolysis has no benefits and a few harmful side-effects compared with stopping $MgSO_4$ abruptly [25].

Mechanism of action. Intracellular calcium antagonist.

Evidence for effectiveness. Compared with placebo, there is insufficient evidence to show if magnesium sulfate reduces the incidence of PTB or perinatal morbidity and mortality [26–28]. Compared with all controls (including other tocolytics), magnesium sulfate did not prevent PTB at 48 hours, PTB at less than 37 weeks or PTB at less than 32 weeks. Perinatal death was higher but very rare, while perinatal morbidities were similar [26]. Dosage of magnesium did not affect efficacy.

Specific contraindications. Myasthenia gravis.

Management. Aim for 4–7 $MgSO_4$ level. Monitor urinary output. Follow deep tendon reflexes: ↓ at ≥8, absent ≥10. ≥10: respiratory depression; ≥15 risk of cardiac arrest.

Side-effects. MATERNAL: Flushing, lethargy, headache, muscle weakness, diplopia, dry mouth, pulmonary edema (1%; Mech: intravenous overhydration), cardiac arrest.

FETAL/NEONATAL: Lethargy, hypotonia, hypocalcemia, respiratory depression. Prolonged use: demineralization.

Oxytocin receptor antagonists

Atosiban (Tractocile in Europe) is not Food and Drug Administration (FDA) approved, and therefore not available in the USA.

Dose. Atosiban 6.75 mg bolus, then 300 μg/min i.v. for 3 hours, then 100 μg/min (max. 45 hours).

Mechanism of action. Competitive inhibitor of oxytocin via blockade of oxytocin receptor.

Evidence for effectiveness. Compared with placebo, atosiban did not reduce incidence of preterm birth or improve neonatal outcome. In one trial, atosiban was associated with an increase in infant deaths at 12 months of age compared with placebo [29]. However, this trial randomized significantly more women to atosiban before 26 weeks' gestation. Use of atosiban resulted in lower infant birthweight and more maternal adverse drug reactions. Compared with betamimetics, atosiban had similar incidences of PTB or perinatal morbidity/mortality. Atosiban was associated with fewer maternal drug reactions requiring treatment cessation [30].

Side-effects. Minimal to none.

There is currently insufficient evidence to support the administration of nitric oxide donors [31], progesterone, or alcohol for prevention of PTB in women with PTL.

Primary tocolysis—multiple agents simultaneously

Indomethacin and ampicillin-sulbactam do not prevent PTB compared with placebo in women in PTL already receiving $MgSO_4$ tocolysis [32].

Refractory tocolysis—primary agent is failing

Indomethacin is similar to sulindac in prevention of PTB in women failing primary $MgSO_4$ tocolysis [33].

Maintenance tocolysis—after successful primary tocolysis

There is evidence that all agents used so far for maintenance tocolysis do not prevent PTB, recurrent PTL, recurrent hospitalizations, or perinatal morbidity and mortality. These include oral betamimetics [34], terbutaline pump [35], CCB [36], COX inhibitors [37,38], magnesium [39], or atosiban [40].

Mode of delivery

There is insufficient evidence to evaluate the use of a policy for uniform elective cesarean delivery (CD) compared with expectant management and selective CD for preterm babies (approximately 24–36 weeks) [41]. Mothers in the elective CD group have higher morbidity, while babies in the ele-ctive CD group show no statistical differences compared with expectant management, except a more frequent low cord pH. The numbers so far are too small for definite conclusions, including for differentiating by fetal presentation [41].

Case presentation

A 25-year-old, African-American, G6P0141 calls her obstetrician at 28w 6d with complaints of vaginal pressure. Upon questioning, she states that she might have intermittent cramps. Based on this history, the attending physician asks her to come to labor and delivery to be evaluated.

Her past obstetric history is significant for two spontaneous abortions, two induced abortions, and one PTB at 30 weeks the year prior. This PTB had been preceded by PTL, unsuccessfully treated with magnesium sulfate. She received steroids for fetal maturation, and her 1484 g (3 lb 4 oz) baby is currently doing well. She denies any other risk factors for PTB. Her prenatal course has been uneventful. Her expected date of confinement has been confirmed by an 18-week ultrasound. Her prenatal laboratory tests were within normal limits, including a negative HIV test.

On physical exam, her blood pressure is 110/74 mmHg, pulse 86 beats/min, temperature 36.9°C (98.4°F), respiratory rate 20. No tenderness or contractions are identified. On speculum exam, pooling, ferning, and nitrazine are negative, and so rupture of membranes is ruled out. Tests for fFN, GBS, gonorrhea and *Chlamydia* are collected. Her cervical exam is 2 cm dilatated, 1 cm long-2 station. The clinical impression is vertex presentation, and size less than dates. Fetal heart and tocomonitoring are initiated.

Twenty minutes after arrival, the fetal heart appears reassuring and appropriate for gestational age. On tocomonitoring, she is contracting every 4 minutes. An ultrasound is performed, and reveals an appropriate for gestational age estimated fetal weight (1498 g), vertex presentation, no placenta previa, and amniotic fluid index of 10. TVU reveals a cervical length of 19 mm.

Based on contraction frequency and cervical exam findings, a diagnosis of PTL is made. Betamethasone 12 mg i.m. is given with a plan to give a second dose at 24 hours. Indomethacin 100 mg p.r. is given, with a plan for continuing indomethacin 50 mg every 6 hours for 48 hours. Extensive counseling is given regarding safety and effectiveness of all interventions, prognosis, and possible complications. A neonatal consult is ordered. The neonatal intensive care unit is level III, and there is availability for care in case of a 28-week PTB.

An hour later, contractions are diminishing in frequency and intensity. Regular nutrition is allowed. Later, the contractions resolve, the FFN result is positive, while GBS, gonorrhea, *Chlamydia* and urine culture are negative. Antibiotics are discontinued. Hospitalization is continued as planned for a total of 48 hours, with tocomonitoring for 1 hour every shift and at the patient's request if she feels symptoms of PTL.

Forty-eight hours after initial assessment, she is discharged home with PTL precautions and close follow-up, aware of her high chance of PTB at less than 35 weeks and its consequences.

References

1 Berghella V, Ness A, Bega G, Berghella M. Cervical sonography in women with symptoms of preterm labor. *Obstet Gynecol Clin North Am* 2005;**32**:383–96.

2 American College of Obsterics and Gynecology. Perinatal care at the threshold of viability. *Obstet Gynaecol* 2002;**79**:181–8. [Review]

3 American College of Obstetrics and Gynecology. Management of preterm labor. *Obstet Gynaecol* 2003;**82**:127–35. [Review]

4 Jobe AH, Soll RF. Choice and dose of corticosteroid for antenatal treatments. *Am J Obstet Gynecol* 2004;**190**:878–81. [Review]

5 Crowley P. Prophylactic corticosteroids for preterm birth. *Cochrane Database Syst Rev* 2005;**3** [Meta-analysis; 18 randomized controlled trials (RCTs); n >3700]

6 Guinn DA, Atkinson MW, Sullivan L, et al. Single vs weekly courses of antenatal corticosteroids for women at risk of preterm delivery: a randomized controlled trial. *JAMA* 2001;**286**:1581–7. [RCT]

7 Crowther CA, Harding, J. Repeat doses of prenatal corticosteroids for women at risk of preterm birth for preventing neonatal respiratory disease. *Cochrane Database Syst Rev* 2005;**3**. [Meta-analysis; 3 RCTs, n=551]

8 Crowther CA, Neilson JP, Verkuyl DAA, Bannerman C, Ashurst HM. Preterm labour in twin pregnancies: can it be prevented by hospital admission? *Br J Obstet Gynaecol* 1989;**96**:850–3. [RCT; n=139]

9 Stan C, Boulvain M, Hirsbrunner-Amagbaly P, Pfister R. Hydration for treatment of preterm labour. *Cochrane Database Syst Rev* 2005;**3**. [2 RCTs, n=228]

10 King J, Flenady V. Prophylactic antibiotics for inhibiting preterm labour with intact membranes. *Cochrane Database Syst Rev* 2005;**3**. [11 RCTs, n=7428]

11 McGregor JA, French JI, Seo K. Adjunctive clindamycin therapy for preterm labor: results of a double-blind, placebo-controlled trial. *Am J Obstet Gynecol* 1991;**165**:867–75. [RCT; clindamycin]

12 Norman K, Pattinson RC, de Souza J, de Jong P, Moller G, Kirsten G. Ampicillin and metronidazole treatment in preterm labour: a multicentre, randomised controlled trial. *Br J Obstet Gynaecol* 1994;**101**:404–8. [RCT; ampicillin/metronidazole]

13 Svare J, Langhoff-Roos J, Andersen LF, et al. Ampicillin-metronidazole treatment in idiopathic preterm labour: a randomised controlled multicentre trial. *Br J Obstet Gynaecol* 1997;**104**:892–7. [RCT; Amp-Metro]

14 Gibbs RS, Schrag S, Schuchat A. Perinatal infections due to group B streptococci. *Obstet Gynecol* 2004;**104**:1062–76. [Review]

15 Anotayanonth S, Subhedar NV, Garner P, Neilson JP, Harigopal S. Betamimetics for inhibiting preterm labour. *Cochrane Database Syst Rev* 2005;**3**. [Meta-analysis; 11 RCTs; n=1332]

16 King JF, Flenady VJ, Papatsonis DNM, Dekker GA, Carbonne B. Calcium channel blockers for inhibiting preterm labour. *Cochrane Database Syst Rev* 2005;**3**. [Meta-analysis; 10 RCTs; n=1029]

17 King J, Flenady V, Cole S, Thornton S. Cyclo-oxygenase (COX) inhibitors for treating preterm labour. *Cochrane Database Syst Rev* 2005;**3**. [Meta-analysis;13 RCTs; n=713]

18 Niebyl JR, Blake DA, White RD, et al. The inhibition of premature labor with indomethacin. *Am J Obstet Gynecol* 1980;**136**:1014–9. [RCT; n=32. Indomethacin 50 mg p.o. then 25 mg q4h for 24 hours vs. placebo]

19 Zuckerman H, Shalev E, Gilad G, Katzuni E. Further study of the inhibition of premature labor by indomethacin. Part II. Double-blind study. *J Perinatal Med* 1984;**12**:25–9. [RCT; n=36. Indomethacin rectal suppository 100 mg then 25 mg p.o. q4h for 24 h. Additional 100 mg suppository if required. Total dose 200–300 mg in 24 h vs. placebo]

20 Abramov Y, Nadjari M, Weinstein D, Ben-Shachar I, Plotkin V, Ezra Y. Indomethacin for preterm labor: a randomized comparison of vaginal and rectal routes. *Obstet Gynecol* 2000;**95**:482–6. [RCT; n=46]

21 Sawdy RJ, Lye S, Fisk NM, Bennett PR. A double-blind randomized study of fetal side effects during and after the short-term maternal administration of indomethacin, sulindac, and nimesulide for the treatment of preterm labor. *Am J Obstet Gynecol* 2003;**188**:1046–51. [RCT; n=30. Sulindac 200 mg orally and a placebo suppository every 12 h; vs. nimesulide 200 mg rectally and a placebo capsule orally every 12 h; vs. indomethacin 100 mg rectally and a placebo capsule orally every 12 h]

22 Stika CS, Gross GA, Leguizamon G, et al. A prospective randomized safety trial of celecoxib for treatment of preterm labor. *Am J Obstet Gynecol* 2002;**187**:653–60. [RCT; n=24. Indomethacin suppository 100 mg then 50 mg p.o. q6h for 48 h plus oral placebo vs. Celecoxib p.o. 100 mg initially then 100 mg q12 h for 48 h plus rectal and oral placebo]

23 Loe SM, Sanchez-Ramos L, Kaunitz A. Assessing the neonatal safety of indomethacin tocolysis: a systematic review with meta-analysis. *Obstet Gynecol* 2005;**106**;173–9. [Meta-analysis of safety of indomethacin; n=1621 fetuses exposed to indomethacin in RCTs and observational studies]

24 Terrone DA, Rinehart BK, Kimmel ES, May WL, Larmon JE, Morrison JC. A prospective randomized controlled trial of high and low maintenance doses of magnesium sulfate for acute tocolysis. *Am J Obstet Gynecol* 2000;**182**:1477–82. [RCT; n=160. All pts: MgSO$_4$ 4 g load; then RCT to 2 g vs. 5 g/h]

25 Lewis DF, Bergstedt S, Edwards MS, et al. Successful magnesium sulfate tocolysis: is "weaning" the drug necessary? *Am J Obstet Gynecol* 1997;**177**:742–5. [RCT; n=140. Stop MgSO$_4$ abruptly vs. wean approx. 1 g q4 h]

26 Crowther CA, Hiller JE, Doyle LW. Magnesium sulfate for preventing preterm birth in threatened preterm labour. *Cochrane Database Syst Rev* 2005;**3**. [Meta-analysis; 23 RCTs; n≥2000]

27 Cotton DB, Strassner HT, Hill LM, Schifrin BS, Paul RH. Comparison of magnesium sulfate, terbutaline and a placebo for inhibition of preterm labor: a randomized study. *J Reprod Med* 1984;**29**.92–7. [RCT; n=56. MgSO$_4$ initial treatment 4 g i.v.;

maintenance 2 g/h. Terbutaline initial treatment 9.2 μg/min i.v.; maintenance: increased 5 μg/min to 25.3 μg/min. Dextrose: 125 mL/h. Duration: therapy continued for 12 h after contractions stopped. Stopped if cervix >7 cm, amnionitis, or side-effects]

28 Cox SM, Sherman ML, Leveno KJ. Randomized investigation of magnesium sulfate for prevention of preterm birth. *Am J Obstet Gynecol* 1990;**163**:767–72. [RCT; *n* = 156. Magnesium sulfate and saline control. Dose: MgSO₄ initial treatment 4 g i.v.. Maintenance: 2 g/h. Increasing to 3 g/h if still contracting after >1 h. Duration: therapy continued for 24 h. Placebo: saline 80 mL/h for 24 h]

29 Romero R, Sibai BM, Sanchez-Ramos L, *et al.* An oxytocin receptor antagonist (atosiban) in the treatment of preterm labor: a randomized, double-blind, placebo-controlled trial with tocolytic rescue. *Am J Obstet Gynecol* 2000;**182**:1173–83. [RCT; *n* = 531. Atosiban group: initial bolus of 6.75 mg atosiban administered over 1 minute. Followed by an infusion of 300 μg/min for 3 h followed by an infusion of 100 μg/min atosiban for 45 h. When uterine quiescence was achieved maintenance therapy was continued subcutaneously with either atosiban or placebo until the end of the 36th week of gestation. Control: initial bolus or placebo administered over 1 minute, followed by an infusion of placebo for 48 hours. Maintenance therapy with subcutaneous placebo until 36 weeks]

30 Papatsonis D, Flenady V, Cole S, Liley H. Oxytocin receptor antagonists for inhibiting preterm labour. *Cochrane Database Syst Rev* 2005;3 [6 RCTs; *n* = 1695]

31 Durckitt K, Thornton S. Nitric oxide donors for the treatment of preterm labour. *Cochrane Database Syst Rev* 2005;3 [Meta-analysis; 5 RCTs; *n* = 466]

32 Newton ER, Shields L, Rigway LE, Berkus MD, Elliott BD. Combination antibiotics and indomethacin in idiopathic preterm labor: a randomized double-blind study. *Am J Obstet Gynecol* 1991;**165**:1753–9. [RCT; *n* = 86]

33 Carlan S, O'Brien WF, O'Leary TD, Mastrogiannis D. Randomized comparative trial of indomethacin and sulindac for the treatment of refractory preterm labor. *Obstet Gynecol* 1992;**79**:223–8. [RCT; *n* = 36]

34 Sanchez-Ramos L, Kaunitz AM, Gaudier FL, Delke I. Efficacy of maintenance therapy for acute tocolysis: a meta-analysis. *Am J Obstet Gynecol* 1999;**181**:484. [5 RCTs terbutaline, 3 RCTs ritodrine]

35 Nanda K, Cook LA, Gallo MF, Grimes DA. Terbutaline pump maintenance therapy after threatened preterm labour for preventing preterm birth. *Cochrane Database Syst Rev* 2005;**3**. [Meta-analysis; 2 RCTs; *n* = 94]

36 Carr DB, Clark AL, Kernek K, Spinnato JA. Maintenance oral nifedipine for preterm labor: a randomized clinical trial. *Am J Obstet Gynecol* 1999;**181**:822–7. [RCT; *n* = 74]

37 Carlan SJ, O'Brien WF, Jones MH, O'Leary TD, Roth L. Outpatient oral sulindac to prevent recurrence of preterm labor. *Obstet Gynecol* 1995;**85**:769–74. [RCT; *n* = 69; sulindac 200 mg for 7 days vs. placebo]

38 Humprey RG, Bartfield MC, Carlan SJ, O'Brien WF, O'Leary TD, Triana T. Sulindac to prevent recurrent preterm labor: a randomized controlled trial. *Obstet Gynecol* 2001;**98**:555–62. [RCT; *n* = 95. Sulindac 100 mg until 34 weeks vs. placebo]

39 Crowther CA, Moore V. Magnesium maintenance therapy for preventing preterm birth after threatened preterm labor. *Cochrane Database Syst Rev* 2005;3 [meta-analysis; 3 RCTs; *n* = 303]

40 Valenzuela GJ, Sanchez-Ramos L, Romero R, *et al.* Maintenance treatment of preterm labor with the oxytocin antagonist atosiban. *Am J Obstet Gynecol* 2000;**182**:1184–90. [RCT; *n* = 503]

41 Grant A, Glazener CMA. Elective caesarean section versus expectant management for delivery of the small baby. *Cochrane Database Syst Rev* 2005;3. [Meta-analysis; 6 RCTs; *n* = 122]

43 Placenta previa and related placental disorders

Yinka Oyelese

The placenta usually implants in the upper uterine segment. However, in some cases, it implants in the lower uterine segment, either covering the internal cervical os, or lying in close proximity to it. This abnormal implantation into the lower segment, called placenta previa, is an important cause of bleeding in the second half of pregnancy and during labor, and is associated with significant maternal and perinatal morbidity and occasionally mortality. Placenta previa may also be associated with two other clinically important conditions, placenta accreta and vasa previa, which are also discussed in this chapter.

Placenta previa

Placenta previa has traditionally been classified into four types (Figs 43.1 and 43.2):
1 *Complete placenta previa*, where the placenta completely overlies the internal os (Fig. 43.2).
2 *Partial placenta previa*, where the placenta partially overlies the internal os.
3 *Marginal placenta previa*, where the placental edge just reaches to the internal os, but does not cover it (Fig. 43.3).
4 *Low-lying placenta*, which reaches into the lower uterine segment but does not reach the internal os.

Incidence and risk factors

Placenta previa complicates approximately 1 in 200 pregnancies (0.5%) [1,2]. Studies have identified several risk factors for placenta previa. These include prior cesarean delivery [3], prior uterine surgery, smoking [2], multifetal gestation [4], cocaine use, increasing parity, and increasing maternal age [1,2,5]. The risk of placenta previa increases with the number of prior cesarean deliveries in a dose–response manner. It is not clear why the placenta in some pregnancies implants in the lower uterine segment. However, it has been established that scarring of the endometrium as a consequence of cesarean

delivery or intrauterine surgery significantly increases the risk of placenta previa.

Clinical presentation

Patients with placenta previa typically present with painless bleeding in the early third trimester. The initial bleed is usually not very heavy, and typically does not lead to delivery, but is frequently sufficient to cause significant alarm. However, approximately one-third of cases of placenta previa will experience no bleeding prior to the onset of labor [6]. Not infrequently, there is a fetal malpresentation or unstable lie. This is because the placenta lies in the lower uterine segment, preventing engagement of the fetal head.

Diagnosis

The diagnosis of placenta previa is usually made by sonography. This typically occurs in one of two scenarios. In the first, the diagnosis is made in asymptomatic women on routine sonography, and the second is when sonography is performed in women who present with vaginal bleeding in the late second trimester or early third trimester. Transabominal sonography will detect the majority of cases of placenta previa. However, transabdominal sonography will produce false positive or false negative diagnoses of placenta previa in 10–20% of cases [7]. A common reason for false positive diagnoses is the approximation of the anterior and posterior walls of the lower uterine segment that occurs with the bladder filling that is necessary for transabdominal sonography; this may give a false impression of a placenta previa [8]. Crucial landmarks such as the internal os and the lower placental edge are frequently not adequately visualized using transabdominal sonography, producing a false negative diagnosis [7]. In addition, the fetal head may prevent adequate visualization of the region over the cervix [8]. Finally, a posterior placenta may be difficult to image transabdominally. Transvaginal sonography places the transducer closer to the region of interest, and because of the

Fig. 43.1 Types of placenta previa. *Complete:* Placental tissue completely overlies the internal os (can be central or noncentral, depending on whether or not the center of the placenta is directly over the os). *Partial:* Placental tissue is situated over part of the os but does not completely overlie it. *Marginal:* Placental tissue approaches the edge of the os but does not overlie any part of it. *Low-lying:* Placental tissue is implanted in the lower uterine segment but does not reach the edge of the os. From Oyelese and Smulian [46] with permission from Lippincott, Williams and Wilkins.

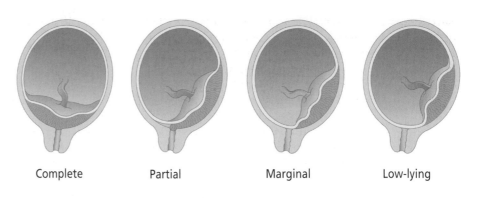

Complete   Partial   Marginal   Low-lying

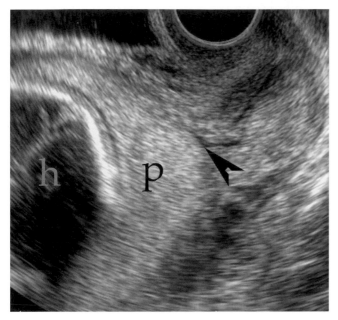

Fig. 43.2 Transvaginal sonogram of a complete placenta previa (placenta marked "p"). The placenta can be seen completely overlying the internal os (indicated by the arrow). The fetal head is marked "h".

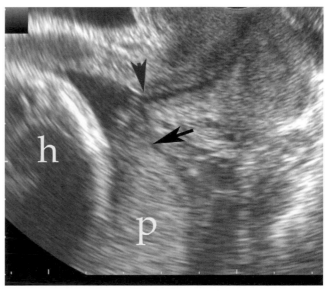

Fig. 43.3 Transvaginal sonogram demonstrating a marginal placenta previa (p). The internal os is again clearly shown (short arrow). There is a prominent sinus at the placental edge. The actual placental edge is indicated by the long arrow. Because this placenta was less than 2 cm from the internal os, the patient required a cesarean delivery. The fetal head is marked "h".

higher frequencies produced by transvaginal transducers, produces images of superior resolution to those obtained by transabdominal sonography [8]. In virtually all cases, the internal os and the placenta can be adequately visualized using this technique (Figs 43.2 and 43.3). Numerous studies have consistently demonstrated that transvaginal sonography is more accurate in the diagnosis of placenta previa than transabdominal sonography [8,9]. Furthermore, the technique is safe and does not lead to an increase in vaginal bleeding [9,10]. When transvaginal sonography is used, false positive diagnoses of placenta previa are avoided; thus, the reported incidence of placenta previa using transvaginal sonography is considerably lower than that obtained by transabdominal sonography. This has several potential benefits, the main one

being that women who do not actually have a placenta previa do not have unnecessary lifestyle restrictions and interventions. Translabial or transperineal sonography and magnetic resonance imaging (MRI) have also been used for placental location. However, these techniques have no benefits over the more readily available transvaginal sonogram.

Placental migration

It has been well documented that the majority of women in whom a placenta previa is detected in the second trimester will no longer have a placenta previa by the third trimester. It is not clear why this occurs. Studies using transvaginal sonography have shown that the incidence of second trimester placenta previa is 1.1–4.9% [11]. Approximately 90% of these will resolve before term [11]. The apparent movement of the placenta away from the cervix is most likely the consequence of the development of the lower uterine segment, leading to a stationary lower placental edge appearing to move away from the cervix. Another proposed mechanism is preferential growth of the placenta towards the better vascularized fundus. The likelihood that a second trimester placenta previa will persist until term can be determined by the degree by which the placenta overlies the internal os in the second trimester. Placentas that do not cover the internal os in the second trimester are unlikely to be placenta previas at term. Conversely, placentas that overlie the internal os by 1.5 cm or more are less likely to resolve by term [11].

Management

Women who present with vaginal bleeding in the late second or third trimester should be considered to have a placenta previa until proven otherwise. However, it must be emphasized that even though this bleeding is classically described as painless, there may be pain, probably the consequence of contractions or placental separation. A digital vaginal examination is contraindicated; this may provoke torrential vaginal bleeding. At least one (and preferably two) wide-bore intravenous cannulae should be inserted and intravenous fluids should be started. Blood should be taken for a complete blood count, blood type, and screen, and at least 2 units of blood should be cross-matched. Sonography, preferably by the transvaginal route, should be performed to confirm or rule out the diagnosis of placenta previa. The patient should be admitted and, initially at least, placed on bed rest. Blood pressure, pulse, and urine output should be monitored closely. Fetal sonography should be performed to rule out fetal anomalies, evaluate fetal growth and amniotic fluid volume. Continuous fetal heart rate monitoring should be commenced. Steroids should be administered to promote fetal lung maturation if the gestational age is between 24 and 32 weeks. In women who are having contractions, cautious use of tocolytics is reasonable [12]. Frequently, the contractions cause further placental separation, which causes further bleeding, which in turn causes more contractions, and thus a vicious cycle is set up. It was traditionally taught that tocolytics should not be used in the presence of vaginal bleeding. However, studies of tocolytic usage in women with placenta previa have demonstrated that they may safely be used with caution, and are associated with significant prolongation of gestation and increased birthweight [12,13].

The subsequent management depends on gestational age, the fetal and maternal status, and the presence of any other coexisting conditions. At a gestational age of less than 36 weeks, conservative management, rather than immediate delivery, is desirable, because prematurity is the cause of most of the perinatal mortality associated with placenta previa. Blood transfusions may be given as required. Cotton et al. [14] found that delivery could be deferred with conservative management in two-thirds of patients with symptomatic placenta previa, and that half of patients with an initial hemorrhagic episode exceeding 500 mL did not require immediate delivery. These authors achieved a mean prolongation of pregnancy of 16.8 days in women with symptomatic previas. Similarly, Silver et al. [15], with conservative aggressive management, prolonged gestation by at least 4 weeks in 50% of patients with a symptomatic previa.

If the mother and fetus are stable, hospitalization for at least 48 hours is justified. When there has been no bleeding for at least 24–48 hours, the patient may be discharged and subsequently managed as an outpatient [16]. However, it is essential that women who are considered for outpatient management live in close proximity to the hospital, have a responsible adult at home, and have access to telephone services and transportation. Outpatient management has been compared with inpatient management in a few studies [16,17]. A randomized controlled study found that stable patients with placenta previa could be safely managed as outpatients with substantial savings in hospital costs, and no worse outcomes (assessed by gestational age at delivery, birthweights, blood transfusions, and neonatal outcomes) than women managed as inpatients [17].

Complications

Fetal

Placenta previa is associated with increased perinatal mortality as well as an excess in neonatal deaths after live births [18,19]. There is a higher risk of preterm birth, and prematurity is the reason for most of the perinatal deaths [18]. Placenta previa is also associated with an increased risk of congenital malformations, respiratory distress syndrome, and intrauterine growth restriction [18]. The perinatal mortality rate associated with placenta previa is approximately three times that of controls [18,19].

Maternal

Women with complete or partial placenta previa require cesarean delivery. In addition, the condition is a major cause of obstetric hemorrhage [20]. Frequently, blood transfusions are necessary. While in almost all cases of placenta previa there is some degree of placental separation, women with placenta previa are also at increased risk of concurrent placental abruption. Prolonged bed rest may put women at greater risk of thromboembolic disease [20]. Morbid adherence of the placenta occurs more frequently in women with placenta previa, and frequently these women will go on to have a hysterectomy [20].

Timing of delivery

Women with a placenta previa should be delivered by cesarean at a time when fetal lung maturation is likely, and before catastrophic bleeding occurs. Doubtless, these patients are better delivered in a controlled scheduled setting, rather than as an emergency for bleeding. A recent study demonstrated that the perinatal mortality for pregnancies complicated by placenta previa started to rise after approximately 37 weeks [19]. For these reasons, scheduled cesarean delivery at 36–37 weeks after documentation of fetal lung maturity by amniocentesis appears reasonable.

Mode of delivery and uterine incisions

There is consensus that women with complete or partial placenta previa require cesarean delivery. What is more controversial is the mode of delivery of women with placentas that lie in close proximity to the internal os, but do not cover it. At least three studies have addressed the mode of delivery in these patients [21–23]. Oppenheimer *et al.* [21] found that a lower placental edge to internal os distance of 2 cm or greater was likely to result in a successful trial of labor. Similar findings were noted by Bhide *et al.* [22]. Women who had a placental edge to os distance in excess of 2 cm did not require cesarean delivery for bleeding, whereas when the distance was less, the patients invariably required cesarean delivery. It must be pointed out that in these studies, the delivering obstetricians were not blinded to the ultrasound results, and thus these results may be significantly biased. Nonetheless, it does appear reasonable to offer women with a placental edge to os distance of 2 cm or greater by transvaginal sonography, who have no other contraindications to vaginal delivery, a trial of labor.

In women with an anterior placenta previa, the surgeon generally has to either incise through the placenta, separate the placenta prior to delivery of the fetus or make an incision that avoids the placenta, such as a vertical fundal incision. Generally, a lower segment transverse incision can be used, but it is useful to determine placental location by sonography prior to the operation, and preferably to avoid the placenta.

Vasa previa

The term vasa previa refers to fetal blood vessels running through the membranes over the cervix, unprotected by umbilical cord or placental tissue (Fig. 43.4) [24]. Consequently, when the membranes rupture, these vessels frequently rupture also, often resulting in fetal exsanguination [24]. Undiagnosed prenatally, this condition carries a perinatal mortality of approximately 56% [25]. Vasa previa can result from velamentous insertion of the umbilical cord into the placenta or from vessels running between lobes of a placenta with accessory lobes [24].

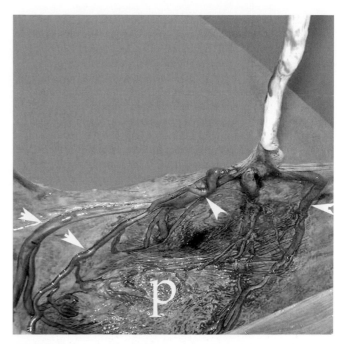

Fig. 43.4 Vasa previa shown after cesarean delivery. In this case, the diagnosis had been made prenatally. Prominent velamentous vessels traverse the membranes (arrows). "p" marks the placenta.

Incidence and risk factors

The diagnosis of vasa previa is often missed, and thus accurate estimates of the frequency of this condition are difficult to make. Nonetheless, studies suggest that the incidence of clinically recognized vasa previa is approximately 1 in 2500 deliveries [24]. Major risk factors for vasa previa include second trimester low-lying placentas or placenta previa [24–27]. This risk exists even when the placenta previa is no longer low-lying by the time of delivery [25,27]. Other risk factors include pregnancies resulting from *in vitro* fertilization [24,28], multifetal gestations, and pregnancies where the placenta has one or more succenturiate lobes [24,25].

Pathophysiology

While the exact reason for developing vasa previa remains unknown, two main hypotheses exist as to the condition's pathogenesis. In the first, it is thought that the portion of the placenta that overlies the cervix early in pregnancy undergoes atrophy because of poor vascularity in that region, leaving blood vessels running exposed through the membranes. The second hypothesis suggests that the placenta grows preferentially toward the better vascularized upper segment, again leaving blood vessels exposed during its differential growth.

Clinical presentation

The classic presentation of vasa previa is of vaginal bleeding at the time of rupture of the membranes followed by fetal death

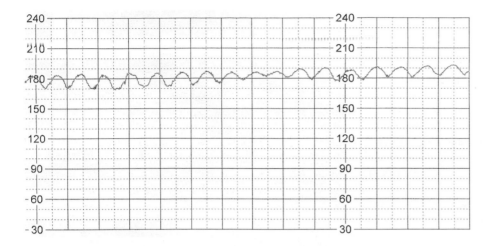

Fig. 43.5 Sinusoidal fetal heart rate tracing in a patient with a ruptured vasa previa. The patient, in labor, ruptured her membranes and had bleeding at the same time. Emergent cesarean delivery was performed. The infant was born extremely pale, was immediately transfused, and did well.

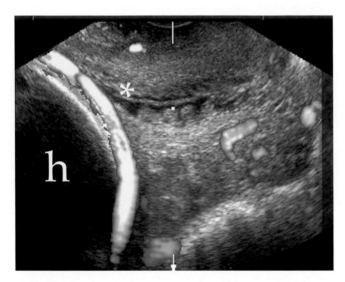

Fig. 43.6 Color Doppler of vasa previa showing flow through a vessel running over the internal os (marked by the asterisk). The fetal head is marked "h".

or distress. A sinusoidal fetal heart rate tracing in this scenario is virtually pathognomonic of vasa previa (Fig. 43.5). Pressure on the exposed vessels by the presenting part may lead to recurrent variable decelerations, even in cases with intact membranes. Rarely, fetal vessels may be palpated in the unruptured membranes during a cervical examination [24]. More recently, vasa previa has been diagnosed during routine second trimester sonography or during sonography in patients presenting with bleeding in the second half of pregnancy or patients having sonography for low-lying placentas [29–32].

Diagnosis

The diagnosis of vasa previa may be made based on a history of fetal death or distress associated with bleeding when the membranes rupture. The delivery of an extremely pale, exsanguinated infant and the finding of ruptured velamentous vessels on placental examination after delivery confirm the diagnosis. The diagnosis of vasa previa may be made in asymptomatic women during second trimester obstetric sonography. Vasa previa has the appearance of linear or tubular structures overlying the cervix. Color Doppler should be employed to demonstrate flow through these vessels, and if pulsed Doppler demonstrates a fetal umbilical or venous waveform, the diagnosis is confirmed (Fig. 43.6). Care must be taken to distinguish a vasa previa from a funic presentation. In a funic presentation, the vessels will move away from the cervix with changes in maternal position, while the position will remain constant.

Several studies have examined the utility of routine screening for vasa previa in asymptomatic patients during the second trimester obstetric sonogram [29–32]. These studies have consistently demonstrated that vasa previa can be diagnosed with accuracy and without excessive extra time over that required for the obstetric examination [29–32]. The strategy for screening for vasa previa consists of identifying the placental cord insertion during the sonographic examination. This essentially excludes a vasa previa unless there is a multilobed placenta. In women with multilobed placentas, those with second trimester low-lying placentas, and those with multifetal gestations, transvaginal sonography with a color Doppler sweep of the region over the cervix should be performed. The diagnosis of vasa previa has been made in women presenting with third trimester bleeding by testing the vaginal blood for fetal blood cells using a test such as the Apt test or Kleihauer–Betke test. However, these tests are rarely used for this purpose, and diagnosis by ultrasound is preferable.

Management

Asymptomatic women with a second trimester diagnosis of vasa previa should be informed about the diagnosis and about the severity of the condition. These women should report to hospital immediately should they experience contractions, bleeding, or loss of fluid. Coitus should be avoided. Consideration should be given to admission to the hospital at approximately 32 weeks' gestation. The major purpose for admission is to ensure quick access to immediate cesarean delivery should the membranes rupture. Because the majority of these women will be delivered preterm, steroids should be administered to promote fetal lung maturation. The patient should be seen by a neonatologist, and facilities for immediate neonatal blood transfusion in the delivery room should be available. Delivery should be by cesarean at 35–36 weeks or after documentation of fetal lung maturation, or if in the third trimester, should significant bleeding, labor, or rupture of the membranes occur. When the membranes have ruptured, immediate cesarean delivery and neonatal blood transfusion may be life-saving [33]. Recently, we have used three-dimensional sonography to map out the course of the vessels prior to surgery in order to plan our incision to avoid transecting the vessels. At cesarean delivery, a transverse uterine incision may be made, but it is important to avoid incising or rupturing the membranes after the uterine incision. Every attempt should be made to deliver the fetus *en caul*.

Outcomes

Perinatal deaths from vasa previa are for the most part preventable; good outcomes depend on prenatal diagnosis and delivery by cesarean before the membranes rupture [24]. Because the fetal blood volume is only approximately 100 mL/kg at term, relatively small amounts of blood loss may prove catastrophic to the fetus, and thus everything must be done to ensure delivery before fetal hemorrhage occurs [24]. A study of 155 cases of vasa previa demonstrated that the most important factor in assuring a good perinatal outcome was prenatal diagnosis; the perinatal mortality in pregnancies in which the prenatal diagnosis had been made was 56% [25]. Furthermore, in survivors in cases where the prenatal diagnosis had not been made, the median Apgar scores were 1 at 1 minute and 4 at 5 minutes [25]. In addition, over half of these survivors required neonatal blood transfusions [25]. Conversely, when the diagnosis was made prenatally, less than 3% of fetuses/neonates died (over 97% survived), and the median Apgar scores were 7 and 9 at 1 and 5 minutes, respectively [25]. In these patients, neonatal blood transfusions were rarely required [25].

Placenta accreta

Placenta accreta refers to a placenta that is abnormally adherent. This condition is caused by a deficiency of the decidua basalis. Invasion into the myometrium is called placenta increta, while invasion through the serosa is termed placenta percreta. In all these entities, the placenta does not separate after delivery and the condition is associated with massive blood loss and high maternal morbidity and mortality. In addition, a placenta percreta may invade into surrounding structures such as the bladder.

Incidence and risk factors

The incidence of placenta accreta is estimated at 1 in 500–2500 pregnancies [34,35]. The most important risk factors for placenta accreta are a prior cesarean delivery and a placenta previa in the current pregnancy [34,35]. Clark *et al.* [36] showed that the incidence of placenta accreta increased with the number of prior cesarean deliveries, rising from 25% in women with one prior cesarean to 68% in women with a low-lying placenta and three prior cesarean deliveries. Consequently, as a result of increasing cesarean rates, the incidence of placenta accreta is rising.

Clinical presentation and diagnosis

Placenta accreta should be suspected, particularly in women with a history of prior cesarean or intrauterine surgery, when the placenta fails to separate after delivery. However, the diagnosis may be made prenatally using sonography [37,38]. Placenta accreta should be suspected in women with a prior cesarean delivery who have a placenta previa in the current pregnancy [37]. These women should have sonographic examination for evidence of placenta accreta [37]. Comstock reviewed the antenatal sonographic diagnosis of placenta accreta and found that the most reliable sign of placenta accreta is the presence of prominent vascular spaces or lacunae in the placenta [37,38]. This may give the placenta a "moth-eaten" appearance (Fig. 43.7). Other sonographic signs of placenta accreta include absence of the retroplacental clear space, the

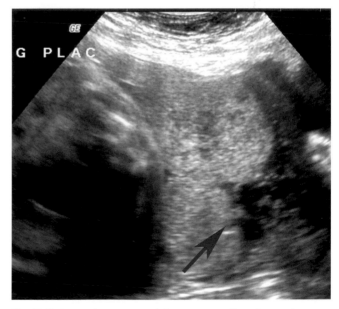

Fig. 43.7 Gray-scale sonogram of placenta accreta. Note the prominent lacunae in the placenta, giving a "moth-eaten" appearance (arrow).

presence of a highly vascular myometrial–bladder interface, and invasion into the bladder [37,38]. These authors found a sensitivity of 93% and a positive predictive value of 92% using gray-scale ultrasound for placenta accreta. Color Doppler imaging has been used in the diagnosis of placenta accreta, with the main finding being turbulent lacunar blood flow extending from the placenta into the surrounding tissues. MRI is useful and accurate in diagnosing placenta accreta, but does not appear to offer any advantages over sonography, except in cases where there is a posterior placenta. Elevated maternal serum alpha-fetoprotein (MSAFP) levels may be found in women with placenta accreta [39], and therefore women with unexplained elevated MSAFP levels should have targeted sonography to rule out placenta accreta.

Management

The standard treatment for placenta accreta is cesarean delivery with immediate hysterectomy. No attempt should be made to separate the placenta, because this may lead to catastrophic hemorrhage. Generally, the fetus is delivered through a fundal incision, avoiding the placenta. Surgery for placenta accreta is associated with massive blood loss, with the average blood loss being approximately 3000–5000 mL [40]. Therefore, these women should be delivered, preferably under controlled scheduled conditions, in a center with skilled personnel and adequate blood transfusion facilities [40]. These women are at risk of disseminated intravascular coagulopathy, and blood components such as fresh frozen plasma and cryoprecipitate should be readily available. Because of the risk of involvement of the bladder and ureters, consulting a urologist is advisable [40]. Preoperative placement of ureteral stents may help minimize the risk of ureteric or bladder injury. Women with placenta accreta should be evaluated preoperatively by the anesthesiologist. Embolization of the internal iliac vessels or the uterine vessels may significantly reduce blood loss, and may aid in performing surgery under more controlled conditions, without catastrophic hemorrhage [41,42].

Several recent reports have documented successfully managing placenta accreta without hysterectomy, leaving the uterus in place after the delivery [43,44]. This approach potentially has several benefits. First, fertility is preserved. Second, it has been proposed that this management modality is associated with less blood loss and lower morbidity. In some cases, methotrexate was administered, and internal iliac artery embolization may be helpful. Adverse outcomes have been reported with conservative management [45]. Massive hemorrhage may occur suddenly, requiring surgery under emergent uncontrolled conditions [45]. Also there is the potential risk of serious intrauterine infection. Nevertheless, it does appear that this may be a viable option in a very few well-selected women who are well informed, motivated, and desire to keep their fertility.

Case presentation

A 40-year-old woman with a history of a prior term cesarean delivery for breech presentation had a routine transabdominal sonogram at 20 weeks which showed a complete placenta previa. She presented to hospital at 30 weeks' gestation with painless vaginal bleeding. Transabdominal and transvaginal sonography demonstrated a complete placenta previa with large lacunae (Fig. 43.7). In addition, color Doppler revealed turbulent blood flow through these lacunae, and was suggestive of absence of the subplacental "clear space." A diagnosis of placenta accreta was made. The patient was admitted to hospital. Two wide-bore intravenous cannulae were inserted, and blood was sent for type and screen. The blood bank was contacted to ensure that at least 4 units of compatible blood as well as blood replacement products could be made available at short notice. The patient was kept on bed rest until the bleeding stopped 48 hours later. Two days later, because she was asymptomatic, she was discharged with instructions to come to the hospital immediately should she experience any bleeding or contractions. At 36 weeks, amniocentesis was performed, and fetal lung maturation was documented. She was delivered by classic cesarean delivery. Prior to the delivery, balloon catheters had been inserted in the internal iliac arteries bilaterally by interventional radiology, and ureteric stents were inserted by urology. Following delivery of the infant, the balloons were inflated. Cesarean hysterectomy was performed. The patient lost 2000 mL blood and was transfused with 2 units of packed red blood cells. Her postoperative course was uncomplicated and she was discharged home on postoperative day 4. Pathologic examination of the uterus revealed a placenta increta.

Management points

1 The patient had been noted on second trimester sonography to have a placenta previa but was not admitted until she was symptomatic. Asymptomatic women with placenta previa do not require admission in the second trimester; most of these cases resolve spontaneously.

2 On admission, intravenous (i.v.) access was established with two 16-gauge i.v. lines and crystalloid infusion was administered to maintain hemodynamic stability and urine output.

3 The blood bank made sure that adequate blood products were readily available.

4 Fetal sonography was performed, as was continuous fetal monitoring.

5 Close monitoring of the maternal hemodynamic status was performed.

6 Because of the history of prior cesarean and a complete previa, targeted sonography was performed which allowed the prenatal diagnosis of placenta accreta.

7 Following resolution of the acute episode, the patient was discharged on bed rest and asked to avoid coitus. She was a candidate for outpatient management because she lived close to the hospital, had a telephone and a car, and had an adult with her at all times.

8 At 36 weeks, amniocentesis was performed, and lung maturity documented.

9 Delivery was by cesarean under scheduled controlled conditions. A multidisciplinary approach with a team including the maternal fetal medicine specialist, anesthesiologist, urologist, interventional radiologist, blood bank team, and neonatologist ensured a good outcome.

10 Blood was replaced liberally as were blood factors in order to prevent disseminated intravascular coagulopathy.

References

1 Iyasu S, Saftlas AK, Rowley DL, Koonin LM, Lawson HW, Atrash HK. The epidemiology of placenta previa in the United States, 1979 through 1987. *Am J Obstet Gynecol* 1993;**168**:1424–9.

2 Faiz AS, Ananth CV. Etiology and risk factors for placenta previa: an overview and meta-analysis of observational studies. *J Matern Fetal Neonatal Med* 2003;**13**:175–90.

3 Ananth CV, Smulian JC, Vintzileos AM. The association of placenta previa with history of cesarean delivery and abortion: a metaanalysis. *Am J Obstet Gynecol* 1997;**177**:1071–8.

4 Ananth CV, Demissie K, Smulian JC, Vintzileos AM. Placenta previa in singleton and twin births in the United States, 1989 through 1998: a comparison of risk factor profiles and associated conditions. *Am J Obstet Gynecol* 2003;**188**:275–81.

5 Zhang J, Savitz DA. Maternal age and placenta previa: a population-based, case–control study. *Am J Obstet Gynecol* 1993;**168**:641–5.

6 Hill DJ, Beischer NA. Placenta praevia without antepartum haemorrhage. *Aust N Z J Obstet Gynaecol* 1980;**20**:21–3.

7 Smith RS, Lauria MR, Comstock CH, *et al.* Transvaginal ultrasonography for all placentas that appear to be low-lying or over the internal cervical os. *Ultrasound Obstet Gynecol* 1997;**9**:22–4.

8 Timor-Tritsch IE, Monteagudo A. Diagnosis of placenta previa by transvaginal sonography. *Ann Med* 1993;**25**:279–83.

9 Leerentveld RA, Gilberts EC, Arnold MJ, Wladimiroff JW. Accuracy and safety of transvaginal sonographic placental localization. *Obstet Gynecol* 1990;**76**:759–62.

10 Timor-Tritsch IE, Yunis RA. Confirming the safety of transvaginal sonography in patients suspected of placenta previa. *Obstet Gynecol* 1993;**81**:742–4.

11 Taipale P, Hiilesmaa V, Ylostalo P. Transvaginal ultrasonography at 18–23 weeks in predicting placenta previa at delivery. *Ultrasound Obstet Gynecol* 1998;**12**:422–5.

12 Sharma A, Suri V, Gupta I. Tocolytic therapy in conservative management of symptomatic placenta previa. *Int J Gynaecol Obstet* 2004;**84**:109–13.

13 Besinger RE, Moniak CW, Paskiewicz LS, Fisher SG, Tomich PG. The effect of tocolytic use in the management of symptomatic placenta previa. *Am J Obstet Gynecol* 1995;**172**:1770–5; discussion 1775–8.

14 Cotton DB, Read JA, Paul RH, Quilligan EJ. The conservative aggressive management of placenta previa. *Am J Obstet Gynecol* 1980;**137**:687–95.

15 Silver R, Depp R, Sabbagha RE, Dooley SL, Socol ML, Tamura RK. Placenta previa: aggressive expectant management. *Am J Obstet Gynecol* 1984;**150**:15–22.

16 Mouer JR. Placenta previa: antepartum conservative management, inpatient versus outpatient. *Am J Obstet Gynecol* 1994;**170**:1683–5; discussion 1685–6.

17 Wing DA, Paul RH, Millar LK. Management of the symptomatic placenta previa: a randomized, controlled trial of inpatient versus outpatient expectant management. *Am J Obstet Gynecol* 1996;**175**:806–11.

18 Crane JM, van den Hof MC, Dodds L, Armson BA, Liston R. Neonatal outcomes with placenta previa. *Obstet Gynecol* 1999;**93**:541–4.

19 Ananth CV, Smulian JC, Vintzileos AM. The effect of placenta previa on neonatal mortality: a population-based study in the United States, 1989 through 1997. *Am J Obstet Gynecol* 2003;**188**:1299–304.

20 Crane JM, Van den Hof MC, Dodds L, Armson BA, Liston R. Maternal complications with placenta previa. *Am J Perinatol* 2000;**17**:101–5.

21 Oppenheimer LW, Farine D, Ritchie JW, Lewinsky RM, Telford J, Fairbanks LA. What is a low-lying placenta? *Am J Obstet Gynecol* 1991;**165**:1036–8.

22 Bhide A, Prefumo F, Moore J, Hollis B, Thilaganathan B. Placental edge to internal os distance in the late third trimester and mode of delivery in placenta praevia. *Br J Obstet Gynaecol* 2003;**110**: 860–4.

23 Dawson WB, Dumas MD, Romano WM, Gagnon R, Gratton RJ, Mowbray RD. Translabial ultrasonography and placenta previa: does measurement of the os–placenta distance predict outcome? *J Ultrasound Med* 1996;**15**:441–6.

24 Oyelese KO, Turner M, Lees C, Campbell S. Vasa previa: an avoidable obstetric tragedy. *Obstet Gynecol Surv* 1999;**54**: 138–45.

25 Oyelese Y, Catanzarite V, Prefumo F, *et al.* Vasa previa: the impact of prenatal diagnosis on outcomes. *Obstet Gynecol* 2004;**103**:937–42.

26 Oyelese Y, Spong C, Fernandez MA, McLaren RA. Second trimester low-lying placenta and *in vitro* fertilization? Exclude vasa previa. *J Matern Fetal Med* 2000;**9**:370–2.

27 Francois K, Mayer S, Harris C, Perlow JH. Association of vasa previa at delivery with a history of second-trimester placenta previa. *J Reprod Med* 2003;**48**:771–4.

28 Schachter M, Tovbin Y, Arieli S, Friedler S, Ron-El R, Sherman D. *In vitro* fertilization is a risk factor for vasa previa. *Fertil Steril* 2002;**78**:642–3.

29 Lee W, Lee VL, Kirk JS, Sloan CT, Smith RS, Comstock CH. Vasa previa: prenatal diagnosis, natural evolution, and clinical outcome. *Obstet Gynecol* 2000;**95**:572–6.

30 Catanzarite V, Maida C, Thomas W, Mendoza A, Stanco L, Piacquadio KM. Prenatal sonographic diagnosis of vasa previa: ultrasound findings and obstetric outcome in ten cases. *Ultrasound Obstet Gynecol* 2001;**18**:109–15.

31 Nomiyama M, Toyota Y, Kawano H. Antenatal diagnosis of velamentous umbilical cord insertion and vasa previa with color Doppler imaging. *Ultrasound Obstet Gynecol* 1998;**12**:426–9.

32 Sepulveda W, Rojas I, Robert JA, Schnapp C, Alcalde JL. Prenatal detection of velamentous insertion of the umbilical cord: a prospective color Doppler ultrasound study. *Ultrasound Obstet Gynecol* 2003;**21**:564–9.

33 Schellpfeffer MA. Improved neonatal outcome of vasa previa with aggressive intrapartum management: a report of two cases. *J Reprod Med* 1995;**40**:327–32.

34 Miller DA, Chollet JA, Goodwin TM. Clinical risk factors for placenta previa–placenta accreta. *Am J Obstet Gynecol* 1997;**177**: 210–4.

35 Wu S, Kocherginsky M, Hibbard JU. Abnormal placentation: twenty-year analysis. *Am J Obstet Gynecol* 2005;**192**: 1458–61.

36 Clark SL, Koonings PP, Phelan JP. Placenta previa/ accreta and prior cesarean section. *Obstet Gynecol* 1985;**66**: 89–92.

37 Comstock CH. Antenatal diagnosis of placenta accreta: a review. *Ultrasound Obstet Gynecol* 2005;**26**:89–96.

38 Comstock CH, Love JJ Jr, Bronsteen RA, *et al*. Sonographic detection of placenta accreta in the second and third trimesters of pregnancy. *Am J Obstet Gynecol* 2004;**190**:1135–40.

39 Zelop C, Nadel A, Frigoletto FD Jr, Pauker S, MacMillan M, Benacerraf BR. Placenta accreta/percreta/increta: a cause of elevated maternal serum alpha-fetoprotein. *Obstet Gynecol* 1992;00.693–4.

40 Hudon L, Belfort MA, Broome DR. Diagnosis and management of placenta percreta: a review. *Obstet Gynecol Surv* 1998;**53**:509–17.

41 Alvarez M, Lockwood CJ, Ghidini A, Dottino P, Mitty HA, Berkowitz RL. Prophylactic and emergent arterial catheterization for selective embolization in obstetric hemorrhage. *Am J Perinatol* 1992;**9**:441–4.

42 Kidney DD, Nguyen AM, Ahdoot D, Bickmore D, Deutsch LS, Majors C. Prophylactic perioperative hypogastric artery balloon occlusion in abnormal placentation. *Am J Roentgenol* 2001;**176**:1521–4.

43 Weinstein A, Chandra P, Schiavello H, Fleischer A. Conservative management of placenta previa percreta in a Jehovah's Witness. *Obstet Gynecol* 2005;**105**:1247–50.

44 Kayem G, Davy C, Goffinet F, Thomas C, Clement D, Cabrol D. Conservative versus extirpative management in cases of placenta accreta. *Obstet Gynecol* 2004;**104**:531–6.

45 Butt K, Gagnon A, Delisle MF. Failure of methotrexate and internal iliac balloon catheterization to manage placenta percreta. *Obstet Gynecol* 2002;**99**:981–2.

46 Oyelese Y, Smulian JC. Placenta previa, accreta, and vasa previa. *Obstet Gynecol* 2006;**107**:927–41.

Complications of Labor and Delivery

44 Prolonged pregnancy

Errol R. Norwitz and Victoria Snegovskikh

The timely onset of labor and delivery is an important determinant of perinatal outcome. Both preterm births (defined as delivery prior to 37 weeks' gestation) and post-term births are associated with increased neonatal morbidity and mortality. Much attention has been paid to the problem of preterm labor and birth. However, despite the high prevalence of post-term pregnancy (10% of all deliveries), the observation that antepartum stillbirths account for more perinatal deaths than either complications of prematurity or sudden infant death syndrome, and the fact that the risks of post-term pregnancy can be easily avoided by earlier induction of labor, relatively less attention has been paid to the management of prolonged pregnancy. This chapter reviews in detail the risks of continuing pregnancy beyond the due date, the option of induction of labor, and the management of low-risk post-term pregnancies.

Definitions

Prolonged (post-term) pregnancy is defined as a pregnancy that continues to or beyond 42w 0d (294 days) from the first day of the last normal menstrual period or 14 days beyond the best obstetric estimate of the date of delivery (EDD) [1,2]. The term 'postdates' is not well defined and, as such, is best avoided.

Incidence

The prevalence of post-term pregnancy depends on the patient population, including such factors as the percentage of primigravid women, women with pregnancy complications, the prevalence of ultrasound assessment of gestational age, and the frequency of spontaneous preterm birth. Local practice patterns such as the rates of scheduled cesarean delivery and routine labor induction will also affect the overall prevalence of post-term birth. In the USA, approximately 18% of all singleton pregnancies continue beyond 41 weeks, 10% (range 3–14%) continue beyond 42 weeks and are therefore post-term, and 4% (2–7%) continue beyond 43 completed weeks in the absence of obstetric intervention [1,3,4].

Etiology

The most common cause of prolonged pregnancy is an error in gestational age dating. Reliance on standard clinical criteria (Table 44.1) contributes to inaccurate diagnosis and tends to overestimate gestational age [5–8]. Uncertainty in dating parameters should prompt ultrasound assessment of gestational age (discussed below). In most cases of "true" post-term pregnancy, the cause is not known. Risk factors include nulliparity and a prior post-term pregnancy [9,10]. Rarer causes include placental sulfatase deficiency (an X-linked recessive disorder characterized by low circulating estriol levels), fetal adrenal insufficiency or hypoplasia [11], and fetal anencephaly (in the absence of polyhydramnios). Recent data have also shown an association with male fetuses [12]. There is no consistent association between post-term pregnancy and maternal age, parity, or ethnicity.

Genetic factors may also have a role in prolonging pregnancy [10,13,14]. In one study, women who were the product of a prolonged pregnancy were more likely themselves to have a prolonged pregnancy (relative risk [RR] 1.3) [10]. Similarly, women who have had a prior post-term pregnancy are more likely to have another such pregnancy [10,14]. For example, after one prolonged pregnancy, the risk of a second such pregnancy in the subsequent birth is increased 2.7-fold (from 10% to 27%). If there have been two successive prolonged pregnancies, the incidence rises to 39% [6]. Paternal genes expressed in the fetoplacental unit also appear to influence length of gestation. In a recent Danish sibling-pair case–control study, the rate of prolonged gestation in a second pregnancy among 21,746 female sibling pairs whose first delivery was post-term was 20% compared to 7.7% among 7009 female sibling pairs whose first delivery was at term [14]. However, the risk of recurrent post-term delivery was reduced to 15% when the first and second child had different fathers (odds ratio [OR] 0.73; 95% confidence interval [CI], 0.63–0.84) [14].

Complications of post-term pregnancy

Recent studies have shown that the risks to the fetus [15–23] and to the mother [20,24–26] of continuing the pregnancy beyond the EDD are greater than originally appreciated.

Table 44.1 Clinical criteria commonly used to confirm gestational age. From ACOG [1].

Reported last normal menstrual period (estimated due date can be calculated by subtracting 3 months and adding 7 days to the first day of the last normal menstrual period [Nägele rule]) or date of assisted reproductive technology (intrauterine insemination or embryo transfer)

The size of the uterus as estimated on bimanual examination in the first trimester should be consistent with dates

The perception of fetal movement ("quickening") usually occurs at 18–20 weeks in nulliparous women and 16–18 weeks in multiparous women

Fetal heart tones can be heard with a nonelectronic fetal stethoscope by 18–20 weeks and with a Doppler ultrasound by 10–12 weeks

At 20 weeks, the fundal height in a singleton pregnancy should be approximately 20 cm above the pubic symphysis (usually corresponding to the umbilicus)

Ultrasound, including crown rump length of the fetus during the first trimester or fetal biometry (biparietal diameter, head circumference, and/or femur length) during the second trimester

Fetal risks

Antepartum stillbirths account for more perinatal deaths than either complications of prematurity or sudden infant death syndrome [19]. Perinatal mortality (defined as stillbirths plus early neonatal deaths) at 42 weeks' gestation is twice that at 40 weeks (4–7 vs. 2–3 per 1000 deliveries, respectively) and increases fourfold at 43 weeks and five- to sevenfold at 44 weeks [17–20,27]. Additionally, recent epidemiologic studies suggest that these calculations may actually underestimate the risk of stillbirth and early neonatal death, because these data used all pregnancies rather than ongoing (undelivered) pregnancies as the denominator (Figs 44.1 and 44.2). Once a fetus is delivered, it is no longer at risk of intrauterine fetal demise (stillbirth). In one retrospective study of over 170,000 singleton births, Hilder et al. [18] demonstrated that the still-birth rate increased sixfold (from 0.35 to 2.12 per 1000 pregnancies) when the denominator was changed from all deliveries to ongoing (undelivered) pregnancies. These data also demonstrate that, when calculated per 1000 ongoing pregnancies, fetal and neonatal mortality rates increase sharply after 40 weeks (Fig. 44.1). Cotzias et al. [19] used the same database to calculate the risk of stillbirth in ongoing pregnancies for each gestational age from 35 to 43 weeks. The risk of stillbirth was 1 in 926 ongoing pregnancies at 40 weeks' gestation, 1 in 826 at 41 weeks, 1 in 769 at 42 weeks, and 1 in 633 at 43 weeks. Uteroplacental insufficiency, asphyxia (with and without meconium), intrauterine infection, and anencephaly all contribute to the excess perinatal deaths, although post-term anencephaly is essentially nonexistent with modern obstetric care [28].

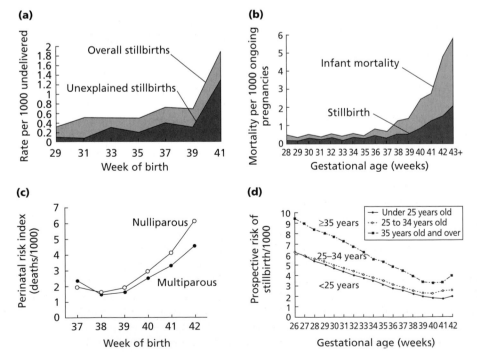

Fig. 44.1 Multiple studies have reported that antepartum stillbirths increase after 38–39 weeks' gestation. This was first demonstrated in 1987 (Yudkin et al. [15] [A]). Subsequent studies showed that this was true not only of antepartum stillbirth, but also of mortality within the first year of life (e.g., Rand et al. [20] [B]). Further studies have shown that the same relationship exists in both nulliparous and multiparous women (Smith [21] [C]) and in women of advanced maternal age (Feldman [17] [D]).

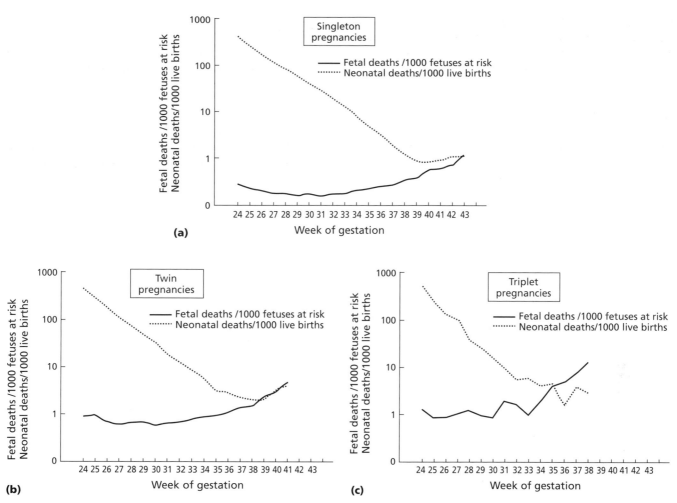

Fig. 44.2 Risk of stillbirths (per 1000 fetuses at risk) and neonatal deaths (per 1000 live births) in singleton (*n*=11,061,599), twin (*n*=297,622), and triplet (*n*=15,375) gestations drawn from the 1995–1998 National Center for Health Statistics linked birth and death files. From Kahn *et al.* [23] with permission.

Post-term infants are larger than term infants (2.5–10% vs. 0.8–1%, respectively), with a higher incidence of fetal macrosomia (defined as an estimated fetal weight of more than 4500 g) [29,30]. Complications associated with fetal macrosomia include prolonged labor, cephalopelvic disproportion, and shoulder dystocia with resultant risks of orthopedic or neurologic injury. Approximately 20% of post-term fetuses have "fetal dysmaturity (postmaturity) syndrome," which describes infants with characteristics of chronic intrauterine growth restriction from uteroplacental insufficiency [31–33]. These pregnancies are at increased risk of umbilical cord compression from oligohydramnios, nonreassuring fetal antepartum or intrapartum assessment, intrauterine passage of meconium, and short-term neonatal complications (e.g., hypoglycemia, seizures, and respiratory insufficiency). Meconium aspiration syndrome refers to respiratory compromise with tachypnea, cyanosis, and reduced pulmonary compliance in newborn infants exposed to meconium *in utero* [34]. It is primarily a disease of post-term infants. Indeed, the fourfold decrease in the incidence of the meconium aspiration syndrome in the USA from 1990 to 1998 has been attributed primarily to a reduction in the post-term delivery rate [35], with very little contribution from conventional interventions designed to protect the lungs from the chemical pneumonitis caused by chronic meconium exposure, such as amnioinfusion [36,37] and routine nasopharyngeal suctioning of meconium-stained neonates [38]. Post-term pregnancy is also an independent risk factor for neonatal encephalopathy [39] and for death in the first year of life [18–20].

Maternal risks

The maternal risks of prolonged pregnancy are often underappreciated. These include an increase in labor dystocia (9–12% vs. 2–7% at term), an increase in severe perineal injury (third and fourth degree perineal lacerations) related to macrosomia (3.3% vs. 2.6% at term), and a doubling in the rate of cesarean delivery (14% vs. 7% at term) [20,24–26]. The latter is associated with higher risks of complications such as endometritis, hemorrhage, and thromboembolic disease [40,41]. In addition to the medical risks, the emotional impact (anxiety and frustration) of carrying a pregnancy 2 weeks beyond the EDD should not be underestimated.

Prevention and management of post-term pregnancy

Appropriate management of post-term pregnancy includes accurate gestational age assessment in early pregnancy, antenatal fetal surveillance, and the timely initiation of delivery if spontaneous labor does not occur.

Accurate gestational age assessment

An accurate EDD should be calculated early in pregnancy. This may be based upon standard clinical criteria, including a known last menstrual period in women with regular, normal menstrual cycles, and confirmatory uterine sizing (Table 44.1). However, uncertainty in dating parameters should prompt ultrasound assessment of gestational age. Some studies suggest that *routine* early ultrasound examination may reduce the rate of false positive diagnoses and thereby the overall rate of post-term pregnancy from 10% to approximately 1–3%, and thereby minimize unnecessary intervention [5–8,42–45]. In one study, the rates of labor induction for post-term pregnancy in low-risk women randomly assigned to routine first or second trimester ultrasound screening were 5% and 13%, respectively [42]. A recent meta-analysis found a similar reduction in the overall rates of induction of labor for post-term pregnancy (OR 0.68; 95% CI, 0.57–0.82) among women who underwent sonographic gestational age assessment before 24 weeks [5]. However, the practice of ultrasound for pregnancy dating has not been recommended as a standard of prenatal care in the USA [46,47].

Antenatal fetal surveillance

Post-term pregnancy is a universally accepted indication for antenatal fetal monitoring [1,48,49]. However, the efficacy of this approach has not been validated by prospective randomized trials. Indeed, because of ethical and medicolegal concerns, there are no studies of post-term pregnancies that include a nonmonitored control group, and it is highly unlikely that such a trial will ever be performed. Options for evaluating fetal well-being include nonstress testing (NST) with or without amniotic fluid volume assessment, the biophysical profile (BPP), the oxytocin challenge test, or a combination of these modalities. There is no consensus in the literature as to which of these modalities is preferred, and no single method has been shown to be superior [1,48–50].

The American College of Obstetricians and Gynecologists (ACOG) has recommended that antepartum fetal surveillance be initiated by 42 weeks (EDD+14 days), without a specific

recommendation regarding type of test or frequency [1,48]. Many investigators would advise twice weekly testing with some evaluation of amniotic fluid volume [49]. Doppler ultrasonography has no benefit in monitoring the post-term fetus and is not recommended for this indication [49,51]. There is insufficient evidence to show that initiating antenatal surveillance at 40–42 weeks' gestation improves pregnancy outcome or confers any benefit to the fetus [1,48]. Therefore, testing should begin at 42 weeks' gestation. If testing cannot be scheduled for 42w 0d, it is preferable (medicolegally) to perform the first test a few days earlier rather than a few days later.

Timing of delivery

Delivery is typically recommended when the risks to the fetus by continuing the pregnancy are greater than those faced by the neonate after birth. High-risk patients (Table 44.2) should not be allowed to progress into the post-term period because in these pregnancies the balance appears to shift in favor of delivery at around 38–39 weeks' gestation. Management of low-risk pregnancies is more controversial. Because delivery cannot always be brought about readily, maternal risks and considerations are more apt to confound this decision. Factors that need to be considered include results of antepartum fetal assessment, favorability of the cervix, gestational age, and maternal preference, after discussion of the risks, benefits, and alternatives to expectant management with antepartum monitoring versus labor induction.

Table 44.2 High-risk pregnancies.

Maternal factors
Preeclampsia (gestational proteinuric hypertension)
Chronic hypertension
Diabetes mellitus (including gestational diabetes)
Maternal cardiac disease
Chronic renal disease
Chronic pulmonary disease
Active thromboembolic disease

Fetal factors
Nonreassuring fetal testing ("fetal distress")
Intrauterine growth restriction
Isoimmunization
Intra-amniotic infection
Known fetal structural anomaly
Prior unexplained stillbirth
Multiple pregnancy

Uteroplacental factors
Premature rupture of fetal membranes
Unexplained oligohydramnios
Prior classic (high vertical) hysterotomy
Placenta previa
Abruptio placenta
Vasa previa

Antepartum fetal assessment

Delivery should be effected immediately if there is evidence of fetal compromise (nonreassuring fetal testing) or oligohydramnios [1,52,53]. Oligohydramnios may result from fetoplacental insufficiency or increased renal artery resistance [54] and may predispose to umbilical cord compression, thus leading to intermittent fetal hypoxemia, meconium passage, or meconium aspiration. Adverse pregnancy outcome (nonreassuring fetal heart rate tracing, neonatal intensive care unit (ICU) admission, low Apgar) is more common when oligohydramnios is present [54–57]. Frequent (twice weekly) screening of post-term patients for oligohydramnios is important because amniotic fluid can become drastically reduced within 24–48 hours [58]. However, a consistent definition of low amniotic fluid volume in the post-term pregnancy has not been established. Options include largest vertical fluid pocket <2 cm, amniotic fluid index (AFI) <5, and a product of length × width × depth of the largest pocket <60 [53,59,60]. A prospective, double blind, cohort study of 1584 women after 40 weeks' gestation found that an AFI <5, but not a largest vertical fluid pocket <2 cm, was associated with birth asphyxia and meconium aspiration, although the sensitivity for adverse outcomes was low [57]. The ability to extrapolate this finding is limited by the relatively early gestational age at testing (almost 60% of tests were performed at 40–41 weeks) and by the absence of repeat testing in patients who did not deliver for 7 or more days after the ultrasound examination (23% of subjects) [57].

Favorability of the cervix

There is insufficient evidence to determine whether expectant management or labor induction in post-term pregnancies with a *favorable* cervical examination yields a better outcome. A favorable cervical examination is defined as a Bishop score ≥6, which has been shown to be superior to transvaginal ultrasound assessment of cervical length at term to predict the time interval from induction to delivery [61,62]. One of the reasons for the lack of data is that the majority of publications comparing induction to expectant management excluded this group of patients or initiated induction at the time the cervix became favorable. In studies that did examine this subgroup, there was no apparent increased risk associated with expectant management [1]. When the ongoing risk of stillbirth (albeit small) is weighed against the very low risk (both in absolute and relative terms) of failed induction leading to cesarean delivery with a favorable cervical examination, common sense suggests that routine induction of labor is a reasonable option for such women at or after 41 weeks' gestation.

In the setting of an *unfavorable* cervical examination, both expectant management and labor induction are associated with low complication rates in low-risk post-term gravida. However, there appears to be a small advantage to labor induction at 41 weeks' gestation using cervical ripening agents, when indicated, regardless of parity or method of induction. The introduction of preinduction cervical maturation has resulted in fewer failed and serial inductions, lower fetal and maternal morbidity, a shorter hospital stay, lower medical cost, and possibly a lower rate of cesarean delivery in the general obstetric population [1,48,63–65].

The largest trial of routine post-term induction compared with expectant management randomly assigned 3407 low-risk women with uncomplicated singleton pregnancies at 41 weeks' gestation to induction of labor (with or without cervical ripening agents) within 4 days of randomization or expectant management until 44 weeks [66]. Elective induction resulted in a lower cesarean delivery rate (21.2% vs. 24.5%), primarily because of fewer surgeries for nonreassuring fetal tracings. A subsequent cost analysis of these data reported a policy of routine labor induction resulted in lower costs compared with expectant management (Canadian $2939 and $3132, respectively) [67]. In addition, a meta-analysis of 19 trials of routine versus selective induction of labor in post-term patients found that routine induction after 41 weeks was associated with a lower rate of perinatal mortality (OR 0.2; 95% CI, 0.06–0.70) and no increase in the cesarean delivery rate (OR 1.02; 95% CI, 0.75–1.38) [50]. The actual risk of stillbirth during the 41st week (41w 0d to 41w 6d) was 1.04–1.27 per 1000 undelivered women compared with 1.55–3.10 at or beyond 42 weeks [68]. These findings, similar to those of other meta-analyses [69], suggest that routine induction at 41 weeks' gestation has fetal benefit without incurring additional maternal risks because of a higher rate of cesarean delivery [20]. However, this conclusion has not been universally accepted [25,68]. An improved ability to identify women who will have a successful induction of labor would allow obstetric care providers to better individualize their recommendations. For example, some [70–74] but not all studies [75,76] have shown that elevated levels of fetal fibronectin (fFN) in cervicovaginal secretions at term are predictive of a shorter interval until delivery and a successful induction of labor, even in nulliparas with an unfavorable cervical examination [71]. More data, including a cost–benefit analysis, are needed before this test can be routinely recommended.

In patients with a prior cesarean delivery who decline elective repeat cesarean at 39 weeks' gestation, failure to go into labor spontaneously by 41 weeks should prompt further discussion about elective repeat cesarean. Every effort should be made to avoid induction of labor in such patients, because of the increased risk of uterine rupture [77].

Gestational age

ACOG no longer describes any specific upper limit of gestational age for expectantly managed pregnancies [1]. Although post-term pregnancy is defined as a pregnancy ≥42 weeks' gestation, the two large multicenter randomized studies of management of prolonged pregnancy reported favorable outcomes with routine induction as early as 41 weeks' gestation [66,78]. Many physicians now induce labor between weeks 41 and 42, and virtually all do not allow pregnancy to extend beyond 43 weeks' gestation (EDD+3 weeks). These practices are supported by recent studies suggesting that the rate of fetal demise is significantly higher than the rate of neonatal death at any time after 283 days' gestation (40 weeks+3 days) [21,79,80].

What is post-term for multiples?

The definition of term (and hence post-term) should incorporate not only the natural history of such pregnancies, but also the effect of gestational age on perinatal mortality. The average length of gestation is 40 weeks in singletons, 36 weeks in twins, 33 weeks in triplets, and 29 weeks in quadruplets [81–84]. To investigate the effect of gestational age on perinatal mortality, Minakami and Sato [85] compared the outcome of 88,936 infants born of multiple pregnancies (96% of which were twins) with that of 6,020,542 infants born of singleton pregnancies after 26 weeks' gestation between 1989 and 1993. In this cohort, the lowest perinatal mortality rate was seen at 38 weeks in multiple pregnancies compared with 40 weeks in singleton pregnancies (10.5 vs. 9.7 deaths per 1000 deliveries, respectively). Thereafter, the perinatal mortality rate increased for both groups, but was more exaggerated in multiple pregnancies. Indeed, the risk of perinatal death was sixfold higher for fetuses of multiple pregnancies born after 37 weeks compared with singleton fetuses born at or after 40 weeks (RR 6.6; 95% CI, 6.1–7.1) [85]. Although no consensus has been reached, these data suggest that that the normal length of gestation for twins should be regarded as 38 rather than 40 weeks. As such, every effort should be made to deliver uncomplicated twins by 40 weeks' gestation (post-term for twins).

Intrapartum management

The post-term fetus is at higher risk of intrapartum fetal heart rate abnormalities and passage of meconium [86]. For this reason, most authors recommend continuous electronic fetal monitoring in labor for these pregnancies. Intrapartum spontaneous or induced fetal heart rate accelerations coupled with adequate fetal heart rate variability are reliable signs of a non-acidotic fetus [87].

Prognosis

At 1 and 2 years of age, the general intelligence quotient, physical milestones, and frequency of intercurrent illnesses is the same for normal term infants and those from prolonged pregnancies [33].

Conclusions

The risks of routine induction of labor (specifically failed induction leading to cesarean delivery) in the era of cervical ripening agents is lower than previously reported. The risk of fetal death is also low, but not zero, with expectantly managed, carefully monitored post-term pregnancies. For these reasons, the authors favor a policy of routine induction of labor for low-risk pregnancies at 41 weeks' gestation.

Case presentation

A 33-year-old Asian woman, gravida 3, para 0, presents for routine prenatal care at 41w 0d gestation. Her prior pregnancies included a first trimester spontaneous abortion and a 20-week preterm and previable delivery as a result of cervical insufficiency. Review of her past medical and surgical histories are otherwise unremarkable. This pregnancy has been uncomplicated to date. Dating criteria include a firm last menstrual period, confirmed by a 6-week ultrasound. An elective Shirodkar cervical cerclage was placed at 14 weeks and removed electively without incident at 37 weeks. Level II ultrasound at 18 weeks' gestation confirmed a structurally normal male fetus and a fundal placenta.

The woman perceives good fetal movements, but reports only irregular uterine contractions and denies symptoms suggestive of rupture of membranes. A perineal culture taken at 36 weeks confirms that she is not a group B streptococcus carrier. Abdominal examination using Leopold maneuver confirms a singleton fetus with an estimated fetal weight of 3500 g. The presentation is cephalic and the vertex is engaged in the maternal pelvis. Pelvic examination confirms a gynecoid pelvis with adequate clinical pelvimetry. The cervix is posterior, firm, and closed. Fetal well-being is confirmed with a baseline fetal heart rate of 140 beats/min and a reactive NST. You explain that up to 30% of all low-risk pregnancies continue beyond 41 weeks' gestation and that there is no proven benefit to routine fetal testing at this gestational age. The patient strongly desires a vaginal delivery, and understands that obstetric intervention in the setting of an unfavorable cervical examination likely increases the risk of cesarean delivery. You review symptoms and signs of labor, and discharge the woman home to follow-up in 1 week.

The patient returns at 42w 0d gestation. She again reports good fetal movements and rare contractions. Estimated fetal weight is 4000 g. Pelvic examination shows the cervix to be 1 cm dilatated, 50% effaced, and posterior. Station is high. You offer the patient cervical ripening and induction for post-term pregnancy, but she declines. Fetal NST is reactive and amniotic fluid index is 12.2 cm. You again discharge the woman home after reviewing symptoms and signs of labor. A follow-up visit is planned in 2 days.

The woman presents the next day to labor and delivery with regular contractions every 3–4 minutes. Initial cervical examination is 4 cm dilatated, 90% effaced, with the vertex at 0 station and membranes bulging. Position is noted to be occiput posterior. Estimated fetal weight is 4200 g. Fetal heart rate tracing is reactive with a baseline of 140–145 beats/min. Intermittent variable decelerations are noted. You again review the options for pain management in labor, and the patient declines analgesia at this time. Over the next 2 hours, the patient's contractions become milder and less frequent and there is no further cervical change or descent of the presenting part. Fetal well-being remains reassuring. After counseling, you rupture the fetal membranes and note moderate meconium staining of the amniotic fluid. You start oxytocin augmentation. Because of a difficulty in tracing the fetal heart rate, you place a fetal scalp electrode. Over the next 4 hours, the contractions are noted to be adequate (>200 Montevideo units), but there is no further cervical dilatation or descent of the presenting part. Moreover, you note increasing caput succedaneum, more exaggerated moulding of the fetal skull bones, and repetitive severe variable decelerations on cardiotocography. You make a diagnosis of cephalopelvic disproportion and recommend cesarean delivery.

An uncomplicated primary cesarean delivery is performed under spinal anesthesia. A viable male infant is delivered in the occiput posterior position without difficulty. Moderate meconium staining of the amniotic fluid is confirmed, and mouth and nose are suctioned on the abdomen. The baby is vigorous at birth. Apgar scores are assigned as 8 at 1 minute and 9 at 5 minutes. Although a segment of umbilical cord was collected at delivery, no cord gases were sent. The birthweight was 4890 g. The baby was discharged home on day 4 of life along with the mother.

References

1 ACOG Committee on Practice Bulletins-Obstetrics. Management of postterm pregnancy. ACOG Practice Bulletin 55. *Obstet Gynecol* 2004;**104**:639–46.

2 WHO. Recommended definitions, terminology and format for statistical tables related to the perinatal period and use of a new certificate for cause of perinatal deaths. *Acta Obstet Gynecol Scand* 1977;**56**:247–53.

3 Ventura SJ, Martin JA, Curtin SC, Mathews TJ, Park MM. Births: final data for 1998. *Natl Vital Stat Rep* 2000;**48**:1–100.

4 Bakketeig LS, Bergsjo P. Post-term pregnancy: magnitude of the problem. In: Chalmers I, Enkin M, Keirse M, (eds). *Effective Care in Pregnancy and Childbirth*. Oxford, Oxford University Press, 1991: 765–86.

5 Neilson JP. Ultrasound for fetal assessment in early pregnancy. *Cochrane Database Syst Rev* 2000;**2**:CD000182.

6 Boyd ME, Usher RH, McLean FH, *et al*. Obstetric consequences of postmaturity. *Am J Obstet Gynecol* 1988;**158**:334–8.

7 Gardosi J, Vanner T, Francis A. Gestational age and induction of labor for prolonged pregnancy. *Br J Obstet Gynaecol* 1997;**104**:792–7.

8 Taipale P, Hiilermaa V. Predicting delivery date by ultrasound and last menstrual period on early gestation. *Obstet Gynecol* 2001;**97**:189–94.

9 Alfirevic Z, Walkinshaw SA. Management of post-term pregnancy: to induce or not? *Br J Hosp Med* 1994;**52**:218–21.

10 Mogren I, Stenlund H, Hogberg U. Recurrence of prolonged pregnancy. *Int J Epidemiol* 1999;**28**:253–7.

11 Naeye RL. Causes of perinatal mortality excess in prolonged gestations. *Am J Epidemiol* 1978;**108**:429–33.

12 Divon MY, Ferber A, Nisell H, Westgren M. Male gender predisposes to prolongation of pregnancy. *Am J Obstet Gynecol* 2002;**187**:1081–3.

13 Laursen M, Bille C, Olesen AW, Hjelmborg J, Skytthe A, Christensen K. Genetic influence on prolonged gestation: a population-based Danish twin study. *Am J Obstet Gynecol* 2004;**190**:489–94.

14 Olesen AW, Basso O, Olsen J. Risk of recurrence of prolonged pregnancy. *Br Med J* 2003;**326**:476.

15 Yudkin PL, Wood L, Redman CW. Risk of unexplained stillbirth at different gestational ages. *Lancet* 1987;**1**:1192–4.

16 Herabutya Y, Prasertsawat PO, Tongyai T, Isarangura NA, Ayudthya N. Prolonged pregnancy: the management dilemma. *Int J Gynecol Obstet* 1992;**37**:253–8.

17 Feldman GB. Prospective risk of stillbirth. *Obstet Gynecol* 1992;**79**:547–53.

18 Hilder L, Costeloe K, Thilaganathan B. Prolonged pregnancy: evaluating gestation-specific risks of fetal and infant mortality. *Br J Obstet Gynaecol* 1998;**105**:169–73.

19 Cotzias CS, Paterson-Brown S, Fisk NM. Prospective risk of unexplained stillbirth in singleton pregnancies at term: population based analysis. *Br Med J* 1999;**319**:287–8.

20 Rand L, Robinson JN, Economy KE, Norwitz ER. Post-term induction of labor revisited. *Obstet Gynecol* 2000;**96**:779–83.

21 Smith GC. Life-table analysis of the risk of perinatal death at term and post term in singleton pregnancies. *Am J Obstet Gynecol* 2001;**184**:489–96.

22 Froen JF, Arnestad M, Frey K, Vege A, Saugstad OD, Stray-Pedersen B. Risk factors for sudden intrauterine unexplained death: epidemiologic characteristics of singleton cases in Oslo, Norway, 1986–1995. *Am J Obstet Gynecol* 2001;**184**:694–702.

23 Kahn B, Lumey LH, Zybert PA, *et al*. Prospective risk of fetal death in singleton, twin, and triplet gestations: implications for practice. *Obstet Gynecol* 2003;**102**:685–92.

24 Campbell MK, Ostbye T, Irgens LM. Post-term birth: risk factors and outcomes in a 10-year cohort of Norwegian births. *Obstet Gynecol* 1997;**89**:543–8.

25 Alexander JM, McIntire DD, Leveno KJ. Forty weeks and beyond: pregnancy outcomes by week of gestation. *Obstet Gynecol* 2000;**96**:291–4.

26 Treger M, Hallak M, Silberstein T, Friger M, Katz M, Mazor M. Post-term pregnancy: should induction of labor be considered before 42 weeks? *J Matern Fetal Neonatal Med* 2002;**11**:50–3.

27 Bakketeig LS, Bergsjo P. Post-term pregnancy: magnitude of the problem. In: Enkin M, Keirse MJ, Chalmers I, (eds). *Effective Care in Pregnancy and Childbirth*. Oxford: Oxford University Press, 1989: 765–75.

28 Hannah ME. Postterm pregnancy: should all women have labour induced? A review of the literature. *Fetal Matern Med Rev* 1993;**5**:3.

29 Spellacy WN, Miller S, Winegar A, Peterson PQ. Macrosomia: maternal characteristics and infant complications. *Obstet Gynecol* 1985;**66**:158 61.

30 Rosen MG, Dickinson JC. Management of post-term pregnancy. *N Engl J Med* 1992;**326**:1628–9.

31 Vorherr H. Placental insufficiency in relation to postterm pregnancy and fetal postmaturity. Evaluation of fetoplacental function: management of the postterm gravida. *Am J Obstet Gynecol* 1975;**123**:67–103.

32 Mannino F. Neonatal complications of postterm gestation. *J Reprod Med* 1988;**33**:271–6.

33 Shime J, Librach CL, Gare DJ, Cook CJ. The influence of prolonged pregnancy on infant development at one and two years of age: a prospective controlled study. *Am J Obstet Gynecol* 1986;**154**:341–5.

34 Kabbur PM, Herson VC, Zaremba S, Lerer T. Have the year 2000 neonatal resuscitation program guidelines changed the delivery room management or outcome of meconium-stained infants? *J Perinatol* 2005;**25**:694.

35 Yoder BA, Kirsch EA, Barth WH, Gordon MC. Changing obstetric practices associated with decreasing incidence of meconium aspiration syndrome. *Obstet Gynecol* 2002;**99**:731.

36 Hofmeyr GJ. Amnioinfusion for meconium-stained liquor in labour. *Cochrane Database Syst Rev* 2002;**1**:CD000014.

37 Fraser WD, Hofmeyr J, Lede R, *et al*. Amnioinfusion for the prevention of the meconium aspiration syndrome. *N Engl J Med* 2005;**353**:909.

38 Vain NE, Szyld EG, Prudent LM, Wiswell TE, Aguilar AM, Vivas NI. Oropharyngeal and nasopharyngeal suctioning of meconium-stained neonates before delivery of their shoulders: multicentre, randomised controlled trial. *Lancet* 2004;**364**:597.

39 Badawi N, Kurinczuk JJ, Keogh JM, *et al*. Antepartum risk factors for newborn encephalopathy: the Western Australian case–control study. *Br Med J* 1998;**317**:1549–53.

40 Alexander JM, McIntire DD, Leveno KJ. Prolonged pregnancy: Induction of labor and cesarean births. *Obstet Gynecol* 2001;**97**:911.

41 Eden RD, Seifert LS, Winegar A, Spellacy WM. Perinatal characteristics of uncomplicated postdate pregnancies. *Obstet Gynecol* 1987;**69**:296–9.

42 Bennett KA, Crane JM, O'Shea P, Lacelle J, Hutchens D, Copel JA. First trimester ultrasound screening is effective in reducing postterm labor induction rates: a randomized controlled trial. *Am J Obstet Gynecol* 2004;**190**:1077–81.

43 Waldenstrom U, Axelsson O, Nilsson S, *et al*. Effects of routine one-stage ultrasound screening in pregnancy: a randomised controlled trial. *Lancet* 1988;**2**:585–8.

44 Saari-Kemppainen A, Karjalainen O, Ylostalo P, Heinonen OP. Ultrasound screening and perinatal mortality: controlled trial of systematic one-stage screening in pregnancy. The Helsinki Ultrasound Trial. *Lancet* 1990;**336**:387–91.

45 Ewigman BG, Crane JP, Frigoletto FD, LeFevre ML, Bain RP, McNellis D. Effect of prenatal ultrasound screening on perinatal outcome. RADIUS Study Group. *N Engl J Med* 1993;**329**:821–7.

46 American College of Obstetricians and Gynecologists. Ultrasonography in pregnancy. ACOG Technical Bulletin 187. Washington, DC: ACOG, 1993.

47 American Academy of Pediatrics and American College of Obstetricians and Gynecologists. Guidelines for perinatal care. Washington, DC: AAP and ACOG, 1997.

48 American College of Obstetricians and Gynecologists. Management of postterm pregnancy. ACOG Practice Pattern 6. Washington, DC: ACOG, 1997.

49 American College of Obstetricians and Gynecologists. Antepartum fetal surveillance. ACOG Practice Bulletin 9. ACOG, Washington, DC. 1999.

50 Crowley P. Interventions for preventing or improving the outcome of delivery at or beyond term. *Cochrane Database Syst Rev* 2000;**2**:CD000170.

51 Stokes HJ, Roberts RV, Newnham JP. Doppler flow velocity waveform analysis in postdate pregnancies. *Aust N Z J Obstet Gynaecol* 1991;**31**:27–30.

52 Phelan JP, Platt LD, Yeh SY, Broussard P, Paul RH. The role of ultrasound assessment of amniotic fluid volume in the management of the postdate pregnancy. *Am J Obstet Gynecol* 1985;**151**:304–8.

53 Crowley P, O'Herlihy C, Boylan P. The value of ultrasound measurement of amniotic fluid volume in the management of prolonged pregnancies. *Br J Obstet Gynaecol* 1984;**91**:444–8.

54 Oz AU, Holub B, Mendilcioglu I, Mari G, Bahado-Singh RO. Renal artery Doppler investigation of the etiology of oligohydramnios in postterm pregnancy. *Obstet Gynecol* 2002;**100**:715–8.

55 Tongsong T, Srisomboon J. Amniotic fluid volume as a predictor of fetal distress in postterm pregnancy. *Int J Gynaecol Obstet* 1993;**40**:213–7.

56 Bochner CJ, Medearis AL, Davis J, Oakes GK, Hobel CJ, Wade ME. Antepartum predictors of fetal distress in postterm pregnancy. *Am J Obstet Gynecol* 1987;**157**:353–8.

57 Morris JM, Thompson K, Smithey J, *et al*. The usefulness of ultrasound assessment of amniotic fluid in predicting adverse outcome in prolonged pregnancy: a prospective blinded observational study. *Br J Obstet Gynaecol* 2003;**110**:989–94.

58 Clement D, Schifrin BS, Kates RB. Acute oligohydramnios in postdate pregnancy. *Am J Obstet Gynecol* 1987;**157**:884–6.

59 Hashimoto B, Filly RA, Belden C, Callen PW, Laros RK. Objective method of diagnosing oligohydramnios in postterm pregnancies. *J Ultrasound Med* 1987;**6**:81–4.

60 Chamberlain PF, Manning FA, Morrison I, Harman CR, Lange IR. Ultrasound evaluation of amniotic fluid volume. I. The relationship of marginal and decreased amniotic fluid volumes to perinatal outcome. *Am J Obstet Gynecol* 1984;**150**:245–9.

61 Rozenberg P, Chevret S, Ville Y. Comparison of pre-induction ultrasonographic cervical length and Bishop score in predicting risk of cesarean section after labor induction with prostaglandins. *Gynecol Obstet Fertil* 2005;**33**:17–22.

62 Roman H, Verspyck E, Vercoustre L, *et al*. The role of ultrasound and fetal fibronectin in predicting the length of induced labor when the cervix is unfavorable. *Ultrasound Obstet Gynecol* 2004;**23**:567–73.

63 Keirse MJNC, Chalmers I. Methods for inducing labour. In: Chalmers I, Enkin M, Keirse MJNC, (eds). *Effective Care in Pregnancy and Childbirth*. Oxford: Oxford University Press, 1989.

64 Poma PA. Cervical ripening: a review and recommendations for clinical practice. *J Reprod Med* 1999;**44**:657–68.

65 Xenakis EM, Piper JM, Conway DL, Langer O. Induction of labor in the nineties: conquering the unfavorable cervix. *Obstet Gynecol* 1997;**90**:235–9.

66 Hannah ME, Hannah WJ, Hellmann J, Hewson S, Milner R, Willan A. Induction of labor as compared with serial antenatal monitoring in post-term pregnancy: a randomized controlled trial. The Canadian Multicenter Post-Term Pregnancy Trial Group. *N Engl J Med* 1992;**326**:1587–92.

67 Goeree R, Hannah M, Hewson S. Cost-effectiveness of induction of labour versus serial antenatal monitoring in the Canadian Multicentre Postterm Pregnancy Trial. *CMAJ* 1995;**152**:1445–50.

68 Menticoglou SM, Hall PF. Routine induction of labour at 41 weeks gestation: nonsensus consensus. *Br J Obstet Gynaecol* 2002;**109**:485–91.

69 Sanchez-Ramos L, Olivier F, Delke I, Kaunitz AM. Labor induction versus expectant management for postterm pregnancies: a systematic review with meta-analysis. *Obstet Gynecol* 2003;**101**:1312–8.

70 Kiss H, Ahner R, Hohlagschwandtner M, *et al.* Fetal fibronectin as a predictor of term labor: a literature review. *Acta Obstet Gynecol Scand* 2000;**79**:3–7.

71 Garite TJ, Casal D, Garcia-Alonso A, *et al.* Fetal fibronectin: a new tool for the prediction of successful induction of labor. *Am J Obstet Gynecol* 1996;**175**:1516.

72 Tam WH, Tai SM, Rogers MS. Prediction of cervical response to prostaglandin E$_2$ using fetal fibronectin. *Acta Obstet Gynecol Scand* 1999; **78**:861.

73 Blanch G, Olah KS, Walkinshaw S. The presence of fetal fibronectin in the cervicovaginal secretions of women at term: its role in the assessment of women before labor induction and in the investigation of the physiologic mechanisms of labor. *Am J Obstet Gynecol* 1996;**174**:262.

74 Ahner R, Egarter C, Kiss H, *et al.* Fetal fibronectin as a selection criterion for induction of term labor. *Am J Obstet Gynecol* 1995;**173**:1513.

75 Ojutiku D, Jones G, Bewley S. Quantitative foetal fibronectin as a predictor of successful induction of labour in post-date pregnancies. *Eur J Obstet Gynecol Reprod Biol* 2002;**101**:143.

76 Reis FM, Gervasi MT, Florio P, *et al.* Prediction of successful induction of labor at term: role of clinical history, digital examination, ultrasound assessment of the cervix, and fetal fibronectin assay. *Am J Obstet Gynecol* 2003;**189**:1361.

77 Lydon-Rochelle M, Holt VL, Easterling TR, Martin DP. Risk of uterine rupture during labor among women with a prior cesarean delivery. *N Engl J Med* 2001;**345**:3–35.

78 National Institute of Child Health and Human Development Network of Maternal-Fetal Medicine Units. A clinical trial of induction of labor versus expectant management in postterm pregnancy. *Am J Obstet Gynecol* 1994;**170**:716–23.

79 Caughey AB, Stotland NE, Escobar GJ. What is the best measure of maternal complications of term pregnancy: ongoing pregnancies or pregnancies delivered? *Am J Obstet Gynecol* 2003;**189**:1047–52.

80 Divon MY, Ferber A, Sanderson M, Nisell H, Westgren M. A functional definition of prolonged pregnancy based on daily fetal and neonatal mortality rates. *Ultrasound Obstet Gynecol* 2004;**23**:423–6.

81 Haning RV, Seifer DB, Wheeler CA, *et al.* Effects of fetal number and multifetal reduction on length of *in vitro* fertilization pregnancy. *Obstet Gynecol* 1996;**87**:964.

82 Melgar CA, Rosenfeld DL, Rawlinson K, *et al.* Perinatal outcome after multifetal reduction to twins compared with nonreduced multiple gestations. *Obstet Gynecol* 1991;**78**:763.

83 Newman RB, Ellings JM. Antenatal management of the multiple gestation: the case for specialized care. *Semin Perinatol* 1995;**19**:387.

84 Kahn B, Lumey LH, Zybert PA, *et al.* Prospective risk of fetal death in singleton, twin, and triplet gestations: implications for practice. *Obstet Gynecol* 2003;**102**:685–92.

85 Minakami H, Sato I. Reestimating date of delivery in multifetal pregnancies. *JAMA* 1996;**275**:1432–4.

86 Knox GE, Huddleston JF, Flowers CE Jr. Management of prolonged pregnancy: results of a prospective randomized trial. *Am J Obstet Gynecol* 1979;**134**:376–84.

87 Shaw K, Clark SL. Reliability of intrapartum fetal heart rate monitoring in the postterm fetus with meconium passage. *Obstet Gynecol* 1988;**72**:886–9.

45 Cesarean delivery

Michael W. Varner

By the mid-20th century, cesarean delivery (CD) was firmly established in Western obstetric practice, primarily as a procedure to improve maternal outcomes in labor. With the evolution of neonatal medicine through the latter half of the century, CD has been increasingly performed for fetal indications.

The 15-year interval from 1970 through 1985 saw an unparalleled increase in the CD rate, both in the USA [1] and elsewhere [2], with the cesarean rate in the USA temporarily peaking at 24.4% in 1987. The ensuing 15-year interval saw a stabilization of this rate (down to 20.6% in 1996), in large part as a result of efforts to encourage vaginal birth following previous CD [3,4], widely abbreviated as VBAC (vaginal birth after cesarean).

The first years of the 21st century have seen a further increase in the CD rate, primarily as a result of evolving pressures against VBAC in community hospitals and an increasing frequency of CD for failure to make adequate progress in labor [5]. An additional factor, the performance of CD on demand, has become more widespread since its endorsement by the American College of Obstetricians and Gynecology (ACOG) [6]. The most recent US CD rate available at the time of this writing is 27.6% (Fig. 45.1).

Maternal and perinatal morbidity and mortality

For the past several decades the maternal mortality ratios in the USA have remained essentially unchanged [7]. However, within that relatively constant prevalence, there has been a gradual shift in etiologies. The historic HIT (hemorrhage, infection, toxemia) maternal mortality triad is being replaced by the TEC triad (trauma, embolism, cardiac). While one might argue that increasing CD rates are decreasing maternal deaths from some of the HIT triad (particularly hemorrhage), one might equally argue that the increasing CD rate is associated with an increased risk of maternal death from some of the TEC triad, particularly thromboembolic disease. What does seem clear, however, is that the dramatic increase in CD rates seen over the past two decades has not been associated with a corresponding decrease in maternal mortality.

Fortunately, maternal mortality is a relatively rare event in the USA. "Near-miss" maternal morbidity, on the other hand, is a more common entity, occurring in 0.4–1.0% of pregnancies in developed countries [8]. Geller et al. [9] have described a useful set of clinical criteria for this definition: organ failure (≥1 organ system), extended intubation (>12 hours), intensive care unit (ICU) admission, surgical intervention, and transfusion (>3 units). While several of these conditions are more likely associated with CD, it is not yet clear that CD per se increases the risk to a previously healthy woman for "near-miss" morbidity.

However, neonatal mortality rates continue to decrease, primarily as a result of continuing advancements in neonatal medicine. Peripartum deaths resulting from birth asphyxia are very uncommon in contemporary US obstetric practice. However, the contribution to these ongoing perinatal improvements has as yet not been proven to be a result of the increasing CD rates. In fact, there is evidence that babies delivered by scheduled elective repeat CD at term are at increased risk of developing respiratory problems (adjusted odds ratio [OR] 2.3; 95% confidence interval [CI], 1.4–3.8) [10].

Evidence-based operative considerations

While debate about indications for CD are ongoing, there has been a substantial body of evidence-based recommendations that address various aspects of the surgical technique.

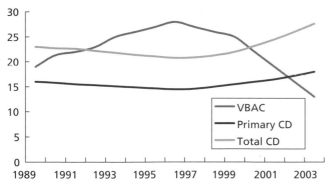

Fig. 45.1 Change in vaginal birth after cesarean (VBAC), total cesarean, and primary cesarean delivery rates, USA, 1989–2003.

Antibiotic prophylaxis

It is clear that women who are delivered abdominally are at increased risk of endometritis and/or wound infection. The Cochrane review of 81 clinical trials confirms that it is beneficial for these women to receive antibiotics either immediately before, during, or immediately after their CD, whether or not they have clinical evidence of infection. Women who receive antibiotic prophylaxis at the time of CD have lower rates of endometritis, whether the CD was performed during labor (relative risk [RR] 0.39; 95% CI, 0.34–0.46) or electively (RR 0.38; 95% CI, 0.22–0.64) [11]. The risk of wound infection was also reduced in women receiving antibiotic prophylaxis at the time of CD, being somewhat greater in those women being delivered nonelectively (RR 0.36; 95% CI, 0.26–0.51) than for women being delivered electively (RR 0.73; 95% CI, 0.53–0.99) [11].

Manual removal of the placenta

Manual removal of the placenta is associated with a clinically important and statistically significant increase in maternal blood loss (weighted mean difference 436 mL; 95% CI, 348–525 mL) [12]. Manual removal was also associated with increased postpartum endometritis (OR 5.44; 95% CI, 1.25–23.75) and trend toward an increase in fetomaternal hemorrhage (OR 2.19; 95% CI, 0.69–6.93).

Extra-abdominal versus intra-abdominal repair of the uterine incision

Six randomized clinical trials, consisting of 1221 participating women, compared uterine exteriorization with intra-abdominal repair. There were no significant differences between the groups in most of the outcomes examined, with the exceptions of febrile morbidity and length of hospital stay. Febrile morbidity was lower (RR 0.41; 95% CI, 0.17–0.97) and length of hospital stay was longer (weighted mean difference 0.24 days; 95% CI 0.08–0.39) with extra-abdominal closure of the hysterotomy [13].

Single versus two-layer hysterotomy closure

There appear to be no perioperative advantages or disadvantages for routine use of single layer closure compared with two-layer closure, expect that of a shorter operation time [14]. However, there are insufficient long-term follow-up data to make any conclusions regarding risks for subsequent pregnancies.

Abdominal wall closure techniques

In a meta-analysis of seven studies involving over 2000 women, Anderson and Gates [15] concluded that the risk of hematoma or seroma was reduced with closure of the subcutaneous tissue compared with nonclosure (RR 0.52; 95% CI, 0.33–0.82). The risk of wound complications (defined as hematoma, seroma, wound infection, or wound separation) was also reduced with subcutaneous tissue closure (RR 0.68; 95% CI, 0.52–0.88). There are no data to address questions of either suture techniques or materials for closure of the rectus sheath.

Thromboprophylaxis

In the developed world, thromboembolic disease is now the most common cause of direct obstetric death, and is more common following CD. ACOG do not have a specific policy statement regarding thromboprophylaxis following CD and there are inadequate randomized controlled trial data on which to make firm recommendations. The National Collaborating Center for Women's and Children's Health does have a policy statement on this issue: 'Women having a CD should be offered thromboprophylaxis, as they are at increased risk of venous thromboembolism. The choice of method of prophylaxis (e.g., graduated stockings, hydration, early mobilization, low molecular weight heparin) should take into account risk of thromboembolic disease and following existing guidelines [16].' Thus, while the optimum regimen(s) have yet to be clearly delineated, it is clear that consideration should be given to the possibility of thromboembolic complications after any CD.

Treatment of postoperative endometritis

In a review of 15 clinical trials, the Cochrane review also confirmed that the combination of gentamycin and clindamycin has fewer treatment failures than other regimens (treatment failure with other regimens RR 1.44; 95% CI, 1.15–1.80) [17]. Drug regimens with poor activity against penicillin-resistant anaerobes were particularly likely to be unsuccessful (RR 1.94; 95% CI, 1.38–2.72) [17]. Three studies that compared continued oral antibiotic therapy after intravenous therapy but with no oral therapy found no differences in recurrent infection or any other adverse outcomes [17].

Potential risks of repeat cesarean delivery

One major contributor to the current increase in the overall CD rate is the dramatic decline in VBAC (Fig. 45.1). A modest decline in VBAC rates had started in 1998 but this was accelerated by a 1999 Technical Bulletin from ACOG [18] that cautioned against VBAC unless the facilities and staff to perform emergency repeat CD were "immediately available."

The VBAC rate in 2003 was only 10.6%, a 16% decline from 12.6% in 2002. Overall, the VBAC rate has decreased 63% since 1996, while the primary cesarean section rate has climbed 31% during this same interval. At the time of this writing, the definitive statements on risks associated with VBAC are the papers produced by the National Institute of Child Health and Human Development (NICHD) funded Maternal-Fetal Medicine Units Network Cesarean Registry [19]. These results are outlined in more detail in Chapter 46. While the magnitude of these risks is small, physician practice patterns and medicolegal concerns will undoubtedly keep interest in VBAC low in the near future.

While substantial attention has been paid to the risks of VBAC, rather less attention has been directed to the risks of repeat CD. In the largest series to address this issue, Silver [20] reviewed the outcomes of 30,132 CDs performed without labor. He found that the risk of accreta, hysterectomy, blood transfusion, cystotomy, bowel injury, ureteric injury, previa, ileus, postoperative ventilation, ICU admission, operative time, and hospital days significantly increased with increasing numbers of CDs. Accreta was present in 15 (0.24%), 49 (0.31%), 36 (0.57%), 31 (2.13%), 6 (2.31%), and 6 (6,74%) women undergoing their first, second, third, fourth, fifth, and sixth or more cesareans. Hysterectomy was required in 40 (0.65%) first, 67 (0.42%) second, 57 (0.90%) third, 35 (2.40%) fourth, 9 (3.46%) fifth, and 8 (8.99%) sixth or more cesareans. In the 723 women with previa, the risk for accreta was 3%, 11%, 40%, 61%, and 67% for first, second, third, fourth, and fifth or more repeat cesareans, respectively. They confirmed that serious maternal morbidity increases with increasing numbers of CD and suggested that the number of intended pregnancies should be factored into consideration of elective repeat CD versus trial of labor in women with prior CD. They also note that over 80,000 women in the USA had their fourth or more cesarean last year, making their recommendations more widely applicable than might often be expected.

In another large series, Gesteland et al. [21] reviewed an electronic database in order to compare the rates of placenta previa, placenta accreta, and placental abruption between women delivered only vaginally and women delivered only by CD. Women delivered by one or more cesareans without any vaginal deliveries were compared with women who had one or more vaginal delivery only. They found that placenta previa and accreta increased with the number of previous CDs. The rate of placenta previa also increases with maternal age, independent of parity and mode of delivery. The rate of accreta increases even more dramatically in patients with prior CDs and placenta previa. Prior CD did not increase the rate of abruption in future pregnancies.

Influence of different patient populations on cesarean delivery rates

CD rates vary substantially between geographic areas in the USA [22] and often vary substantially between hospitals in the same community [23]. Numerous factors contribute to these differences, including the availability of ancillary staff (e.g., anesthesia, pediatrics), training and experience of the surgeon(s), and characteristics of particular patient populations. The latter observation has been frequently cited as an explanation for these observed differences. Although not widely utilized in the USA, the Robson CD classification system [24] allows comparison of cesarean rates within specific subsets of an obstetric population and thereby obviates many of the historic arguments that have arisen when comparing overall cesarean rates between different populations. In this system, any CD can be placed in one, but only one, of 10 mutually exclusive patient population categories (Table 45.1). This classification system could be of value for defining and comparing optimum CD rates for different patient populations. Fischer et al. [25] demonstrated significant practice pattern differences in Robson group 1 women (term primigravidas, vertex presentation, spontaneous labor; see Table 45.1) between hospitals in the same geographic area with high (16.3%) and low (7.8%) CD rates. Although women delivering in the low CD rate hospital were not more likely to receive oxytocin augmentation, their mean maximum oxytocin dosage was higher (14.5 vs. 11.5 units; $P < 0.001$) and they were more

Table 45.1 Robson cesarean classification [24].

Group	Description
1	Nullipara, >37 weeks, single, cephalic presentation, spontaneous labor
2	Nullipara, >37 weeks, single, cephalic presentation, induced labor or CD before labor
3	Multipara, no previous CD, >37 weeks, single, cephalic presentation, spontaneous labor
4	Multipara, no previous CD, >37 weeks, single, cephalic presentation, induced labor
5	Multipara, previous CD, >37 weeks, single, cephalic presentation
6	Nullipara, single breech presentation
7	Multipara, single breech presentation
8	Multiple gestation (with or without previous CD)
9	Singleton pregnancy, oblique or transverse lie (excluding breech, with or without previous CD)
10	Single, cephalic pregnancy, <37 weeks (including previous CD)

likely to receive both fetal scalp electrodes (60.9% vs. 37.3%; *P* <0.001) and intrauterine pressure catheters (63.8% vs. 26.0%; *P* <0.001) compared with an equivalent population in a high CD rate hospital with a similar patient population. They concluded that such benchmarking practices could be considered in obstetric practices interested in long-term reductions of their CD rates.

Current indications for cesarean delivery

Failure to progress in labor

The most common indication for primary CD is failure to progress in labor. The landmark papers of Friedman [26,27] have defined the expectations of normal labor progress for the past generation of obstetric practitioners in the USA.

In the 1980s, there was hope that the active management of labor, as initially championed by the National Maternity Hospital in Dublin [28], might reverse the increasing CD rates. Unfortunately, this management approach has ultimately failed to stop a rising CD rate in Ireland [29].

There has been no suggestion that maternal pelves or uterine activity has changed appreciably in the USA over the past several decades. Likewise, mean birthweight has not increased in recent years (1990, 3365 g; 2003, 3325 g) [22]. However, the frequency of CD for failure to progress in labor has continued to increase during the same interval.

Researchers at the University of Alabama at Birmingham have put forth convincing data that extending the minimum period of oxytocin augmentation for active-phase labor arrest from 2 to at least 4 hours is effective and safe [30]. Following the diagnosis of a 2-hour active-phase arrest, oxytocin was initiated with an intent to achieve a sustained uterine contraction pattern of greater than 200 Montevideo units. CD was not performed for labor arrest until at least 4 hours of a sustained uterine contraction pattern of greater than 200 Montevideo units, or a minimum of 6 hours of oxytocin augmentation if this contraction pattern could not be achieved. A total of 542 women were managed by this protocol and 92% delivered vaginally. They have subsequently demonstrated that oxytocin-augmented labor proceeds at a slower rate than spontaneous labor [31]. During oxytocin augmentation, nulliparas who were delivered vaginally dilated at a median rate of 1.4 cm/hour versus 1.8 cm/hour for parous women. In both groups, the 5th percentile of cervical dilatation rate was 0.5 cm/hour.

Another contributor to the increased rate of CD because of failure to progress in labor is the epidemic increase in obesity seen in the USA over the past two decades. LaCoursiere *et al.* [32] have shown that a 40% increase in prepregnancy overweight (body mass index [BMI] 25.0–29.9) and obesity (BMI ≥30) over a recent 10-year interval in Utah (1991–2001) was accompanied by an attributable fraction of CD of 0.388 (0.369–0.407). Put differently, among all women undergoing CD at the end of this interval, 1 in 7 was attributable to overweight and/or obesity.

Fetal distress

The Cochrane systematic review demonstrated that women followed in labor were more likely to be delivered abdominally and their babies were less likely to suffer neonatal asphyxial seizure (RR 0.52; 95% CI, 0.32–0.82) [33]. However, the majority of babies delivered abdominally for "nonreassuring fetal heart rate patterns" or "fetal distress" suffered no perinatal complications and long-term follow-up of the Dublin population revealed no difference in any neuropsychiatric or developmental landmarks by age 5 years [34].

Earlier attempts to reduce false positive interventions focused on fetal scalp blood sampling for fetal pH determination and did demonstrate a reduced CD rate for this indication [35]. However, the difficulties of maintaining this equipment, as well as the invasive nature of the procedure, precluded its widescale use, particularly in the community sector. More recently, fetal pulse oximetry has been evaluated as a less invasive technique for assessment of fetal oxygenation during labor, with convincing animal and human data to suggest that a fetal oxygen saturation of greater than 30% was almost never associated with a pH of <7.15 [36–38]. An initial evaluation demonstrated a convincing reduction in CD rates for the diagnosis of "fetal distress" but interestingly demonstrated that those fetuses with nonreassuring fetal heart rates plus reassuring pulse oximetry were more likely to require CD eventually for the diagnosis of failure to progress in labor [39]. More recently, a large randomized controlled trial failed to show any benefit to fetal pulse oximetry when applied prospectively to primigravidas at term in labor [40].

Malpresentation

In 3–4% of laboring patients, the fetus is in breech presentation. Current practice calls for CD, except in unusual circumstances. The only ways to lower this figure would be to reduce the frequency of CD for breech presentation (not likely in early 21st century Western obstetrics in view of the Term Breech Trial results [41]) or to reduce the incidence of breech, which can be accomplished by external cephalic version (ECV). Because breech presentation is more common in primigravidas and because ECV is less likely to be successful near term in this same group, several studies have confirmed that ECV is more likely to be effective if performed at 34–36 weeks in primigravidas. ECV can be deferred to 37–38 weeks in multiparous women. Although historic concerns about complications such as cord entanglement, placental abruption, fetomaternal transfusion, and ruptured uterus have limited the use of ECV is some areas, these problems seem to be more theoretic than real [42]. Nonetheless, ECV should only be performed in a hospital setting where emergency CD is "immediately available."

Repeat cesarean

Safe reduction in CD rates for primigravidas will proportionately reduce the number of repeat CDs required. In view of the aforementioned dominant indications for primary CD, a modern definition of failure to progress in labor, a critical distinction between "fetal distress" versus "fetal stress" and/or "provider distress," and timely correction of breech presentation can all contribute to a lower rate of repeat CD. Higher order repeat CDs are clearly associated with increased maternal morbidity. While it is less clear that a single repeat CD is associated with significant maternal risk, the admonition that "today's primigravidas are tomorrow's multigravidas" is still germane inasmuch as the subgroup of women with the lowest risk of peripartum complications are multiparous women undergoing normal vaginal delivery with a surgically intact uterus.

Case presentation 1

A 33-year-old primigravida is admitted at 41w 2d gestation for induction of labor with the diagnosis of postdates pregnancy. Her Bishop score is 3 and she initially receives 25 µg misoprostol per vaginam every 4 hours for a total of three doses, at which time her Bishop score has improved to 7. She is begun on oxytocin and her contractions increase in frequency and intensity. She declines an offer of epidural anesthesia. The fetal heart rate tracing remains reassuring. After 6 hours her cervix is 4 cm dilatated and completely effaced, with the vertex estimated at −2 station. An amniotomy is performed for augmentation of labor with return of a large amount of clear fluid. With the next contraction sustained fetal bradycardia is noted on the fetal monitor. A sterile vaginal examination is performed and reveals umbilical cord prolapsing through the cervix. The presenting part is elevated, the oxytocin discontinued, and she is urgently transferred to the operating room where she initially received 0.25 mg terbutaline subcutaneously for uterine relaxation. Following induction of general anesthesia, an emergency CD is performed via a transverse suprapubic abdominal incision.

She was delivered of a 3600-g female whose Apgar scores were 4 and 8 and whose cord artery pH was 7.07 and who thereafter did well. She received 1 g cefazolin intravenously following delivery of the baby. She remained afebrile after delivery and was nursing her baby on the third postpartum day when she developed shortness of breath and left-sided chest pain. A chest spiral CT revealed a pulmonary embolism in the lower lobe of the right lung. She was begun on intravenous heparin and oral coumadin. After 2 days her symptoms were greatly improved and the heparin discontinued. She was discharged on the sixth postpartum day on oral coumadin. She was advised to use condoms and foam for contraception.

Case presentation 2

An 18-year-old primigravida who is 1.68 m (5 feet 6 inches) tall and whose late-pregnancy BMI is 28.6, presents at 39w 4d gestation for evaluation of labor. She is found to be 3 cm dilatated and completely effaced and is contracting painfully every 3 minutes. She is admitted with the diagnosis of spontaneous labor. After 2 hours there has been no change in her cervix yet she remains quite uncomfortable. The decision is made to provide an epidural for pain relief and to proceed thereafter with amniotomy. Both are accomplished uneventfully, the latter revealing clear amniotic fluid. The fetal heart rate pattern remains reactive.

After another 2 hours there has still been no change in her cervical examination. Internal heart rate and pressure catheters are placed, revealing a reactive fetal heart rate with a baseline of 130–140 beats/min and contractions whose total Montevideo units average 140. Oxytocin augmentation is begun with resultant increase of her average Montevideo units to 210.

She progresses to 6 cm dilatation but thereafter fails to make any further change in either cervical dilatation or station of the vertex in the ensuing 2 hours. As a result, she is taken to the operating room where a primary CD is performed for the diagnosis of failure to progress in labor. A male infant weighing 3280 g is delivered whose Apgar scores are 8 and 9 at 1 and 5 minutes, respectively.

Her intraoperative course is complicated by uterine atony that responds to 250 mg carboprost given intramuscularly. The estimated blood loss is 1200 mL. She has a single temperature elevation to 38.6°C in the recovery room, is started on broad-spectrum antibiotics, and remains afebrile thereafter. Her postoperative course is thereafter uncomplicated and she is discharged with her baby on postoperative day 3.

Case presentation 3

A 34-year-old gravida 3, para 2-0-0-2 woman is admitted at 39w 0d gestation for scheduled repeat CD. Her first cesarean was performed because of breech presentation diagnosed at the time of labor. Her second delivery was a repeat cesarean at term and she is admitted now for scheduled repeat cesarean and tubal ligation. She is known to be Rh-negative and received 300 µg RhoGAM intramuscularly at 28 weeks in all three pregnancies and had also received RhoGAM following delivery of her first child. Her second baby was Rh-negative and RhoGAM had not been administered following delivery.

A repeat cesarean is performed following induction of adequate spinal anesthesia. At the time of surgery, multiple dense adhesions are encountered between the omentum and the lower uterine section. After these are removed, further difficulty is encountered dissecting the bladder from the anterior lower uterine segment. Because she has requested permanent sterilization, the decision is made to perform a transverse hysterotomy in the lower contractile portion of the uterus. This is performed and a 3760-g male is delivered with some difficulty. The placenta is delivered spontaneously and subsequent inspection reveals a 4-cm extension of the hysterotomy inferiorly on the left side. This is repaired with running, locking, absorbable sutures and the hysterotomy repaired in two layers with similar suture materials. A Pomeroy tubal ligation is performed and segments of fallopian tube submitted for histologic confirmation.

Prior to closure of the abdomen the bladder is distended with sterile milk and none is seen intra-abdominally. The remainder of the procedure is accomplished uneventfully. The estimated blood loss is 1000 mL.

Analysis of a cord blood sample reveals the baby to be Rh-positive. Although a tubal ligation had been performed, she received 300 μg RhoGAM intramuscularly.

References

1 Sachs BP. Is the rising rate of cesarean sections a result of more defensive medicine? *Medical Professional Liability and the Delivery of Obstetrical Care*. Vol. II, *An Interdisciplinary Review*. Washington, DC: 1989, 27–40.

2 Fauendes A, Cecatti JG. Which policy for caesarean sections in Brazil? An analysis of trends and consequences. *Health Policy Plan* 1993;**8**:33–42.

3 Menard MK. Cesarean delivery rates in the United States: the 1990s. *Obstet Gynecol Clin North Am* 1999;**26**:275–86.

4 Clarke SC, Taffel S. Changes in cesarean delivery in the United States, 1988 and 1993. *Birth* 1995;**22**:63–7.

5 Sheiner E, Levy A, Feinstein U, Hallak M, Mazor M. Risk factors and outcome of failure to progress during the first stage of labor: a population-based study. *Acta Obstet Gynecol Scand* 2002;**81**:222–6.

6 American College of Obstetricians and Gynecologists. Surgery and patient choice: Ethics of decision making. Committee Opinion No. 289. *Obstet Gynecol* 2003;**102**:1101–6.

7 Berg CJ, Chang J, Callaghan WM, Whitehead SM. Pregnancy-related mortality in the United States, 1991–1997. *Obstet Gynecol* 2003;**101**:289–96.

8 Say L, Pattinson RC, Gulmezoglu AM. WHO systematic review of maternal morbidity and mortality: the prevalence of severe acute maternal morbidity (near miss). *Reprod Health* 2004;**1**:3.

9 Geller SE, Rosenberg D, Cox S, Brown M, Simonson L, Kilpatrick S. A scoring system identified near-miss maternal morbidity during pregnancy. *J Clin Epidemiol* 2004;**57**:716–20.

10 Hook B, Kiwi R, Amini SB, Fanaroff A, Hack M. Neonatal morbidity after elective repeat cesarean section and trial of labor. *Pediatrics* 1997;**100**:348–53.

11 Smaill F, Hofmeyr GJ. Antibiotic prophylaxis for cesarean section. *Cochrane Database Syst Rev* 2002;**3**:CD000933.

12 Wilkinson C, Enkin MW. Manual removal of placenta at caesarean section. *Cochrane Database Syst Rev* 1996;**1**:CD000130.

13 Jacobs-Jokhan D, Hofmeyr GJ. Extra-abdominal versus intra-abdominal repair of the uterine incision at caesarean section. *Cochrane Database Syst Rev* 2004;**4**:CD000085.

14 Enkin MW, Wilkinson C. Single versus two layer suturing for closing the uterine incision at caesarean section. *Cochrane Database Syst Rev* 1996;**1**:CD000192.

15 Anderson ER, Gates S. Techniques and materials for closure of the abdominal wall at caesarean section. *Cochrane Database Syst Rev* 2004;**18**:CD004663.

16 National Collaborating Center for Women's and Children's Health. *Caesarean Section*. RCOG Press, 2004: 71–2.

17 French LM, Smaill FM. Antibiotic regimens for endometritis after delivery. *Cochrane Database Syst Rev* 2004;**4**:CD001067.

18 American College of Obstetricians and Gynecologists. *Vaginal Birth After Previous Cesarean Delivery*. Practice Bulletin 5. Washington, DC, July 1999.

19 Landon MB, Hauth JC, Leveno KJ, *et al.* The MFMU cesarean registry: Maternal and perinatal outcome in women undergoing trial of labor after cesarean delivery. *N Engl J Med* 2004;**351**:2581–9.

20 Silver RM, for the NICHD Maternal-Fetal Medicine Units Network. Morbidity associated with multiple repeat cesarean deliveries. *Am J Obstet Gynecol* 2004;**191**:S17.

21 Gesteland K, Oshiro B, Henry E, Andres R, French T, Varner M. Rates of placenta previa and placental abruption in women delivered only vaginally or only by cesarean section. *J Soc Gynecol Invest* 2004;**11**:208A.

22 Martin JA, Hamilton BE, Sutton PD, Ventura SJ, Menacker F, Munson ML. Births: final data for 2003. *Natl Vital Stat Rep* 2005;**54**:85.

23 Varner MW, Shah G, Bloebaum L. Toward optimum cesarean rates in Utah. *Am J Obstet Gynecol* 2002;**187**:S106.

24 Robson MS. Classification of caesarean sections. *Fetal Matern Rev* 2001;**12**:123–9.

25 Fischer A, LaCoursiere DY, Barnard P, Bloebaum L, Varner M. Differences in cesarean rates and indications between hospitals for term primigravidas with vertex presentation. *Obstet Gynecol* 2005;**105**:816–21.

26 Friedman EA. Primigravid labor; a graphicostatistical analysis. *Obstet Gynecol* 1955;**6**:567–89.

27 Friedman EA. Labor in multiparas; a graphicostatistical analysis. *Obstet Gynecol* 1956;**8**:691–703.

28 O'Driscoll K, Foley M, MacDonald D. Active management of labor as an alternative to cesarean section for dystocia. *Obstet Gynecol* 1984;**63**:485–90.

29 Farah N, Geary M, Connolly G, McKenna P. The caesarean section rate in the Republic of Ireland in 1998. *Ir Med J* 2003;**96**:242–3.

30 Rouse DJ, Owen J, Hauth JC. Active-phase labor arrest: oxytocin augmentation for at least 4 hours. *Obstet Gynecol* 1999;**93**:323–8.

31 Rouse DJ, Owen J, Savage KG, Hauth JC. Active phase labor arrest: revisiting the 2-hour minimum. *Obstet Gynecol* 2001;**98**:550–4.

32 LaCoursiere DY, Bloebaum L, Duncan JD, Varner MW. Population-based trends and correlates in maternal overweight and obesity, Utah, 1991–2001. *Am J Obstet Gynecol* 2005;**192**: 832–9.

33 Thacker SB, Stroup D, Chang M. Continuous electronic heart rate monitoring for fetal assessment during labor. *Cochrane Database Syst Rev* 2001;2:CD000063.

34 MacDonald D, Grant A, Sheridan-Pereira M, Boylan P, Chalmers I. The Dublin randomized controlled trial of intrapartum fetal heart rate monitoring. *Am J Obstet Gynecol* 1985;**152**:524–39.

35 Zalar RW Jr, Quilligan EJ. The influence of scalp sampling on the cesarean section rate for fetal distress. *Am J Obstet Gynecol* 1979; **135**:239–46.

36 Luttkus AK, Friedmann W, Homm-Luttkus C, Dudenhausen JW. Correlation of fetal oxygen saturation to fetal heart rate patterns: evaluation of fetal pulse oximetry with two different oxisensors. *Acta Obstet Gynecol Scand* 1998;**77**:307–12.

37 Carbonne B, Langer B, Goffinet F, *et al.* Multicenter study on the clinical value of fetal pulse oximetry. II. Compared predictive values of pulse oximetry and fetal blood analysis. *Am J Obstet Gynecol* 1997;**177**;593–8.

38 Dildy GA, Thorp JA, Yeast JD, Clark SL. The relationship between oxygen saturation and pH in umbilical blood: implications for intrapartum fetal oxygen saturation monitoring. *Am J Obstet Gynecol* 1996;**175**:682–7.

39 Garite TJ, Dildy GA, McNamara H, *et al.* A multicenter controlled trial of fetal pulse oximetry in the intrapartum management of nonreassuring fetal heart rate patterns. *Am J Obstet Gynecol* 2000;**183**:1049–58.

40 Bloom SL, for the NICHD Maternal-Fetal Medicine Units Network. The MFMU Network Randomized Trial of Fetal Pulse Oximetry. Oral Presentation, 2006 Society for Maternal-Fetal Medicine, Miami Beach, FL, February 2006.

41 Hannah ME, Hannah WJ, Hewson SA, Hodnett ED, Saigal S, Willan AR. Planned caesarean section versus planned vaginal birth for breech presentation at term: a randomized multicenter trial. Term Breech Trial Collaborative Group. *Lancet* 2000;**356**:1375–83.

42 Ranney B. The gentle art of external cephalic version. *Am J Obstet Gynecol* 1973;**116**:239–51.

46 Vaginal birth after cesarean delivery

Mark B. Landon

Trends in VBAC-TOL

Over 25 year ago, Bottoms *et al.* [1] concluded that primary emphasis should be placed on reducing cesarean deliveries for dystocia and repeat operations as these two indications were the primary causes of the increased national rate of cesarean deliveries. This sentiment was expressed by the 1981 National Institute of Child Health and Human Development (NICHD) sponsored conference which also recognized the importance of decreasing elective repeat operations as a means of curtailing the rising overall cesarean rate [2]. A modest decline in cesarean delivery followed from 1988 to 1996, which was largely the result of an increased trial of labor (TOL) rate in women with prior cesareans. However, by 2004, only 9.2% of women with prior cesarean underwent a TOL in the USA [3]. Remarkably, nearly two-thirds of women with a prior cesarean are actually candidates for a TOL [4]. Thus, the majority of repeat operations can be considered elective and are clearly influenced by physician discretion [5]. TOL rates are consistently lower in the USA when compared with European nations, suggesting significant underutilization of TOL in the USA [6]. As 8–10% of the obstetric population has had previous cesarean delivery, more widespread use of TOL could decrease the overall cesarean delivery rate by approximately 5% [7].

The evolution in management of the woman with prior cesarean delivery is apparent through review of several American College of Obstetricians and Gynecologists (ACOG) documents and key studies over the last 15 years. In 1988, ACOG published "Guidelines for vaginal delivery after a previous cesarean birth," recommending VBAC-TOL (vaginal birth after cesarean delivery–trial of labor), as it became clear that this procedure was safe and did not appear to be associated with excess perinatal morbidity compared with elective cesarean delivery. They recommended that each hospital develop its own protocol for the management of VBAC-TOL patients and that a woman with one prior low transverse cesarean delivery should be counseled and encouraged to attempt labor in the absence of a contraindication such as a prior classic incision. This recommendation was supported by several large case series attesting to the safety and effectiveness of TOL [8–12]. Driven by this encouraging information, VBAC rates reached a peak of 28.3% by 1996. Third-party payers and managed care organizations embraced these data and began to encourage TOL for women with prior cesarean delivery by tracking provider and institutional VBAC rates. Physicians, feeling pressure to lower cesarean delivery rates, began to offer TOL liberally and may have included less than optimal candidates.

With greater utilization of VBAC-TOLs, reports surfaced suggesting a possibly greater than previously appreciated risk for uterine rupture and its maternal and fetal consequences [13–17]. Descriptions of uterine rupture with maternal hemorrhage, hysterectomy, and adverse perinatal outcomes including death and brain injury set the stage for the precipitous decline in VBAC witnessed during the last decade [18–21].

Eventually, ACOG acknowledged the apparent statistically small but significant risks of uterine rupture with poor outcomes for both women and their infants during TOL [22]. It was also recognized that such adverse events during a TOL might precipitate malpractice litigation. A more conservative approach to TOL has thus been adopted by even ardent supporters of VBAC. Nonetheless, in its updated 2004 bulletin ACOG states clearly that most women with one previous cesarean delivery with a low transverse incision are candidates for VBAC and should be counseled about VBAC and offered TOL [23].

Candidates for TOL

Women who have had low transverse uterine incision with prior cesarean delivery and have no contraindications to vaginal birth can be considered candidates for TOL. The following are criteria suggested by ACOG [23] for identifying candidates for VBAC:

* One previous low transverse cesarean delivery;
* Clinically adequate pelvis;
* No other uterine scars or previous rupture; and
* Physicians immediately available throughout active labor capable of monitoring labor and performing an emergency cesarean delivery.

Additionally, several retrospective studies would indicate that it may be reasonable to offer TOL to women in other clinical situations. These would include: two previous low transverse cesarean deliveries, gestation beyond 40 weeks, previous low vertical incision, unknown uterine scar type, and twin gestation [23].

TOL is *contraindicated* in women at high risk for uterine rupture and should not be attempted in the following circumstances:

* Previous classic or T-shaped incision or extensive transfundal uterine surgery;
* Previous uterine rupture;
* Medical or obstetric complications that preclude vaginal delivery; or
* Inability to perform emergency cesarean delivery because of unavailable surgeon, anesthesia, sufficient staff or faculty.

Success rates for TOL

The overall success rate for VBAC appears to be in the 70–80% range according to published reports [24–26]. In published series with the highest TOL rates, success was only present in 60% of cases [27]. More recently, selective criteria resulting in TOL rates in the 30% range have been associated with a higher number of vaginal births, 70–75% [28,29]. Several predictors of successful TOL have been well described (Table 46.1). The

Table 46.1 Success rates for trial of labor. After Landon *et al.* [28].

	VBAC Success (%)
Prior indication	
CPD/FTP	63.5
NRFWB	72.6
Malpresentation	83.8
Prior vaginal delivery	
Yes	86.6
No	60.9
Labor type	
Induction	67.4
Augmented	73.9
Spontaneous	80.6

CPD, cephalopelvic disproportion; FTP, failure to progress; NRFWB, nonreassuring fetal well-being; VBAC, vaginal birth after cesarean delivery.

prior indication for the cesarean delivery clearly impacts on the likelihood of successful VBAC. A history of prior vaginal birth or a nonrecurring condition such as breech or fetal distress is associated with the highest success rates for VBAC (Table 46.1) [10]. Understanding that there is no reliable method to predict success of TOL for an individual woman, a number of factors have been studied which influence success and these are summarized in the following sections.

Maternal demographics

Race, age, body mass index, and insurance status have all been demonstrated to impact the success of TOL [28]. In a multicenter study of 14,529 term pregnancies undergoing TOL, Caucasian women had an overall 78% success rate compared with 70% in non-Caucasian women [28]. Obese women are more likely to fail TOL as are women older than age 40 [28]. Conflicting data exist with regard to payer status (uninsured versus private patients).

Prior indication for cesarean delivery

Success rates for women whose first cesarean delivery was performed for a nonrecurring indication (breech, nonreassuring fetal well-being) are similar to vaginal delivery rates among nulliparous women [30]. Prior cesarean for breech presentation is associated with the highest reported success rate of 89% [28,30]. In contrast, prior operative delivery for cephalopelvic disproportion or failure to progress is associated with success rates in the range 50–67% [31–33]. If dystocia was diagnosed between 5 and 9 cm in a prior labor, 67–73% of VBAC attempts are successful compared with only 13% if prior cesarean delivery was performed during the second stage of labor [34].

Prior vaginal delivery

Prior vaginal delivery including prior successful VBAC is apparently the best predictor for a successful TOL [28]. In one series, a prior vaginal delivery was associated with an 87% success rate compared with 61% success in women without prior vaginal delivery [28]. Caughey *et al.* [35] reported patients with a prior VBAC had a 93% success rate compared with 85% for women with a vaginal delivery prior to their cesarean birth that were without prior VBAC.

Birthweight

Large for gestational age or fetal macrosomia is associated with a lower likelihood of VBAC success [29]. Birthweight greater than 4000 g in particular is associated with a significantly higher risk of failed TOL [28]. Nonetheless, Flamm and Goings [36] reported that 60–70% of women who attempt VBAC with a macrosomic fetus are successful.

Labor status and cervical examination

Both labor status and cervical examination upon admission influence VBAC success [37]. An 86% VBAC success rate has been reported in women presenting with cervical dilatation ≥4 cm [38]. Conversely, the success rate drops to 67% if the cervical examination is less than 4 cm upon admission.

Women who undergo induction of labor are at higher risk for a failed TOL or repeat cesarean delivery compared with those who enter spontaneous labor [28,38]. This risk is approximately 1.5- to 2.0-fold higher. Landon *et al.* [28] reported a 67.4% successful VBAC rate in women undergoing induction versus 80.6% in those entering spontaneous labor. Remarkably, Grinstead and Grobman [39] reported a surprisingly high success rate (78%) in 429 women undergoing induction with prior cesarean delivery. These authors noted several factors in addition to past obstetric history, including indication for induction and need for cervical ripening as determinants of VBAC success [39].

Previous incision type

Previous incision type may be unknown in certain patients. It appears that women with unknown scar have VBAC success rates similar to those of women with documented prior low transverse incisions [28]. Similarly, women with previous low vertical incisions do not appear to have lower VBAC success rates [40].

Multiple prior cesarean deliveries

Women with more than one prior cesarean have been demonstrated to consistently have a lower likelihood of achieving VBAC [41–43]. Caughey *et al.* [41] reported a 75% success rate for women with one prior cesarean compared with 62% in women with two prior operations. In contrast, Macones *et al.*'s [44] large multicenter study of 13,617 women undergoing TOL revealed a 75.5% success rate for women with two prior cesareans, which was not statistically different from the 75% success rate in women with one prior operation (Table 46.3).

Risks of VBAC-TOL

Uterine rupture

The principal risk associated with VBAC-TOL is uterine rupture. This complication is directly attributable to attempted VBAC, as symptomatic rupture is a rare observation at the time of elective repeat operations [45,46]. An important distinction exists between uterine rupture and uterine scar dehiscence. This difference is clinically relevant as dehiscence most often represents an occult scar separation observed at laparotomy in women with a prior cesarean delivery. The serosa of

Table 46.2 Success rates for trial of labor with two prior cesarean deliveries.

Author	*n*	Success Rate (%)
Miller *et al.* [42]	2936	75.3
Caughey *et al.* [41]	134	62.0
Macones *et al.* [44]	1082	74.6
Landon *et al.* [43]	876	67.0

the uterus is intact with most cases of dehiscence and hemorrhage is absent. In contrast, uterine rupture is a thorough disruption of all uterine layers with consequences of hemorrhage, cord compression, potential abruption, fetal compromise, and significant maternal morbidity. The VBAC literature varies with respect to terminology, definitions, and ascertainment for uterine rupture [47]. A review of 10 observational studies providing the best evidence on the occurrence of symptomatic rupture with TOL revealing rupture rates ranging from 0 in 1000 in a small study to 7.8 in 1000 in the largest study, with a pooled rate of 3.8 per 1000 TOL [47,48]. The large, multicenter, prospective, observational Maternal Fetal Medicine Units (MFMU) Network study reported a 0.69% incidence with 124 symptomatic ruptures occurring in 17,898 women undergoing TOL [49].

The rate of uterine rupture depends on both the type and location of the previous uterine incision (Table 46.2). Uterine rupture rates are highest with previous classic or T-shaped incisions, with a reported range of 4–9% [50]. The risk for rupture with a previous low vertical incision is difficult to determine. Distinguishing this incision type from classic incision can be arbitrary and low vertical incision is relatively uncommon. Two reports suggest a rupture rate of 0.8–1.1% for prior low vertical scar [50,51].

Women with unknown scar type may not be at increased risk for uterine rupture. This may simply be because most cases are undocumented prior low transverse incisions. Among 3206 women with unknown scar in the MFMU Network report, uterine rupture occurred in 0.5% of TOL [49].

The most serious sequelae of uterine rupture include perinatal death, fetal hypoxic brain injury, and hysterectomy. Guise *et al.* [48] calculated a rate of 0.14 additional perinatal deaths per 1000 TOL related to uterine rupture. This figure is similar to the NICHD-MFMU Network study in which there were two neonatal deaths among 124 ruptures, for an overall rate of rupture-related perinatal death of 0.11 per 1000 TOL [49]. Chauhan *et al.* [52], in reviewing 880 maternal uterine ruptures during a 20-year period, calculated 40 perinatal deaths in 91,039 TOL for a rate of 0.4 per 1000.

In most studies, perinatal hypoxic brain injury has been an underreported adverse outcome related to uterine rupture. Landon *et al.* [49] found a significant increase in the rate of hypoxic ischemic encephalopathy (HIE) related to uterine rupture among the offspring of women who underwent TOL at term, compared with the children of women who underwent elective repeat cesarean delivery (0.46 per 1000 TOL versus no cases, respectively). In 114 cases of uterine rupture at term, seven infants (6.2%) sustained HIE and two of these infants died in the neonatal period.

Maternal hysterectomy may be a complication of uterine rupture, particularly if the defect is unrepairable or is associated with uncontrollable hemorrhage. In five studies reporting on hysterectomies related to rupture, seven cases occurred in 60 symptomatic ruptures (13%; range 4–27%), indicating that 3.4 per 10,000 women electing TOL sustain a rupture that necessitates hysterectomy [47]. The NICHD-MFMU Network study included 5/124 (4%) rupture cases requiring hysterectomy in which the uterus could not be repaired [49].

Risk factors for uterine rupture

Rates of uterine rupture vary significantly depending on a variety of associated risk factors. In addition to uterine scar type, obstetric history characteristics including number of prior cesareans, prior vaginal delivery, interdelivery interval, and uterine closure technique have all been reported to affect the risk of uterine rupture. Similarly, factors related to labor management including induction and the use of oxytocin augmentation have all been studied.

Number of prior cesarean deliveries

Miller et al. [42] reported uterine rupture in 1.7% of women with two or more previous cesarean deliveries compared with a frequency of 0.6% in those with one prior operation (odds ratio [OR] 3.06; 95% confidence interval [CI], 1.95–4.79). Interestingly, the risk for uterine rupture was not increased further for women with three prior cesareans. Caughey et al. [41] conducted a smaller study of 134 women with two prior cesareans and controlled for labor characteristics as well as obstetric history. These authors reported a rate of uterine rupture of 3.7% among these 134 women compared with 0.8% in the 3757 women with one previous scar (OR 4.5; 95% CI, 1.18–11.5). This information led to the ACOG recommendation that TOL for women with two prior cesarean deliveries be limited to those with a history of prior vaginal delivery [23]. Recently, Macones et al. [44] reported a uterine rupture rate of 20/1082 (1.8%) in women with two prior cesareans compared with 113/12,535 (0.9%) in women with one prior operation (adjusted OR 2.3; 95% CI, 1.37–3.85). In contrast, an analysis from the MFMU Network Cesarean Registry found no significant difference in rupture rates in women with one prior cesarean; 115/16,916 (0.7%) versus multiple prior cesareans 9/982 (0.9%) [43]. Thus, it appears that if multiple prior cesarean section is associated with an increased risk for uterine rupture, the magnitude of any additional risk is fairly small.

Table 46.3 Risk of uterine rupture with trial of labor.

Prior Incision Type	Rupture Rate (%)
Low transverse	0.5–1.0
Low vertical	0.8–1.1
Classic or T-shaped	4–9

Prior vaginal delivery

Prior vaginal delivery is protective against uterine rupture following TOL. Zelop et al. [53] noted the rate of uterine rupture among women with prior vaginal birth to be 0.2% (2/1021) compared with 1.1% (30/2762) among women with no prior vaginal deliveries. A similar protective effect of prior vaginal birth has been reported in two large multicenter studies [43,54]. There is currently no information as to whether a history of successful VBAC is also protective against uterine rupture.

Uterine closure technique

Single-layer uterine closure technique has gained popularity as it may be associated with shorter operating time with similar short-term complications compared with the traditional two-layer technique. A retrospective study of 292 women undergoing TOL found similar rates of uterine rupture for women with one- and two-layer closures [55]. Chapman et al. [56] conducted a randomized trial that compared the incidence of uterine rupture in 145 women who received either one- or two-layer closure at their primary cesarean delivery. No cases of uterine rupture were found in either group; however, the study is of insufficient size to detect a potential difference. A large observational cohort study identified an approximate fourfold increased rate of rupture following single-layer closure technique when compared with previous double-layer closure [56,57]. These authors conducted detailed review of operative reports in which the rate of rupture was 15/1489 (3.1%) with single-layer closure versus 8/1491 (0.5%) with previous double-layer closure. A large randomized study will be necessary to resolve whether single-layer closure increases the risk of subsequent uterine rupture.

Interpregnancy interval

Short interpregnancy intervals have been studied as a risk factor for uterine rupture during TOL [58–60]. Shipp et al. [58] reported an incidence of rupture of 2.3% (7/311) in women with an interdelivery interval less than 18 months compared with 1.1% (22/2098) with a longer interdelivery interval. In contrast, Huang et al. [59] found no increased risk for uterine rupture with an interdelivery interval of less than 18 months. Bujold et al. [60] have reported an interdelivery interval of less than 24 months to be independently associated with an almost threefold increased risk for uterine rupture. These authors reported a rate of rupture of 2.8% in women with a short interval versus 0.9% in women with more than 2 years since the prior cesarean birth.

Labor induction

Induction of labor appears be associated with an increased risk of uterine rupture [49,54,61]. Lydon-Rochelle *et al.* [61] reported a uterine rupture rate of 24/2326 (1.0%) for women undergoing induction compared with 56/10,789 (1.5%) women with spontaneous onset of labor. In the prospective MFMU Network cohort analysis, Landon *et al.* [49] noted the risk for uterine rupture to be nearly threefold elevated (OR 2.86; 95% CI, 1.75–4.67) with uterine rupture occurring after 48/4708 (1.0%) of induced TOL versus 24/6685 (0.4%) of spontaneous labors. After controlling for various potential confounders, the risk of uterine rupture in women undergoing oxytocin labor induction has been reported to be increased 4.6-fold compared with spontaneous labor (rupture rate of 2.0% versus 0.7%) [53]. Despite these analyses, it remains unclear whether induction causes uterine rupture or whether an associated risk factor such as cervical status is the ultimate cause.

Conflicting data also exist whether various induction methods increase the risk for uterine rupture [62]. Lydon-Rochelle *et al.*'s [61] study suggested an increased risk for uterine rupture with use of prostaglandins for labor induction. Uterine rupture was noted in 15/1960 (0.8%) of women induced without prostaglandin use compared with 9/366 (2.5%) induced with prostaglandin use. Two recent large studies have failed to confirm the findings of Lydon-Rochelle *et al.* of an increased risk of rupture associated with the use of prostaglandin agents alone for induction [49,54]. Macones *et al.* [54] did report an increased risk for rupture in women undergoing induction only if they received a combination of prostaglandins and oxytocin. In the MFMU Network study, there were no cases of uterine rupture when prostaglandin alone was used for induction, including 52 cases of misoprostol use [49]. The safety of this medication, which is popular for cervical ripening and labor induction, has been challenged for women attempting VBAC. Despite several studies that did not demonstrate an increased risk for rupture with prostaglandins and the fact that no studies or meta-analyses of sufficient size have detected a statistically increased risk for rupture with misoprostol use, ACOG has issued a committee opinion discouraging the use of prostaglandins for cervical ripening or induction in women attempting VBAC-TOL until this issue is further clarified [63].

Labor augmentation

Excessive use of oxytocin may be associated with uterine rupture such that careful labor augmentation should be practiced in women attempting TOL [20]. In a case–control study, Leung *et al.* [20] reported an odds ratio of 2.7 for uterine rupture in women receiving oxytocin augmentation. In contrast, a meta-analysis concluded that oxytocin does not increase the risk for uterine rupture [10]. Dysfunctional labor including arrest disorders actually increased the risk sevenfold and thus may actually be the primary factor responsible for rupture. In support of this concept, Zelop *et al.* [53] found that labor aug-

mentation with oxytocin did not significantly increase the risk for rupture. In the MFMU Network study, the rate of uterine rupture with oxytocin augmentation was 52/6009 (0.9%) compared with 24/6685 (0.4%) without oxytocin use [49]. In summary, oxytocin augmentation *may* marginally increase the risk for uterine rupture in women undergoing TOL. It follows that judicious use of oxytocin should be employed in this population.

Management of VBAC-TOL

Because uterine rupture may be catastrophic, it is recommended that TOL after prior cesarean delivery should only be attempted in institutions equipped to respond to emergencies, with physicians immediately available to provide emergent care [23]. Thus, an obstetrician and anesthesia personnel must both be available to comply with this recommendation.

Recommendations for management of women undergoing a TOL after prior cesarean delivery are primarily based upon expert opinion. Women attempting VBAC should be encouraged to contact their health care provider promptly when labor or ruptured membranes occur. Continuous electronic fetal heart rate (FHR) monitoring is prudent, although the need for intrauterine pressure catheter monitoring is debatable. Studies that have examined FHR patterns prior to uterine rupture consistently report that nonreassuring signs, particularly significant variable decelerations or bradycardia, are the most common finding accompanying uterine rupture [64,65]. Despite the presence of adequate personnel to proceed with emergency cesarean delivery, prompt intervention does not always prevent fetal neurologic injury or death [48,66]. In one study, significant neonatal morbidity occurred when 18 minutes or longer elapsed between the onset of FHR deceleration and delivery [20]. If prolonged deceleration is preceded by variable or late decelerations, fetal injury may occur as early as 10 minutes from the onset of the terminal deceleration.

TOL is not a contraindication to the use of epidural analgesia. Moreover, epidural use does not appear to affect success rates [28]. Epidural analgesia also does not mask the signs and symptoms of uterine rupture. Oxytocin augmentation is employed as necessary, understanding that hyperstimulation should be avoided. In a case–control study, Goetzl *et al.* [67] reported no association between uterine rupture and oxytocin dosing intervals, total dose utilized, and the mean duration of oxytocin administration.

Vaginal delivery is conducted as in cases without a history of prior cesarean. Most individuals do not routinely explore the uterus in order to detect asymptomatic scar dehiscences because these generally heal well. However, excessive vaginal bleeding or maternal hypotension should be promptly evaluated including assessment for possible uterine rupture. Of 124 cases of uterine rupture accompanying TOL, 14 (11%) were identified *following* vaginal delivery [49].

Complication	Trial of Labor (*n* = 17,898)	Elective Repeated Cesarean Delivery (*n* = 15,801)	Odds Ratio (98% CI)
Uterine rupture	124 (0.7)	0	–
Hysterectomy	41 (0.2)	47 (0.3)	0.77 (0.51–1.17)
Thromboembolic disease	7 (0.04)	10 (0.1)	0.62 (0.24–1.62)
Transfusion	304 (1.7)	158 (1.0)	1.71 (1.41–2.08)
Endometritis	517 (2.9)	285 (1.8)	1.62 (1.40–1.87)
Maternal death	3 (0.02)	7 (0.04)	0.38 (1.10–1.46)
One or more of the above	978 (5.5)	563 (3.6)	1.56 (1.41–1.74)

Table 46.4 Comparison of maternal complications in trial of labor vs. elective repeat cesarean delivery. After Landon *et al.* [49].

Table 46.5 Risks associated with trial of labor (TOL).

Uterine rupture and related morbidity
Uterine rupture   (0.5–1.0/100 TOL)
Perinatal death and/or encephalopathy   (0.5/1000 TOL)
Hysterectomy   (0.3/1000 TOL)

Increased maternal morbidity with failed trial of labor
Transfusion
Endometritis
Length of stay

Potential risk for perinatal asphyxia with labor (cord prolapse, abruption)

Potential risk for antepartum stillbirth beyond 39 weeks' gestation

Table 46.6 Risks associated with elective repeat cesarean delivery.

Increased maternal morbidity compared with successful trial of labor
Increased length of stay and recovery
Increased risks for abnormal placentation and hemorrhage with successive cesarean operations

Counseling for VBAC-TOL

A pregnant woman with prior cesarean delivery is at risk for both maternal and perinatal complications whether undergoing TOL or choosing elective repeat operation (Table 46.4). Complications of both procedures should be discussed and an attempt should be made to individualize risk for both uterine rupture and the likelihood of successful VBAC (Tables 46.1 and 46.5). For example, a woman who might require induction of labor may be at slight increased risk for uterine rupture and is also less likely to achieve vaginal delivery. Future childbearing and the risks of multiple cesarean deliveries including risks of placenta previa and accreta should also be considered (see Chapter 45).

It is important to make every possible effort to obtain the operative records of a prior cesarean delivery in order to determine previous uterine incision type. This is particularly relevant to cases of prior preterm breech delivery in which vertical uterine incision or a low transverse incision in an undeveloped lower uterine segment might preclude TOL. There may be an increased rate of subsequent uterine rupture in women with a prior preterm cesarean attempting TOL [68]. If previous uterine incision type is unknown, the implications of this missing information should also be discussed.

Following complete informed consent detailing the risks and benefits for the individual woman, the delivery plan should be formulated by both the patient and physician. Documentation of counseling is advisable and some practitioners prefer to use a specific VBAC consent form. Many women will elect repeat operation after thorough counseling. However, VBAC-TOL should continue to remain an option for most women with prior cesarean delivery (Tables 46.5 and 46.6). The magnitude of risks accompanying TOL must be conveyed to the women undergoing counseling. The attributable risk for a serious adverse perinatal outcome (perinatal death or HIE) at term appears to be approximately 1 in 2000 TOL [49]. Combining an independent risk for hysterectomy attributable to uterine rupture at term with the risk for newborn HIE indicates the chance of one of these adverse events occurring to be approximately 1 in 1250 cases [49].

The decision to elect TOL may also increase the risk for perinatal death and HIE unrelated to uterine rupture. For women awaiting spontaneous labor beyond 39 weeks, there is a small possibility of unexplained stillbirth which might be avoidable with scheduled repeat operation. A risk for fetal hypoxia and its sequelae may also accompany labor events unrelated to the uterine scar. In the MFMU Network study, five cases of nonrupture-related HIE occurred in term infants in the TOL group compared with none in the elective repeat cesarean population [49].

Case presentation

A 31-year-old gravida 2 para 1 at 40 weeks' gestation presents for continued prenatal care. This woman underwent a low transverse cesarean delivery for breech presentation 2 years previously. She has been planning to attempt TOL and, having reached 40 weeks' gestation, is considering her options. Her cervical examination reveals a long closed cervix.

Prior to reaching term, this woman will have undergone complete counseling regarding benefits and risks of TOL. The counseling should include a detailed discussion of risks of TOL including potential uterine rupture and its sequelae. The benefits of VBAC including faster recovery and shorter hospital stay will be reviewed. Providing this woman is not interested in having a large family, the option of scheduled repeat cesarean delivery should also be presented. If she is considering several future pregnancies, multiple repeat operations may pose additional risk for her of accreta and hysterectomy.

As this woman has a history of prior breech as an indication for cesarean, her overall chance for successful TOL is approximately 80%. However, she may be forced to consider induction if she does not enter spontaneous labor in the next week. If her cervix remains unfavorable, her chance for successful VBAC may only be 50–60%. In addition, induction may slightly increase her risk for uterine rupture from 0.4% to approximately 1%. This information should be considered in planning the mode of delivery. A reasonable approach provided the woman still desires TOL after discussion, might be to wait 1 week (41 weeks) and assess the cervical status at that time. If the cervix ripens, induction may be planned whereas if the cervix remains unfavorable, a repeat cesarean could be scheduled.

References

1 Bottoms SF, Rosen MG, Sokol RJ. The increase in the cesarean birth. *N Engl J Med* 1980;**302**:559–63.

2 Cesarean Childbirth: NICHD Consensus Development Conference. Washington, DC: DHHS Publication No. 81-2067, 1981.

3 Martin JA, Hamilton BE, Menachker F, Sutton PD, Matthews TJ. Preliminary births for 2004. Health E-Stats. National Center for Health Statistics. www.cdc.gov/nchs/products/pubs/pubd/hestats/prelimbirths/prelimbirths04.htm

4 Flamm BL. Vaginal birth after cesarean section: controversies old and new. *Clin Obstet Gynecol* 1985;**28**:735–44.

5 Goldman G, Pineault R, Potvin L, Blais R, Bilodeau H. Factors influencing the practice of vaginal birth after cesarean section. *Am Public Health* 1993;**83**:1104–8.

6 Shiono PH, Fielden JR, McNellis D, et al. Recent trends in cesarean birth and trial of labor rates in the United States. *JAMA* 1987;**257**:494–7.

7 American College of Obstetricians and Gynecologists. *Vaginal delivery after previous cesarean birth. practice patterns*, No. 1. Washington, DC: ACOG, 1995.

8 Flamm BL, Newman LA, Thomas SJ, et al. Vaginal birth after cesarean delivery: results of a 5-year multicenter collaborative study. *Obstet Gynecol* 1990;**76**:750–4.

9 Flamm B, Goings J, Liu Y, Wolde-Tsadik G. Elective repeat cesarean section delivery versus trial of labor: a prospective multicenter study. *Obstet Gynecol* 1994;**83**:927–32.

10 Rosen MG, Dickinson JC, Westhoff CL. Vaginal birth after cesarean: a meta-analysis of morbidity and mortality. *Obstet Gynecol* 1991;**77**:465–70.

11 Paul RH, Phelan JP, Yeh S. Trial of labor in the patient with a prior cesarean birth. *Am J Obstet Gynecol* 1985;**151**:297–304.

12 Martin JN Jr, Harris BA Jr, Huddleston JF, et al. Vaginal delivery following previous cesarean birth. *Am J Obstet Gynecol* 1983;**146**:255–63.

13 Beall M, Eglinton GS, Clark SL, et al. Vaginal delivery after cesarean section in women with unknown types of uterine scars. *J Reprod Med* 1984;**29**:31–5.

14 Pruett K, Kirshon B, Cotton D. Unknown uterine scar in trial of labor. *Am J Obstet Gynecol* 1988;**159**:807–10.

15 Scott J. Mandatory trial of labor after cesarean delivery: an alternative viewpoint. *Obstet Gynecol* 1991;**77**:811–4.

16 Pitkin RM. Once a cesarean? *Obstet Gynecol* 1991;**77**:939.

17 Sachs BP, Kobelin C, Castro MA, Frigoletto F. The risks of lowering the cesarean-delivery rate. *N Engl J Med* 1990;**340**:54–7.

18 Farmer RM, Kirschbaum T, Potter D, Strong TH, Medaris AL. Uterine rupture during a trial of labor after previous cesarean section. *Am J Obstet Gynecol* 1991;**165**:996–1001.

19 Boucher M, Tahilramaney MP, Eglinton GS, et al. Maternal morbidity as related to trial of labor after previous cesarean delivery: a quantitative analysis. *J Reprod Med* 1984;**29**:12–6.

20 Leung AS, Farmer RM, Leung EK, et al. Risk factors associated with uterine rupture during trial of labor after cesarean delivery: a case controlled study. *Am J Obstet Gynecol* 1993;**168**:1358–63.

21 Arulkumaran S, Chua S, Ratnam SS. Symptoms and signs with scar rupture: value of uterine activity measurements. *Aust N Z J Obstet Gynaecol* 1992;**32**:208–12.

22 American College of Obstetricians and Gynecologists. *Vaginal birth after previous cesarean delivery: clinical management guidelines for obstetricians-gynecologists*. ACOG Practice Bulletin 5. Washington DC: July 1999.

23 American College of Obstetricians and Gynecologists. *Vaginal birth after previous cesarean delivery: clinical management guidelines for obstetrician-gynecologists*. ACOG Practice Bulletin 54. Washington DC: July 2004.

24 Whiteside DC, Mahan CS, Cook JC. Factors associated with successful vaginal delivery after cesarean section. *J Reprod Med* 1983;**28**:785–8.

25 Silver RK, Gibbs RS. Prediction of vaginal delivery in patients with a previous cesarean section who require oxytocin. *Am J Obstet Gynecol* 1987;**156**:57–60.

26 Flamm BL. Vaginal birth after cesarean section. In: Flamm BL, Quilligan EJ, (eds). *Cesarean Section: Guidelines for Appropriate Utilization*. New York: Springer-Verlag, 1995: 51–64.

27 Gregory KD, Korst LM, Cane P, Platt LD, Kahn K. Vaginal birth after cesarean and uterine rupture rates in California. *Obstet Gynecol* 1999;**93**:985–9.

28 Landon MB, Leindecker S, Spong CY, for the National Institute of Child Health and Human Development Maternal-Fetal Medicine Units Network. The MFMU Cesarean Registry. Factors affecting the success and trial of labor following prior cesarean delivery. *Am J Obstet Gynecol* 2005;**193**:1016–23.

29 Elkousky MA, Samuel M, Stevens E, Peipert JF, Macones G. The effect of birthweight on vaginal birth after cesarean delivery success rates. *Am J Obstet Gynecol* 2003;**188**:824–30.

30 Coughlan C, Kearney R, Turner MJ. What are the implications for the next delivery in primigravidae who have an elective cesarean

section for breech presentation? *Br J Obstet Gynaecol* 2002;**109**:624–6.

31 Abitbol MM, Castillo I, Taylor UB, *et al.* Vaginal birth after cesarean section: the patient's point of view. *Am Fam Physician* 1993;**47**:129–34.

32 Ollendorff DA, Goldberg JM, Minoque JP, Socol ML. Vaginal birth after cesarean section for arrest of labor: is success determined by maximum cervical dilatation during the prior labor? *Am J Obstet Gynecol* 1988;**159**:636–9.

33 Jongen VHWM, Halfwerk MGC, Brouwer WK. Vaginal delivery after previous cesarean section for failure of second stage of labour. *Br J Obstet Gynecol* 1998;**195**:1079.

34 Hoskins IA, Gomez JL. Correlation between maximum cervical dilation at cesarean delivery and subsequent vaginal birth after cesarean delivery. *Obstet Gynecol* 1997;**89**:591–3.

35 Caughey AB, Shipp TD, Repke JT, *et al.* Trial of labor after cesarean delivery: the effects of previous vaginal delivery. *Am J Obstet Gynecol* 1998;**179**;938–41.

36 Flamm BL, Goings JR. Vaginal birth after cesarean section: is suspected fetal macrosomia a contraindication? *Obstet Gynecol* 1989;**74**:694–7.

37 Weinstein D, Benshushan A, Tanos V, *et al.* Predictive score for vaginal birth after cesarean section. *Am J Obstet Gynecol* 1996;**174**:192–8.

38 Shipp TD, Zelop CM, Repke JT, Cohen A, Caughey AB, Lieberman E. Labor after previous cesarean: influence of prior indication and parity. *Obstet Gynecol* 2000;**95**:913–6.

39 Grinstead J, Grobman WA. Induction of labor after one prior cesarean: predictors of vaginal delivery. *Obstet Gynecol* 2004;**103**:534–8.

40 Rosen MG, Dickinson JC. Vaginal birth after cesarean: a meta-analysis of indicators for success. *Obstet Gynecol* 1990;**76**:865–9.

41 Caughey AB, Shipp TD, Repke JT, *et al.* Rate of uterine rupture during a trial of labor in women with one or two prior cesarean deliveries. *Am J Obstet Gynecol* 1999;**181**:872–6.

42 Miller DA, Diaz FG, Paul RH. Vaginal birth after cesarean: a 10 year experience. *Obstet Gynecol* 1994;**84**:255–8.

43 Landon MB, Spong CY, Thom E, for the National Institute of Child Health and Human Development Maternal-Fetal Medicine Units Network. Maternal morbidity associated with multiple repeat cesarean deliveries. *Obstet Gynecol* 2006;**107**:1226–32.

44 Macones GA, Cahill A, Para E, *et al.* Obstetric outcomes in women with two prior cesarean deliveries: is vaginal birth after cesarean delivery a viable option? *Am J Obstet Gynecol* 2005;**192**:1223–9.

45 Kieser KE, Baskett TF. A 10-year population-based study of uterine rupture. *Obstet Gynecol* 2002;**100**:749–53.

46 Mozurkewich EL, Hutton EK. Elective repeat cesarean delivery versus trial of labor: a meta-analysis of the literature from 1989 to 1999. *Am J Obstet Gynecol* 2000;**183**:1187–97.

47 *Vaginal birth after cesarean (VBAC)*. Rockville, MD: Agency for Health Care Research and Quality. March 2003. (AHRQ publication no. 03-E018.)

48 Guise JM, McDonagh MS, Osterweil P, *et al.* Systematic review of the incidence and consequences of uterine rupture in women with previous cesarean section. *Br Med J* 2004;**329**:19–25.

49 Landon MB, Hauth JC, Leveno KJ, *et al.* for the National Institute of Child Health and Human Development Maternal-Fetal Medicine Units Network. Maternal and perinatal outcomes associated with a trial of labor after prior cesarean delivery. *N Engl J Med* 2004;**351**:2581–9.

50 Naif RW 3rd, Ray MA, Chauhan SP, *et al.* Trial of labor after cesarean delivery with a lower-segment, vertical uterine incision: is it safe? *Am J Obstet Gynecol* 1995;**172**:1666–73.

51 Shipp TD, Zelop CM, Repke TJ, *et al.* Intrapartum uterine rupture and dehiscence in patients with prior lower uterine segment vertical and transverse incisions. *Obstet Gynecol* 1999;**94**:735–40.

52 Chauhan SP, Martin JN Jr, Henrichs CE, Morrison JC, Magann EF. Maternal and perinatal complications with uterine rupture in 142,075 patients who attempted vaginal birth after cesarean delivery: a review of the literature. *Am J Obstet Gynecol* 2003;**189**:408–17.

53 Zelop CM, Shipp TD, Repke JT, *et al.* Uterine rupture during induced or augmented labor in gravid women with one prior cesarean delivery. *Am J Obstet Gynecol* 1999;**181**:882–6.

54 Macones G, Peipert J, Nelson D, *et al.* Maternal complications with vaginal birth after cesarean delivery: a multicenter study. *Am J Obstet Gynecol* 2005;**193**:1656–62.

55 Tucker JM, Hauth JC, Hodgkins P, *et al.* Trial of labor after a one- or two-layer closure of a low transverse uterine incision. *Obstet Gynecol* 1993;**168**:545–6.

56 Chapman SJ, Owen J, Hauth JC. One-versus two-layer closure of a low transverse cesarean: the next pregnancy. *Obstet Gynecol* 1997;**89**:16–8.

57 Bujold E, Bujold C, Hamilton EF, *et al.* The impact of a single-layer or double-layer closure on uterine rupture. *Am J Obstet Gynecol* 2002;**186**:1326–30.

58 Shipp TD, Zelop CM, Repke JT, *et al.* Interdelivery interval and risk of symptomatic uterine rupture. *Obstet Gynecol* 2001;**97**:175–7.

59 Huang WH, Nakashima DK, Rummey PJ, *et al.* Interdelivery interval and the success of vaginal birth after cesarean delivery. *Obstet Gynecol* 2002;**99**:41–4.

60 Bujold E, Mehta SH, Bujold C, Gauthier RJ. Interdelivery interval and uterine rupture. *Am J Obstet Gynecol* 2002;**187**:199–202.

61 Lydon-Rochelle M, Holt V, Easterling TR, Martin DP. Risk of uterine rupture during labor among women with a prior cesarean delivery. *N Engl J Med* 2001;**345**:36–8.

62 Stone JL, Lockwood CJ, Berkowitz G, *et al.* Use of cervical prostaglandin E$_2$ gel in patients with previous cesarean section. *Am J Perinatol* 1994;**11**:309–12.

63 American College of Obstetricians and Gynecologists. *Induction of labor*. ACOG Practice Bulletin No 10, 1999.

64 Jones R, Nagashima A, Hartnett-Goodman M, Goodlin R. Rupture of low transverse cesarean scars during trial of labor. *Obstet Gynecol* 1991;**77**:815–7.

65 Rodriguez M, Masaki D, Phelan J, Diaz F. Uterine rupture: are intrauterine pressure catheters useful in the diagnosis? *Am J Obstet Gynecol* 1989;**161**:666–9.

66 Clark SL, Scott JR, Porter TF, *et al.* Is vaginal birth after cesarean less expensive than repeat cesarean delivery? *Am J Obstet Gynecol* 2000;**182**:599–602.

67 Goetzl L, Shipp TD, Cohen A, Zelop CM, Repke JT, Lieberman E. Oxytocin dose and the risk of uterine rupture in trial of labor after cesarean. *Obstet Gynecol* 2001;**97**:381–4.

68 Scissione A, for the MFMU Network, NICDH, Bethesda, Maryland. The MFMU Cesarean Registry: Previous preterm low transverse cesarean delivery and risk of subsequent uterine rupture [Abstract]. *Am J Obstet Gynecol* 2005;**193**:S20.

47 Breech delivery

Edward R. Yeomans and Larry C. Gilstrap

Previous editions of this textbook have chronicled the unprecedented change in the conduct of breech delivery in the USA: the rate of cesarean breech delivery rose sharply from 5–20% in the 1950s to 80% by 1980 [1]. In 1999 it was 84.5% [2]. This change is even more significant because the highly publicized Term Breech Trial [3], a multinational, multisite, randomized controlled trial, was not published until 2000. Based on the results of this trial, as well as other retrospective studies the American College of Obstetricians and Gynecologists (ACOG) issued a committee opinion [4] which stated that planned vaginal delivery of a singleton term breech may no longer be appropriate. However, it is the conviction of the authors of this chapter, and the editors of this textbook [5], that teaching the techniques of vaginal breech delivery is both necessary and appropriate. Evidence has accumulated since the publication of the Term Breech Trial that supports offering an attempt at vaginal breech delivery in very carefully selected and consenting women [6–11].

The objectives of this chapter are to review this recent evidence, to present reasonable and prudent selection criteria for women at term with breech presentation, and to describe proper technique for breech vaginal and abdominal delivery. Finally, it is stressed that the critical step between candidate selection and vaginal breech delivery is the astute management of labor in a woman with breech presentation at term.

Epidemiology

The incidence of term breech presentation is approximately 3–4%. Accurate determination of breech presentation during prenatal care, followed by referral for and successful completion of external cephalic version (ECV) may lower that incidence somewhat. The approximate breakdown by type of breech is: frank (65–70%), complete (5–10%), and footling (20–30%). In 2003, 87% of breech presentations underwent cesarean delivery [12]. It is not possible to determine how many of the vaginal deliveries were planned, nor to analyze the cesarean delivery rate by type of breech.

Maternal/perinatal outcomes following vaginal breech delivery (2000–06)

The Term Breech Trial [3] compared planned cesarean delivery with planned vaginal delivery for breech presentation at term. Maternal morbidity and mortality was not found to be different between groups. The impact of a uterine scar in a subsequent pregnancy, such as uterine rupture, placenta accreta, and the need for repeat cesarean delivery, was not considered. The salient and highly publicized conclusion of this trial was that planned cesarean delivery reduced perinatal mortality and serious neonatal morbidity by one-third. However, many of the deaths in the vaginal delivery arm were unrelated to the mode of delivery. Moreover, the definitions used for "serious neonatal morbidity" are at least debatable. Multiple letters to the editor and editorials have been written that take issue with either the conduct of the Term Breech Trial or the interpretation of the results. Such *post hoc* discussion is interesting but not germane to the readers of this textbook. The cesarean delivery rate prior to the publication of the Term Breech Trial was already high and it was predicted that more cesarean breech deliveries would occur after the trial. However, this has not been the case in all centers. Shown in Table 47.1 are data that have accumulated since the Term Breech Trial [6–11], demonstrating that vaginal breech delivery is still being conducted at individual centers. In addition, the success rate for attempted vaginal delivery at these centers is greater than or equal to that in the Term Breech Trial and morbidity and mortality in the vaginal breech group is significantly less than that reported in the trial though generally higher in the trial of labor/vaginal delivery groups. For each of the studies cited, the elective cesarean delivery rate was well below that in the USA. However, as noted in Table 47.1, none of the data came from centers in the USA. Importantly, relatively few reports of

Table 47.1 Summary of maternal and perinatal outcomes following vaginal breech delivery. All reports were published after the Term Breech Trial and all came from centers outside the USA.

Reference	Total breech (n)	Elective C/S	Allowed TOL	Successful TOL	Serious morbidity		Mortality	
					Vag	C/S	Vag*	C/S
[6]	841	349 (41.5%)	492 (58.5%)	254 (52%)	–	–	2	0
[7]†	809	427 (52.8%)	382 (47.2%)	284 (74.3%)	0.5%	0%	0	0
[8]	1433	552 (38.5%)	881 (61.5%)	416 (47.2%)	5.9%	0.9%	3	1
[9]	986	396 (40.2%)	590 (59.8%)	455 (77.1%)	1.2%	0.5%	1	1
[10]	699	218 (31.2%)	481 (68.8%)	352 (71%)	2.3%	0.5%	0	0
[11]	641	343 (53.5%)	298 (46.5%)	146 (49%)	0.7%	0%	3	0

C/S, cesarean section; TOL, trial of labor; Vag, vaginal.
* Of the total of nine deaths with vaginal delivery, only one [8] was related to mode of delivery.
† 73 cases were excluded from the 882 breeches reported by the authors.

vaginal breech delivery after the Term Breech Trial are expected to come from the USA, given the litigation risk, and those that do will have very small numbers. A report from the authors' institution illustrates this [13].

One exception to the small numbers is a population-based study from California where approximately 5000 vaginal breech deliveries were compared with 60,000 prelabor cesarean breech deliveries [14,15]. Neonatal mortality was lower than that reported in the Term Breech Trial. Morbidity was still increased for vaginal breech deliveries compared to elective cesarean deliveries. However, this report was based on birth certificate and maternal and neonatal hospital discharge data. Such methodology imposes significant limitations on the conclusions drawn: selection criteria for vaginal breech delivery were not reported, skill of the operator could not be assessed, and even the type of breech could not be verified. The following section elaborates on the importance of selection criteria, labor management, and delivery technique because they dramatically affect outcome.

Selection criteria for attempted vaginal breech delivery

The success rate for vaginal breech delivery is defined as the number delivering vaginally divided by the number attempting vaginal delivery. This rate varies between centers, but for the series of articles referenced in Table 47.1, it ranged between 49% and 77%. However, to compute the overall vaginal breech delivery rate, the success rate has to be multiplied by a "first term" which reflects the proportion of term breeches offered an attempt at vaginal breech delivery (see the equation below). This "first term" is also variable. In Table 47.1, this variability is in the range 46–69%, but the reader should recall that these reports all came from centers with a strong interest in vaginal

Table 47.2 Selection criteria for vaginal breech delivery.

Estimated fetal weight 2000–4000 g*
Complete or frank breech presentation
Fetal head flexed or military†
Adequate maternal pelvis‡
Normal fetal morphology
Experienced operator
Informed consent

* By either clinical or ultrasound estimation. Others [11] have suggested 2500–3800 g.
† Ultrasound or radiographic determination, not clinical.
‡ As determined by an experienced examiner or radiographically.

breech delivery. In the USA, the variability of this term is undoubtedly greater, because the low end of the range is lower (near zero in some centers). In other words, the fact that 87% of breeches are delivered abdominally in the USA implies that only a small minority of women actually attempt vaginal breech delivery. Of the two terms, it is the one most affected by selection criteria. It should be apparent to the reader that it is also the one that is influenced by the informed consent process.

$$\frac{\text{Vaginal breech}}{\text{delivery (VBD) rate}} = \frac{\text{Attempted VBD}}{\text{No. term breeches}} \times \frac{\text{Successful VBD}}{\text{Attempted VBD}}$$

In general, selection criteria for vaginal breech delivery can be considered lax or stringent. The more stringent the criteria, the smaller the proportion of term breech presentations allowed a trial of labor. So what are considered reasonable selection criteria? Those cited in Table 47.2 are open to criticism but they do provide a framework for clinicians to adapt to their local practice environments. These criteria are the ones in use at the authors' institutions. Two of the listed criteria are deserving of special emphasis: an experienced operator and a consenting patient. Operator experience will eventually diminish without training during residency, and experience affects all three areas covered in this section: selection criteria, management of labor, and conduct of vaginal breech delivery. Finally, the manner in which consent is obtained, the discussion of risks and benefits, along with alternatives, is often biased by the perception of medicolegal risk to the person obtaining the consent and caring for the patient.

Labor management

Once an appropriate candidate for vaginal breech delivery is identified, careful labor management is essential in order to achieve a good outcome. All studies report a 20–50% incidence of intrapartum cesarean delivery, commonly attributed to either nonreassuring fetal status or failure to progress. With regard to the former, electronic fetal heart rate monitoring (EFM) is recommended, although EFM has not been shown to be a clear benefit for vertex or breech presentations. If the fetal heart rate tracing is concerning enough to consider fetal blood sampling, prompt cesarean delivery is reasonable instead. The use of oxytocin for induction or augmentation has long been a point of contention in vaginal breech delivery. Alarab *et al.* [11] allowed neither but still achieved a respectable rate of vaginal breech delivery. At the authors' institutions, use of oxytocin for either induction or augmentation is permitted, but is individualized and used sparingly. In contrast, the Term Breech Trial had a combined rate of induction and augmentation of more than 60%.

The management of labor in breech presentations is more complex than simply interpreting fetal heart rate information and monitoring labor progress. Attention must be paid to position of the patient, timing and type of anesthesia, and emotional support and encouragement. In the second stage, the importance of coached pushing [16] has not been evaluated, nor has the incidence of second stage cesarean delivery. Timing and type of episiotomy may also be important factors. It is noteworthy that episiotomy is not necessary in all cases.

Technique of vaginal breech delivery

Once careful selection of candidates and astute labor management have allowed for the possibility of vaginal breech delivery, proper conduct of the delivery will minimize trauma and optimize overall outcome. Listed in Table 47.3 are a number of complications associated with, but not unique to, vaginal breech delivery. While not guaranteed to eliminate complications, the suggestions that appear in Table 47.4 should produce the best possible results. Despite the time-honored use of the

Table 47.3 Morbidity associated with breech delivery.

Intracranial hemorrhage	Pharyngeal diverticulum
Cervical spine injury	Brachial plexus palsy
Liver	Scrotal/testicular/labial trauma
Adrenal —— Blunt trauma	Skull fracture
Spleen	Long bone fracture
Bladder rupture	

Table 47.4 Suggestions for vaginal breech delivery.

Do	Do Not
Await spontaneous delivery to the umbilicus*	Pull on the fetus prematurely
Perform episiotomy as indicated	Grasp the fetal abdomen
Grasp the fetal pelvis over bony prominences (sacrum and iliac crests)	Put transverse pressure on long bones (risk of fracture)
Apply finger pressure parallel to long bones	Allow the fetus to rotate ventrally
Use forceps for the aftercoming head	Attempt vaginal delivery though an incompletely dilated cervix
If forceps not available, maintain flexion of aftercoming head with suprapubic pressure	Panic

* Except under unusual circumstances.

Mauriceau–Smellie–Veit maneuver, the authors favor the *routine* application of either Piper or Laufe forceps to the aftercoming head. Both Laufe and Piper forceps have a reverse pelvic curve to facilitate application to the aftercoming head from below. The low neonatal morbidity and mortality associated with vaginal breech delivery that we and others (Table 47.1) have reported make it feasible to continue to teach this technique to residents in training. The effectiveness of simulation training to acquire skill is intriguing but requires further evaluation [16].

Cesarean delivery for term breech presentation

Most of the suggestions for vaginal breech delivery listed in Table 47.4 apply equally to cesarean delivery of a breech. Proper placement of the hands of the operator on the bony pelvis of the infant can prevent some of the abdominal trauma listed in Table 47.3. Given that the current cesarean to vaginal delivery ratio is nearly 9:1, residents can be trained in the application of Laufe forceps to the aftercoming head at cesarean delivery [17]. Almost all cesarean deliveries for breech presentation are performed for fetal indications; that is, to prevent either birth injury or hypoxia/acidemia that are, albeit infrequently, associated with vaginal breech delivery. With that purpose in mind it is very important that the uterine incision be adequate to deliver the infant atraumatically.

Conclusions

Some women will still desire to attempt a vaginal delivery of a breech fetus. Other women with breech presentation will be seen for the first time in either advanced labor or with imminent delivery. Physicians will still be called upon to manage labor and vaginal delivery in these circumstances. Finally, some physicians remain unconvinced by the evidence against planned vaginal delivery and prefer to offer selected women a trial of labor and vaginal breech delivery. At some centers, additional experience with vaginal breech delivery can be gained via delivery of the second twin, but there are important distinctions between breech singleton and breech second twin. Total breech extraction is permissible for second twin but is rarely performed for a singleton. Continuing to train the next generation of obstetricians in the principles and conduct of vaginal breech delivery is imperative.

Case presentation

A 26-year-old G1P0, was admitted in active labor at 39 weeks' gestation. On examination, she was completely effaced, 5-cm dilated, and had a frank breech presentation confirmed by ultrasound. The fetal head was noted to be flexed and the ultrasound estimated fetal weight of 3150 g was consistent with a clinical estimate of 3400 g. Ultrasound examination revealed a morphologically normal fetus. Clinical pelvimetry was performed by two residents and an attending and the pelvis was deemed to be adequate for breech delivery. Radiographic pelvimetry was not obtained. The patient had received prenatal care from a midwife and was highly motivated to avoid cesarean delivery. She consented to vaginal breech delivery and requested and received epidural analgesia. She reached complete dilatation in 4 hours and her second stage lasted 45 minutes. Assisted vaginal breech delivery was performed by a second-year resident and a fourth-year resident placed Piper forceps to deliver the aftercoming head. A faculty with 25 years of experience supervised the labor and delivery. Apgar scores were 7 at 1 minute and 9 at 5 minutes. Mother and infant were discharged home on postpartum day 2, doing well.

References

1 Gimovsky ML, Petrie RH. Breech delivery: In: Queenan JT, ed. *Management of High-Risk Pregnancy*, 4th edn. Oxford; Blackwell Science, 1999: 495–500.

2 Ventura SJ, Martin JA, Curtin SC, Menacker F, Hamilton BE. Births: final data for 1999. *Natl Vital Stat Rep* 2001;**49**:1–100.

3 Hannah ME, Hannah WJ, Hewson SA, Hodnett ED, Saigal S, Willan AR, for the Term Breech Trial Collaborative Group. Planned caesarean section versus planned vaginal birth for breech presentation at term: a randomized multicentre trial. *Lancet* 2000;**356**:1375–83.

4 ACOG Committee Opinion. *Mode of Term Singleton Breech Delivery*. Number 265, December 2001.

5 Queenan JT. (Editorial) Teaching infrequently used skills: vaginal breech delivery. *Obstet Gynecol* 2004;**103**:405–6.

6 Lashen H, Fear K, Strudee D. Trends in the management of the breech presentation at term; experience in a District General hospital over a 10-year period. *Acta Obstet Gynecol Scand* 2002;**81**:1116–22.

7 Krupitz H, Arzt W, Ebner T, Sommergruber M, Steininger E, Tews G. Assisted vaginal delivery versus caesarean section in breech presentation. *Acta Obstet Gynecol Scand* 2005;**84**:588–92.

8 Pradhan P, Mohajer M, Deshpande S. Outcome of term breech births: 10-year experience at a district general hospital. *Br J Obstet Gynaecol* 2005;**112**:218–22.

9 Uotila J, Tuimala R, Kirkinen P. Good perinatal outcome in selective vaginal breech delivery at term. *Acta Obstet Gynecol Scand* 2005;**84**:578–83.

10 Giuliani A, Scholl WMJ, Basver A, Tamussino KF. Mode of delivery and outcome of 699 term singleton breech deliveries at a single center. *Am J Obstet Gynecol* 2002;**187**:1694–8.

11 Alarab M, Regan C, O'Connell MP, Keane DP, O'Herlihy C, Foley ME. Singleton vaginal breech delivery at term: still a safe option. *Obstet Gynecol* 2004;**103**:407–12.

12 Martin JA, Hamilton BE, Sutton PD, Ventura SJ, Menacker F, Munson ML. Births: final data for 2003. *Natl Vital Stat Rep* 2005;**54**:116.

13 Doyle NM, Riggs JW, Ramin SM, Sosa MA, Gilstrap LC. Outcomes of term vaginal breech delivery. *Am J Perinatol* 2005;**22**:325–8.

14 Gilbert WM, Hicks SM, Boe NM, Danielson B. Vaginal versus cesarean delivery for breech presentation in California: a population-based study. *Obstet Gynecol* 2003;**102**:911–7.

15 Bloom SL, Casey BM, Schaffer JI, McIntire DD, Leveno KJ. A randomized trial of coached versus uncoached maternal pushing during the second stage of labor. *Am J Obstet Gynecol* 2006;**194**:10–3.

16 Deering S, Brown J, Hodor J, Satin AJ. Simulation training and resident performance of singleton vaginal breech delivery. *Obstet Gynecol* 2006;**107**:86–9.

17 Locksmith GJ, Gei AF, Rowe TF, Yeomans ER, Hankins GD. Teaching the Laufe–Piper forceps technique at cesarean delivery. *J Reprod Med* 2001;**46**:457–61.

48 Obstetric analgesia and anesthesia

Gilbert J. Grant

The first "modern" recorded use of pain relief for childbirth was in 1847, when Dr. James Young Simpson administered ether to facilitate vaginal delivery for a woman with a deformed pelvis. Since that time, obstetric anesthesia practice has evolved from the use of systemic routes for analgesic administration (inhalation, intravenous, intramuscular) to regional administration of analgesics by the epidural and spinal routes. Currently, in the USA, more than 60% of parturients receive regional analgesia to manage their pain of childbirth. An advantage of the regional approach is that relatively low doses of analgesics reliably provide pain relief. Thus, the fetus is spared exposure to the relatively large doses of medication required when the systemic approach is used. Although the systemic route remains an option, it is currently used for a minority of parturients. This review describes current practices in obstetric anesthesia.

Labor and vaginal delivery

Consequences of unrelieved pain

The pain of childbirth, which is likely to be the most severe pain that a woman experiences [1], results in untoward physiologic effects [2]. The hyperventilation that accompanies labor pain causes profound hypocarbia, which may suppress the ventilatory drive between contractions and produce maternal hypoxemia and loss of consciousness [3]. The accompanying respiratory alkalosis interferes with fetal oxygenation by shifting the oxyhemoglobin dissociation curve in favor of the mother and by producing uteroplacental vasoconstriction [4]. The neurohumoral responses to stress and pain also conspire to adversely affect placental perfusion and fetal oxygenation. These changes are mediated by increases in circulating catecholamines, which decrease uterine blood flow [5]. Epidural analgesia lowers circulating maternal epinephrine, and effectively inhibits the respiratory [6] and neurohumoral [7] responses to pain, with a resultant increase in oxygen tension

in the parturient and fetus [8]. There is also evidence that unrelieved pain during childbirth may contribute to the development of postpartum psychologic problems including postpartum depression [9] and post-traumatic stress disorder (PTSD) [10].

Multimodal regional analgesia

Current methods for providing pain relief for labor and vaginal delivery are considerably different from the techniques that were used as recently as 15 years ago. Regional analgesia for childbirth has been transformed from a one-drug approach using a local anesthetic, to an approach in which different classes of analgesics are administered concurrently; most commonly, a local anesthetic and an opioid. Although local anesthetics produce profound analgesia, they indiscriminately block conduction in all nerves with which they come in contact, and therefore also produce unwanted effects: hypotension and motor block. Hypotension may decrease fetal oxygen delivery by reducing placental perfusion. Motor block may cause profound lower extremity weakness, which can be very distressing for the parturient. Moreover, profound motor and sensory block may interfere with effective pushing during the second stage, particularly if the parturient is unable to perceive rectal or vaginal pressure, as the presence of this pressure facilitates expulsive efforts.

The traditional approach to regional analgesia, in which a local anesthetic was used as the sole agent, changed when clinicians recognized the analgesic efficacy of opioids administered into the neuraxis. Unlike local anesthetics, which act by blocking nerve conduction, opioids injected into the neuraxis inhibit pain by binding to specific spinal opioid receptors. Opioids and local anesthetics act synergistically, so relatively low doses of each agent are required. This synergism is the rationale for the concurrent use of a combination of different types of analgesics, and is known as multimodal analgesia [11]. Some clinicians combine other classes of analgesics such as those that stimulate adrenergic (e.g., epinephrine, clonidine) and cholinergic (e.g., neostigmine) receptors to further potentiate analgesia.

A distinct advantage of multimodal analgesia is that it produces fewer side-effects than typically occur when a local anesthetic is used alone. The different classes of analgesics act through different mechanisms, and they also have distinct side-effect profiles. Furthermore, the likelihood of side-effects is reduced because with the multimodal approach, a relatively low dose of each component is used. The profound motor block that was a frequent accompaniment of high concentrations of local anesthetic does not occur with the low concentrations of local anesthetics that are part of the multimodal approach. Hypotension, which commonly occurred with epidural administration of high concentrations of local anesthetic, is also less likely to occur when low concentrations are administered.

Pruritus and nausea are the most common untoward effects that occur with neuraxial multimodal analgesic regimens, and are caused by the opioid component. These side-effects may be dose-related, and are more likely to occur with the relatively water-soluble opioid morphine, and less likely to occur with relatively lipophilic opioids such as fentanyl and sufentanil. Opioid side-effects may be treated by intravenous administration of specific opioid receptor antagonists such as naloxone, naltrexone, nalmefene, or nalbuphine. Fortunately, low doses of opioid antagonists selectively reverse the unwanted effects without appreciably affecting the analgesia. Another side-effect that may occur after intrathecal injection of opioid alone is fetal bradycardia or late decelerations of the fetal heart rate, as a result of uterine hyperactivity. This effect is twice as likely to occur after intrathecal administration of opioid alone than after epidural administration of local anesthetic and opioid (24% vs. 11%) [12]. The fetal bradycardia may be reversed by administration of a tocolytic, such as terbutaline or nitroglycerine.

For patients, the improved lower extremity mobility is perhaps the most noticeable effect of multimodal analgesia. Although commonly described as a "walking epidural," this term is a poor descriptor, as few parturients walk much during labor after their pain is relieved. Furthermore, the lack of motor block is not a result of the epidural approach per se, but may also be achieved with a spinal approach, or a combined spinal and epidural (combined spinal–epidural, CSE) approach. The primary determinant of motor block intensity is the concentration of local anesthetic, not its site of administration.

Epidural, spinal, and combined spinal–epidural analgesia

Safe and effective multimodal regional analgesia may be achieved by using the epidural or spinal routes, or a combination of both. An advantage of the epidural approach is that a catheter may be inserted into the epidural space to facilitate continuous and/or intermittent analgesic dosing to prolong the duration of pain relief. With spinal techniques, the duration of analgesia is limited to the duration of action of a single dose, as catheterization of the intrathecal space is rarely performed. The onset of analgesia is more rapid with the spinal approach (3–5 minutes) than it is with the epidural approach (approximately 10 minutes). The CSE approach offers the advantages of both the spinal and epidural techniques; rapid onset of analgesia and prolonged duration if needed.

The type of regional analgesia chosen for a particular patient depends on many factors. One of the most important determinants is the anticipated duration of labor. In early labor, when delivery is not expected for many hours, catheterization of the epidural space is indicated (epidural or CSE technique) to establish a conduit for administering multiple doses of analgesics. For an epidural technique, the analgesic medication is typically administered using a continuous infusion pump, perhaps with patient-controlled epidural analgesia (PCEA; see below). For a CSE technique, a dose of analgesics is administered intrathecally and then a catheter is inserted into the epidural space. The epidural analgesics may be administered either immediately after the intrathecal injection, or when the pain relief from the initial intrathecal dose begins to wane.

Epidural catheterization is a sensible approach at any time during labor for parturients who have a high likelihood of an instrumental or operative delivery, as it permits administration of additional anesthetics, should they be needed. If delivery is imminent, a single-shot spinal is a reasonable choice, because analgesia onset is rapid. However, these patients may benefit more from a CSE technique, as it requires little additional time compared to an epidural technique, and an indwelling epidural catheter may be quite helpful. The epidural catheter may be used to administer additional analgesics if delivery does not occur as quickly as anticipated, if the intrathecal medication does not produce adequate analgesia, or if an instrumental or operative delivery is required.

Patient-controlled epidural analgesia

Programmable, microprocessor-controlled infusion pumps facilitate precise administration of analgesics into the epidural space. Continuous infusion of analgesics is advantageous, as it avoids the peaks and valleys of pain and relief that occur with intermittent bolus dosing. PCEA is a further refinement of this technology. Originally introduced for intravenous use, PCEA enables the parturient to "fine-tune" her pain relief. PCEA may be administered using intermittent boluses exclusively, or intermittent boluses superimposed on a background infusion, which appears to be a superior strategy [13]. PCEA has many advantages over non-PCEA techniques including better analgesia and decreased anesthetic requirement, as well as improved patient satisfaction [14], because the patient feels empowered by having some control over her pain relief.

Ideally, PCEA is used to provide analgesia for the duration of labor and delivery. For some patients, the low dose delivered from the infusion pump may not be adequate for the late first stage and second stage of labor, when a somatic pain component is superimposed on the visceral pain input. Breakthrough pain that occurs during continuous epidural infusion is treated by increasing the rate of the infusion or by administration of a more concentrated dose of anesthetic as a "rescue dose." Ideally, with PCEA, the parturient titrates the analgesia to experience a sensation of pressure during the second stage of labor, while maintaining lower extremity motor strength. PCEA may be continued to provide analgesia through delivery. However, many practitioners prefer to halt the epidural administration of analgesics during the second stage of labor. These practitioners believe that curtailing epidural analgesia will increase the likelihood of spontaneous vaginal delivery. Although conclusive data are not yet available, a meta-analysis showed that discontinuing epidural analgesia did not decrease the incidence of instrumental deliveries, but did result in significant increases in pain [15].

Timing of regional pain relief

The optimal time for administering regional pain relief has been an issue plagued by misunderstanding and controversy for decades. Those opposed to "early" administration of epidural analgesia have claimed that it would somehow interfere with the progress and outcome of labor. Proponents of "early" administration of epidural analgesia have maintained that there is no proven deleterious effect on labor's progress or outcome, and that parturients should not be denied the right to have their pain relieved. Two recently published studies found that administration of regional analgesia prior to 4 cm cervical dilatation in nulliparous women did not influence the outcome of labor. Vahratian *et al.* [16] reviewed data during two 1-year intervals: before and after epidural use increased from 2% to 92% at Tripler Army Medical Center in Hawaii. They found that the timing of epidural administration did not affect the incidence of forceps or cesarean deliveries. In a prospective study, Wong *et al.* [17] compared the effect of CSE analgesia administered prior to 4 cm cervical dilatation to epidural analgesia initiated after 4 cm dilatation on the progress and outcome of labor. The women randomized to receive epidural analgesia had their initial pain managed with intravenous opioids. The rate of cesarean delivery was not statistically different whether the women received CSE analgesia prior to 4 cm (18%) or epidural analgesia after 4 cm dilatation (21%). Interestingly, labor progressed more rapidly in the women who received early regional analgesia. That group reached full cervical dilatation 89 minutes before the group that had their regional analgesia delayed until after 4 cm cervical dilatation [17]. These studies support the principle of allowing women to have pain relief whenever they choose, as the American College of Obstetricians and Gynecologists has noted "In the absence of a medical contraindication, maternal request is a sufficient medical indication for pain relief during labor" [18].

Cesarean delivery

Most cesarean deliveries in the USA are performed under regional anesthesia. Spinal anesthesia is most commonly used for planned cesarean deliveries, although epidural anesthesia and CSE anesthesia are also used. If the decision to perform a cesarean delivery is reached after labor has commenced, and the parturient is receiving epidural analgesia, surgical anesthesia is readily achieved by injecting a more concentrated dose of local anesthetic through the epidural catheter. Currently, in the USA, general anesthesia is used for 3–5% of planned and 15–30% of emergent cesarean deliveries [19]. The unconsciousness that accompanies general anesthesia increases the risk of pulmonary aspiration of gastric contents. A large survey found that maternal mortality associated with general and regional anesthesia was 32 and 2 per million cases, respectively [20], reinforcing the belief that regional anesthesia is inherently safer. In addition to the potential safety issues, general anesthesia-induced unconsciousness prevents the mother from experiencing the moment of birth. However, regional anesthesia is associated with its own unique potential side-effects, such as postspinal headache and, rarely, spinal hematoma, epidural abscess, meningitis, or nerve damage.

The status of the fetus is an important factor in determining the anesthetic choice. If urgent delivery of the fetus is indicated, and if there is no indwelling epidural catheter, general anesthesia is preferred. However, in some circumstances there may be sufficient time to induce spinal anesthesia. Epidural anesthesia is the least desirable choice if time is of the essence because of the prolonged latency of block onset compared to the spinal approach. Ultimately, the choice of anesthetic technique is influenced by a variety of factors including the urgency of the procedure, maternal and fetal status, and physician and patient preference.

Cesarean delivery requires a denser anesthetic block than labor analgesia, as surgical stimulation causes more intense pain than occurs during labor. A denser block is achieved by administering a relatively high concentration of local anesthetic, as much as 10-fold greater than is used to provide labor analgesia. This dose predictably produces a profound motor block. In addition, cesarean delivery necessitates a higher dermatomal anesthetic level than does labor analgesia. Whereas sensory block to the 10th thoracic dermatome is sufficient to provide labor analgesia, the anesthetic level must be extended to at least the 4th thoracic dermatome for cesarean delivery, lest the parturient perceives pain from intraoperative peritoneal manipulation.

Physiologic changes of pregnancy have important clinical implications for providing anesthesia for cesarean delivery. The gastroesophageal sphincter is relatively incompetent, increasing the risk of pulmonary aspiration of gastric contents when upper airway reflexes are compromised during induction of general anesthesia. Pain, anxiety, sedatives, and opiates contribute by prolonging intestinal transit time, increasing the risk of aspiration of gastric contents. Edema of upper airway tissues, especially in preeclamptic parturients, may render tracheal intubation more difficult. The greater basal metabolic rate and reduced pulmonary functional residual capacity predispose to the development of hypoxemia during the apneic interval that accompanies the induction of general anesthesia. Compression of the aorta and vena cava by the gravid uterus decreases venous return, cardiac output, and blood pressure. Thus, when the parturient is in the supine position, the uterus must be displaced off the great vessels by placing a wedge under the right hip (left uterine displacement).

Left uterine displacement does not eliminate the occurrence of maternal hypotension during induction of anesthesia. In contrast to the low concentrations of local anesthetic used for labor analgesia, which are unlikely to cause maternal hypotension, the higher concentrations used for cesarean delivery are very likely to produce hypotension. The reduction in blood pressure is caused by sympathetic block mediated vasodilatation, which causes pooling of blood in capacitance vessels. Hypotension is particularly likely to occur with spinal anesthesia (55–71% of women) [21]. Interestingly, spinal anesthesia is also associated with relatively greater fetal acidemia than epidural or general anesthesia [22]. Strategies to mitigate regional anesthesia-induced hypotension include prophylactic volume expansion with intravenous fluids and administration of vasopressors. Although prophylactic intravenous fluid administration does not prevent maternal hypotension resulting from regional anesthesia, it does reduce its incidence. Vasopressors, such as ephedrine and phenylephrine, reverse the regional anesthesia-induced hypotension. Mixed alpha- and beta-agonists such as ephedrine produce a greater degree of fetal acidosis than a pure alpha-agonist such as phenylephrine [23].

Postoperative analgesia

The pain that accompanies cesarean delivery has pathophysiologic consequences that may result in medical complications. For example, discomfort induced by moving about may limit ambulation and lead to the formation of venous thrombi. Remaining at bed rest promotes atelectasis, makes clearing of pulmonary secretions more difficult, and predisposes to pneumonia. Good pain relief may help to prevent these effects.

Systemically administered opiates have been the mainstay of postoperative pain relief regimens. On-demand intramuscular techniques have been largely replaced by intravenous patient-controlled analgesia (PCA). In comparison with intramuscular administration, intravenous PCA results in more reliable plasma levels and a more rapid onset of analgesia. Various opiates may be used for intravenous PCA, including morphine, fentanyl, and its congeners. For patients receiving regional anesthesia for cesarean delivery, postoperative analgesia is often provided by administration of opioids into the intrathecal or epidural space. Morphine (0.2–0.4 mg intrathecal; 2–4 mg epidural) is the most popular opioid for this application because of its relatively prolonged duration of action. A single morphine dose in the neuraxis provides analgesia for up to 24 hours. Bothersome side-effects, including pruritus and nausea, are treated with opioid antagonists (as outlined above). Respiratory depression, a feared side-effect of neuraxial opioids, is not likely to occur during the postpartum period, because of the persistence of pregnancy-associated increases in respiratory drive. Another option to provide excellent postoperative analgesia is PCEA. Whether an intravenous or neuraxial approach is used after cesarean delivery, administration of a nonsteroidal anti-inflammatory drug (NSAID) such as ibuprofen or ketorolac is helpful in potentiating the analgesia [24]. Furthermore, NSAIDs are particularly effective in relieving the cramping pain of postpartum uterine involution.

Case presentation

A 42-year-old G3P0 presents to the labor and delivery suite at 39 weeks' gestation with presumed rupture of membranes. She states she is experiencing severe pain in her lower abdomen with each uterine contraction. A pelvic examination confirms rupture of membranes, and finds cervical dilatation to be 2 cm; fetal head not engaged. The patient indicates her desire for pain relief. Her obstetrician and the anesthesiologist on duty are consulted. They agree that the patient is a candidate for regional analgesia, as rupture of membranes and a diagnosis of labor have committed the patient to delivery. The patient is offered and accepts epidural analgesia. An epidural catheter is sited at the L3–L4 interspace, and analgesia is initiated with 20 mL 0.06% bupivacaine and 0.4 µg/mL sufentanil. Analgesia is maintained with an infusion of the same solution at 6 mL/hour. PCEA is instituted giving the parturient the option of self-dosing 5 mL every 10 minutes. When her cervical dilatation reaches 8 cm, she states that her self-administered doses are no longer sufficient to relieve her pain, so the anesthesiologist administers a rescue dose of 5 mL 0.125% bupivacaine. Within 10 minutes, this provides relief of her pain, and afterwards she only senses rectal pressure with each contraction. After reaching full dilatation, she delivers a 3430 g baby boy over an intact perineum after a 78-minute second stage. Although she sensed pressure while she was pushing, she denied experiencing pain.

References

1 Melzack R. The myth of painless childbirth (the John J. Bonica lecture). *Pain* 1984;**19**:321–37.

2 Brownridge P. The nature and consequences of childbirth pain. *Eur J Obstet Gynecol Reprod Biol* 1995;**59**(Suppl):S9–15.

3 Burden RJ, Janke EL, Brighouse D. Hyperventilation-induced unconsciousness during labour. *Br J Anaesth* 1994;**73**:838–9.

4 Ralston DH, Shnider SM, DeLorimier AA. Uterine blood flow and fetal acid–base changes after bicarbonate administration to the pregnant ewe. *Anesthesiology* 1974;**40**:348–53.

5 Shnider SM, Wright RG, Levinson G, *et al*. Uterine blood flow and plasma norepinephrine changes during maternal stress in the pregnant ewe. *Anesthesiology* 1979;**50**:524–7.

6 Reynolds F, Sharma SK, Seed PT. Analgesia in labour and fetal acid–base balance: a meta-analysis comparing epidural with systemic opioid analgesia. *Br J Obstet Gynaecol* 2002;**109**:1344–53.

7 Shnider SM, Abboud TK, Artal R, *et al*. Maternal catecholamines decrease during labor after lumbar epidural anesthesia. *Am J Obstet Gynecol* 1983;**147**:13–5.

8 Bergmans MG, van Geijn HP, Hasaart TH, *et al*. Fetal and maternal transcutaneous PCO_2 levels during labour and the influence of epidural analgesia. *Eur J Obstet Gynecol Reprod Biol* 1996;**67**:127–32.

9 Hiltunen P, Raudaskoski T, Ebeling H, Moilanen I. Does pain relief during delivery decrease the risk of postnatal depression? *Acta Obstet Gynecol Scand* 2004;**83**:257–61.

10 Soet JE, Brack GA, DiIorio C. Prevalence and predictors of women's experience of psychological trauma during childbirth. *Birth* 2003;**30**:36–46.

11 Kehlet H, Dahl JB. The value of "multimodal" or "balanced analgesia" in postoperative pain treatment. *Anesth Analg* 1993;**77**:1048–56.

12 Van de Velde M, Teunkens A, Hanssens M, Vandermeersch E, Verhaeghe J. Intrathecal sufentanil and fetal heart rate abnormalities: a double-blind, double placebo-controlled trial comparing two forms of combined spinal epidural analgesia with epidural analgesia in labor. *Anesth Analg* 2004;**98**:1153–9.

13 Bremerich DH, Waibel HJ, Mierdl S, *et al*. Comparison of continuous background infusion plus demand dose and demand-only parturient-controlled epidural analgesia (PCEA) using ropivacaine combined with sufentanil for labor and delivery. *Int J Obstet Anesth* 2005;**14**:114–20.

14 Saito M, Okutomi T, Kanai Y, *et al*. Patient-controlled epidural analgesia during labor using ropivacaine and fentanyl provides better maternal satisfaction with less local anesthetic requirement. *J Anesth* 2005;**19**:208–12.

15 Torvaldsen S, Roberts CL, Bell JC, Raynes-Greenow CH. Discontinuation of epidural analgesia late in labour for reducing the adverse delivery outcomes associated with epidural analgesia. *Cochrane Database Syst Rev* 2004;CD004457.

16 Vahratian A, Zhang J, Hasling J, Troendle JF, Klebanoff MA, Thorp JM Jr. The effect of early epidural versus early intravenous analgesia use on labor progression: a natural experiment. *Am J Obstet Gynecol* 2004;**191**:259–65.

17 Wong CA, Scavone BM, Peaceman AM, *et al*. The risk of cesarean delivery with neuraxial analgesia given early versus late in labor. *N Engl J Med* 2005;**352**:655–65.

18 Goetzl LM. ACOG Committee on Practice Bulletins–Obstetrics. ACOG Practice Bulletin. Clinical Management Guidelines for Obstetrician-Gynecologists, Number 36, July 2002. Obstetric analgesia and anesthesia. *Obstet Gynecol* 2002;**100**:177–91.

19 Bucklin BA, Hawkins JL, Anderson JR, Ullrich FA. Obstetric anesthesia workforce survey: twenty-year update. *Anesthesiology* 2005;**103**:645–53.

20 Hawkins JL, Koonin LM, Palmer SK, Gibbs CP. Anesthesia-related deaths during obstetric delivery in the United States, 1979–1990. *Anesthesiology* 1997;**86**:277–84.

21 Rout CC, Rocke DA, Levin J, Gouws E, Reddy D. A reevaluation of the role of crystalloid preload in the prevention of hypotension associated with spinal anesthesia for elective cesarean section. *Anesthesiology* 1993;**79**:262–9.

22 Reynolds F, Seed PT. Anaesthesia for Caesarean section and neonatal acid–base status: a meta-analysis. *Anaesthesia* 2005;**60**:636–53.

23 Cooper DW, Carpenter M, Mowbray P, Desira WR, Ryall DM, Kokri MS. Fetal and maternal effects of phenylephrine and ephedrine during spinal anesthesia for cesarean delivery. *Anesthesiology* 2002;**97**:1582–90.

24 Pavy TJ, Paech MJ, Evans SF. The effect of intravenous ketorolac on opioid requirement and pain after cesarean delivery. *Anesth Analg* 2001;**92**:1010–4.

Procedures

A local anesthetic (e.g., 2–3 mL 1% lidocaine) may be used, but in most cases this is not necessary. We use a 22-gauge spinal needle and recommend a needle no larger than a 20-gauge. During the entire procedure, ultrasonographic monitoring with continuous visualization of the needle should be performed. Needle insertion should be performed with one smooth continuous motion until the tip is within the amniotic cavity (Fig. 49.1).

After the needle tip is satisfactorily positioned in the amniotic cavity, the stylet is removed. The first 1–2 mL which theoretically contain maternal cells from blood vessels, the abdominal wall, or the myometrium are usually discarded.

Twenty to 30 mL amniotic fluid is aspirated into sterile, disposable plastic syringes. It is preferable to use 10- or 20-mL syringes because only gentle traction on the barrel of the syringe is desirable or necessary. Overly vigorous traction in search of fluid, especially with a 30–50-mL syringe, can result in the amniotic membranes being drawn into the needle, obstructing flow. Once the amniotic fluid is obtained, it is either left in the labeled syringes or transferred into labeled flasks that are either transported at ambient temperature directly to the laboratory or are prepared for shipping.

Fetal heart activity should be documented again by ultrasonographic visualization following amniocentesis. Patients should be alerted that occasional cramping and loss of a small amount of amniotic fluid may occur shortly after the proce-

dure. Instructions to report excessive vaginal fluid loss, bleeding, or fever should be given. We recommend that strenuous exercise (e.g., jogging or aerobic exercises) and coitus be avoided for a day. Most other normal activities may be resumed immediately following the procedure.

Fetomaternal transfusion caused by disruption of the fetoplacental circulation might occur and have an immunizing effect. While the magnitude of the risk has not been determined, the American College of Obstetricians and Gynecologists recommends that 300 µg Rh-immunoglobulin (RhIG) be administered to all Rh negative woman. This should be carried out irrespective of whether the needle has traversed the placenta [6].

Multiple gestations

Amniocentesis can be performed on each fetus in a multiple gestation, provided the amniotic fluid volume is adequate [7]. In addition to the ultrasound evaluation performed for singletons, the location of the placentas and identification of the dividing membrane is observed and documented. Aspiration of amniotic fluid from the first sac is performed as for a singleton. Prior to removing the needle, 2–3 mL indigo carmine or Evans blue dye is injected, diluted 1 : 10 in bacteriostatic water. After the membrane separating the two sacs has been revisualized, a second amniocentesis is performed into the sac of the second fetus. Aspiration of clear fluid confirms that the second sac has truly been entered (Fig. 49.2). Methylene blue should never be used as an indicator because it has been associated with jejunoileal atresia and fetal death following intra-amniotic injection [8]. Amniocentesis can be performed successfully in almost all twin pregnancies with apparently no increased risks over that of amniocentesis in singleton pregnancies [7,9].

Triplets (and presumably gestations of greater multiplicity) can be managed by sequentially injecting dye into successive sacs following withdrawal of clear amniotic fluid from each sac. The number of aspirations of clear amniotic fluid should equal the number of fetuses. As long as clear fluid can be aspirated, one can be reassured that a new amniotic sac has been entered.

Safety

Risks of mid-trimester amniocentesis can be divided into those affecting the mother and those affecting the fetus. Maternal risks are quite low, with amnionitis occurring only rarely. However, cases of maternal sepsis, some of which have led to maternal death, have been reported [10]. These are usually associated with bowel flora such as *Escherichia coli* and underscore the importance of avoiding inadvertent bowel penetration during the procedure. Minor maternal complications such as transient vaginal spotting and minimal amniotic fluid leakage occur after 1% or less of procedures and almost always

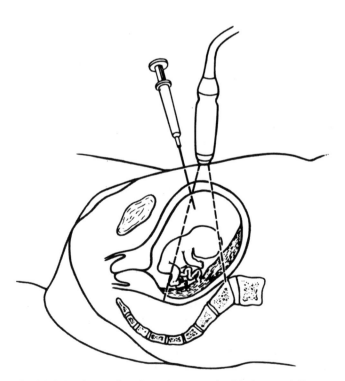

Fig. 49.1 Amniocentesis performed concurrently with ultrasound. (From Simpson and Elias [59] with permission.)

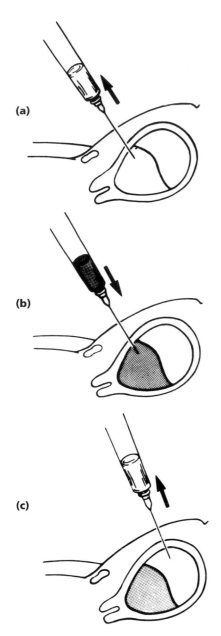

Fig. 49.2 Technique of amniocentesis in twin gestations, performed under concurrent ultrasound guidance. (a) Fluid aspirated from the first amniotic sac. (b) Indigo carmine injected into the first amniotic sac. (c) Second tap in the ultrasonographically determined location of the second fetus. Clear fluid confirms that the second amniotic sac was successfully aspirated. (From Elias *et al.* [7] with permission.)

are self-limited. Even significant fluid leakage will usually spontaneously resolve with bed rest [11]. Other very rare complications include intra-abdominal viscous injury and hemorrhage.

The most concerning complication of amniocentesis is the risk of procedure-induced miscarriage. Only one study has evaluated this in a prospective randomized fashion, compar-

ing woman having amniocentesis with those having no procedure. This trial involved 4606 women aged 25–34 years who were without known risk factors for fetal genetic abnormalities [12]. Women with three or more previous spontaneous abortions, diabetes mellitus, multiple gestation, uterine anomalies, or intrauterine contraceptive devices were excluded. Maternal age, social group, smoking history, number of previous induced and spontaneous abortions, stillbirths, live births, and low-birthweight infants were comparable in the study and control groups, as was gestational age at the time of entry into the study. Amniocentesis was performed under real-time ultrasound guidance with a 20-gauge needle by experienced operators. The total spontaneous abortion rate after 16 weeks was 1.7% in the amniocentesis patients compared with 0.7% in control subjects ($P=0.01$) (95% confidence interval [CI], 0.3–1.5; relative risk [RR] 2.3). Respiratory distress syndrome was diagnosed more often (RR 2.1) in the study group and more infants were treated for pneumonia (RR 2.5).

Recently, Seeds [13] performed a meta-analysis of studies evaluating the pregnancy loss risk associated with second trimester amniocentesis. Overall, 68,119 amniocenteses from both controlled and uncontrolled studies were included and provided a substantive basis for several conclusions:

1 Contemporary amniocentesis with concurrent ultrasound guidance in controlled studies appears to be associated with a procedure-related rate of excess pregnancy loss of 0.6% (95% CI, 0.31–0.90).

2 The use of concurrent ultrasound guidance appears to reduce the number of punctures and the incidence of bloody fluid.

3 Direct fetal needle trauma is rare, but may occur more frequently than is reported because of a failure to diagnose and a failure of consistent production of sequelae.

4 There is no additional risk of pregnancy loss if placental puncture is required.

Based on this information, patients undergoing second trimester amniocentesis should be counseled that there is approximately a 1.5% pregnancy loss rate following the procedure. Of these, approximately 1 in 3 are procedure-induced; so the risk of a procedure-induced pregnancy loss is approximately 1 in 200 to 1 in 300 sampled pregnancies.

Early amniocentesis (<14 weeks' gestation)

In recent years some obstetricians have recommended earlier amniocentesis (<14 weeks' gestation) as an alternative to CVS for patients who desire prenatal diagnosis. However, recent randomized controlled studies have shown that these earlier procedures have an increased procedure-induced pregnancy loss rate and a 10-fold increased risk of club foot [14–21]. Accordingly, it is currently recommended that amniocentesis not be performed prior to 14 weeks and preferably be deferred until 15 weeks or later.

Chorionic villus sampling

Chorionic villus sampling involves suction aspiration of individual villi from the site of the developing placenta (chorion frondosum). The procedure can be performed by either a transcervical approach using a catheter or transabdominally using a needle. Studies have shown that the sampling routes are equally safe [22], with the best results coming from centers skilled in both procedures. This assures sampling of any placental location and allows the operator to choose the safest approach for each patient.

Technique

Transcervical chorionic villus sampling

The optimal time for transcervical sampling is 11–13 weeks 6 days. Prior to CVS, fetal viability and normal fetal growth are confirmed by ultrasound. In addition, ultrasound is used to identify the location of the placenta, evaluate uterine position, assure appropriate bladder filling, eliminate the possibility of additional demised gestational sacs that could contaminate the sample, locate uterine contractions that may distort the sampling path, and image the cervix as it enters into the uterine cavity.

The procedure is performed with a plastic catheter with a 1.5-mm external diameter which encloses a metal obturator ending in a blunt tip which extends just distal to the tip of the cannula. Absolute contraindications include maternal blood group sensitization and active cervical infection with gonorrhea or herpes.

The patient is placed in the lithotomy position. The vagina is cleansed with povidone-iodine solution, a speculum inserted sterilely and the cervix and vagina further cleansed. A catheter with its encased obturator is curved slightly and introduced transcervically under concurrent ultrasonographic visualization. The device is directed into the placenta, parallel to its long axis (Fig. 49.3). It is important that the catheter is inserted into the chorion frondosum and avoids injury to the membranes or decidua. This is assured by choosing a tissue plane that offers no resistance as the catheter is advanced. Once the catheter is well within the placenta, the obturator is withdrawn and the catheter connected to a 20- or 30-mL syringe containing approximately 5 mL tissue culture medium and a small amount of heparin. Chorionic villi are obtained by slowly removing the catheter as negative pressure is created by retracting the syringe plunger. An adequate sample is at least 5 mg (approximately five moderate-sized villi), but 10–25 mg is preferred.

Adequacy of the sample should be confirmed immediately after retrieval by direct visualization of the villi floating in the syringe. It is important to differentiate villi from the small amount of decidua that is usually also present. Villi have a

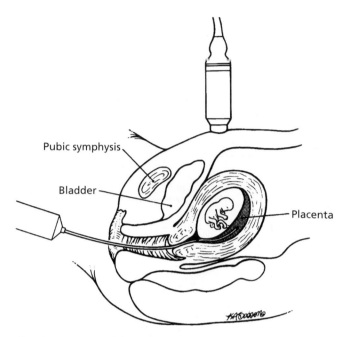

Fig. 49.3 Transcervical chorionic villus sampling.

branching frond-like appearance whereas decidua is amorphous. If necessary, a dissecting microscope can be used to confirm the adequacy of the sample. If additional villi are required, a second attempt is performed with a new catheter. In general, two aspirations can be safely performed. On rare occasions, three attempts may be required but the risk of pregnancy loss is slightly increased when this is necessary.

Villi are retained in a transport medium and transferred to the laboratory, where they are dissected free of decidua and blood clots using fine forceps. Cytogenetic studies are performed either by direct harvest (cytotrophoblast cells) after an overnight incubation or after establishment of *in situ* cultures (mesenchymal core cells) that are harvested at 5–8 days. Chorionic villi can also be processed for DNA or enzymatic analyses.

Following CVS, fetal heart activity is verified by ultrasonography and the patient discharged. Patients are informed that a small amount of bleeding or spotting is not unusual and is without consequence. They should notify the physician of heavy bleeding, leakage of fluid, or fever. Unsensitized Rh-negative patients are given RhIG. Maternal serum AFP screening for fetal neural tube defects or a detailed ultrasound is necessary at 15–18 weeks' gestation; AFP assay results are not affected by the prior invasive procedure.

Transabdominal chorionic villus sampling

Transabdominal CVS is now widely used as a complement to transcervical sampling. Placentas especially amenable to this approach include those located in the fundus or anteriorly in a slightly anteflexed uterus. Samples retrieved transabdominally are usually smaller, making the transcervical approach preferable when larger samples are required for complex laboratory analysis.

The patient is placed in the supine position. An insertion path that avoids the bowel and bladder and allows the needle to be placed within the placenta, parallel to the chorionic membrane, is chosen by ultrasonographic examination. The abdominal skin is cleansed with povidone-iodine solution, and the abdominal area draped in a fashion similar to amniocentesis. The skin may be infiltrated with local anesthetic but this is usually not necessary because any discomfort usually occurs secondary to uterine puncture. A standard 20-gauge spinal needle with stylet is inserted percutaneously through the maternal abdominal wall and myometrium. The tip is advanced into the long axis of the placenta under concurrent ultrasound monitoring (Fig. 49.4). Once in place, the stylet is withdrawn and a 20-mL syringe containing approximately 5 mL of media and heparin is attached to the needle and the plunger pulled back until moderate pressure is felt. Some centers will attach a biopsy aspiration device (Cook Ob/Gyn, Spencer, IN) to the syringe to facilitate one-handed retrieval.

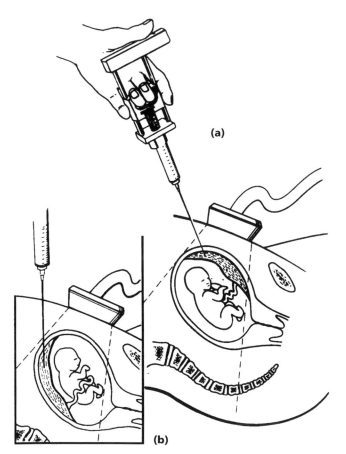

Fig. 49.4 Transabdominal chorionic villus sampling performed: (a) in an anterior placenta; and (b) in a posterior placenta.

We have found this to be unnecessary. Chorionic villi are obtained by performing approximately 3–7 passes through the placenta remaining parallel to the membrane. With each of these passes the needle is slightly redirected to sample different sites. The needle is then withdrawn under continuous negative pressure. The amount of villi obtained by transabdominal CVS is about half that usually obtained by transcervical aspiration [23]. However, such smaller amounts are still adequate for diagnostic testing. If a repeat sampling is required, a new needle is used.

Variations in technique for transabdominal CVS have been proposed. In addition to the "freehand technique" described above, others have used needles with cutting abilities and double-needle systems with an 18-gauge, thin-walled, outer needle guide and a 20-gauge sampling needle. In our center we find that a biopsy guide is quite helpful in defining the exact site and angle for needle insertion.

Transabdominal CVS may also be used in the late second and third trimesters for performing rapid fetal karyotype analysis, thus offering an alternative to cordocentesis and late amniocentesis. Transcervical CVS cannot be used for this purpose.

Safety comparisons

Pregnancy loss after chorionic villus sampling

Although post-CVS loss rates (calculated from the time of the procedure until 28 weeks' gestation) are approximately 1% greater than those after amniocentesis (2.5% vs. 1.5%), this comparison fails to take into consideration that the background miscarriage rate at 11–13 weeks is approximately 1% greater than at 15–16 weeks. To compare the two procedures appropriately, studies must enroll all patients in the first trimester, assign them to either approach, and then calculate the frequency of all subsequent losses, including spontaneous and induced abortions. In 1989, the Canadian Collaborative CVS/Amniocentesis Clinical Trial Group [24] reported such a prospective randomized trial and demonstrated equivalent safety of CVS and second trimester amniocentesis. In over 2650 patients assigned to either procedure, there was a 7.6% loss rate in the CVS group and a 7.0% loss rate in the amniocentesis group (95% CI, 0.92–1.30; RR 1.10). No significant differences were noted in the incidence of preterm birth, low birthweight, or rate of maternal complication. The investigators concluded that these data "may reassure women on the safety of first trimester CVS" [24].

A multicenter, prospective, nonrandomized study has been performed in the USA and enrolled 2235 women in the first trimester who chose either transcervical CVS or second trimester amniocentesis [25]. An excess pregnancy loss rate of 0.8% in the CVS group over the amniocentesis group was calculated, which was not statistically significant. Repeated catheter insertions were significantly associated with pregnancy loss, with cases requiring three or more passes having a 10.8% spontaneous abortion rate, compared with 2.9% in cases that required only one pass.

Eight US centers later participated in a second National Institute of Child Health and Human Development (NICHD) sponsored collaborative study to address the relative safety of transcervical and transabdominal CVS [22]. Subjects in whom either procedure was technically feasible were randomized into transabdominal and transcervical arms. Loss rates were nearly identical in the two groups. With availability of both transcervical and transabdominal CVS, total loss rates decreased over the rate seen in the initial trial described above, which only included transcervical CVS, obliterating even the nonsignificant arithmetic difference between amniocentesis and CVS loss rates.

Further information comes from a Danish randomized trial [26] which assigned 1068 patients to transcervical CVS, 1078 to transabdominal CVS, and 1158 to second trimester amniocentesis. There was no difference in loss rates between transabdominal CVS and amniocentesis (95% CI, 0.66–1.23; RR 0.9). Overall, there was a slight increased risk of pregnancy loss following CVS (95% CI, 1.01–1.67; RR 1.30) compared with amniocentesis which was completely accounted for by an excess of losses in the group sampled transcervically (95% CI, 1.30–2.22; RR 1.70); the technique with which this group of investigators had the least experience. Excess loss following transcervical CVS has not been replicated in four other direct comparisons [22,27–29].

A prospective, randomized, collaborative comparison of more than 3200 pregnancies, sponsored by the European Medical Research Council, reported that CVS had a 4.6% greater pregnancy loss rate than amniocentesis (95% CI, 1.24–1.84; RR 1.51) [30]. The present consensus is that operator inexperience with CVS accounts for the discrepancy between this trial in which operators were only required to perform 30 "practice procedures" and the other major studies performed by physicians already performing CVS in clinical practice. The US trial consisted of seven experienced centers and the Canadian trial 11, whereas the Medical Research Council trial used 31. There were, on average, 325 cases per center in the US study, 106 in the Canadian study, and 52 in the European trial.

CVS, particularly the transcervical approach, has a relatively prolonged learning curve. Saura et al. [31] suggested that over 400 cases may be required before safety is maximized. The role of experience as demonstrated by three sequential NICHD sponsored trials is of interest. In three sequential studies in which the majority of operators remained relatively constant, the post-procedure loss rate following CVS fell from 3.2% in the initial trial performed 1985–87, [25] to 2.4% for the trial performed 1987–89 [22] to only 1.3% in their most recent experience of 1997–2001 [19]. These data strongly suggest the value of operator experience.

Limb reduction defects

Firth et al. [32,33] reported five occurrences of severe limb abnormalities out of 289 pregnancies sampled by CVS between 56 and 66 days. Four of these cases had the unusual but severe oromandibular-limb hypogenesis syndrome, which occurs in the general population at a rate of 1 in 175,000 births [34]. Burton et al. [35] then reported on 14 more post-CVS cases of limb reduction defects (LRD) ranging from mild to severe, only two of which occurred when sampling was performed beyond 9.5 weeks. Alternatively, the World Health Organization (WHO) gathered data and concluded that CVS was not associated with LRD when performed after 8 completed weeks of pregnancy [34,36]. The infrequent occurrence of LRD after CVS was echoed by the American College of Obstetricians and Gynecologists, who stated that a risk for LRD of 1 in 3000 would be a prudent upper limit for counseling patients [37]. The WHO experience has been expanded and now contains information on 216,381 procedures [38]. These data have been used to analyze the frequency of limb anomalies, their pattern, and their associated gestational age at sampling. No overall increased risk of LRD or any difference in the pattern of defects was identified when compared with the general population. To investigate a possible temporal relationship between CVS and LRD, a subset of 106,383 cases was stratified by the week at which the procedure was performed. The incidence of LRD was 11.7, 4.9, 3.8, 3.4, and 2.3 per 10,000 CVS procedures in weeks 8, 9, 10, 11, and more than 12, respectively. Only the rate at week 8 exceeded the background risk of 6.0 per 10,000 births. The association of LRD and early gestational age sampling has been further supported in reports by Brambati et al. [39] and Wapner et al. [40]. Brambati et al. [39] had a LRD incidence of 1.6% for procedures performed in weeks 6 and 7, 0.1% in week 8, and 0.059% (population frequency) in week 9. The association of structural anomalies with early CVS as well as early amniocentesis demonstrates that gestational age "windows of vulnerability" exist for any prenatal diagnostic procedure and should serve as a warning when any new test is developed. Patients can be reassured that performing CVS in the gestational window of 10–13 weeks does not increase the risk of any type of LRD. CVS sampling before 10 weeks is not recommended, except in very unusual circumstances, such as when a patient's religious beliefs may preclude a pregnancy termination beyond a specific gestational age [4]. However, these patients must be informed that the incidence of severe LRD could be as high as 1–2%.

Finally, the Committee on Genetics of the American College of Obstetricians and Gynecologists [37] considered all the above data and rendered the following conclusions and recommendations:

• Transcervical and transabdominal CVS, when performed at 10–12 weeks' gestation, are relatively safe and accurate procedures and may be considered acceptable alternatives to mid-trimester genetic amniocentesis.

- Until further information is available, CVS for clinical application should not be performed before 10 weeks' gestation.
- CVS requires appropriate genetic counseling before the procedure is performed, an operator experienced in performing the technique, and a laboratory experienced in processing the villus specimen and interpreting the results. Counseling should include comparing and contrasting the risks and benefits of amniocentesis and CVS.
- Although further studies are needed to determine whether there is an increased risk of transverse digital deficiency following CVS performed at 10–12 weeks' gestation, it is prudent to counsel patients that such an outcome is possible and that the estimated risk may be in the order of 1 in 3000 births.

Diagnostic studies

Cytogenetics

Analysis of either chorionic villi or amniotic fluid cells has certain pitfalls that should be recognized by the obstetrician [41–43]. First, cells may not grow, or growth may be insufficient to perform analyses. Although now uncommon, failure of amniotic cell cultures still occurs. Chorionic villus cultures are likewise usually successful and in fact, may require fewer days for growth than amniotic fluid cell cultures.

A second potential laboratory problem is that *in vitro* chromosome aberrations may arise in amniotic fluid or villus cultures. In fact, cells containing at least one additional structurally abnormal chromosome are detected in 1–3% of all amniotic cell cultures [42]. If such cells are confined to a single culture flask or clone, the phenomenon is termed pseudomosaicism and is not considered clinically important. If a chromosome abnormality is detected in more than one flask or clone, true mosaicism is said to exist, and is considered clinically significant.

While amniocentesis has been available for over three decades, CVS is a relatively new procedure and has required almost 10 years to understand the unique aspects of evaluating placental tissue. As opposed to cells retrieved by amniocentesis, which are predominantly extravasated fetal cells, chorionic villi have three major components: an outer layer of hormonally active syncytiotrophoblast, a middle layer of cytotrophoblast from which syncytiotrophoblast cells are derived, and an inner mesodermal core containing fetal blood capillaries. The cytotrophoblast has a high mitotic index, with many spontaneous mitoses available for immediate chromosome analysis, whereas the mesenchymal core requires culture. Because these multiple tissue sources arise from slightly different lineages, the reliability of CVS results needed to be confirmed.

We now know with certainty that genetic evaluation of chorionic villi provides a high degree of accuracy; particularly in regard to the diagnosis of common trisomies. The US collaborative study revealed a 99.7% rate of successful cytogenetic diagnosis, with only 1.1% of the patients requiring a second diagnostic test, such as amniocentesis or fetal blood analysis, to further interpret the results [43,44]. In most cases, the additional testing was required to delineate the clinical significance of mosaic or other ambiguous results (76%), whereas laboratory failure (21%) and maternal cell contamination (3%) also required follow-up testing. As laboratories have become more familiar with handling and interpreting villus material and operators have become more skilled in obtaining adequately sized samples, the need for additional evaluation has continued to decrease.

Maternal cell contamination

Chorionic villus samples typically contain a mixture of placental villi and maternally derived decidua. Although specimens are thoroughly cleaned and separated under a microscope, some maternal cells may occasionally remain and grow in culture. As a result, two cell lines, one fetal and the other maternal, may be identified. In other cases, the maternal cell line may completely overgrow the culture, thereby leading to diagnostic errors, including incorrect sex determination [43,44], and potentially to false negative diagnoses, although there are no published reports of the latter. Direct preparations of chorionic villi are generally thought to prevent maternal cell contamination, whereas long-term culture has a rate varying from 1.8% to 4%. Fortunately, when this occurs, the contaminating cells are easily identified as maternal and should not lead to clinical errors. Contamination of samples with significant amounts of maternal decidual tissue occurs more frequently with a small sample size, making selection of appropriate tissue by the laboratory difficult. In experienced centers in which adequate quantities of villi are available and laboratory personnel are skilled in villus preparation, this problem has disappeared [44,45]. Choosing only whole, clearly typical villus material and discarding any atypical fragments, small pieces, or fragments with adherent decidua will avoid confusion. Therefore, if at the time of sampling the initial aspiration is small, a second pass should be performed rather than risk inaccurate results. When proper care is taken and good cooperation and communication exist between the sampler and the laboratory, prevention of even small amounts of contaminating maternal tissue can be accomplished.

Confined placental mosaicism

Another potential associated with CVS is mosaicism confined to the placenta [46]. Although the fetus and placenta have a common ancestry, chorionic villus tissue will not always reflect fetal genotype [44]. Although initially there was concern that this might invalidate CVS as a prenatal diagnostic tool, subsequent investigations have led to a clearer understanding of villus biology, so that accurate clinical interpretation is now possible and may in some cases add clinically relevant information. It should be recalled that mosaicism also occurs in 0.25% of amniotic cell cultures and is only confirmed in 70–80% of abortuses or live births [42,47].

Discrepancies between the cytogenetics of the placenta and fetus can occur because early in development the cells contributing to the chorionic villi become separate and distinct from those forming the embryo. Specifically, at approximately the 32–64-cell stage, only 3–4 cells become the inner cell mass and form the embryo, whereas the remainder become precursors of the extra embryonic tissues. Mosaicism can then occur through two possible mechanisms [48].

An initial meiotic error in one of the gametes can lead to a trisomic conceptus that normally would spontaneously abort. However, if during subsequent mitotic divisions one or more of the early aneuploid cells loses one of the trisomic chromosomes through anaphase lag, the embryo can be "rescued" by reduction of a portion of its cells to disomy. This will result in a mosaic morula with the percentage of normal cells dependent on the cell division at which rescue occurred. Because only a small proportion of cells are incorporated into the inner cell mass and perhaps because the embryo is less tolerant of aneuploid cells than the placenta, the abnormal cells are frequently isolated in the extra fetal tissues resulting in "confined placental mosaicism."

In the second mechanism, mitotic postzygotic errors produce a mosaic morula or blastocyst with the distribution and percent of aneuploid cells dependent on the timing of nondisjunction. If mitotic errors occur early in the development of the morula, they may segregate to the inner cell mass and have the same potential to produce an affected fetus as do meiotic errors. Mitotic errors occurring after primary cell differentiation and compartmentalization has been completed lead to cytogenetic abnormalities in only one lineage.

The mechanism of meiotic (trisomy) rescue can lead to uniparental disomy (UPD). This occurs when the original trisomic cell containing two chromosomes from one parent and one from the other expels the unmatched chromosome, resulting in progenitor cells containing a pair of chromosomes from a single parent. UPD has clinical consequences when the chromosome pair involved carries imprinted genes in which expression is based on the parent of origin. For example, Prader–Willi syndrome may result from uniparental maternal disomy for chromosome 15. Therefore, a CVS diagnosis of confined placental mosaicism for trisomy 15 may be the initial clue that UPD may be present. Because of this, when trisomy 15 (either complete or mosaic) is confined to the placenta, evaluation for UPD by amniotic fluid analysis is required [49,50]. In addition, chromosomes 7, 11, 14, and 22 are believed to be imprinted and require similar follow-up [51].

Confined placental mosaicism unassociated with UPD has been shown to alter placental function and lead to fetal growth failure or perinatal death [52–54]. Although the effect is limited to specific chromosomes, the exact mechanism by which the presence of an abnormal cell line within the placenta alters function is unknown. The most striking example of the clinical impact of confined placental mosaicism occurs with trisomy 16. Confined placental mosaicism for chromosome 16 most often leads to severe intrauterine growth restriction, prematurity, or perinatal death, with less than 35% of pregnancies resulting in normal, appropriate-for-gestational-age, full-term infants [53,55–57].

Enzymatic and DNA analyses

Most biochemical diagnoses that can be made from amniotic fluid or cultured amniocytes can also be made from chorionic villi [5]. In many cases, the results are available more rapidly and efficiently when villi are used because sufficient enzyme or DNA is present to allow direct analysis rather than requiring tissue culture. However, for certain rare biochemical diagnosis, villi will not be an appropriate or reliable diagnostic source [58]. To ensure that appropriate testing is possible, the laboratory should be consulted before sampling.

Because many of these disorders are autosomal recessive or X-linked and have a 25% or greater risk of resulting in an affected pregnancy, performing prenatal diagnosis by amniocentesis is not recommended because:

1 The procedure is usually not carried out until 15 weeks' gestation or later, compared to 10–12 weeks' gestation for CVS; and

2 Amniocentesis does not yield sufficient DNA for many analyses without additional weeks of cell culture [41].

There are potential pitfalls of CVS including maternal cell contamination, failure to optimize laboratory conditions for chorionic villi analyses (e.g., appropriate controls matched for gestational age), or investigator inexperience with a particular assay.

Case presentation

Mrs Smith is a 29-year-old G1P0 presenting for genetic counseling at 12 weeks' gestation because of a first trimester combined screen giving her a 1 in 100 risk of fetal Down syndrome.

After a complete pedigree is performed and no other genetic risks are identified, the patient is informed that because of her increased risk of aneuploidy she may wish to consider undergoing invasive prenatal diagnosis. At 12 weeks' gestation the preferred procedure is CVS. She is informed that although there is approximately a 2.5% risk of pregnancy loss following the procedure, most of these miscarriages are unrelated to the sampling. The procedure-induced risk of loss is approximately 1 in 200. This is a similar risk compared to amniocentesis so there is no advantage to waiting until 16 weeks to have an amniocentesis performed. She is also informed that previous concerns that CVS may cause fetal LRD do not apply because this does not occur if the procedure is performed after the 10th week.

Other potential risks include a small chance of bleeding and spotting. Rare complications include leakage of fluid and maternal infections. She is informed that the results of the CVS karyotype are very accurate but in approximately 1% of cases an extra cell line may be present in the placenta which may require further evaluation including amniocentesis.

The patient decides to undergo the CVS procedure. Prior to the procedure her physician performs a cervical culture for gonococcus which is negative. Her blood type is checked and she is found to be A negative with a negative antibody screen. She has a transcervical CVS procedure without difficulty and receives 300 µg RhIG immediately following the CVS. In 7 days, she receives a call from the genetic counselor telling her that she is having a chromosomally normal son. She is advised that CVS does not test for spina bifida so that at 16 weeks she should have a maternal serum AFP drawn and an ultrasound to evaluate fetal anatomy.

References

1 Wapner R, Thom E, Simpson JL, *et al*. First-trimester screening for trisomes 21 and 18. *N Engl J Med* 2003;**349**:1405–13.

2 Malone FD, Carnick JA, Ball RH, *et al*. First and second trimester evaluation of risk for fetal anueploidy (FASTER): principal results of NICHD multicenter Down syndrome screening study. *N Engl J Med* 2005;**353**:2001–11.

3 Nicolaides KH. Nuchal translucency and other first-trimester sonographic markers of chromosomal abnormalities. *Am J Obstet Gynecol* 2004;**191**:45–67.

4 Wald NJ, Rodeck C, Hackshaw AK, *et al*. First and second trimester antenatal screening for Down's syndrome: the results of the Serum, Urine and Ultrasound Screening Study (SURUSS). *Health Technol Assess* 2003;**7**:1–77.

5 Poenaru L. First trimester prenatal diagnosis of metabolic diseases: a survey in countries from the European community. *Prenat Diagn* 1987;**7**:333–41.

6 American College of Obstetricians and Gynecologists. *Prevention of D isoimmunization*. ACOG Technical Bulletin No. 147, October 1990.

7 Elias S, Gerbie AB, Simpson JL, *et al*. Genetic amniocentesis in twin gestations. *Am J Obstet Gynecol* 1980;**138**:169–74.

8 Wapner RJ. Genetic diagnosis in multiple pregnancies. *Prenat Diagn* 1995;**19**:351–62.

9 Anderson RL, Goldberg JD, Goldbus M. Prenatal diagnosis in multiple gestations: 20 years experience with amniocentesis. *Prenat Diagn* 1991;**11**:263–70.

10 Thorp JA, Helfgott AW, King EA, King AA, Minyard AN. Maternal death after second-trimester genetic amniocentesis. *Obstet Gynecol* 2005;**105**:1213–5.

11 Crane JP, Rohland BM. Clinical significance of persistent amniotic fluid leakage after genetic amniocentesis. *Prenat Diagn* 1986;**6**:25–31.

12 Tabor A, Philip J, Madsen M, *et al*. Randomized controlled trial of genetic amniocentesis in 4606 low-risk women. *Lancet* 1986;**1**:1287–93.

13 Seeds JW. Diagnostic mid trimester amniocentesis: how safe? *Am J Obstet Gynecol* 2004;**191**:607–15.

14 Johnson J, Wilson RD, Winsor EJ, *et al*. The Early Amniocentesis Study: a randomized clinical trial of early amniocentesis versus midtrimester amniocentesis. *Fetal Diagn Ther* 1996;**11**:85–93.

15 Canadian Early and Mid-trimester Amniocentesis Trial Group. Randomised trial to assess safety and fetal outcome of early and midtrimester amniocentesis. *Lancet* 1998;**351**:242–7.

16 Vandenbussche FP, Kanhai HH, Keirse MJ. Safety of early amniocentesis. *Lancet* 1994;**344**:1032.

17 Brumfield CG, Lin S, Conner W, *et al*. Pregnancy outcome following genetic amniocentesis at 11–14 versus 16–19 weeks' gestation. *Obstet Gynecol* 1996;**88**:114–8.

18 Cederholm M, Axelsson O. A prospective comparative study on transabdominal chorionic villus sampling and amniocentesis performed at 10–13 weeks' gestation. *Prenat Diagn* 1997;**17**:311–7.

19 Philip J, Silver RK, Wilson RD, *et al*. NICHDEATA Trial Group: late first-trimester invasive prenatal diagnosis: results of an international randomized trial. *Am J Obstet Gynecol* 2004;**103**:1164–73.

20 Nicolaides KH, Brizot ML, Patel F, *et al*. Comparison of chorionic villus sampling and amniocentesis for fetal karyotyping at 10–13 weeks' gestation. *Lancet* 1994;**344**:435–9.

21 Sundberg K, Bang J, Smidt-Jensen S, *et al*. Randomized study of risk of fetal loss related to early amniocentesis versus chorionic villus sampling. *Lancet* 1997;**350**:697–703.

22 Jackson LG, Zachary JM, Fowler SE, *et al*. A randomized comparison of transcervical and transabdominal chorionic villus sampling. *N Engl J Med* 1992;**327**:594–8.

23 Elias S, Simpson JL, Shulman LP, *et al*. Transabdominal chorionic villus sampling for first-trimester prenatal diagnosis. *Am J Obstet Gynecol* 1989;**160**:879–84.

24 Canadian Collaborative CVS/Amniocentesis Clinical Trial Group. Multicentre randomized clinical trial of chorion villus sampling and amniocentesis. First report. *Lancet* 1989;**1**:1–6.

25 Rhoads GG, Jackson LG, Schlesselman SE, *et al*. The safety and efficacy of chorionic villus sampling for early prenatal diagnosis of cytogenetic abnormalities. *N Engl J Med* 1989;**320**:609–17.

26 Smidt-Jensen S, Permin M, Philip J, *et al*. Randomized comparison of amniocentesis and transabdominal and transcervical chorionic villus sampling. *Lancet* 1992;**340**:1237–44.

27 Bovicelli L, Rizzo N, Montacuti V, *et al*. Transabdominal vs. transcervical routes for chorionic villus sampling. *Lancet* 1986;**2**:290.

28 Brambati B, Terizian F, Tognoni G. Randomized clinical trial of transabdominal vs. transcervical chrionic villus sampling methods. *Prenat Diagn* 1991;**11**:285–93.

29 Tomassini A, Campagna G, Paolucci M, *et al*. Transvaginal CVS vs. transabdominal CVS (our randomized cases. XI European Congress of Prenat Med 1988; 1104.

30 MRC Working Party on the Evaluation of Chorionic Villus Sampling. Medical Research Council European Trial of Chorion Villus Sampling. *Lancet* 1991;**337**:1491–99.

31 Saura R, Gauthier B, Tame L, *et al*. Operator experience and fetal loss rate in transabdominal CVS. *Prenat Diagn* 1994;**14**:70–1.

32 Firth HV, Boyd PA, Chamberlin P, *et al*. Severe limb abnormalities after chorion villus sampling at 55–66 days' gestation. *Lancet* 1991;**337**:762–63.

33 Firth HV, Boyd PA, Chamberlain P, *et al*. Limb abnormalities and chorion villus sampling. *Lancet* 1991;**338**:51.

34 Froster UG, Jackson L. Safety of chorionic villous sampling: limb defects and chorionic villous sampling: results from an international registry (1992 to 1994). *Lancet* 1996;**347**:489–94.

35 Burton BK, Schulz CJ, Burd L. Limb anomalies associated with chorionic villus sampling. *Obstet Gynecol* 1992;**79**:726–30.

36 Kuliev A, Jackson L, Froster U, *et al*. Chorionic villus sampling safety. Report of World Health Organization/EURO Meeting in association with the Seventh International Conference on Early Prenatal Diagnosis of Genetic Disease, Tel-Aviv, Israel, May 21, 1994. *Am J Obstet Gynecol* 1996;**174**:807–11.

37 ACOG Committee Opinion No. 160. *Chorionic villus sampling*. American College of Obstetricians and Gynecologists, 409 12th Street, SW, Washington, DC 20024-2188. October 1995.

38 WHO/PAHO Consultation on CVS. Evaluation of chorionic villus sampling safety. *Prenat Diagn* 1999;**19**:97–9.

39 Brambati B, Simoni G, Travi M, *et al*. Genetic diagnosis by chorionic villus sampling before 8 gestational weeks: efficiency, reliability, and risk on 317 completed pregnancies. *Prenat Diagn* 1992;**12**:689–799.

40 Wapner RJ, Evans Ml, Davis G, *et al*. Procedural risks versus theology: chorionic villus sampling for Orthodox Jews at less than 8 weeks' gestation. *Am J Obstet Gynecol* 2002;**186**:1133–6.

41 Tharapel AT, Elias S, Shulman LP, *et al*. Resorbed co-twin as an explanation for discrepant chorionic villi results: non-mosaic 47, XX, 116 in villi (direct and culture) with normal (46, XX) amniotic fluid and neonatal blood. *Prenat Diagn* 1989;**9**:467–72.

42 Hsu LYF, Perlis TE. United States survey on chromosome mosaicism and pseudomosaicism in prenatal diagnosis. *Prenat Diagn* 1980;**4**:97–130.

43 Ledbetter DH, Zachary JM, Simpson JL, *et al*. Cytogenetic results from the US collaborative study on CVS: high diagnostic accuracy in over 11 000 cases. *Prenat Diagn* 1992;**12**:317–45.

44 Ledbetter DH, Martin AO, Verlinsky Y, *et al*. Cytogenetic results of chorionic villus sampling: high success rate and diagnostic accuracy in the US collaborative study. *Am J Obstet Gynecol* 1990;**162**:495–501.

45 Elles RG, Williamson R, Niazi M, *et al*. Absence of maternal contamination of chorionic villi used for fetal-gene analysis. *N Engl J Med* 1983;**308**:1433–5.

46 Kalousek DK, Dill FJ, Pantzar T, *et al*. Confined chorionic mosaicism in prenatal diagnosis. *Hum Genet* 1987;**77**:163–7.

47 Karkut I, Zakrzewski S, Sperling K. Mixed karyotypes obtained by chorionic villi analysis: mosaicism and maternal contamination. In: Fraccaro M, *et al*. (eds): *First Trimester Fetal Diagnosis*. Heidelberg: Springer-Verlag, 1985.

48 Wolstenholmec J. Confined placental mosaicism for trisomies 2, 3, 7, 8, 9, 16, and 22: their incidence, likely origins, and mechanisms for cell lineage compartmentalization. *Prenat Diagn* 1996;**16**:511–24.

49 Cassidy SB, Lai LW, Erickson RP, *et al*. Trisomy 15 with loss of the paternal 15 as a cause of Prader–Willi syndrome due to maternal disomy. *Am J Hum Genet* 1992;**51**:701–8.

50 Purvis-Smith SG, Saville T, Manass S, *et al*. Uniparental disomy 15 resulting from "correction" of an initial trisomy 15. *Am J Hum Genet* 1992;**50**:1348–50.

51 Ledbetter DH, Engel F. Uniparental disomy in humans: development of an imprinting map and its implication for prenatal diagnosis. *Hum Mol Genet* 1995;**4**:1757–64.

52 Johnson A, Wapner RJ, Davis GH, *et al*. Mosaicism in chorionic villus sampling: an association with poor prenatal outcome. *Obstet Gynecol* 1990;**75**:573–7.

53 Breed AS, Mantingh A, Vosters R, *et al*. Follow-up and pregnancy outcome after a diagnosis of mosaicism in CVS. *Prenat Diagn* 1991;**11**:577–80.

54 Wapner RJ, Simpson JT, Golbus MS, *et al*. Chorionic mosaicism: association with fetal loss but not with adverse perinatal outcome. *Prenat Diagn* 1992;**12**:347–55.

55 Post JG, Nijhuis JG. Trisomy 16 confined to the placenta. *Prenat Diagn* 1992;**12**:1001–7.

56 Kalousek DK, Langlois S, Barrett I, *et al*. Uniparental disomy for chromosome 16 in humans. *Am J Hum Genet* 1992;**52**:8–16.

57 Benn P. Trisomy 16 and trisomy 16 mosaicism: a review. *Am J Med Genet* 1998;**9**:121–33.

58 Gray RG, Green A, Cole T, *et al*. A misdiagnosis of X-linked adrenoleukodystrophy in cultured chorionic villus cells by the measurement of very long chain fatty acids. *Prenat Diagn* 1995;**15**:486–90.

59 Simpson JL, Elias S. Prenatal diagnosis of genetic disorders. In: Creasy RK, Resnik R, eds. *Maternal-Fetal Medicine: Principles and Practice*, 3rd edn. Philadelphia: WB Saunders, 1994: 61–88.

50 Direct fetal blood sampling: cordocentesis

Alessandro Ghidini and Caterina Bocchi

Cordocentesis is the ultrasound-guided technique of choice used to gain access to fetal blood. Because it provides direct access to fetal blood, it can be used for diagnostic purposes, offering unique insights for the diagnosis and clinical management of some important fetal pathologic conditions. Moreover, cordocentesis can be the initial step prior to transfusion of blood or platelets.

Indications

During the period since its original description in 1982, cordocentesis has seen a change in its indications, as many conditions that required diagnosis by cordocentesis can now be diagnosed using DNA analysis of material obtained by chorionic villus sampling or amniocentesis. Nevertheless, the conditions shown in Table 50.1 remain as examples of possible indications for cordocentesis. The most common ones are discussed in this chapter.

Cytogenetic diagnosis

Diagnostic cordocentesis for karyotype analysis is indicated when results are required within a few days, such as when the time limit for legal termination is near or when delivery is imminent. Such situations may be encountered when fetal anatomy survey detects structural abnormalities. In a series of 936 fetuses with structural anomalies identified by ultrasound, the prevalence of chromosome anomalies was 12% in fetuses with an isolated structural anomaly and 29% in fetuses with multiple anomalies [1]. Trisomies 21, 18, 13, and monosomy X accounted for 80% of all anomalies [1], suggesting that fluorescence *in situ* hybridization (FISH) on amniocytes could be an important alternative to cordocentesis in such cases. A controversial indication for rapid fetal karyotype may be diagnosis of polyhydramnios (amniotic fluid index of 25 cm or more) in absence of sonographically detected anomalies, maternal diabetes, or isoimmunization. The rate of chromosomal abnormalities in such cases ranges from 0.3% to 3.2% [2,3]. Cordocentesis can be helpful in identifying karyotype anomalies as a cause of early onset and severe fetal growth restriction (FGR). The risk of aneuploidy is higher with more severe growth disorders, earlier gestational age at diagnosis, and when FGR is associated with polyhydramnios (27%), structural anomalies (31%), or both (50%) [1].

Cordocentesis may also have a role in confirmation of fetal involvement of true mosaicism at genetic amniocentesis, which has been reported in 0.1–0.3% of cases [4]. However, parents should be informed that the absence of abnormal cells in fetal blood does not exclude the possibility that a mosaic cell line may be present in fetal tissues other than blood; that the proportion of the abnormal cell line in amniotic fluid or fetal blood does not necessarily correspond to the proportion in other fetal tissues.

Congenital infections

Cordocentesis has only a limited role in the prenatal diagnosis and treatment of congenital infections. In fact, when performed in cases of documented maternal infection, it has the potential of facilitating transplacental passage of infectious agents. Amniocentesis is currently the primary tool used to diagnose fetal infection. However, cordocentesis retains an important role in the management of fetal parvovirus infection, which can lead to fetal hydrops resulting from severe anemia with or without direct myocardial injury [5]. In a series of 539 fetuses with parvovirus-induced hydrops who were not transfused, 34% resolved spontaneously and 30% died [6]. Noninvasive monitoring of fetal anemia can now be accomplished with Doppler velocimetry of the middle cerebral artery [7,8]. Suspicion of fetal anemia at Doppler velocimetry is an indication of cordocentesis in preparation for blood transfusion. Elevated fetal reticulocyte count at cordocentesis may help to identify those fetuses with resolving anemia, thus indicating that fetal transfusion is not required. Since these fetuses may also be profoundly thrombocytopenic, platelets

Table 50.1 Indications for cordocentesis.

Rapid karyotype analysis
Fetal structural anomalies
Idiopathic polyhydramnios
Unexplained fetal growth restriction
Abnormalities at amniocentesis

Congenital infections

Fetal growth restriction

Twin–twin transfusion syndrome
Fetal thyroid disorders
Coagulopathies (e.g., hemophilia)

Suspected fetal anemia
Immune
Nonimmune

Suspected fetal thrombocytopenia
Alloimmune thrombocytopenia

should be available for transfusion if confirmed by coulter counter or if there is excess bleeding.

Acid–base balance in fetal growth restriction

Cordocentesis has been proposed in the assessment of fetal acid–base status and to assist in the identification of the optimal timing for delivery in severe FGR. However, cordocentesis carries a 9–14% rate of procedure-related loss among FGR fetuses [9,10]. Moreover, its value for longitudinal assessment of fetal well-being is currently unproven.

Severe twin–twin transfusion syndrome

Cordocentesis has been proposed to assess severity of inter-twin discrepancy in hematocrit in cases of twin–twin transfusion syndrome (TTTS), which may assist in choosing the optimal timing for delivery [11]. However, the evidence is lacking that cordocentesis for this indication may improve perinatal outcome. Following a co-twin death, cordocentesis may allow identification of severe fetal anemia in the surviving twin. However, it is unknown whether prompt correction of the fetal anemia may ameliorate the outcome. Moreover, pertinent information can be obtained noninvasively using Doppler velocimetry of the fetal middle cerebral artery (personal observation) [12].

Fetal anemia

Suspicion of fetal anemia either in the setting of an alloimmunologic process (e.g., maternal immunization to Rh or Kell incompatible fetus), or from other reasons (parvovirus, homozygous alpha-thalassemia, nonimmune hydrops, feto-maternal hemorrhage) is an indication for cordocentesis in preparation for fetal transfusion. Less common indications for fetal blood sampling include detection of thalassemia major or sickle cell disease in the presence of carrier parents and when rapid diagnosis is desired.

Fetal thrombocytopenia

Cordocentesis may have a role in the management of immune thrombocytopenias to assist in the decision to initiate or change therapy, and in preparation for platelet transfusion.

Technique

Cordocentesis should not be attempted without considerable experience in sonographically guided invasive procedures. The skill should be acquired under the guidance and supervision of someone skilled in the procedure. Prior to fetal viability, cordocentesis can be performed in any room used for sonographic examinations or in a labor room. After viability, the procedure should be performed in proximity to an operating room because an emergency cesarean delivery may be required if nonreassuring fetal heart rate patterns develop during or after the procedure.

Preparation

A sample of maternal blood should be drawn before the procedure for subsequent quality control of the fetal samples obtained. An obstetric ultrasound examination should be performed to determine fetal viability, position, biometry, location of the placenta, and to select the optimal site for aspiration (i.e., cord insertion on an anterior or posterior placenta or a free loop of cord). The maternal abdomen should be cleaned with an antiseptic solution and draped. We use sterile gowns, caps, and masks to minimize the risk of field contamination. The probe is covered with a sterile probe cover that extends along the cable to the ultrasound machine.

Equipment and medications (Table 50.2)

The use of an antibiotic prophylaxis is based on evidence that up to 40% of procedure-related fetal losses are associated with intrauterine infection [13]. The risk of chorioamnionitis far outweighs the risk of adverse drug reactions. On the contrary, the risk–benefit ratio of the use of corticosteroids to enhance fetal lung maturity has yet to be evaluated, given the small risk of procedure-related preterm delivery. If steroids are considered, they should be administered at least 24 hours prior to the procedure. Most operators prefer to insert the needle while holding the transducer themselves; once the needle tip is in place, an assistant is necessary either to hold the transducer or to draw the blood samples. Other operators prefer to be guided throughout the procedure by an assistant. The use of a needle

Table 50.2 Equipment and medications needed for cordocentesis.

48 hours prior to the procedure
Corticosteroids (optional between 24 and 34 weeks' gestation)

On the day of the procedure
Identify optimal insertion site for the needle in relation to fetal and
    placental position (using color Doppler if necessary)
Maternal intravenous access (recommended)
Antibiotics (broad-spectrum prophylaxis, 30–60 min prior to the
    procedure)

On the sterile cart
Local anesthesia (e.g. lidocaine 1% solution in 10 mL syringe)
Needle guide (optional)
Needles (20- to 22-gauge spinal needles, 8.9–15 cm)
Aspiration syringes (1 or 2 mL) primed with anticoagulant (e.g., heparin)
Aspiration syringes (10–20 mL) if amniocentesis is necessary
3 or 5 mL syringes with normal saline

guide to target the sampling site may decrease the risk of cord laceration or needle displacement [14], but it restricts the lateral motion of the needle and hampers the procedure if the needle needs repositioning. This problem can be resolved by removing the guiding device during the procedure, if it becomes necessary. A "free-hand technique" is also commonly employed because it provides flexibility for adjusting the needle path. The length of the needle should take into account the thickness of the maternal panniculus, location of the target segment of cord, and the possibility of intervening events (e.g., contractions). The standard length of a spinal needle is 8.9 cm but longer needles are available (15 cm). Priming the needle with sodium citrate solution or heparin immediately before the procedure helps to prevent clot formation.

Sampling procedure

Identification of a fixed segment of the cord or the insertion site of the umbilical cord in the placenta is essential. Color Doppler can be used to assist in site identification. Cordocentesis is easiest when the placenta is anterior; such an approach also decreases the vulnerability of the needle to fetal movements. When the placenta is posterior, manipulation of the maternal abdomen may be necessary to move the fetus away from the sampling site. Because crossing the amniotic cavity makes the needle vulnerable to fetal movements, administration of paralytic agents to the fetus may be necessary. Alternatively, the intrahepatic portion of the umbilical vein can be accessed. It may be necessary to perform a therapeutic amniocentesis to gain access to the cord insertion in cases complicated by polyhydramnios with a posterior placenta. Oligohydramnios can also interfere with visualization of the insertion site of the cord; amnioinfusion or needling of a fixed loop of cord may overcome the difficulty.

Some important additional considerations are as follow:
1 Amniocentesis, if indicated, should be performed prior to

cordocentesis to avoid blood contamination of the fluid specimen. After aspiration of amniotic fluid, the needle is either advanced into the cord or, in cases with an anterior placenta, withdrawn within the placental mass, reoriented, and advanced into the cord.

2 It is easier and safer to sample the umbilical vein than an artery; puncture of the artery has been associated with a greater incidence of bradycardia and longer post-procedural bleeding [15,16]. The vessels can be distinguished by their relative size and by the direction of blood flow using Doppler color flow mapping. Distinction of the origin of the sample (arterial vs. venous) is crucial for interpretation of the acid–base and oxygenation status of the fetus.

3 Upon entering the umbilical cord, the stylet is removed and blood is withdrawn into a syringe attached to the hub of the needle. Proper positioning of the needle can be confirmed by injection of physiologic saline solution into the cord and observation of turbulent flow along the vessel. After umbilical blood flow is documented by color Doppler, an initial sample should be submitted to distinguish fetal from maternal cells (see below). RhIg should be used in unsensitized Rh negative women.

Post-procedure monitoring

After the sample is obtained, the needle is withdrawn and the puncture site monitored for bleeding. If an intrauterine transfusion is performed after sampling, the fetal heart rate should be monitored intermittently by interrogating an umbilical artery near the sampling area using pulse Doppler. If the patient has a viable fetus, the fetal heart rate is also monitored for at least 1–2 hours after the procedure using an external fetal heart rate monitor. RhIg should be used in unsensitized Rh negative women.

Quality control

Contamination with maternal blood or amniotic fluid can alter the diagnostic value of the fetal blood specimen. The purity of the fetal blood sample is commonly assessed using the red blood cell size determination (mean corpuscular volume, MCV) because fetal red blood cells are larger than maternal ones. On occasion, this parameter can be misinterpreted (e.g., in the presence of macrocytic anemia or after repeated fetal transfusions of adult donor blood). Other methods to differentiate maternal from fetal blood include Apt test, Kleihauer–Betke test, human chorionic gonadotropin (hCG) determination, or blood typing (I antigen present only on adult red blood cells). The hCG determination is the best marker for detection of maternal blood contamination [17]. The fetal blood : amniotic fluid : maternal blood ratio of hCG is 1 : 100 : 400. The HCC determination can detect as little as 0.2%

contamination with maternal blood or 1% contamination with amniotic fluid [17]. In Apt test, 0.1 mL sampled blood is added to a glass tube containing alkali reagent (5 mL water and 0.3 mL, 10% potassium hydroxide) and the tube is gently shaken for 2 minutes. The sample is considered contaminated with maternal blood if the colour of the mixture changes from red to green–brown [18,19]. The utility of Kleihauer–Betke test is limited during the late third trimester because fetal erythrocytes contain increasing amounts of haemoglobin A near term.

Dilution with amniotic fluid can be inferred by a similarly proportional decrease in the number of red blood cells, white blood cells, and platelets in the specimen. Confirmation can be obtained by observing an amniotic fluid arborization pattern or multiple desquamated epithelial cells on a smear [20,21].

Samples

Fetal blood samples are placed into tubes containing ethylenediaminetetra-acetic acid (EDTA) or heparin and mixed well to prevent clotting. The appropriate tubes and minimum required amount of blood for specific studies are listed in Table 50.3. The maximal volume of blood removed should not exceed 6–7% of the fetoplacental blood volume for the gestational age, which can be calculated as 100 mL/kg of estimated fetal weight [22].

Normal values

The distribution of the most common hematologic and acid–base parameters in fetal blood in relation to gestational age are available in the literature (www.uptodate.com).

Table 50.3 Collection tubes for laboratory studies.

Tube Content	Tests
EDTA	Complete blood cell count
	Reticulocyte count
	Kleiheuer–Betke test
	Polymerase chain reaction
Citrate	Coagulation studies
Dry tube	Blood group typing
	Coombs (direct or indirect)
	Total and specific IgM
	Serum chemistry
Sodium heparin	Molecular biology analysis
	Blood gas analysis
	Karyotype or fluorescence *in situ* hybridization

EDTA, ethylenediaminetetra-acetic acid; IgM, immunoglobulin M.

Complications

Bleeding, bradycardia, and infection are the major fetal complications associated with cordocentesis. Maternal complications unrelated to the pregnancy are unusual.

Bleeding from the puncture site is the most common complication of cordocentesis, occurring in up to half of cases [15,23]. Puncture of the umbilical artery is associated with a significantly longer duration of bleeding than venipuncture [15,16]. Post-procedural bleeding appears to carry a more ominous prognosis when it occurs at less than 21 weeks' gestation [24]. Fetuses with defects in platelet number or function are at significant risk for potentially fatal bleeding from the puncture site [25]. Thus, it is prudent to slowly transfuse the fetus with concentrated, washed maternal platelets while awaiting the fetal platelet count when cordocentesis is performed to diagnose a fetal platelet disorder. Dislodgement of the needle before platelet transfusion can have fatal consequences for the fetus affected with a platelet abnormality.

Cord hematoma is generally asymptomatic, but can be associated with a transient or prolonged sudden fetal bradycardia [23,26,27]. Expectant management is recommended in the presence of reassuring fetal monitoring and a nonexpanding hematoma.

Fetomaternal hemorrhage (FMH) is more common with an anterior rather than a posterior placenta, with procedures lasting longer than 3 minutes, and with those requiring two or more needle insertions [28–30]. A significant FMH occurs in approximately 40% of cases [28–30] and can be defined by either a more than 50% post-procedural increase in maternal serum alpha-fetoprotein concentration from blood taken immediately before and after cordocentesis, or Kleihauer–Betke staining of the maternal blood showing a calculated FMH of more than 1 mL. The main consequence of FMH is increase in maternal antibody titers when the procedure is performed for red blood cell isoimmunization [28,29].

Transient fetal bradycardia is reported in 3–12% of fetuses [13,15,16,31]. A higher incidence of bradycardia is described in cases involving puncture of an umbilical artery [16] and among growth restricted fetuses (17%). The greatest risk of bradycardia is in the growth-restricted fetus with absent diastolic flow in the umbilical artery by Doppler analysis (21%) [16].

Maternal infections from cordocentesis are rare and mainly limited to chorioamnionitis when procedures are performed without antibiotic prophylaxis. Infection occurs in less than 1% of procedures but is responsible for up to 40% of pregnancy losses associated with the procedure [9,13,16,31].

Procedure-related pregnancy loss risks are difficult to assess. Losses that occur within a short time after the procedure are usually considered to be procedure-related. A review of the published series of low-risk cases found an overall risk of fetal loss of 1.4% before 28 weeks' gestation, and an additional 1.4% risk of perinatal death after 28 weeks [32]. This loss rate is significantly greater than that related to amniocentesis (0.5–1.0%) and about six times higher than that of a general obstetric population near term. Another study compared pregnancy outcome in 1020 women with no known fetal anomalies undergoing cordocentesis at 16–24 weeks' gestation with matched control subjects [33]. The pregnancy loss rates before 28 weeks in the cordocentesis and control groups were 1.8% and 0.7%, respectively, and 1.5% and 1.1%, respectively, after 28 weeks.

The risk of fetal loss is higher in presence of fetal pathology. The total spontaneous pregnancy loss rate within 2 weeks of the procedure is 1% when it is performed for diagnosis of genetic disorders or karyotyping, 7–13% in the presence of structural fetal anomalies, 9–14% among growth restricted fetuses, and 25% in fetuses with nonimmune hydrops [9,10]. There is a higher frequency of fetal loss in smaller series, suggesting that operator experience affects the complication rate [13]. Both puncture of the intrahepatic portion of the umbilical vein and cardiocentesis carry an increased risk of fetal death.

Case presentation

A 26-year-old gravida 4 Para 2012 had a history of the second child with jaundice requiring phototherapy. An indirect Coombs test at 11 weeks was positive for anti-Kell with titer of 1:8. At amniocentesis at 20 weeks, DNA studies by polymerase chain reaction (PCR) on amniocytes predicted a Kell-positive fetus. Maternal titers monitored serially revealed an increase to 1:32 at 32 weeks accompanied by an elevation in peak systolic velocity in the middle cerebral artery (70 cm/s). Cordocentesis documented a fetal hematocrit of 15.5%. After transfusion of 120 mL packed red blood cells, the fetal hematocrit increased to 36.4%. The fetus was delivered 1 week later because of nonreassuring fetal testing and the baby did well. Three years later the same patient was pregnant again. Indirect Coombs titers were stable at 1:4. In light of the experience with the previous pregnancy, fetal status was monitored with serial Doppler velocimetry of the middle cerebral artery. At 31 weeks, a sudden increase was noted in peak systolic velocity (89 cm/s). Cordocentesis revealed a Kell-positive fetus with an initial hematocrit of 22.3%. After transfusion of 90 mL Kell-negative blood, the hematocrit increased to 37.7%. Serial transfusions were continued and delivery effected at 36.5 weeks, when fetal lung maturity was documented. The baby was delivered and did well.

This case illustrates how information provided by noninvasive testing (Doppler velocimetry of the fetal middle cerebral artery), amniocentesis, and cordocentesis can successfully be combined to assist in the management, minimize risks of unnecessary procedures, and ensure an optimal outcome.

References

1 Eydoux P, Choiset A, Le Porrier N, *et al.* Chromosomal prenatal diagnosis: study of 936 cases of intrauterine abnormalities after ultrasound assessment. *Prenat Diagn* 1989;**9**:255–69.
2 Brady K, Polzin WJ, Kopelman JN, Read JA. Risk of chromosomal abnormalities in patients with idiopathic polyhydramnios. *Obstet Gynecol* 1992;**79**:234–8.
3 Biggio JR Jr, Wenstrom KD, Dubard MB, Cliver SP. Hydramnios prediction of adverse perinatal outcome. *Obstet Gynecol* 1999;**94**:773–7.
4 Hsu LYF. Prenatal diagnosis of chromosomal abnormalities through amniocentesis. In: Milunsky A, (ed.) *Genetic Disorders and the Fetus*, 4th edn. Baltimore: Johns Hopkins University Press, 1998: 179.
5 Schild RL, Bald R, Plath H, *et al.* Intrauterine management of fetal parvovirus B19 infection. *Ultrasound Obstet Gynecol* 1999;**13**:161–6.
6 Rodis JF, Borgida AF, Wilson M, *et al.* Management of parvovirus infection in pregnancy and outcomes of hydrops: a survey of the Society of Perinatal Obstetricians. *Am J Obstet Gynecol* 1998;**179**:985–8.
7 Cosmi E, Mari G, Delle Chiaie L, *et al.* Noninvasive diagnosis by Doppler ultrasonography of fetal anemia resulting from parvovirus infection. *Am J Obstet Gynecol* 2002;**187**:1290–3.
8 Delle Chiaie L, Buck G, Grab D, Terinde R. Prediction of fetal anemia with Doppler measurement of the middle cerebral artery peak systolic velocity in pregnancies complicated by maternal blood group alloimmunization or parvovirus B19 infection. *Ultrasound Obstet Gynecol* 2001;**18**:232–6.
9 Maxwell DJ, Johnson P, Hurley P, *et al.* Fetal blood sampling and pregnancy loss in relation to indication. *Br J Obstet Gynaecol* 1991;**98**:892–7.
10 Antsaklis A, Daskalakis G, Papantoniou N, Michalas S. Fetal blood sampling: indication-related losses. *Prenat Diagn* 1998;**18**:934–40.
11 Denbow M, Fogliani R, Kyle P, *et al.* Haematological indices at fetal blood sampling in monochorionic pregnancies complicated by feto-fetal transfusion syndrome. *Prenat Diagn* 1998;**18**:941–6.
12 Senat MV, Loizeau S, Couderc S, Bernard JP, Ville Y. The value of middle cerebral artery peak systolic velocity in the diagnosis of fetal anemia after intrauterine death of one monochorionic twin. *Am J Obstet Gynecol* 2003;**189**:1320–4.
13 Boulot P, Deschamps F, Lefort G, *et al.* Pure fetal blood samples obtained by cordocentesis: technical aspects of 322 cases. *Prenat Diagn* 1990;**10**:93–100.
14 Weiner CP, Okamura K. Diagnostic fetal blood sampling-technique related losses. *Fetal Diagn Ther* 1996;**11**:169–75.
15 Weiner CP. Cordocentesis for diagnostic indications: two years' experience. *Obstet Gynecol* 1987;**70**:664–8.
16 Weiner CP, Wenstrom KD, Sipes SL, Williamson RA. Risk factors for cordocentesis and fetal intravascular transfusion. *Am J Obstet Gynecol* 1991;**165**:1020–5.
17 Forestier F, Cox WL, Daffos F, Rainaut M. The assessment of fetal blood samples. *Am J Obstet Gynecol* 1988;**158**:1184–8.
18 Ogur G, Gul D, Ozen S, *et al.* Application of the 'Apt test' in prenatal diagnosis to evaluate the fetal origin of blood obtained

by cordocentesis: results of 30 pregnancies. *Prenat Diagn* 1997;**17**:879–82.

19 Sepulveda W, Be C, Youlton R, *et al*. Accuracy of the haemoglobin alkaline denaturation test for detecting maternal blood contamination of fetal blood samples for prenatal karyotyping. *Prenat Diagn* 1999;**19**:927–9.

20 Lazebnik N, Hendrix PV, Ashmead GG, *et al*. Detection of fetal blood contamination by amniotic fluid obtained during cordocentesis. *Am J Obstet Gynecol* 1990;**163**:78–80.

21 Chao A, Herd JP, Tabsh KM. The ferning test for detection of amniotic fluid contamination in umbilical blood samples. *Am J Obstet Gynecol* 1990;**162**:1207–13.

22 Nicolaides KH, Clewell WH, Rodeck CH. Measurement of human fetoplacental blood volume in erythroblastosis fetalis. *Am J Obstet Gynecol* 1987;**157**:50–3.

23 Hogge WA, Thiagarajah S, Brenbridge AN, Harbert GM. Fetal evaluation by percutaneous blood sampling. *Am J Obstet Gynecol* 1988;**158**:132–6.

24 Orlandi F, Damiani G, Jakil C, *et al*. The risks of early cordocentesis (12–21 weeks): analysis of 500 procedures. *Prenat Diagn* 1990;**10**:425–8.

25 Daffos F, Forestier F, Kaplan C, Cox W. Prenatal diagnosis and management of bleeding disorders with fetal blood sampling. *Am J Obstet Gynecol* 1988;**158**:939–46.

26 Jauniaux E, Donner C, Simon P, *et al*. Pathologic aspects of the umbilical cord after percutaneous umbilical blood sampling. *Obstet Gynecol* 1989;**73**:215–8.

27 Chenard E, Bastide A, Fraser WD. Umbilical cord hematoma following diagnostic funipuncture. *Obstet Gynecol* 1990;**76**:994–6.

28 Nicolini U, Kochenour NK, Greco P, *et al*. Consequences of feto-maternal hemorrhage following intrauterine transfusion. *Br Med J* 1988;**297**:1379–81.

29 Weiner C, Grant S, Hudson J, *et al*. Effect of diagnostic and therapeutic cordocentesis on maternal serum α-fetoprotein concentration. *Am J Obstet Gynecol* 1989;**161**:706–8.

30 Chitrit Y, Caubel P, Lusina D, *et al*. Detection and measurement of fetomaternal hemorrhage following diagnostic cordocentesis. *Fetal Diagn Ther* 1998;**13**:253–6.

31 Ludomirsky A, Weiner S, Ashmead GG, *et al*. Percutaneous fetal umbilical blood sampling: procedure safety and normal fetal hematologic indices. *Am J Perinatol* 1988;**5**:264–6.

32 Ghidini A, Sepulveda W, Lockwood CJ, Romero R. Complications of fetal blood sampling. *Am J Obstet Gynecol* 1993;**168**:1339–44.

33 Tongsong T, Wanapirak C, Kunavikatikul C, *et al*. Fetal loss rate associated with cordocentesis at midgestation. *Am J Obstet Gynecol* 2001;**184**:719–23.

51 Amnioinfusion: indications and controversies

Catherine Y. Spong

Amnioinfusion was first described in 1957 at a postgraduate course in obstetrics and gynecology [1]. Despite this early report, amnioinfusion was not widely accepted until the late 1980s. A recent survey of amnioinfusion practices in US academic obstetric gynecologic departments revealed that 96% of responding centers use amnioinfusion and 79% have a formal protocol [2].

Amnioinfusion is defined as the insertion of fluid into the amniotic cavity. This procedure can be performed transcervically through an intrauterine pressure catheter when membranes are ruptured, or transabdominally in those with intact membranes. Amnioinfusion is used for a variety of indications, including relief of repetitive fetal heart rate decelerations during labor or to improve sonographic visualization in the setting of oligohydramnios, among other indications which are described below.

Inclusion and exclusion criteria

Patients with contraindications for vaginal delivery (e.g., placenta previa) are not candidates for transcervical amnioinfusion; however, they may receive a transabdominal amnioinfusion if indicated. Patients with prior cesarean section, myomectomy with entry into the endometrium, or history of a vertical uterine scar were not initially considered to be candidates for amnioinfusion during labor. However, studies have shown that amnioinfusion is safe in these patients because most of the fluid leaks and thus minimizes uterine distention [3]; however, it is important to monitor that fluid is leaking out. The presence of chorioamnionitis has been a relative contraindication to amnioinfusion. Support for this view rests on the following findings: with amnioinfusion, a foreign body is introduced into the infected cavity and fluid is inserted into a potentially weakened, infected uterus. The infusion washes out the amniotic fluid, which has bacteriolytic properties [4]. However, amnio-infusion used in the presence of chorioamnionitis also washes out the bacteria present within the uterus. No randomized controlled trials have been performed to clarify this situation.

Amount infused

There are many different protocols for amnioinfusion. For a transcervical infusion, the infusate can be given as a bolus of 250–500 mL of fluid and repeated until the indication resolves. Alternatively, a constant infusion of 180 mL/h can be started after the bolus. In a transabdominal amnioinfusion, 250–800 mL saline solution can be infused, depending on the indication. The change in amniotic fluid volume after amnioinfusion was studied by one team. In 30 women with oligohydramnios at 37 weeks' gestation or later, a bolus of 250 mL increased the amniotic fluid index (AFI) 4.3 cm with a standard deviation of 1.5 cm [5].

Route of administration

For a transcervical infusion, a sterile catheter, either single or double lumen, is placed transcervically and infusion of sterile physiologic fluid is started. Transabdominal infusion is performed through a sterile needle inserted into the amniotic cavity (similar to an amniocentesis) under ultrasonographic guidance.

The type of solution used for amnioinfusion does not affect the outcome. One team of investigators compared effects of normal saline with those of lactated Ringer solution [6]. No differences were identified in neonatal outcome, duration of labor, neonatal serum electrolytes, or cord blood gas values among the groups. Another study showed that the temperature of the infusate, warmed versus room temperature, is not associated with detectable differences in neonatal outcome [7].

Studied indications

The studied indications for amnioinfusion can be divided into two groups: treatment and prophylaxis. Therapeutic indications include the following:

1 Relief of repetitive variable decelerations.
2 Treatment of chorioamnionitis.
3 Improvement of visualization of fetal anatomy for prenatal diagnosis of congenital anomalies in the setting of oligohydramnios.
4 Improvement of the odds of success after a failed version.

Prophylactic amnioinfusion has been proposed for the prevention of fetal heart rate decelerations in term or preterm patients in labor with oligohydramnios and for patients with meconium-stained amniotic fluid.

Relief of repetitive variable decelerations

Variable decelerations are usually caused by umbilical cord compression resulting from oligohydramnios, entrapment of the cord, or a true knot in the cord. Variable decelerations observed after amniotomy were probably caused by oligohydramnios [8]. The initial treatment for variable decelerations consists of changing the maternal position to shift the fetus off of the umbilical cord and administering oxygen to the mother to increase oxygen delivery to the fetus. Because amnioinfusion can replace fluid, studies were designed to evaluate whether this procedure could relieve variable decelerations by providing a "cushion" for the umbilical cord.

In 1983, Miyazaki and Taylor [9] treated 42 patients who had repetitive or prolonged variable decelerations with transcervical amnioinfusion. Amnioinfusion effectively resolved the fetal heart rate pattern in 68% of patients with repetitive variable decelerations and in 86% of those with prolonged decelerations. In 1985, Miyazaki and Nevarez [10] randomized 96 patients with repetitive variable decelerations not relieved by changes in position or administration of oxygen to either receive or not receive amnioinfusion. Relief of variable decelerations occurred in 51% of patients treated with amnioinfusion compared with only 4% of the control (noninfused) group. These results demonstrated that amnioinfusion is beneficial for the treatment of repetitive or prolonged variable decelerations.

Because variable decelerations are often associated with oligohydramnios, a study was performed to evaluate whether an AFI obtained before amnioinfusion can predict the success of amnioinfusion in the presence of repetitive variable decelerations [11]. The AFI was measured in 67 patients prior to amnioinfusion. Amnioinfusion was considered successful if there was a 50% or greater decrease in total number of variable decelerations or a 50% decrease in atypical or severe variable decelerations. The probability of amnioinfusion success decreased with higher preamnioinfusion AFI. A preamnioinfusion AFI of more than 8 cm was associated with a less than 50% chance for relief of the decelerations with amnioinfusion. If the index prior to amnioinfusion was more than 8 cm, the cause of the fetal heart rate pattern was commonly either a tight nuchal cord or a true knot in the cord—conditions that are not relieved with amnioinfusion. This suggests that obtaining an AFI prior to initiating an amnioinfusion for repetitive variable heart rate decelerations may predict the success, with greater success likely if the initial AFI is low.

Treatment or prophylaxis of chorioamnionitis

Amnioinfusion with an antibiotic infusate has potential to deliver locally high levels of antibiotics while avoiding toxicity to the mother and fetus. Antibiotics in the amniotic fluid are in direct contact with the fetus and could inhibit bacterial growth on fetal skin and in the respiratory and gastrointestinal tracts. In 1981, Goodlin [1] performed transcervical amnioinfusions with ampicillin (1 g in 500 mL saline solution) in 53 laboring patients with documented chorioamnionitis. Of the patients, 96% had negative amniotic fluid cultures after infusion. In 1988, another team studied 64 term patients with premature rupture of membranes (PROM) and no clinical evidence of infection in an attempt to determine the best antibiotic method for preventing ascending infection [12]. Patients received infusion of two doses of latamoxef, cefoperazone, or cefotaxime sodium through a transcervical catheter. All three antibiotics maintained concentrations above 10 μg/mL even 24 hours after infusion.

Amnioinfusion studies have also been performed to determine whether the infusion can dilute pathogens associated with amnionitis. Patients with ruptured membranes for longer than 6 hours and no evidence of infection were randomized to a routine amnioinfusion or a noninfused control group [13]. Patients receiving amnioinfusion had significantly less chorioamnionitis or endometritis than did the controls (25% vs. 50%; $P = 0.03$). In a retrospective study, investigators evaluated 97 laboring patients who were at 35 weeks' gestation or later, did not receive antibiotics, and delivered by cesarean section [14]. Of the 97 patients, 23 received amnioinfusion in labor and the 74 noninfused patients were controls. The incidence of postpartum endometritis was significantly lower in the amnioinfused patients (13%) compared with control subjects (38%, $P = 0.03$).

For the treatment or prophylaxis of chorioamnionitis, an antibiotic infusate appears safe. However, the studies are too different and few in numbers to permit drawing definitive conclusions. Some studies suggested that amnioinfusion decreases the incidence of infectious morbidity;

other studies reported this as a complication [15,16]. Further studies are needed to establish the role, if any, for amnioinfusion in the prophylaxis or treatment of chorioamnionitis.

Congenital anomalies in the setting of oligohydramnios

Congenital anomalies can be associated with oligohydramnios [17]. However, decreased amniotic fluid volume can impair ultrasonographic visualization of the fetus. Transabdominal amnioinfusion has been proposed to aid in the visualization of fetal anatomy by increasing the amount of amniotic fluid.

In 1991, one group evaluated 61 pregnancies with oligohydramnios [18]. Amnioinfusion with saline stained with blue dye (indigo carmine) improved visualization in all cases and allowed confirmation and identification of fetal malformations in 23 patients and membrane rupture in 15. Results after amnioinfusion led to a change in diagnosis in 13% of patients. Reaspiration of the amniotic-infused fluid mixture also aided in karyotype analysis. Other reports showed similar results [19–25]. Complications associated with transabdominal amnioinfusion include procedure-related rupture of membranes, preterm labor, and amnionitis.

Transabdominal amnioinfusion allows improved fetal evaluation and karyotyping in the presence of oligohydramnios. However, this procedure is not without complications and should be performed only if management would be affected by the results.

Failed version

External cephalic version in breech presentation is beneficial for both the mother and the neonate. At term, 4% of presentations are breech; of these, fewer than 25% will spontaneously change to vertex presentation. Because the odds of a successful version increase with the volume of amniotic fluid, transabdominal amnioinfusion has been considered after an unsuccessful external cephalic version, to improve the chances of success for a reattempt at version.

In a series of six patients in whom three unsuccessful external cephalic versions had been attempted, transabdominal infusion of 800 mL of warmed saline solution over 10 minutes led to successful version after infusion in all patients [26]. Version was performed on the day after amnioinfusion. All patients had transient uterine contractions immediately after the procedure. In this series, the postinfusion version was performed 24 hours after infusion; however, because the turnover rate of amniotic fluid is rapid (24–72 hours), the benefit of waiting 24 hours after infusion is uncertain.

Prophylaxis in laboring patients with oligohydramnios

Because amnioinfusion can treat variable decelerations caused by cord compression resulting from oligohydramnios, prophylactic use of amnioinfusion in the setting of oligohydramnios has been proposed to avoid developing variable decelerations in both term and preterm infants [27].

In 1990, one group randomized 60 patients at more than 37 weeks' gestation with oligohydramnios, defined as an AFI of 5 cm or less [28]. Thirty patients without variable decelerations received amnioinfusion to keep their AFI above 8 cm; the remaining 30 did not receive amnioinfusion. In the amnioinfusion group there were significant improvements with respect to variable decelerations, operative delivery, fetal distress, and umbilical artery pH. Other studies reported similar results (Table 51.1) [5,16,29–32]. However, the control groups in these studies were not given amnioinfusion even if they developed repetitive variable decelerations, an action that may have created a bias.

In a randomized study carried out in 1994, term patients with oligohydramnios receiving prophylactic amnioinfusion for oligohydramnios were compared with a control group in whom therapeutic amnioinfusion was given to control patients only if they developed repetitive moderate or severe variable decelerations [15]. No significant differences in variable decelerations, operative delivery, fetal distress, or umbilical artery pH were identified between the two groups. Only 22% of the control group developed moderate or severe variable decelerations and required amnioinfusion. Thus, in four of five term patients with oligohydramnios, neither prophylactic nor therapeutic amnioinfusion was indicated.

The use of prophylactic amnioinfusion for oligohydramnios appears beneficial when compared with no amnioinfusion. However, when compared with therapeutic amnioinfusion (amnioinfusion for the development of repetitive variable decelerations), prophylactic amnioinfusion has no apparent benefit in term patients with oligohydramnios.

Amnioinfusion to prevent decelerations in preterm premature rupture of membranes

When there is preterm premature rupture of membranes (PPROM), during labor fetuses may have higher risks associated with variable decelerations. The premature fetus without the amniotic fluid cushion may be unable to withstand uterine contractions. Amnioinfusion increases the amount of fluid in the amniotic cavity. The increased fluid may provide a cushion during labor, and in the antepartum period allows for fetal movement and may improve fetal development in patients with PPROM.

Table 51.1 Amnioinfusion prophylaxis for oligohydramnios.

Study	Definition	GA	AI Method	No. of AIs	No. of Controls	Findings
Amnioinfusion vs. no amnioinfusion						
Strong *et al.* [5]	AFI ≤ 5 cm	> 37 wk	Bolus to AFI > 8 cm	30	30	↓Operative del ↓Severity of VD ↓Mec passage ↑Umbil art pH
Nageotte *et al.* [28]	AFI < 8 cm	> 42 wk or IUGR	Continuous	26	50	↓Frequency and severity of VD No Δ C/S No Δ umbil art pH
Schrimmer *et al.* [29]	AFI < 5 cm	NS, 41-wk mean	Bolus to AFI ≥ 10 cm	175	130	↓Operative del ↓C/S ↑Umbil art pH
MacGregor *et al.* [30]	<1 × 1 cm pocket	> 26 wk	Continuous	19	16	↓Frequency of VD No Δ C/S No Δ umbil art pH
Chauhan *et al.* [31]	AFI ≤ 5 cm	≥ 37 wk	Bolus to AFI ≥ 5.1	21	17	No Δ C/S No Δ umbil art pH
Amnioinfusion vs. standard care						
Ogundipe *et al.* [15]	AFI < 5 cm	≥ 36 wk	Continuous	56	60	No Δ fetal distress No Δ C/S No Δ umbil art pH ↑Intrapartum fever

AFI, amniotic fluid index; AI, amnioinfusion; C/S, cesarean section; del, delivery; GA, gestational age; IUGR, intrauterine growth restriction; mec, meconium; NS, not specified; Oligo, oligohydramnios; umbil art, umbilical artery; VD, variable decelerations; Δ, change.

A 1985 study involved 61 patients with PPROM with gestational ages between 26 and 35 weeks [32]. Patients were randomized to receive prophylactic amnioinfusion during labor or no amnioinfusion. In the amnioinfused group, umbilical artery and venous pH were improved and there were significantly fewer severe and total variable decelerations in both the first and second stages of labor. However, the control group did not receive amnioinfusion even in the presence of repetitive variable decelerations.

A nonrandomized study of amnioinfusion in 49 women at less than 26 weeks' gestation with PPROM for more than 4 days found that women with persistent oligohydramnios despite amnioinfusion had the worst outcome with 20% neonatal survival, 62% pulmonary hypoplasia and, of the survivors, 60% had abnormal neurologic outcomes as compared with those in whom amnioinfusion was not necessary or was successful [33]. Others have reported similar findings [34].

Amnioinfusion may be beneficial in laboring patients with PPROM because the increase in amniotic fluid cushions the preterm fetus during contractions. However, there are no studies evaluating prophylactic versus therapeutic amnioinfusion in PPROM patients in labor and the data are inadequate

to recommend either prophylactic amnioinfusion to improve pregnancy outcome in women with PPROM.

Prophylactic amnioinfusion for meconium-stained amniotic fluid

An important complication of meconium-stained amniotic fluid is the development of meconium aspiration syndrome in the neonate. This syndrome occurs in 1–4% of infants who have meconium-stained amniotic fluid. The mortality rate is 25% [35]. Amnioinfusion can dilute meconium in the amniotic fluid and thus has the potential to prevent meconium aspiration syndrome [36]. However, amnioinfusion may also make very thick meconium soluble and thus may increase the risk for meconium aspiration syndrome. Furthermore, studies have suggested that meconium aspiration syndrome predates labor, thus limiting the utility of amnioinfusion for prevention [37]. Studies were performed to evaluate whether prophylactic amnioinfusion for meconium would be beneficial and if it would decrease the incidence of meconium aspiration syndrome.

In a 1989 study, 85 patients with thick meconium were randomized to receive prophylactic amnioinfusion or no amnioinfusion [38]. The patients receiving amnioinfusion had significantly less fetal distress, less meconium below the cords, and operative deliveries. However, amnioinfusion was not offered to the patients in the control group who developed variable decelerations. These results were confirmed in other studies with the same design (Table 51.2) [36,39–43]. It is unclear whether the worse obstetric outcome in the control groups could have been averted by therapeutic amnioinfusions.

In 1994, 93 term patients with moderate to thick meconium were randomized to receive prophylactic amnioinfusion or standard care, which included therapeutic amnioinfusion for variable decelerations occurring after enrollment [44]. No significant differences in operative deliveries, fetal distress, Apgar scores, meconium below the cords, or umbilical pH values were identified between the prophylactic and therapeutic amnioinfusion groups. There were four cases of meconium aspiration syndrome; three occurred in the prophylactic amnioinfusion group and one in the standard care group. Of the patients receiving standard care, eight (16%) required therapeutic amnioinfusion for repetitive severe variable decelerations. In this study, prophylactic amnioinfusion did not improve perinatal outcome compared with standard management.

Indirect evidence in support of this conclusion comes from two retrospective studies. In 1992, investigators evaluated a protocol of routine prophylactic amnioinfusion for thick meconium and found that meconium aspiration syndrome continued to occur at the same rate [45]. Six patients with amnioinfusion developed meconium aspiration syndrome. In 1995, another team evaluated their policy of routine prophylactic amnioinfusion for meconium in 937 patients with moderately thick meconium [16]. No amnioinfusion was performed in 53% of the patients because of imminent delivery, occult meconium, or cesarean section. There was no improvement in neonatal outcome between those who received amnioinfusion and those who did not. Specifically, there were no changes in Apgar scores, in the amount of meconium below the cords, or in the incidence of meconium aspiration syndrome.

Two meta-analyses have been performed [46,47] including over 2000 patients which found that amnioinfusion was beneficial in patients with meconium-stained amniotic fluid in reducing meconium below the cords and meconium aspiration syndrome. However, these analyses were compromised by large differences in the trial designs and did not account for the presence of oligohydramnios or abnormalities in the fetal heart rate patterns. A large international multicenter trial at 56 centers in 13 countries randomized 1998 patients with thick meconium at term to amnioinfusion or no amnioinfusion [48]. This trial stratified according to the presence or absence of fetal heart rate variable decelerations.

In the overall group, amnioinfusion did not improve perinatal death or meconium aspiration syndrome (4.5% in amnioinfused vs. 3.4% in the control group; relative risk [RR] 1.3). Amnioinfusion did not reduce the risk of meconium aspiration syndrome (4.4% vs. 3.1%), cesarean delivery (31.8% vs. 29%), or other major indicators of maternal or neonatal morbidity. The study did not have the power to evaluate if the procedure might be beneficial in the subgroup of patients with decelerations.

Prophylactic amnioinfusion for meconium is not indicated and is not beneficial as the data demonstrate that amnioinfusion for this indication does not reduce meconium-related morbidity. Data are not available on whether therapeutic amnioinfusion in this setting decreases meconium aspiration syndrome or other meconium-related morbidities. However, amnioinfusion is a reasonable approach to treatment of repetitive variable decelerations irrespective of amniotic fluid meconium status. Thus, in the setting of meconium-stained fluid in the presence of repetitive fetal heart rate variable decelerations, amnioinfusion may be beneficial.

Complications of amnioinfusion

Of the centers that responded to an amnioinfusion survey, 26% reported at least one associated complication. The most frequent complication was uterine hypertonus (14%), followed by abnormal fetal heart tracing (9%) [2]. In a case report of uterine overdistention, the intrauterine pressure reached 50 mmHg, and the fetus developed decelerations and bradycardia that were relieved by draining amniotic fluid [49]. Two other teams also have published case reports of uterine overdistention [50,51]. This potential complication emphasizes the importance of monitoring the amount infused as well as the amount of amniotic fluid leaking out.

The incidence of amnionitis or endometritis in relationship with amnioinfusion is unclear. Two randomized controlled trials showed an association between amnioinfusion and higher rates of maternal infection [5,15]. One retrospective study confirmed the association [16]. However, eight randomized controlled studies demonstrated no change in the incidence of maternal infection with amnioinfusion [28,29,34–39]. It is known that amnioinfusion washes out amniotic fluid, which has bacteriolytic properties. This action possibly explains an increase in the incidence of infection. However, amnioinfusion also washes out bacteria and cleanses the amnion and fetus, which may lower infectious morbidity. Whether the association represents a causal relationship remains to be proven.

Other complications described in association with amnioinfusion include dehiscence of uterine scar, umbilical cord prolapse, and maternal pulmonary embolus [9,52,53]. Whether the rate of these rare complications is increased by amnioinfusion remains to be proven.

Table 51.2 Amnioinfusion prophylaxis for meconium.

Study	Type	Meconium Classification	GA	n	Findings in Amnioinfused Group
Amnioinfusion vs. no amnioinfusion					
Wenstrom and Parsons [38]	P–R	Thick	NS 39 wk (mean)	80	↓Operative delivery ↓Mec below cords ↓Fetal distress No Δ mec aspiration No Δ umbil art pH
Sadovsky *et al.* [36]	P–R	>Trace	≥34 wk	40	↓Thickness of mec ↓Mec below cords ↑Umbil art pH No mec aspiration
Macri *et al.* [39]	P–R	Thick oligohydramnios (AFI ≤ 5)	>37 wk	160	↓Operative delivery ↓Mec below cords ↓Mec aspiration ↑Umbil art pH ↑1 and 5 Apgar scores
Cialone *et al.* [40]	P–R	Moderate–thick	>36 wk	105	↑Birthweight ↓Fetal distress ↓Mec aspiration ↑Umbil art pH
Eriksen *et al.* [41]	P–R	Thick	>36 wk	124	No Δ operative delivery No Δ fetal distress No Δ umbil art pH ↓Mec below cords
Puertas *et al.* [42]	P–R	>Mod mec	Term	206	↓Cesarean delivery (fetal distress) ↓Mec below cords ↑pH
Rathore *et al.* [43]	P–R	>Mod mec	≥37 wks	200	↓Cesarean delivery ↓Mec below cords ↑1 min Apgar score
Fraser *et al.* [48]	P–R	Thick mec	>36 wks	1998	No Δ MAS No Δ cesarean delivery No Δ perinatal death No Δ maternal or neonatal morbidity
Amnioinfusion vs. standard care					
Parsons *et al.* [45]	R	Thick	NS	NS	No Δ mec aspiration No Δ NICU admissions No Δ umbil art pH for mec aspiration
Spong *et al.* [44]	P–R	Moderate–thick	≥37 wk	93	No Δ operative delivery No Δ fetal distress No Δ umbil art pH No Δ mec below cords No Δ mec aspiration
Usta *et al.* [16]	R	Moderate–thick	NS	937	No Δ mec below cords No Δ mec aspiration ↑Operative delivery ↑Endometritis

AFI, amniotic fluid index; GA, gestational age; mec, meconium; MAS, meconium aspiration syndrome; NICU, neonatal intensive care unit; NS, not specified; P–R, prospective randomized; R, retrospective (evaluation of policy of routine AI in all cases with meconium); umbil art, umbilical artery; wk, weeks; Δ, change.

Table 51.3 Indications for amnioinfusion.

	Beneficial	Uncertain	No Benefit
Therapeutic			
Repetitive variable decelerations	■		
Chorioamnionitis		■	
Severe oligohydramnios	■		
Failed version		■	
Prophylaxis			
Preterm premature rupture of membranes		■	
Term oligohydramnios			■
Meconium			■

Conclusions

Amnioinfusion, an easy procedure to perform, can increase the amniotic fluid volume and relieve variable decelerations. Table 51.3 summarizes the indications for amnioinfusion and its relative usefulness.

Case presentation

A 32-year-old nulliparous woman presents to labor and delivery in active labor. Review of medical records and examination reveals she is in labor (4 cm dilatated, 80% effaced, −1 station) with a singleton term baby and no other medical complications. The clinically estimated fetal weight is 3400 g. She was monitored and then allowed to ambulate. After several hours she complained of leaking fluid and is found to have ruptured membranes. The fetal heart tracing has had a steady baseline of 140 beats/min with good accelerations and uterine contractions every 3–4 minutes. After rupture of membranes, repetitive variable decelerations are noted, reaching a nadir of 50–60 beats/min with a "v" pattern. Alteration of the maternal position did not alleviate the variable decelerations. Assessment of the amniotic fluid index found oligohydramnios with an AFI of 1.2 cm. Internal monitors were placed including a double lumen intrauterine pressure catheter to allow infusion of fluid along with monitoring of intrauterine pressure. Amnioinfusion was started with room temperature normal saline with a 500-mL bolus followed by a constant infusion of 180 mL/h (3 mL/min). Monitoring of the bed pads was assessed to confirm leaking of fluid. The fetal heart rate tracing improved after the bolus of fluid was complete with resolution of the repetitive variable decelerations. After several hours she complained of pressure and examination revealed she was completely dilatated and +2 station. The amnioinfusion was stopped. After 45 minutes of pushing, she delivered a 3250 g female with Apgar scores of 8 and 9.

References

1 Goodlin RC. Intra-amniotic infusion. *Am J Obstet Gynecol* 1981;**139**:975 (letter).

2 Wenstrom K, Andrews WW, Maher JE. Amnioinfusion survey: prevalence, protocols, and complications. *Obstet Gynecol* 1995;**86**:572–6.

3 Strong TH Jr, Vega JS, O'Shaughnessy MJ, *et al.* Amnioinfusion among women attempting vaginal birth after cesarean delivery. *Obstet Gynecol* 1992;**79**:673–4.

4 Bratlid D, Lindback T. Bacteriolytic activity of amniotic fluid. *Obstet Gynecol* 1978;**51**:63–6.

5 Strong TH Jr, Hetzler G, Paul RH. Amniotic fluid volume increase after amnioinfusion of a fixed volume. *Am J Obstet Gynecol* 1990;**162**:746–8.

6 Puder KS, Sorokin Y, Bottoms SF, *et al.* Amnioinfusion: does the choice of solution adversely affect neonatal electrolyte balance? *Obstet Gynecol* 1994;**84**:956–9.

7 Nageotte MP, Bertucci L, Towers CV, *et al.* Prophylactic amnioinfusion in pregnancies complicated by oligohydramnios: a prospective study. *Obstet Gynecol* 1991;**77**:677–80.

8 Gabbe SG, Ettinger BB, Freeman RK. Umbilical cord compression associated with amniotomy: laboratory observations. *Am J Obstet Gynecol* 1976;**126**:353–5.

9 Miyazaki FS, Taylor NA. Saline amnioinfusion for relief of variable or prolonged decelerations. *Am J Obstet Gynecol* 1983;**146**:670–8.

10 Miyazaki FS, Nevarez F. Saline amnioinfusion for relief of repetitive variable decelerations: a prospective randomized study. *Am J Obstet Gynecol* 1985;**153**:301–6.

11 Spong CY, McKindsey FM, Ross MG. Amniotic fluid index predicts the relief of variable decelerations following amnioinfusion bolus. *Am J Obstet Gynecol* 1996;**175**:1066–70.

12 Ogita S, Imanaka M, Matsumoto M, *et al.* Transcervical amnioinfusion of antibiotics: a basic study for managing premature rupture of membranes. *Am J Obstet Gynecol* 1988;**158**:23–7.

13 Monahan E, Katz VL, Cox RL. Amnioinfusion for preventing puerperal infection: a prospective study. *J Reprod Med* 1995;**40**:721–3.

14 Moen MD, Besinger RE, Tomich PG, *et al.* Effect of amnioinfusion on the incidence of postpartum endometritis in patients undergoing cesarean delivery. *J Reprod Med* 1995;**40**:383–6.

15 Ogundipe OA, Spong CY, Ross MG. Prophylactic amnioinfusion for oligohydramnios: a reevaluation. *Obstet Gynecol* 1994;**84**:544–8.

16 Usta IM, Mercer BM, Aswad NK, *et al.* The impact of a policy of amnioinfusion for meconium-stained amniotic fluid. *Obstet Gynecol* 1995;**85**:237–41.

17 Chamberlain PF, Manning FA, Morrison L, *et al.* The relationship of marginal and decreased amniotic fluid volumes to perinatal outcome. *Am J Obstet Gynecol* 1984;**150**:245.

18 Fisk NM, Ronderos-Dumit D, Soliani A, *et al.* Diagnostic and therapeutic transabdominal amnioinfusion in oligohydramnios. *Obstet Gynecol* 1991;**78**:270–8.

19 Nicolini U, Fisk NM, Talbert DG, *et al.* Intrauterine manometry: technique and application to fetal pathology. *Prenat Diagn* 1989;**9**:243–54.

20 Quetel TA, Mejides AA, Salman FA, *et al*. Amnioinfusion: an aid in the ultrasonographic evaluation of severe oligohydramnios in pregnancy. *Am J Obstet Gynecol* 1992;**167**:333–6.

21 Reuss A, Wladimiroff JW, van den Wijngaard JA, *et al*. Fetal renal anomalies, a diagnostic dilemma in the presence of intrauterine growth retardation and oligohydramnios. *Ultrasound Med Biol* 1987;**13**:619–24.

22 van den Wijngaard JA, Pijpers L, Reuss A, *et al*. Effect of amnioinfusion on the umbilical Doppler flow velocity waveform: a case report. *Fetal Ther* 1987;**2**:27–30.

23 Sherer DM, McAndrew JA, Liberto L, *et al*. Recurring bilateral renal agenesis diagnosed by ultrasound with the aid of amnioinfusion at 18 weeks' gestation. *Am J Perinatol* 1992;**9**:49–51.

24 Haeusler MC, Ryan G, Robson SC, *et al*. The use of saline solution as a contrast medium in suspected diaphragmatic hernia and renal agenesis. *Am J Obstet Gynecol* 1993;**168**:1486–92.

25 Gembruch U, Hansmann M. Artificial instillation of amniotic fluid as a new technique for the diagnostic evaluation of cases of oligohydramnios. *Prenat Diagn* 1988;**8**:33–5.

26 Benifla JL, Goffinet F, Darai E, *et al*. Antepartum transabdominal amnioinfusion to facilitate external cephalic version after initial failure. *Obstet Gynecol* 1994;**84**:1041–2.

27 Strong TH Jr, Hetzler G, Sarno AP, *et al*. Prophylactic intrapartum amnioinfusion: a randomized clinical trial. *Am J Obstet Gynecol* 1990;**162**:1370–5.

28 Nageotte MP, Bertucci L, Towers CV, *et al*. Prophylactic amnioinfusion in pregnancies complicated by oligohydramnios: a prospective study. *Obstet Gynecol* 1991;**77**:677–80.

29 Schrimmer DB, Macri CJ, Paul RH. Prophylactic amnioinfusion as a treatment for oligohydramnios in laboring patients: a prospective, randomized trial. *Am J Obstet Gynecol* 1991;**165**:972–5.

30 MacGregor SN, Banzhaf WC, Silver RK, *et al*. A prospective randomized evaluation of intrapartum amnioinfusion. *J Reprod Med* 1991;**36**:69–73.

31 Chauhan SP, Rutherford SE, Hess LW, *et al*. Prophylactic intrapartum amnioinfusion for patients with oligohydramnios: a prospective randomized study. *J Reprod Med* 1992;**37**:817–20.

32 Nageotte MP, Freeman RK, Garite TJ, *et al*. Prophylactic intrapartum amnioinfusion in patients with preterm premature rupture of membranes. *Am J Obstet Gynecol* 1985;**153**:557–62.

33 Locatelli A, Vergani P, DiPirro G, *et al*. Role of amnioinfusion in the management of premature rupture of the membranes at <26 weeks' gestation. *Am J Obstet Gynecol* 2000;**183**:78–82.

34 Tan LK, Kumar S, Jolly M, Gleeson C, Johnson P, Fisk NM. Test amnioinfusion to determine suitability for serial therapeutic amnioinfusion in midtrimester premature rupture of membranes. *Fetal Diagn Ther* 2003;**18**:183–9.

35 Katz VL, Bowes WA. Meconium aspiration syndrome: reflections on a murky subject. *Am J Obstet Gynecol* 1992;**166**;171–83.

36 Sadovsky Y, Amon E, Bade ME, *et al*. Prophylactic amnioinfusion labor complicated by meconium: a preliminary report. *Am J Obstet Gynecol* 1989;**161**:613–7.

37 Ghidini A, Spong CY. Severe meconium aspiration syndrome is not caused by aspiration of meconium. *Am J Obstet Gynecol* 2001;**185**:931–8.

38 Wenstrom KD, Parsons MT. The prevention of meconium aspiration in labor using amnioinfusion. *Obstet Gynecol* 1989;**73**:647–51.

39 Macri CJ, Schrimmer DB, Leung A, *et al*. Prophylactic amnioinfusion improves outcome of pregnancy complicated by thick meconium and oligohydramnios. *Am J Obstet Gynecol* 1992;**167**:117–21.

40 Cialone PR, Sherer DM, Ryan RM, *et al*. Amnioinfusion during labor complicated by particulate meconium-stained amniotic fluid decreases neonatal morbidity. *Am J Obstet Gynecol* 1994;**170**:842–9.

41 Eriksen NL, Hostetter M, Parisi VM. Prophylactic amnioinfusion in pregnancies complicated by thick meconium. *Am J Obstet Gynecol* 1994;**171**:1026–30.

42 Puertas A, Carrillo MP, Molto L, Alvarez M, Sedeno S, Miranda JA. Meconium-stained amniotic fluid in labor: a randomized trial of prophylactic amnioinfusion. *Eur J Obstet Gynecol Reprod Biol* 2001;**99**:33–7.

43 Rathore AM, Singh R, Ramji S, Tripathi R. Randomized trial of amnioinfusion during labour with meconium stained amniotic fluid. *Br J Obstet Gynaecol* 2002;**109**:17–20.

44 Spong CY, Ogundipe OA, Ross MG. Prophylactic amnioinfusion for meconium-stained amniotic fluid. *Am J Obstet Gynecol* 1994;**171**:931–5.

45 Parsons MT, Parsons AK, Angel JL. The failure of routine amnioinfusion in patients with thick meconium to eliminate the occurrence of meconium aspiration syndrome. *Am J Obstet Gynecol* 1992;**166**:405.

46 Pierce J, Gaudier FL, Sanchez-Ramos L. Intrapartum amnioinfusion for meconium-stained fluid: meta-analysis of prospective clinical trials. *Obstet Gynecol* 2000;**95**:1051.

47 Hofmeyr GJ. Amnioinfusion for meconium-stained liquor in labor. *Cochrane Database Syst Rev* 2000; CD000014.

48 Fraser WD, Hofmeyr J, Lede R, *et al*. Amnioinfusion for the prevention of the meconium aspiration syndrome. *N Engl J Med* 2005;**353**:909.

49 Tabor BL, Maier JA. Polyhydramnios and elevated intrauterine pressure during amnioinfusion. *Am J Obstet Gynecol* 1987;**156**:130–1.

50 Posner MD, Ballagh SA, Paul RH. The effect of amnioinfusion on uterine pressure and activity: a preliminary report. *Am J Obstet Gynecol* 1990;**163**:813–8.

51 Sorensen T, Sobeck J, Benedetti T. Intrauterine pressure in acute iatrogenic hydramnios. *Obstet Gynecol* 1991;**78**:917–9.

52 Dragich DA, Ross AF, Chestnut DH, *et al*. Respiratory failure associated with amnioinfusion during labor. *Anesth Analg* 1991;**72**:549–51.

53 Maher JE, Wenstrom KD, Hauth JC, *et al*. Amniotic fluid embolism after saline amnioinfusion: two cases and review of the literature. *Obstet Gynecol* 1994;**83**:851–4.

52 Fetal surgery

Robert H. Ball, Hanmin Lee, and Michael R. Harrison

Over the last decade, technologic advances have allowed a transition towards less invasive procedures. Initial fetal surgical procedures depended on maternal laparotomy and hysterotomy. This approach evolved into maternal laparotomy with uterine endoscopy and most recently into percutaneous approaches. It appears that the less invasive approaches are associated with a less complicated postoperative recovery for the mother, but morbidity is not eliminated [1].

As the proposed indications for fetal surgical interventions and the number of procedures performed have expanded, so too have the centers at which they are performed and the number of physicians performing them. Nevertheless, the availability and proven utility of these procedures remain very limited when compared with the number of fetuses with malformations. One of the responsibilities of physicians with an interest in prenatal diagnosis and intervention is to determine training needs and oversight for operators and centers involved in this field. It is unclear how many centers would be needed given the rarity of these malformations in which a fetal surgical approach may be effective and the even smaller proportion of those with malformation that may need fetal intervention. We must achieve a delicate balance between the ease of accessibility and surgical experience.

Open fetal surgery (hysterotomy)

The feasibility of performing a hysterotomy with subsequent closure of the gravid human uterus was tested in the primate. The safety profile in this series of primate fetal surgeries was reassuring, including subsequent fertility [2]. The human experience is now quite extensive, both from our own center and others [1,3,4], and has been primarily associated with the large numbers of fetal spina bifida repairs. We currently reserve hysterotomies for repair of spina bifida, resection of sacrococcygeal teratomas (SCTs) and other tumors, and lobectomies for congenital cystic adenomatoid malformations (CCAM).

Risks and benefits

We have recently reviewed our experience at the University of California, San Francisco (UCSF) with maternal hysterotomy (Table 52.1) [1]. Eighty-seven hysterotomies were performed between 1989 and 2003. There were significant postoperative complications. In the early experience, pulmonary edema related to multiple tocolytic use, particularly nitroglycerin, and aggressive fluid management were significant problems [5]. Transfusion for intraoperative blood loss was not uncommon. Pregnancy outcomes were also adversely impacted by high rates of premature rupture of membrane and preterm labor. The mean time from hysterotomy to delivery was 4.9 weeks (range 0–16 weeks). The mean gestational age at the time of delivery was 30.1 weeks (range 21.6–36.7 weeks). Others have similar experiences with respect to an increased risk of preterm delivery following hysterotomy [6,7]. Most of the morbidity associated with hysterotomy has decreased with experience. Significant pulmonary edema or blood loss is now rare, and the mean gestational age at the time of delivery following *in utero* repair of myelomeningocele (MMC) is now around 34 weeks.

The practical aspects of hysterotomy and postoperative management have evolved since the early years of experience. The following is a description of our current approach. Lengthy discussions regarding the risks, benefits, and alternatives of the procedure are important, including the experimental nature of the surgery. We generally differentiate the risks to the mother, the fetus, and the pregnancy in our counseling. The risks to the mother are similar to other major abdominal surgery, although in this case there is no direct physical benefit to her. In addition, there are the risks associated with aggressive tocolytic therapy and bed rest in a hypercoagulable state. The risks to the fetus are primarily vascular instability and hypoperfusion intraoperatively, leading to injury or death, and prematurity resulting from postoperative complications. The risks to the pregnancy are primarily preterm labor, premature rupture of membranes, and preterm delivery.

Table 52.1 Maternal morbidity and mortality for 178 interventions at University of California, San Francisco (UCSF) with postoperative continuing pregnancy and divided into operative subgroups.

Operative Technique	Open Hysterotomy	Endoscopy FETENDO/ Lap-FETENDO	Percutaneous FIGS/ Lap-FIGS	All Interventions
Patients with postop continuing pregnancy	79	68	31	178
Gestational age at surgery (weeks)	25.1	24.5	21.1	24.2
Range (weeks)	17.6–30.4	17.9–32.1	17.0–26.6	17.0–32.1
Gestational age at delivery (weeks)	30.1	30.4	32.7	30.7
Range (weeks)	21.6–36.7	19.6–39.3	21.7–40.4	19.6–40.4
Interval surgery to delivery (weeks)	4.9	6.0	11.6	6.5
Range (weeks)	0–16	0–19	0.3–21.4	0–21.4
Pulmonary edema	22/79 (27.8%)	17/68 (25.0%)	0/31 (0.0%)	39/178 (21.9%)
Bleeding requiring blood transfusion	11/87 (12.6%)	2/69 (2.9%)	0/31 (0.0%)	13/187 (7.0%)
PTL leading to delivery	26/79 (32.9%)	18/68 (26.5%)	4/31 (12.9%)	48/178 (27.0%)
Premature rupture of membranes (PROM)	41/79 (51.9%)	30/68 (44.1%)	8/31 (25.8%)	79/178 (44.4%)
Chorioamnionitis	7/79 (8.9%)	1/68 (1.5%)	0/31 (0.0%)	8/178 (4.5%)

PTL, Preterm labor.

Infectious complications are rare, except when premature rupture of membranes leads to chorioamnionitis. An important additional counseling point is that all subsequent deliveries, including the index pregnancy, must be by cesarean section. Data regarding future fertility is reassuring, with no increased incidence of infertility in the UCSF experience in those patients subsequently attempting pregnancy [8]. Experience from Children's Hospital of Philadelphia (CHOP) suggests a substantial risk of uterine rupture in subsequent pregnancies that may be as high as 17%. This is higher than the risk after previous low transverse cesarean delivery (1% or less) or classic cesarean delivery (4–5%). Another potential risk in subsequent pregnancies is placenta accreta. The reason for this is that the uterine location of the hysterotomy incision performed in the second trimester is not in the same area as a cesarean delivery uterine entry site. There is an increased risk of placenta accreta in any setting where implantation occurs in an area of uterine scarring. Multiple incisions will increase the likelihood of implantation in such an area. To our knowledge there has not been a case of placenta accreta in a fetal surgical patient of ours in a subsequent pregnancy (approximately 80 patients and 40 subsequent pregnancies).

Technique

The following is our usual management scheme. Prior to surgery, the patients are premedicated with indomethacin and a cephalosporin. Compression stockings and pneumatic antithrombotic boots are placed on the lower extremities. General anesthesia is initiated, with high levels of a halogenated inhalational agent to maximize uterine relaxation. A Foley catheter is placed to drain the bladder. An epidural catheter is placed for postoperative pain control. Following prepping and draping, ultrasound transducers with sterile covers are used to identify fetal lie and placental location. The latter will determine the need for exteriorization of the uterus to allow access to the posterior aspect in cases of an anterior placenta. The transverse skin incision is generally a third of the way between the pubic symphysis and the umbilicus, lower with an anterior placenta, so that the uterus can more easily be exteriorized. Usually, the rectus muscles need to be at least partially transected to allow appropriate exposure. Once the peritoneal cavity is entered, the ultrasound transducer is placed directly on the myometrium and the edge of the placenta identified and marked. The general strategy is to place the hysterotomy as far from the placenta as possible, with the direction of the incision parallel to its edge. This will minimize the risk of extension towards the placenta, as placental bed bleeding cannot generally be controlled. The additional determinant for the site of the hysterotomy is the fetal surgical site and fetal position. Frequently, transuterine (hands on serosal surface of uterus) fetal manipulation will achieve successful position.

Initial uterine entry can be performed either using the Bruner–Tulipan trochar, or direct cut-down. The initial entry is then extended using the Harrison uterine stapler. Use of ultrasound is critical to confirm that the stapler compresses no fetal part or loop of cord, and is definitively intra-amniotic. The stapler fires a line of dissolvable staples 8 cm long and cuts in between them. This produces a hemostatic myometrial incision with the membranes tacked to the myometrium, minimizing the risk of dissection. Occasionally, bleeding from the myometrial edge, particularly at the apices, requires placement of atraumatic clamps or a figure of eight stitch. Specially designed Harrison–Moran backbiting retractors provide further hemostasis and exposure (Figs 52.1 and 52.2).

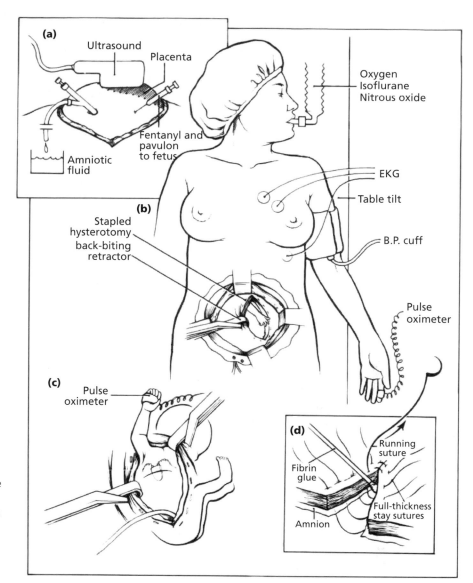

Fig. 52.1 Summary of open fetal surgery techniques. (a) The uterus is exposed through a low transverse abdominal incision. Ultrasonography is used to localize the placenta, inject the fetus with narcotic and muscle relaxant, and aspirate amniotic fluid. (b) The uterus is opened with staples that provide hemostasis and seal the membranes. Maternal anesthesia, and monitoring are shown. (c) Absorbable staples and backbiting clamps facilitate hysterotomy exposure of the pertinent fetal part. A miniaturized pulse oximeter records pulse rate and oxygen saturation intraoperatively. (d) After fetal repair the uterine incision is closed with absorbable sutures and fibrin glue. Amniotic fluid is restored with warm lactated Ringer solution.

Once the hysterotomy incision is appropriately hemostatic, attention can be turned to the fetus. Only that part of the fetus needed to perform the procedure should be exteriorized. This is important for fetal temperature control, and to avoid tissue desiccation and abruption secondary to uterine decompression. The fetus can be monitored using either a pulse oximeter and/or sonographic surveillance of the fetal heart. During the surgery, continued relaxation of the uterus is monitored by palpation, and the serosal surfaces are irrigated with warm saline. If the uterus begins to contract, options include increasing inhalational agents, use of nitroglycerin or loading with magnesium sulfate, or a combination of the above.

Following the procedure on the fetus, the uterine closure begins. This is usually the time we initiate the bolus of magnesium sulfate, followed by a maintenance dose. The uterus is closed in two layers of No. 0 polyglycolic monofilament suture.

Full-thickness interrupted stay sutures are placed first but not tied, then the continuous suture is placed. Prior to tying the continuous suture, a catheter is used to refill the amniotic cavity under ultrasound guidance with lactated Ringer solution. The fluid is replenished to a level of low normal fluid, then the stay sutures are tied. When it is assured that the suture line is hemostatic and hydrostatic, the abdominal wall is closed in layers in the usual fashion.

Postoperative recovery in our unit is accomplished in the labor and delivery suite. For pain control, the preoperatively placed epidural catheter is used for the first 48 hours. Intravenous magnesium sulfate is continued for 24 hours and oral nifedipine then initiated. Indomethacin is continued for a total of 48 hours, with ductal constriction surveillance performed by fetal echocardiography daily. The nifedipine is continued long term. Activity is limited to bed rest for the first 48 hours

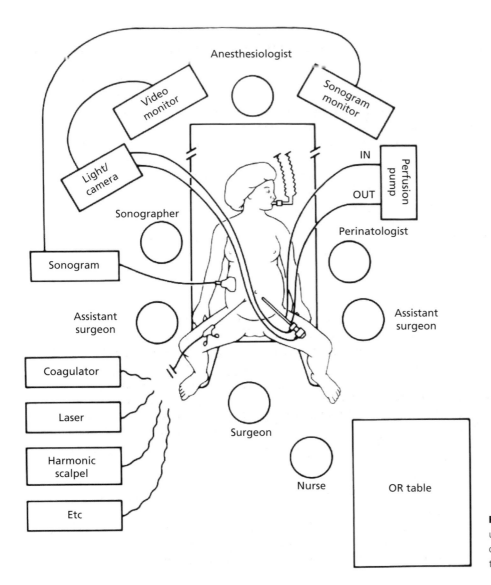

Fig. 52.2 Drawing of the operating room set-up. Note that there are two monitors at the head of the table: one for the fetoscopic picture and the other for the real-time ultrasound image.

postoperatively and then liberalized. Upon discharge, patients are still encouraged to limit activity. Close outpatient follow-up with weekly visits and ultrasounds is our routine.

Indications for open fetal surgery

Myelomeningocele (MMC)

The most common indication for hysterotomy-based fetal intervention currently in our center is MMC. This is a birth defect with sequelae that affect both the central and peripheral nervous systems. A change in cerebrospinal fluid (CSF) dynamics results in the Arnold–Chiari II malformation and hydrocephalus. The abnormally exposed spinal cord results in lifelong lower extremity neurologic deficiency, fecal and urinary incontinence, sexual dysfunction, and skeletal deformities. This defect carries enormous personal, familial, and societal costs, as the near normal lifespan of the affected child is characterized by hospitalization, multiple operations, disability, and, occasionally, institutionalization. Although it has been assumed that the spinal cord itself is intrinsically malformed in children with this defect, recent work suggests that the neurologic impairment after birth may be caused by exposure and trauma to the spinal cord *in utero*, and that covering the exposed cord may prevent the development of the Chiari malformation [9].

Since 1997, more than 200 fetuses have had *in utero* closure of MMC by open fetal surgery. Preliminary clinical evidence suggests this procedure reduces the incidence of shunt-dependent hydrocephalus and restores the cerebellum and brainstem to a more normal configuration. However, clinical results of fetal surgery for MMC are based on comparisons with historical controls, examine only efficacy not safety, and lack long-term follow-up.

The National Institutes of Health (NIH) has funded a multicenter randomized clinical trial (Management of Myelomeningocele Study or "MOMS") of 200 patients that will be conducted at three centers: UCSF; CHOP; and Vanderbilt University Medical Center, along with an independent Data and Study Coordinating Center, the George Washington University Biostatistics Center. There is a moratorium on performing this surgery outside the trial until the results are reported.

Congenital cystic adenomatoid malformation

Congenital cystic adenomatoid malformation (CCAM) leading to hydrops is another indication for hysterotomy. Although CCAM often presents as a benign pulmonary mass in infants and children, some fetuses with large lesions die *in utero* or at birth from hydrops and pulmonary hypoplasia [10]. The pathophysiology of hydrops and the feasibility of resecting the fetal lung have been studied in animals [10,11]. Experience managing more than 200 cases suggests that most lesions can be successfully treated after birth, and that some lesions resolve before birth [12]. Although only a few fetuses with very large lesions develop hydrops before 26 weeks' gestation, these lesions may progress rapidly and the fetuses die *in utero*. Careful sonographic surveillance of large lesions is necessary to detect the first signs of hydrops, because fetuses developing hydrops can be successfully treated by emergency resection of the abnormal lobe *in utero*. Fetal pulmonary lobectomy has proven to be surprisingly simple and quite successful at UCSF and CHOP. For lesions with single large cysts, thoracoamniotic shunting has also been successful [13]. Percutaneous ablation techniques are being investigated. We have seen regression of very large lesions with hydrops after maternal steroid treatment.

Sacrococcygeal teratoma

Hysterotomy is the most common fetal surgical approach to treat fetuses in high output failure and hydrops with large SCTs. Most neonates with SCT survive, and malignant invasion is unusual. However, the prognosis of patients with SCT diagnosed prenatally (by sonogram or elevated alphafetoprotein [AFP]) may be less favorable. There is a subset of fetuses (fewer than 20%) with large tumors who develop hydrops from high-output failure secondary to extremely high blood flow through the tumor. Because hydrops may progress quite rapidly to fetal death, close sonographic follow-up is critical. Attempts to interrupt the vascular steal phenomenon by sonographically guided or fetoscopic techniques have not yet been successful. Excision of the tumor reverses the pathophysiology if it is performed before "mirror syndrome" (maternal preeclampsia) develops in the mother. Hysterotomies in these cases may involve quite large incisions because of the size of the masses.

Fetoscopic surgery (FETENDO)

With advances in technology and familiarity with endoscopic techniques, application of this technique to fetal surgery was natural. Common sense would suggest that the smaller the incision in the uterus, the lower the risk of subsequent pregnancy complications. At UCSF, endoscopic approaches were first applied to pregnancies complicated by diaphragmatic hernia, urinary tract obstruction, and twin–twin transfusion (Lap-FETENDO).

The initial pioneering approach involved maternal minilaparotomies, with direct exposure of the uterus. Ultrasound is used to determine the point of entry and the laparotomy site, depending on placental location and fetal lie. Once the uterus has been exposed, stay sutures are placed and a 3- to 5-mm step trocar advanced into the amniotic cavity under direct ultrasound visualization. Initially, several trocars were required for *in utero* dissections, placement of staples, etc. Later, many procedures could be performed through a single trocar using an endoscope with an operating channel. Initial caution regarding this approach led to similar perioperative management compared with hysterotomy cases. This included general anesthesia, use of multiple tocolytics, and prolonged hospitalization. One important difference even initially was that patients could labor following FETENDO procedures. Since these initial cases, endoscopic procedures have become less invasive with smaller instruments passed through 3-mm ports. This may explain why pregnancy outcomes and pulmonary edema rates were initially similar comparing the hysterotomy and endoscopy groups, although transfusions were required less frequently in the latter cases (Table 52.1) [1]. The interval from procedure to delivery was also little changed as was the gestational age at delivery. In our experience, many of the deliveries still required cesarean section to accommodate EXIT procedures [1,13]. This is essentially a cesarean delivery in which the cord is not clamped until airway management is secure. It involves strategies similar to those used for open surgery, including uterine relaxation with general anesthesia, myometrial incision hemostasis with staples, and fetal monitoring. The endoscopic procedures that necessitated EXITs were balloon tracheal occlusions for congenital diaphragmatic hernias. This was also amongst the most frequent indication for an endoscopic fetal surgical approach at UCSF.

Percutaneous FETENDO

Currently, we rarely use the more invasive Lap-FETENDO and have since progressed towards a percutaneous approach using a smaller 2.0-mm endoscope with an operating channel (Micro-FETENDO). We have used this technique for balloon tracheal occlusions, fetal cystoscopies, and for laser ablation in monochorionic twin gestations complicated by severe twin–twin transfusion. We anticipate based on our early experience and that of others [13] that the risk profile with percutaneous micro-endoscopy will be similar to percutaneous sonography-guided procedures (see below). The perioperative management is very different compared to the more invasive procedures. Although patients are treated with prophylactic indomethacin and antibiotics, uterine relaxation from inhalational agents is not required and may in fact be detrimental. Therefore, we generally use regional anesthesia. Ultrasound is again critical for safe uterine access to determine the best entry point. This is based on fetal position, placental location, membrane position in multiple gestations, and uterine vascularity. Postoperative tocolytic therapy is usually based on contraction activity. A 24–48-hour course of indomethacin or nifedipine is often all that is required. In cases where there are significant postoperative changes in uterine size, such as with interventions for twin–twin transfusion syndrome (TTTS), prophylactic intravenous magnesium sulfate may be helpful. This has to be balanced against the risk of port site hemorrhage, which may be more likely in our experience with a greater degree of uterine relaxation.

Indications for fetoscopic surgery (FETENDO)

Congenital diaphragmatic hernia

The fundamental problem in babies born with a congenital diaphragmatic hernia (CDH) is pulmonary hypoplasia. Research in experimental animal models and later in human patients over two decades has aimed to improve growth of the hypoplastic lungs before they are needed for gas exchange at birth. Anatomic repair of the hernia by open hysterotomy proved feasible but did not decrease mortality and was abandoned. Fetal tracheal occlusion was developed as an alternative strategy to promote fetal lung growth by preventing normal egress of lung fluid. Occlusion of the fetal trachea was shown to stimulate fetal lung growth in a variety of animal models. Techniques to achieve reversible fetal tracheal occlusion were explored in animal models and then applied clinically, evolving from external metal clips placed on the trachea by open hysterotomy or fetoscopic neck dissection, to internal tracheal occlusion with a detachable silicone balloon placed by fetal bronchoscopy through a single 5-mm uterine port, as described above.

Our initial experience suggested that fetal endoscopic tracheal occlusion improved survival in human fetuses with severe CDH. To evaluate this novel therapy, we conducted a randomized controlled trial comparing tracheal occlusion with standard care. Survival with fetal endoscopic tracheal occlusion (73%) met expectations (predicted 75%) and appeared better than that of historic controls (37%), but proved no better than that of concurrent randomized controls. The higher than expected survival in the standard care group may be because the study design mandated that patients in both treatment groups be delivered, resuscitated, and intensively managed in a unit experienced in caring for critically ill newborns with suspected pulmonary hypoplasia. Attempts to improve outcome for severe CDH by treatments either before or after birth have proven to be double-edged swords. Intensive care after birth has improved survival but has increased long-term sequelae in survivors, and is expensive. Intervention before birth may increase lung size, but prematurity caused by the intervention itself can be detrimental. In our study, babies with severe CDH who had tracheal occlusion before birth were born on average at 31 weeks, as a consequence of the intervention. The observation that their rates of survival and respiratory outcomes (including duration of oxygen requirement) were comparable to infants without tracheal occlusion who were born at 37 weeks, suggests that tracheal occlusion improved pulmonary hypoplasia, but the improvement in lung growth was adversely affected by pulmonary immaturity related to earlier delivery.

The current results underscore the role of randomized trials in evaluating promising new therapies. This is the second NIH-sponsored trial comparing a new prenatal intervention for severe fetal CDH. The first trial showed that complete surgical repair of the anatomic defect (which required hysterotomy), although feasible, was no better than postnatal repair in improving survival and was ineffective when the liver as well as the bowel were herniated [15]. That trial led to the abandonment of open complete repair at our institution and subsequently around the world. Information derived from that trial regarding measures of severity of pulmonary hypoplasia (including liver herniation and the development of the lung : head ratio [LHR], area of contralateral lung in axial plane at level of four chamber view of heart, normalized to head circumference) led to the development of an alternative physiologic strategy to enlarge the hypoplastic fetal lung by temporary tracheal occlusion and to the development of less-invasive fetal endoscopic techniques that did not require hysterotomy to achieve temporary, reversible tracheal occlusion [16,17].

Our ability to accurately diagnose and assess severity of CDH before birth has improved dramatically. Fetuses with CDH who have associated anomalies do poorly, whereas fetuses with isolated CDH, no liver herniation, and an LHR above 1.4 have an excellent prognosis (100% in our experience). In this study, fetuses with an LHR between 0.9 and 1.4 had a chance of survival greater than 80% when delivered at a tertiary care center. The small number of fetuses with LHR below 0.9 had a poor prognosis in both treatment groups, and should be the focus of further studies [18].

Because tracheal occlusion does work in enlarging hypoplastic lungs, approaches to tracheal occlusion other than that used here might be beneficial. Although the duration of occlusion in this study (36.2 ± 14.7 days) is comparable with that studied in animal models [18,19], the optimal timing and duration of occlusion is not known in humans. Short-term occlusion later in gestation and earlier occlusion (with possible reversal *in utero*) have been studied in animal models [21,22] and applied in humans. It is also possible that the risk of premature rupture of membranes leading to preterm labor and delivery might be reduced by using smaller 2-mm fetoscopes percutaneously and by newly developed techniques to seal membranes. Fetuses with an LHR less than 0.9 have poor survival and remain the focus for new treatment strategies either before or after birth.

Twin–twin transfusion syndrome

TTTS was one of the first entities to be treated endoscopically at UCSF. It is a complication of monochorionic multiple gestations resulting from an imbalance in blood flow through vascular communications, such that one twin is compromised and the other favored. It is the most common serious complication of monochorionic twin gestations, affecting between 4% and 35% of monochorionic twin pregnancies, or approximately 0.1–0.9 per 1000 births each year in the USA. Yet, despite the relatively low incidence, TTTS disproportionately accounts for 17% of all perinatal mortality associated with twin gestations [23]. Standard therapy has been limited to serial amnioreduction, which appears to improve the overall outcome but has little impact on the more severe end of the spectrum in TTTS. In addition, survivors of TTTS treated by serial amnioreduction have an 18–26% incidence of significant neurologic and cardiac morbidity. Selective fetoscopic laser photocoagulation of communicating vessels has emerged as an alternative treatment strategy with at least comparable, if not superior, survival to serial amnioreduction, as demonstrated in a randomized trial in Europe [24].

Urinary tract obstruction

As a group at UCSF we are particularly enthusiastic about the potential of fetal intervention in bladder outlet obstruction by percutaneous fetal cystoscopy. Fetal urethral obstruction produces pulmonary hypoplasia and renal dysplasia, and these often-fatal consequences can be ameliorated by urinary tract decompression before birth. The natural history of untreated fetal urinary tract obstruction is well documented, and selection criteria based on fetal urine electrolyte and B_2 microglobulin levels and the sonographic appearance of fetal kidneys have proven reliable [24–27]. Of all fetuses with urinary tract dilatation, the vast majority do not require intervention. However, fetuses with bilateral hydronephrosis and bladder distension resulting from urethral obstruction subsequently developing oligohydramnios require treatment. Depending on the gestational age, the fetus can be delivered early for postnatal decompression. Alternatively, the bladder can be decompressed *in utero* by a catheter vesicoamniotic shunt (e.g., Harrison shunt) placed percutaneously under sonographic guidance [29], by fetoscopic vesicostomy [30,31], or

more recently by fetocystoscopic ablation of urethral valves [32]. Treatment with shunting has been relatively disappointing, as shunts often migrate or do not remain patent. Even when adequately decompressed, the obstructed bladder may not cycle correctly, resulting in a severe bladder dysfunction requiring surgery after birth. We have now developed a percutaneous fetal cystoscopic technique to disrupt posterior urethral valves through a single 3-mm port.

Fetal intervention guided by sonography

The first fetal procedure, developed in the early 1980s, was percutaneous sonographically guided placement of fetal bladder catheter shunt. Many other catheter-shunt procedures have been developed and described [33]. More recently, we have developed percutaneous sonographically guided radiofrequency ablation procedures for management of anomalous multiple gestations. All these procedures we now group as 'fetal intervention guided by sonography' (FIGS). Very complicated procedures may still require laparotomy (Lap-FIGS).

Percutaneous or micro-FIGS is used to sample or drain fetal blood, urine, and fluid collection, to sample fetal tissue, to place catheter shunts in the fetal bladder, chest, abdomen, or ventricles, and to perform radiofrequency ablation (RFA). The most common indication at UCSF is RFA for acardiac twins/ twin reversed arterial perfusion (TRAP) sequence or monochorionic twins for selective reduction. Other operators have used bipolar coagulation or umbilical cord ligation for similar indications. Compared with the 17-gauge RFA needles we use, these techniques are more invasive, using at least 3-mm trochars. Additionally, the length of the cord or its position may preclude use of these instruments. The perioperative management of these patients is similar to the current micro-FETENDO patients. The procedures are performed under spinal anesthesia, with prophylactic antibiotics and indometacin. Postoperative tocolysis is rarely necessary and the patients are frequently discharged within hours of the procedure. Ultrasound is critical both for the planning and execution of the procedure. We attempt to avoid entry into the sac of a normal twin if at all possible. The RFA needle is guided into the abdominal cord insertion of the abnormal twin under ultrasound guidance. The tines (thin wires protruding out of the needle like hooks) are then deployed and energy delivered to the device to create thermal injury to the tissue. The device we currently use measures the temperature at the tines. This allows us to use an energy level to provide the quickest obliteration of the vascular communications possible. This is of benefit as there are theoretical concerns regarding the differential obliteration of arterial and venous vessels, which might place the normal twin at risk for exsanguination. Ultrasound is also used to monitor the procedure and welfare of the normal twin. Thermal injury can be monitored by watching for the characteristic out-gassing in the tissue. Once active energy delivery to the device has ceased, color-flow Doppler can be used to detect any residual flow, both in the cord and the abnormal fetus. Once absence of blood flow is confirmed, the tines are retracted and the device then withdrawn. We have not found an increased frequency of adverse outcomes with a transplacental approach. We have had good success with this approach with a survival rate of close to 95% and a mean gestational age at delivery of over 35 weeks and an average time from procedure of over 11 weeks. There has been no maternal pulmonary edema or blood loss.

There are a few complicated FIGS procedures that may require maternal laparotomy to allow fetal positioning and sonography directly on the uterus (Lap-FIGS). A few simple structural cardiac defects that interfere with development may benefit from prenatal correction. For example, if obstruction of blood flow across the pulmonary or aortic valve interferes with development of the ventricles or pulmonary or systemic vasculature, relief of the anatomic obstruction may allow normal development with an improved outcome. Alternatively, congenital aortic stenosis may lead to hypoplastic left heart syndrome. Stenotic aortic valves have been dilated by a balloon catheter placed using both FIGS and Lap-FIGS, with some promising results [33]. The procedure is technically difficult. Several centers are developing experimental techniques to correct fetal heart defects [34].

In summary, fetal surgery has evolved considerably since its birth at UCSF two decades ago. The indications remain quite limited, but numerically have the potential to expand as patients and providers become increasingly informed. Recent advances in the development of less invasive fetal endoscopic (FETENDO) and sonography-guided techniques (FIGS) have extended the indications for fetal intervention.

Case presentation

The patient is a 36-year-old G3P2 at 18 weeks' gestation. She was referred to a perinatologist for evaluation because an ultrasound was suspicious for a twin pregnancy with demise of an anomalous fetus with a cystic hygroma.

The perinatologist performed a detailed ultrasound and identified a monochorionic diamnionic twin pregnancy. One twin is morphologically normal and the other has a torso with edematous skin and no heart and is of similar size to the normal twin. The blood flow in the cord is reversed with flow in the single artery towards the anomalous twin. This therefore is an acardiac twin and the situation represents TRAP. The perinatologist discusses with the patient and her partner that in cases of TRAP, the normal or pump twin is at risk of cardiac failure, hydrops, and stillbirth. They discuss the management options including observation or intervention with bipolar cord coagulation or RFA.

The family is seen for evaluation. Ultrasound documents the previous findings and also identifies polyhydramnios and an enlarged intra-abdominal umbilical vein in the pump twin sac, and significant blood flow into the acardiac twin. Fetal echocardiography shows increased biventricular output in the pump twin with some increased pulsatility in the ductus venosus. The multidisciplinary team meets with the patient and her family and discusses the management options and risks and benefits of each. They decide to proceed with RFA.

The procedure is performed the next day, under spinal anesthesia in the operating room. The RFA device is deployed percutaneously under ultrasound guidance into the abdomen of the acardiac twin at the level of the cord insertion. The device is energized, and the tissue is heated acutely. After cool down, ultrasound documents cessation of blood flow based on color flow and pulse Doppler. The patient stays hospitalized overnight. The next day a repeat ultrasound confirms no acute changes in the pump twin without residual flow into the acardiac twin. She is discharged home to return to the care of her referring perinatologist and primary obstetrician. Several months later she delivers a healthy infant at term by induced vaginal delivery.

References

1 Golombeck K, Ball RH, Lee H, *et al*. Maternal morbidity after fetal surgery. *Am J Obstet Gynecol* 2006;**194**:834–9.

2 Adzick NS, Harrison MR, Glick PL, *et al*. Fetal surgery in the primate. III. Maternal outcome after fetal surgery. *J Pediatr Surg* 1986;**21**:477–80.

3 Bruner JP, Tulipan N, Reed G, *et al*. Intrauterine repair of spina bifida: preoperative predictors of shunt-dependent hydrocephalus. *Am J Obstet Gynecol* 2004;**190**:1305–12.

4 Johnson MP, Sutton LN, Rintoul N, *et al*. Fetal myelomeningocele repair: short-term clinical outcomes. *Am J Obstet Gynecol* 2003;**189**:482–7.

5 DiFederico EM, Burlingame JM, Kilpatrick SJ, Harrison MR, Matthay MA. Pulmonary edema in obstetric patients is rapidly resolved except in the presence of infection or of nitroglycerin tocolysis after open fetal surgery. *Am J Obstet Gynecol* 1998;**179**:925–33.

6 Wilson RD, Johnson MP, Crombleholme TM, *et al*. Chorioamniotic membrane separation following open fetal surgery: pregnancy outcome. *Fetal Diagn Ther* 2003;**18**:314–20.

7 Bruner JP, Tulipan NB, Richards WO, Walsh WF, Boehm FH, Vrabcak EK. *In utero* repair of myelomeningocele: a comparison of endoscopy and hysterotomy. *Fetal Diagn Ther* 2000;**15**:83–8.

8 Farrell JA, Albanese CT, Jennings RW, Kilpatrick SJ, Bratton BJ, Harrison MR. Maternal fertility is not affected by fetal surgery. *Fetal Diagn Ther* 1999;**14**:190–2.

9 Bouchard S, Davey MG, Rintoul NE, Walsh DS, Rorke LB, Adzick NS. Correction of hindbrain herniation and anatomy of the vermis after *in utero* repair of myelomeningocele in sheep. *J Pediatr Surg* 2003;**38**:451–8.

10 Adzick NS, Harrison MR, Glick PL, *et al*. Fetal cystic adenomatoid malformation: prenatal diagnosis and natural history. *J Pediatr Surg* 1985;**20**:483–8.

11 Adzick NS, Glick PL, Harrison MR, *et al.* Compensatory lung growth after pneumonectomy in the fetus. *Surg Forum* 1986;**37**:648–9.

12 MacGillivray TE, Harrison MR, Goldstein RB, Adzick NS. Disappearing fetal lung lesions. *J Pediatr Surg* 1993;**28**:1321–4.

13 Blott M, Nicolaides KH, Greenough A. Postnatal respiratory function after chronic drainage of fetal pulmonary cyst. *Am J Obstet Gynecol* 1988;**159**:858–65.

14 Hirose S, Farmer DL, Lee H, Nobuhara KK, Harrison MR. The *ex utero* intrapartum treatment procedure: looking back at the EXIT. *J Pediatr Surg* 2003;**39**:375–80.

15 Harrison MR, Adzick NS, Bullard KM, *et al.* Correction of congenital diaphragmatic hernia *in utero* VII: a prospective trial. *J Pediatr Surg* 1997;**32**:1637–42.

16 Harrison MR, Adzick NS, Flake AW, *et al.* Correction of congenital diaphragmatic hernia *in utero* VIII: response of the hypoplastic lung to tracheal occlusion. *J Pediatr Surg* 1996;**31**:1339–48.

17 Skarsgard ED, Meuli M, VanderWall KJ, Bealer JF, Adzick NS, Harrison MR. Fetal endoscopic tracheal occlusion ('Fetendo-PLUG') for congenital diaphragmatic hernia. *J Pediatr Surg* 1996;**31**:1335–8.

18 Lipshutz GS, Albanese CT, Feldstein VA, *et al.* Prospective analysis of lung-to-head ratio predicts survival for patients with prenatally diagnosed congenital diaphragmatic hernia. *J Pediatr Surg* 1997;**32**:1634–6.

19 Papadakis K, De Paepe ME, Tackett LD, Piasecki GJ, Luks FI. Temporary tracheal occlusion causes catch-up lung maturation in a fetal model of diaphragmatic hernia. *J Pediatr Surg* 1998;**33**:1030–7.

20 VanderWall KJ, Bruch SW, Meuli M, *et al.* Fetal endoscopic ('Fetendo') tracheal clip. *J Pediatr Surg* 1996;**31**:1101–3.

21 Luks FI, Wild YK, Piasecki GJ, De Paepe ME. Short-term tracheal occlusion corrects pulmonary vascular anomalies in the fetal lamb with diaphragmatic hernia. *Surgery* 2000;**128**:266–72.

22 Flageole H, Evrard VA, Piedboeuf B, Laberge JM, Lerut TE, Deprest JA. The plug–unplug sequence: an important step to achieve type II pneumocyte maturation in the fetal lamb model. *J Pediatr Surg* 1998;**33**:299–303.

23 Quintero RA. Twin–twin transfusion syndrome. *Clin Perinatol* 2003;**30**:591–600.

24 Senat MV, Deprest J, Boulvain M, Paupe A, Winer N, Ville Y. Endoscopic laser surgery versus serial amnioreduction for severe twin-to-twin transfusion syndrome. *N Engl J Med* 2004;**351**:136–44.

25 Adzick NS, Harrison MR, Glick PL, Flake AW. Fetal urinary tract obstruction: experimental pathophysiology. *Semin Perinatol* 1985;**9**:79–90.

26 Crombleholme TM, Harrison MR, Golbus MS, *et al.* Fetal intervention in obstructive uropathy: prognostic indicators and efficacy of intervention. *Am J Obstet Gynecol* 1990;**162**:1239–44.

27 Manning FA, Harrison MR, Rodeck C. Catheter shunts for fetal hydronephrosis and hydrocephalus. Report of the International Fetal Surgery Registry. *N Engl J Med* 1986;**315**:336–4.

28 Nicolaides KH, Cheng HH, Snijders RJ, Moniz CF. Fetal urine biochemistry in the assessment of obstructive uropathy. *Am J Obstet Gynecol* 1992;**166**:932–7.

29 Glick PL, Harrison MR, Adzick NS, Noall RA, Villa RL. Correction of congenital hydronephrosis in utero IV: *in utero* decompression prevents renal dysplasia. *J Pediatr Surg* 1984;**19**:649–5.

30 Johnson MP, Bukowski TP, Reitleman C, Isada NB, Pryde PG, Evans MI. *In utero* surgical treatment of fetal obstructive uropathy: a new comprehensive approach to identify appropriate candidates for vesicoamniotic shunt therapy. *Am J Obstet Gynecol* 1994;**170**:1770–6.

31 Crombleholme TM, Harrison MR, Langer JC, *et al.* Early experience with open fetal surgery for congenital hydronephrosis. *J Pediatr Surg* 1988;**23**:1114–21.

32 MacMahon RA, Renou PM, Shekelton PA, Paterson PJ. *In utero* cystostomy. *Lancet* 1992;**340**:123.

33 Wilson RD, Baxter JK, Johnson MP, *et al.* Thoracoamniotic shunts: fetal treatment of pleural effusions and congenital cystic adenomatoid malformations. *Fetal Diagn Ther* 2004;**19**:413–2.

34 Allan LD, Maxwell D, Tynan M. Progressive obstructive lesions of the heart: an opportunity for fetal therapy. *Fetal Ther* 1991;**6**:173–6.

35 Hanley FL. Fetal cardiac surgery. *Adv Cardiac Surg* 1994;**5**:47–74.

53 Problems in the newborn

Avroy A. Fanaroff

Background—the population; statistical definitions: infant mortality

More than half of neonatal deaths in the USA still occur in the approximately 60,000 very low birth weight (VLBW) infants born each year, but advances in neonatal and perinatal care have improved the chances of survival for such infants. Hence, in 2006, in excess of 80% of low birthweight (LBW) infants were the beneficiaries of antenatal corticosteroids with an attendant survival rate of approximately 85%. Factors influencing survival rate include antenatal corticosteroids, birthweight, gestational age, gender, race, mode, and site of delivery. There is improved survival with advancing birthweight and gestational age. Almost 60% of infants with a birthweight of 501–750 g, 90% of 751–1000 g infants, and in excess of 95% of infants who weigh 1001–1500 g survive to hospital discharge. Survival almost doubles at 23–24 weeks (30–60%), increasing steadily between 25 and 27 weeks, and leveling off thereafter (80% at 25 weeks, 85% at 26 weeks, 90% at 27 weeks, and 92% at 28 weeks). Although there were dramatic increases in survival following the introduction of surfactant and widespread use of antenatal corticosteroids, mortality rates appear to have leveled off.

Whether the dramatic improvements in survival of extremely preterm infants have resulted in increased rates and absolute numbers of disabled survivors has been a matter of much debate and concern for physicians caring for these infants. Interpretation of the literature on long-term outcome of extremely preterm infants is limited by small sample sizes, lack of population- and gestational age-based samples, differing proportions of inborn infants, different times of assessment and outcome measures, inconsistent classification of neurodevelopmental impairment, and excessive loss to follow-up [1,2].

The rate of preterm survival without major sensorineural disability at 2 years, based on infants who had survived to initial hospital discharge, was 80%. Twenty percent of the children had a major sensorineural disability (bilateral blindness, deafness, cerebral palsy of such severity that the child did not walk or walked with great difficulty, or had an intelligence quotient greater than 2 standard deviations below the mean); 11% had cerebral palsy. Risk factors during the initial hospitalization for major disability at 5 years of age were grade 3 or 4 intraventricular hemorrhage (IVH), cystic periventricular leukomalacia, postnatal steroid therapy, and surgery before discharge. Among the almost half of the cohort who had none of these risk factors, the rate of survival without major sensorineural disability was 93%, similar to the rate among the normal birthweight controls [3–5].

Parents and physicians of extremely preterm neonates require reliable information on their prognosis for survival and survival without disability in order to make informed decisions about how to best provide for their care. This information is, of necessity, offset in time from current practice and is often not specific to the institution caring for the infant or to the individual infant. Current estimates of the range in survival without impairment (calculated from the product of the lowest survival and the lowest survival without impairment rates vs. the highest survival and highest survival without impairment rates) at 23 weeks is 4–28%; at 24 weeks 12–49%; and at 25 weeks 23–78%. Moreover, although preterm infants may not be neurodevelopmentally impaired at follow-up, they are at significant risk of academic difficulties so that they are more likely to be enrolled in special education classes and are at increased risk for developing attention deficit hyperactivity disorder (ADHD) compared with the term controls. Fewer VLBW infants ultimately graduate from high school compared with their term peers.

In summary, advances in perinatal care have led to the survival of increasing numbers of children born at the lower limits of viability. VLBW children have poorer outcomes relative to normal birthweight term controls in neurologic and health status, cognitive-neuropsychological skills, school performance, academic achievement, and behavior. Outcomes are highly variable but are related to medical risk factors, neonatal medical complications of prematurity, and social risk factors. Attention is increasingly focused on long-term outcome as an indicator of the individual infant's medical and social risk factors, as well as the quality of the medical care the infant received. Systematic evaluation of risk factors (e.g., inflammatory exposures, nutritional status, brain injury on magnetic resonance imaging), and care practices (e.g., ventilatory management) may identify strategies and interventions needed to achieve further improvements in the outcome of babies born at the limits of viability.

Thermoregulation

Thermoregulation of the fetus

The metabolic rate of the fetus per tissue weight is relatively high when compared with that of an adult. Moreover, heat is transferred to the fetus via the placenta and the uterus, resulting in a 0.5°C higher temperature than that of the mother. Also, any changes in the maternal temperature are closely followed in the fetus to maintain this gradient. The maternal arterial temperature is the single most important factor in thermoregulation of the fetus. The fetus does not independently regulate its body temperature. If the pregnant woman develops prolonged and high fever, it reduces the efficiency of the placenta in dissipating the heat generated by the fetus. This causes hyperthermia of the fetus, which could result in teratogenesis, spontaneous abortion, stillbirth, or premature delivery. Maternal fever early in pregnancy is potentially teratogenic.

The umbilical circulation transfers 85% of the heat produced by the fetus to the maternal circulation. The remaining 15% is dissipated through the fetal skin to the amnion, and is then transferred through the uterine wall to the maternal abdomen. As long as fetal heat production and loss are appropriately balanced, the temperature differential between the fetus and the mother remains constant. However, if the umbilical circulation is interrupted for any reason, the fetal temperature will rise and the fetus may become profoundly hyperthermic which may adversely affect brain development. Whereas the neonate will generate extra heat by nonshivering thermogenesis, this mechanism is inhibited in the fetus by adenosine and prostaglandin E_2 derived from the placenta. Both these agents have strong antilipolytic actions.

Thermal regulation after birth

At birth neonates rapidly drop their temperature in response to the relatively cold extrauterine environment together with large convective, radiant, and evaporative heat loss. That is why it is critically important to rapidly dry and warm high risk neonates. The neonate must accelerate heat production which occurs predominantly by nonshivering thermogenesis as shivering is rarely seen in term infants and never in preterm infants. Nonshivering thermogenesis is initiated by lipolysis in the richly vascular brown adipose tissue. Thermogenesis must begin shortly after birth and continue for several hours. Because thermogenesis requires adequate oxygenation, a distressed neonate with hypoxemia cannot produce an adequate amount of heat to increase its temperature and body temperature falls. This is notable in preterm infants where the inability to accommodate to cold stress has long been recognized as a major difference between the preterm and the term neonate.

Thermal regulation under special circumstances

The delivery room

At delivery, newborn infants rapidly lose heat by evaporative, radiant, and convective heat losses. Heat losses by conduction are minimal unless the infant is placed on a cold surface. Heat losses may be minimized by immediately drying infants with dry, prewarmed towels, and wrapping and placing them under a radiant warmer. The delivery room should be kept reasonably warm (more than 25°C) and both term and preterm infants should be dried with prewarmed blankets, wrapped, and placed under a radiant warmer.

Preterm infants are especially prone to hypothermia immediately following birth. Excessive evaporative heat loss and the relatively cool ambient temperature of the delivery room may be important contributing factors. It is important to keep the delivery room warm and in controlled trials which evaluate the effect of placing infants <29 weeks gestation in polyurethane bags up to their necks immediately after delivery even before being dried, the infants had higher mean admission temperatures upon arrival in the nursery and the conclusion is that polyurethane occlusive skin wrapping prevents rather than delays heat loss at delivery in very preterm infants.

Radiant warmers

Rapid, safe warming of hypothermic infants can be accomplished with radiant warmers. These heating devices maintain body temperature by providing radiant heat. Radiant warmers allow for easy accessibility to the infant and are used predominantly in the delivery room and in the care of ill infants who need intensive monitoring and frequent interventions. The optimal skin temperature for the control of radiant heaters is undetermined, but radiant warmers should be used only with a servocontrol and an abdominal skin temperature set at 36.5°C. Such constraints as possible dislodgement of the probe and the need for the thermistor to be covered by an aluminum patch should be clearly understood by those who operate radiant warmers. Radiant warmers significantly increase insensible water loss, especially in preterm infants (50% or more). This can result in rapid dehydration unless there is sufficient water replacement.

Transport

Newborn infants, especially those who are preterm, are at risk of hypothermia while being transported from delivery room to nursery, from one hospital to another, or to and from the operating room. Formerly, a prewarmed, double-walled transport incubator or a single-walled transporter with the infant dressed and/or covered by a blanket or silver swaddler helped prevent a fall in body temperature. More recently, the infants are immediately covered with plastic bags. Transport by aircraft increases the risk of hypothermia by radiant heat loss, so the use of a double-walled transporter is recommended to decrease the loss of body temperature. For procedures, the infant should be placed under a radiant warmer with servocontrol on a continuously warmed mattress, in a draft-free, humidified (50%) room to minimize heat loss.

Induced cooling

Hypothermia is protective against brain injury after asphyxiation in animal models. Recent randomized trials of hypothermia have been completed in infants with a gestational age of at least 36 weeks who were admitted to the hospital at or before 6 hours of age with either severe acidosis or perinatal complications and resuscitation at birth and who had moderate or severe encephalopathy [6,7]. In both trials, death or moderate or severe disability was reduced with cooling. Also there were no differences noted in the frequency of clinically important complications. Shankaran *et al*. [6] reported no increase in major disability such as cerebral palsy among survivors. Moderate cooling offers a new therapy for asphyxia neonatorum.

Anemia

Anemia is defined as a hemoglobin level less than 12 g/100 mL in the first week of life. The hemoglobin and hematocrit peak at 3–12 hours of age as levels both rise 2–3 g/100 mL and 3–6%, respectively. The capillary values for both hemoglobin and hematocrit are consistently higher than venous or arterial measurements.

There are many causes of anemia in the neonatal period. Anemia may result from one of three causes: hemorrhage, hemolysis, and failure of red blood cell production. The presence of severe anemia at the time of delivery or on the first day of life is usually the result of hemorrhage or hemolysis resulting from isoimmunization. When the anemia is secondary to acute blood loss at the time of birth, there may be evidence of

circulatory insufficiency. Causes of anemia in the neonatal period include the following.

Obstetric accidents and malformations of the placenta and cord

This subgroup includes rupture of a normal or abnormal umbilical cord. Rupture of the normal umbilical cord is rare and may result from an unattended precipitous delivery. Severe fetal hemorrhage may accompany placenta previa, abruptio placentae, or incision of the placenta or umbilical cord during cesarean delivery. Failure of the infant to receive the usual placental transfusion during the cesarean delivery and clamping the cord with the infant above the placenta aggravates the situation, because fetoplacental hemorrhage will occur. It may be extremely difficult to distinguish the infant with hypovolemic shock from the severely asphyxiated newborn; both may be extremely pale with evidence of poor perfusion and circulatory insufficiency.

Occult hemorrhage prior to birth

Although some degree of hemorrhage from the fetus into the maternal circulation occurs during 50% of pregnancies, it has been estimated that in only 1% will the amount of fetal loss exceed 40 mL and cause anemia in the newborn. Massive fetal–maternal hemorrhage, defined as more than 150 mL fetal blood in the maternal circulation, is said to account for 3% of perinatal mortality and occurs in approximately 1 in 800 deliveries. Some of the causes of fetal–maternal hemorrhage include amniocentesis, external version, fundal pressure during the second stage of labor, the use of intravenous oxytoxics, trauma, placenta previa, and abruptio placentae [8].

The clinical manifestations of fetal–maternal hemorrhage depend on the timing and acuity. Chronic bleeding results in a very pale infant, not necessarily in distress or manifesting any features of shock but with enlargement of the liver and spleen. The blood smear is typically microcytic and hypochromic, and there is no evidence of hemolysis. Fetal cells can be demonstrated in the maternal circulation, usually by means of the acid elution technique of Kleihauer and Betke. If fetal–maternal hemorrhage of significant proportions has occurred acutely, the clinical features of shock and hypoperfusion predominate. The red blood cell morphology is normocytic and normochromic, and no hepatosplenomegaly is present. In contrast with the infants with chronic loss, who require only iron supplementation, these latter infants are in dire need of fluid replacement to restore intravascular volume, and then blood transfusion.

Internal hemorrhage

There are many potential sites for blood loss in the newborn. The detection of anemia during the first days of life should initiate a careful evaluation to determine the source of blood loss. The finding of a large cephalohematoma or extensive swelling of the scalp associated with a subaponeurotic collection of blood is a common site of blood loss. Infants delivered in the breech position may have significant blood loss into the muscles and manifest bruising but not necessarily swelling. The advent of ultrasonography and computed tomography (CT) has facilitated the search for intracranial and intra-abdominal sites of blood loss.

Traditionally, adrenal hemorrhage, rupture of the liver, and rupture of the spleen all accompany difficult and traumatic deliveries of both macrosomic and premature infants, and are more likely to be noted with breech presentation. The usual clinical manifestations of shock are accompanied by specific abdominal findings, which includes periumbilical discoloration.

Iatrogenic blood loss

Iatrogenic blood loss is associated with excessive blood withdrawal, bleeding from inadequate clamping of the umbilical cord, bleeding associated with improper management of the umbilical arterial catheters, or excessive bleeding following procedures such as circumcision. It is important to monitor closely the volume of blood withdrawn from sick neonates, to restrict the number of laboratory investigations, and to draw the minimal volume of blood necessary. Strict adherence to protocols regarding care of catheters diminishes the risks of hemorrhage from this source.

Hemolytic anemias

There are many causes of hemolytic disease in the newborn. The presence of jaundice distinguishes hemolytic anemia from that characterized by blood loss. Major categories of hemolysis of significance in the neonatal period are as follows:
1 Isoimmunization
2 Congenital defects of the red blood cell
3 Acquired defects of the red blood cell

The problem of isoimmunization is dealt with in Chapter 36. Congenital defects of the red blood cell, which include the enzymatic defects, are characterized by specific morphology of the red blood cell or the presence of abnormal hemoglobin. Among the causes of acquired defects of the red blood cell are a variety of bacterial and viral infections (notably parvovirus which may cause aplastic anemia) and a multitude of drugs and toxins.

In summary, hemorrhage is the most common cause of early anemia. The cause is usually apparent from the history. The initial evaluation requires a complete blood count with smear and reticulocyte count, total and direct bilirubin, blood type and Coombs' test, and the Kleihauer–Betke test on maternal blood. TORCH titers (for a group of infections comprising

Toxoplasma gondii, other viruses, rubella, cytomegalovirus, and herpes simplex), a full coagulation profile, red blood cell enzymes, and hemoglobin electrophoresis are analyzed as indicated by the history and physical examination.

If significant hemorrhage has occurred and the neonate manifests shock with reduced blood pressure and metabolic acidosis, arrangements should be made for immediate blood transfusion. In the meantime, circulation is supported with fluid pushes to expand the intravascular volume, and mechanical ventilation to optimize oxygenation.

Respiratory disorders

Respiratory distress syndrome

Clinical features

Respiratory distress syndrome (RDS) remains a major cause of morbidity in newborn babies. The greatest risk factor appears to be low gestational age, whereas other risk factors include maternal diabetes, hydrops fetalis, and perinatal asphyxia. Although the diagnosis can be established biochemically by documentation of surfactant deficiency in amniotic fluid or in tracheal or gastric aspirate, this is rarely performed and a clinical diagnosis is made, hence statistical data on the prevalence must be interpreted with caution. Nonetheless, the incidence of RDS probably exceeds 80% at a gestation of less than 27 weeks, although severity varies widely. With improved survival, sequelae have increased dramatically, especially bronchopulmonary dysplasia (BPD), because of the disease process as well as modes of treatment [26–29].

Impaired or delayed surfactant synthesis superimposed on a structurally immature lung appears to be key to the pathogenesis of RDS. The resultant decrease in lung compliance leads to alveolar hypoventilation and ventilation–perfusion imbalance. This in turn leads to hypoxemia, which may cause metabolic acidosis, and both may contribute to pulmonary vasoconstriction and aggravate hypoxemia. Meanwhile, high inspired oxygen and barotrauma from assisted ventilation initiate an inflammatory process in the immature lung that paves the way for development of chronic neonatal lung disease or BPD.

Infants with RDS typically present with a combination of tachypnea, nasal flaring, subcostal and intercostal retractions, cyanosis, and expiratory grunting. Retractions are prominent and are the result of the very compliant ribcage being drawn in on inspiration as the infant generates high intrathoracic pressures to expand the poorly compliant lungs. The typical expiratory grunt is thought to result from partial closure of the glottis during expiration and, in this way, acts as a means of trapping alveolar air and maintaining an adequate end-expiratory lung volume (or functional residual capacity, FRC). Although these signs are characteristic of neonatal respiratory disease, they may result from a wide variety of nonpulmonary causes, such as hypothermia, hypoglycemia, anemia, polycythemia, or metabolic acidosis. Furthermore, such nonpulmonary conditions may complicate the clinical course of RDS.

A constant feature of RDS in the pre-surfactant era was the early onset of clinical signs of the disease, typically within 1–2 hours of delivery. The uncomplicated natural course of clinical disease was characterized by a progressive worsening of symptoms, with a peak severity by days 2–3 and onset of recovery by 72 hours. This is now rare because all but the mildest cases of RDS are treated with exogenous surfactant. RDS requiring assisted ventilation may be complicated by the development of air leaks, significant shunting through a patent ductus arteriosus, or BPD, and the infant's recovery may be delayed for days to months.

The typical radiographic features consist of a diffuse reticulogranular pattern in both lung fields with superimposed air bronchograms. These findings cannot be reliably differentiated from those of neonatal pneumonia, most commonly caused by group B streptococci. This problem has been the major reason for the widespread use of antibiotics in the initial management of infants with RDS.

Management

In an infant with respiratory symptoms (especially if preterm), there is a tendency to conclude that underlying pulmonary parenchymal disease is present; however, the differential diagnosis is extensive. Disorders of the upper airway (e.g., choanal atresia, micrognathia), larynx, trachea, intrathoracic airway, chest wall, central nervous system, cardiovascular system, and musculoskeletal system—together with hematologic and metabolic problems or sepsis—may be easily confused with lung disorders. Analysis of simple laboratory data includes blood gases, hematocrit, blood sugar, and white blood cell count with differential, together with appropriate radiographic studies.

General measures

Infants with respiratory difficulty require an optimal thermal environment to minimize oxygen consumption and oxygen requirements. The ability to supply an adequate caloric intake to the critically ill infant receiving respiratory assistance is facilitated by intravenous hyperalimentation including lipid solutions commencing on the first day after birth.

Metabolic acidosis is most often encountered when the infant has been depressed at birth and required resuscitation. A subsequent metabolic acidosis out of proportion to the degree of respiratory distress may signify hypoperfusion, sepsis, or an IVH. It is not necessary to correct metabolic or respiratory acidosis if the pH is greater than 7.25, whereas a pH of less than 7.20 typically requires intervention. In the case of respiratory acidosis, alkali therapy is not indicated until some form of assisted ventilation has been initiated.

It is customary to maintain a venous hematocrit of at least 40% during the acute phase of RDS to support an adequate oxygen-carrying capacity. Arterial oxygen tension (PaO_2) is maintained at 50–80 mmHg. Although umbilical arterial catheters still form the basic means of arterial sampling in infants with RDS, the list of catheter-related thrombotic, embolic, and ischemic complications is formidable. Saturation is monitored continuously, with efforts made to keep the saturation at 89–94%.

Surfactant therapy

Surfactant therapy has been a major advance in the care of infants with RDS. All regimens of surfactant therapy appear to decrease the incidence of air leaks and improve oxygenation of ventilated preterm infants. More strikingly, mortality from RDS, and even overall mortality of preterm infants, is significantly reduced, especially when multiple-dose surfactant therapy is used for these infants. In contrast with the impressive improvement in mortality, the incidence of BPD, IVH, sepsis, and symptomatic patent ductus arteriosus appears unaltered in most studies [9–17].

The overall incidence of BPD has not been reduced by the use of surfactant therapy. This may be a consequence of enhanced survival, and there is evidence that surfactant has increased the rate of survival without BPD. Presumably, BPD is more likely to be a direct consequence of barotrauma in the preterm survivors of neonatal intensive care who have a more advanced gestational age, and such diverse factors as impaired respiratory drive, nutritional compromise, intercurrent infection, and congestive heart failure are less of a problem than in the smallest survivors of assisted ventilation.

Transient tachypnea

Transient tachypnea typically presents as respiratory distress in term infants or preterm infants who are close to term. The clinical features comprise various combinations of mild cyanosis, grunting, flaring, retracting, and tachypnea in the first few hours after birth associated with a modest requirement for supplemental oxygen. The chest radiograph shows prominent perihilar streaking which may represent engorgement of the periarterial lymphatics that participate in the clearance of alveolar fluid. The radiographic appearance can usually be readily distinguished from the diffuse reticulogranular pattern with air bronchograms that is characteristic of RDS.

Patchy infiltrates that clear within 48 hours and are associated with perihilar streaking are probably also manifestations of transient tachypnea. Differentiation from neonatal pneumonia or meconium aspiration can be extremely difficult, especially if antenatal or postnatal history includes risk factors for these disorders. Transient tachypnea of the newborn by definition is self-limiting with no risk of recurrence or residual pulmonary dysfunction.

Extracorporeal membrane oxygenation

Indications and patient selection

Because of the invasive nature of extracorporeal membrane oxygenation (ECMO), most notably the need to ligate the right common carotid artery in many patients and the risk of major hemorrhage resulting from systemic heparinization, ECMO continues to be reserved for neonates who do not respond to maximal conventional support and are believed to have a chance of survival of 20% or less [18]. Because of the high risk of intracranial hemorrhage in babies born before 34 weeks' gestation, ECMO is currently applicable only to term or near-term infants. In general, to be considered for ECMO therapy, a baby must have completed 34 weeks' gestation, weigh at least 2 kg, and have a reversible cause of pulmonary or cardiac failure. Meconium aspiration syndrome is the most frequent cause of respiratory failure leading to ECMO. Other common underlying conditions are diaphragmatic hernia, sepsis, congenital pneumonia, RDS, and perinatal asphyxia. Persistent pulmonary hypertension of the newborn (PPHN) is almost always a major contributing factor, usually accompanied by varying degrees of myocardial dysfunction. Primary cardiac failure is a relatively rare indication for ECMO and the success of the procedure in these patients is limited.

The survival rate for ECMO patients listed in the Extracorporeal Life Support Organization (ELSO) Registry based at the University of Michigan as of July 1997 is 80.4% [19]. For the years 1973–82 the survival rate was 57.8%, rising to 82.2% in 1983–89. The survival rate has declined slightly in 1990–97 to 79.8%, reflecting a change in the patient mix toward a greater proportion of more difficult cases. The prognosis for survival depends mainly on birthweight, gestational age, and the underlying diagnosis (Fig. 53.1). Admission pH may also be a useful prognostic feature.

Serious complications of ECMO are not frequent but can be devastating. Of greatest concern are those related to systemic heparinization and to the ligation of the carotid and perhaps jugular vessels. Intracranial hemorrhage occurs in approximately 16% of patients and is more frequent in babies of 34–35 weeks' gestation. Other significant complications include internal hemorrhage, renal failure, and seizures. Cerebral infarction, predominantly involving the right hemisphere, is an occasional occurrence in patients who were hypotensive at the time of carotid artery ligation. Follow-up data suggest that despite the extreme severity of their neonatal illness, most ECMO graduates survive the experience without apparent neurologic or developmental impairment. Transient feeding problems are a frequent occurrence and may delay discharge. However, they rarely persist beyond a few weeks, except in

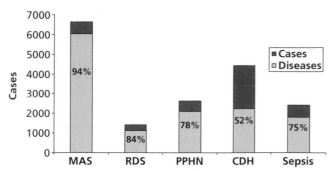

Figure 53.1 ELSO registry – outcomes with ECMO according to diagnosis. Modified from Martin RJ, Fanaroff AA, Walsh MC (eds). Fanaroff and Martin's Neonatal-Perinatal Medicine, 8th edn. Philadelphia: Mosby Elsevier, 2006 with permission. CDH, congenital diaphragmatic hernia; MAS, meconium aspiration syndrome; PPHN, persistent pulmonary hypertension of the newborn; RDS, respiratory distress syndrome.

children with diaphragmatic hernia. Sensorineural hearing loss is a common complication of ECMO and was noted in 29 of 111 (26%) ECMO graduates. The need for early, routine, audiologic evaluations throughout childhood for all ECMO graduates is apparent.

Jaundice

Bilirubin is produced from breakdown of hemoglobin, myoglobin cytochromes, and other heme-containing compounds mainly in the liver, spleen, and bone marrow. The indirect bilirubin so formed is water-insoluble but fat-soluble, and hence potentially toxic to the central nervous system. Beta-glucuronidase present in human milk enhances the reabsorption of bilirubin from the gut [20]. In the fetus, the indirect bilirubin is transported across the placenta. Hyperbilirubinemia is observed either when production of bilirubin is enhanced (e.g., hemolysis) or when elimination is reduced.

An elevated bilirubin level (hyperbilirubinemia) is the most common problem encountered in the full-term neonate and is a significant problem in the late preterm infant (36–38 weeks). Hyperbilirubinemia is clinically relevant in the neonate because it has been associated with kernicterus (yellow staining of the basal ganglia and hippocampus). Most reports indicate that in term infants, without evidence of hemolysis, kernicterus is unlikely to occur if the serum bilirubin is maintained below 25 mg/dL, although kernicterus has been reported at autopsy in low birthweight infants when the serum bilirubin never exceeded 10 mg/dL. There has been a resurgence of kernicterus in term and near-term infants attributable to early discharge, poorly supervised breast feeding, and inadequate follow-up most notably of late preterm infants (13–15 weeks' gestation) [21,22].

Clinical manifestations of kernicterus in the full-term infant include temperature instability, lethargy, poor feeding, high-pitched cry, vomiting, and hypotonia. Subsequently, irritability, opisthotonus, sun-setting appearance of the eyes, and seizures may occur. "Wind-milling" movements of the extremities have been reported. Pulmonary or gastric hemorrhage may occur as a terminal event. Long-term sequelae include the spastic or athetoid form of cerebral palsy, hearing loss (especially high-tone), paralysis of upward gaze, and enamel hypoplasia. In the preterm infant, fisting, apnea, and increased tone may be the only acute manifestations. The search continues for a method of identifying infants at greatest risk to determine if and when encephalopathy is imminent.

Jaundice usually progresses from the head and neck to the trunk and limbs. It disappears in the reverse direction. The onset of significant jaundice within the first 36 hours of life, persistence beyond the first week of life, a serum bilirubin that is rapidly rising or has exceeded the 90th percentile for age in hours according to the Bhutani nomogram or a combination thereof, is an indication for investigation of the jaundice [23]. Generally, the serum bilirubin ranges between 6 and 7 mg/dL between days 2 and 4 and infants with bilirubin levels above the 90th percentile for their age (in hours) require investigation and treatment [23].

Bilirubin can now be detected noninvasively via transcutaneous monitors. Maisels and Kring [24] sequentially followed infants' bilirubin levels using the transcutaneous technology. They concluded that infants who require closer evaluation and observation initially are those whose bilirubin levels are ≥95th percentile (i.e., increasing more rapidly than 0.22 mg/dL/hour in the first 24 hours, 0.15 mg/dL/hour at 24–48 hours, and 0.06 mg/dL/hour after 48 hours).

In determining the cause of jaundice the important historical data include the blood types of the parents and the isoimmune status, ethnic origin of parents, maternal drug history, gestation, mode of delivery, past history with regard to jaundiced neonates, stooling pattern, and method of feeding. Jaundice associated with breastfeeding is the most common cause of hyperbilirubinemia in the otherwise healthy full-term infant.

The presence of plethora, bruising, and cephalohematoma should be sought. Hepatosplenomegaly accompanied by pallor, purpura, and rashes may indicate congenital infection or hemolytic disease. The initial evaluation should always include a complete blood count with smear and reticulocyte count, blood type of mother and infant, direct antibody test, total and direct bilirubin level, and urinalysis to rule out infection and galactosemia. If the infant is sick with the jaundice, a blood culture, spinal tap, and chest radiograph are also indicated. If the direct bilirubin exceeds 10% of the total, this indicates either biliary obstruction or hepatocellular damage. Therefore, in addition to the aforementioned studies, serum protein and protein electrophoresis, serum transaminases, α_1-antitrypsin concentration, hepatitis-associated antigens and titers, TORCH titers, sweat chloride, and clotting profile may

be indicated. An abdominal ultrasonograph may prove extremely productive, as may CT scan of the liver. A liver biopsy may be indicated.

Persistent elevation of the indirect bilirubin occurs predominantly with hemolytic disease, hypothyroidism, or breastmilk jaundice. The latter has been attributed at various times to hormones in the breastmilk, to nonesterified fatty acids in the breastmilk that inhibit glucuronyl transferase, and to the presence of β-glucuronidase in human milk, which enhances the enterohepatic circulation of bilirubin. ABO incompatibility is the most common cause of hemolytic disease in the newborn. A very high anti-A or anti-B antibody titer may be found in the maternal serum; the infant's blood smear reveals abundant spherocytes, and the reticulocyte count may be elevated. Hemolytic disease of the newborn, secondary to Rh incompatibility, has become extremely rare with the widespread screening and use of Rh immunoglobulin, so that g6PD deficiency has become more important [25].

Treatment

It is important to ensure adequate hydration of jaundiced neonates. This has generated considerable controversy because proponents of breastfeeding are convinced that supplementation with formula or water decreases the success of breastfeeding. Evidence is strongly mounting to indicate that a reduced calorie or fluid intake is responsible for the early elevated bilirubin levels noted among breastfed infants. Breastfeeding should not be discontinued during the first days of life.

Phototherapy has been extensively used for the treatment of jaundice [26]. Light reduces bilirubin levels predominantly by photoisomerization and, to a lesser extent, photo-oxidation. Essentially during photoisomerization, bilirubin is rapidly converted from a relatively insoluble state to water-soluble photoisomers. When bilirubin is exposed to light, native bilirubin is converted to photobilirubin and the structural isomer lumirubin. Lumirubin appears to be the principal route of pigment elimination during phototherapy. Before phototherapy is ordered, the cause of the hyperbilirubinemia should be investigated. Most recent studies on the natural history of jaundice reveal that the early use of phototherapy offers no advantage, and prophylactic phototherapy, even in tiny immature infants, has not proved to be necessary.

Guidelines for the use of phototherapy and exchange transfusions are outlined in guidelines published by the American Academy of Pediatrics [27]. It is important to recognize that these are only guidelines. Therapy should always be dictated by the clinical condition and clinical evaluation, not merely by laboratory tests. In bruised, asphyxiated, acidotic, or potentially septic infants, more liberal indications for treatment are often used (Fig. 53.2).

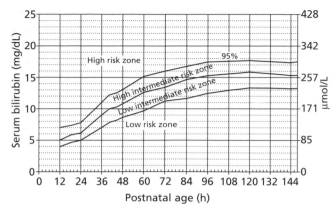

Figure 53.2 Nomogram for designation of risk in 2840 well newborns at 36 or more weeks' gestational age with birthweight 2000 g or more, or 35 or more weeks' gestational age and birthweight 2500 g or more based on the hour-specific serum bilirubin values. From Subcommittee on Hyperbilirubinemia, *Pediatrics* 2004;**114**:297–316 with permission.

Lactation

A mother's decision to breastfeed her baby, and facilitating her lactation success, commences during pregnancy and is heavily influenced by all her caregivers. In view of the unique content of human milk together with the short- and long-term benefits of feeding human milk to the neonate, every effort should be made to encourage breastfeeding.

When discussing nutritional support the clinician should mention the psychosocial aspects of breastfeeding as well as the compelling nutritional and immunologic advantages of breastmilk over formula. Breastfed infants have improved general health, growth, and development, with fewer and less severe episodes of diarrhea, less sudden infant deaths, fewer lower respiratory infections or otitis media, less bacteremia, bacterial meningitis, urinary tract infection, and necrotizing enterocolitis. Breastfeeding has also been related to possible enhancement of cognitive development. There are also considerable emotional and physical benefits for the mother.

Properties of human milk

The major component of human milk is water, making up approximately 50% of the milk by volume. There is a balance of proteins (the major components of which are alpha-lactalbumin and whey), carbohydrates (lactose), and fats [28]. The fats are composed of cholesterol, triglycerides, short-chain fatty acids and long-chain polyunsaturated (LCP) fatty acids. The LCP fatty acids (16- to 22-carbon length) are needed for brain and retinal development. Large amounts of omega-6 and omega-3 LCP fatty acids, predominantly the 20-carbon arachidonic acid (AA) and the 22-carbon docosahexaenoic acid (DHA), are deposited in the developing brain and retina

during prenatal and early postnatal growth [29–34]. As an infant may have a limited ability to synthesize optimal levels of AA and DHA from linoleic and linolenic acid, these two fatty acids may be essential. Infant formulas in the USA have only recently been supplemented with AA and DHA.

The majority of proteins in milk are blood plasma derived. Other proteins such as alpha-lactalbumin are unique to the mammary gland and are synthesized *de novo* upon stimulation by prolactin, insulin, and cortisol. Enzymes and bioactive substances, which may have both local and systemic effects, add credence to the concept of human milk as a dynamic substance with nutritive as well as nonnutritive functions.

Human milk is a dynamic substance, its characteristics evolving as the infant matures. For example, early milk or colostrum has higher concentrations of protein and minerals than does mature milk, but lower concentrations of fat. This relationship reverses as the infant matures. Also, within a given breastfeeding session, the milk first ingested by the infant has a lower fat content (fore milk), and as the infant continues to nurse over the next several minutes, the fat content increases (hind milk), facilitating satiety in the infant. There are various enzymes in human milk, some specific for the biosynthesis of milk components in the mammary gland (e.g., lactose synthetase, fatty acid synthetase, and thioesterase) and some specific for the digestion of proteins, fats, and carbohydrates that facilitate food breakdown and absorption of human milk by the infant. In addition, certain enzymes serve as transport moieties for other substances such as zinc, selenium, and magnesium.

Human milk also contains a host of hormones, enzymes, cytokines, growth factors, and a myriad of nutrients including immunoglobulins, lactoferrin, lysozyme, glycoconjugates, oligosaccharides, and various types of white blood cells that protects the intestine from infectious pathogens and intact dietary antigens. Indeed, there is a wide repertoire of antibacterial, antiviral, antifungal, and food antibodies in human milk that reflect the antigenic repertoire of the mother's intestine and respiratory tract. Therefore mother's milk is a significant source of passively provided secretory immunoglobulin A (sIgA)-specific antibody for the infant during the time of reduced neonatal gut immune function. Assuming mother and infant, who are closely associated, share common gut flora, then the antigen specificity of mother's milk sIgA will be directed against the same antigens present in the neonate's gut.

Whereas human milk is a unique species-specific nutritive fluid, commercially available formulas are not. In fact, formulas are inert nutritive fluids whose composition is modeled after human milk. Each provides adequate amounts of protein, fat, carbohydrate, minerals, and vitamins for the growth of normal infants. Further, long-term epidemiologic studies demonstrated a number of interesting differences between breastfed and formula-fed infants. More specifically, studies of infants during the first years of life demonstrated a protective effect of human milk against infectious disease [35–40]. Human milk is the preferred feeding for all infants, including premature and sick newborns, with rare exceptions. When direct breastfeeding is not possible, expressed human milk, fortified when necessary for the premature infant, should be provided. Before advising against breastfeeding or recommending premature weaning, the practitioner should weigh thoughtfully the benefits of breastfeeding against the risks of not receiving human milk [41].

Neonates, especially those born prematurely with an immature or unsensitized immune system, are highly dependent on the delivery of substances to the gut to help stimulate gut epithelial cell proliferation and closure from the outside world. In addition, there appears to be a critical period in brain development when diet influences later outcome; as a consequence, preterm infants who receive mother's milk are afforded a lower risk of adverse neurodevelopmental sequelae. It is recommended then that premature infants receive mother's milk with fortification [42,43].

There are a few situations where feeding human milk to neonates is contraindicated. Galactosemia is one of the few absolute contraindications to the use of human milk. Other situations include maternal chemotherapy; illegal drug use by the mother or radioactive isotopes that mandate temporary interruption of breastfeeding; untreated active tuberculosis; and the infant in the USA whose mother has been infected with the human immunodeficiency virus. Most prescribed and over the counter medications are safe for the breastfed infant [44].

Case presentation

A term infant, birthweight 3700 g, who is exclusively breastfed becomes lethargic and is noted to be jaundiced on the fourth day of life. His weight is 3367 g (down 9% from birthweight), the hematocrit is 60%, and the infant's serum sodium is 147 meq/L. There is no history of vomiting, diarrhea, or excessive voiding. He has only had two wet diapers in the past 24 hours.

Whereas weight loss and jaundice are common in breastfed babies, this combination of severe dehydration with hypernatremia and jaundice is not very common. These findings reflect usually an inadequate intake of milk. Normal babies lose 1–2% of their body weight per day until the mother's milk comes in (usually by day 3); and thereafter they rapidly gain weight. Infants receiving insufficient breastmilk often appear to be content (i.e., they cry less in contrast to the irritable formula-fed infants who are not getting sufficient milk).

The condition known as "hypernatremic dehydration" results when newborn infants are unable to establish a sufficient transfer of breastmilk during nursing, either because they do not latch on well or there is inadequate milk production. The condition is more common amongst first time mothers.

Breastmilk jaundice refers to an elevation of indirect bilirubin in a breastfed newborn that develops following the first 4–7 days of life, persists, and has no other identifiable cause. In contrast, breastfeeding jaundice occurs before the first 4–7 days of life and is caused by insufficient production or intake of breastmilk.

Breastmilk jaundice is thought to be caused by a substance or substances in the breastmilk that inhibits uridine diphosphoglucuronic acid (UDPGA) glucuronyl transferase resulting in a prolonged unconjugated hyperbilirubinemia. Lipoprotein lipase, found in some breastmilk, produces non-esterified long-chain fatty acids, is one such substance. Another mechanism is enhanced enterohepatic circulation of bilirubin induced by beta glucuronidase which is abundant in breastmilk and not found in formula.

References

1 Lorenz JM, Paneth N, Jetton JR, den Ouden L, Tyson JE. Comparison of management strategies for extreme prematurity in New Jersey and the Netherlands: outcomes and resource expenditure. *Pediatrics* 2001;**108**:1269–74.
2 Marlow N, Wolke D, Bracewell MA, Samara M, EPICure Study Group. Neurologic and developmental disability at six years of age after extremely preterm birth. *N Engl J Med* 2005;**352**:9–19.
3 Doyle LW, Victorian Infant Collaborative Study Group. Neonatal intensive care at the borderline viability—is it worth it? *Early Hum Dev* 2004;**80**:103–13.
4 Doyle LW, Victorian Infant Collaborative Study Group. Evaluation of neonatal intensive care for extremely low birth weight infants in Victoria over two decades: I. Effectiveness. *Pediatrics* 2004;**113**:505–9.
5 Doyle LW, Victorian Infant Collaborative Study Group. Evaluation of neonatal intensive care for extremely low birth weight infants in Victoria over two decades: II. Efficiency. *Pediatrics* 2004;**113**:510–4.
6 Shankaran S, Laptook AR, Ehrenkranz RA, *et al.* National Institute of Child Health and Human Development Neonatal Research Network. Whole-body hypothermia for neonates with hypoxic-ischemic encephalopathy. *N Engl J Med* 2005;**353**:1574–84.
7 Gluckman PD, Wyatt JS, Azzopardi D *et al.* Selective head cooling with mild systemic hypothermia after neonatal encephalopathy: multicentre randomised trial. *Lancet* 2005;**365**:663–70.
8 Malcus P, Bjorklund LJ, Lilja M, Teleman P, Laurini R. Massive feto-maternal hemorrhage: Diagnosis by cardiotocography, Doppler ultrasonography and ST waveform analysis of fetal electrocardiography. *Fetal Diagn Ther* 206;**21**:8–12.
9 Horbar JD, Wright LL, Soll RF, *et al.* A multicenter randomized trial comparing two surfactants for the treatment of neonatal respiratory distress syndrome. National Institute of Child Health and Human Development Neonatal Research Network. *J Pediatr* 1993;**123**:757–66.

10 Malloy CA, Nicoski P, Muraskas JK. A randomized trial comparing beractant and poractant treatment in neonatal respiratory distress syndrome. *Acta Paediatr* 2005;**94**:779–84.

11 Reininger A, Khalak R, Kendig JW *et al*. Surfactant administration by transient intubation in infants 29 to 35 weeks' gestation with respiratory distress syndrome decreases the likelihood of later mechanical ventilation: a randomized controlled trial. *J Perinatol* 2005;**25**:703–8.

12 Sinha SK, Lacaze-Masmonteil T, Valls i Soler A, *et al*. Surfaxin Therapy Against Respiratory Distress Syndrome Collaborative Group. A multicenter, randomized, controlled trial of lucinactant versus poractant alfa among very premature infants at high risk for respiratory distress syndrome. *Pediatrics* 2005;**115**:1030–8.

13 Lam BC, Ng YK, Wong KY. Randomized trial comparing two natural surfactants (Survanta vs. bLES) for treatment of neonatal respiratory distress syndrome. *Pediatr Pulmonol* 2005;**39**:64–9.

14 Horbar JD, Carpenter JH, Buzas J, *et al*. Collaborative quality improvement to promote evidence based surfactant for preterm infants: a cluster randomized trial. *Br Med J* 2004;**329**:1004.

15 Stevens TP, Blennow M, Soll RF. Early surfactant administration with brief ventilation vs selective surfactant and continued mechanical ventilation for preterm infants with or at risk for respiratory distress syndrome. *Cochrane Database Syst Rev* 2004;**3**: CD003063.

16 Escobedo MB, Gunkel JH, Kennedy KA, *et al*. Early surfactant for neonates with mild to moderate respiratory distress syndrome: a multicenter, randomized trial. *J Pediatr* 2004;**144**:804–8.

17 Dani C, Bertini G, Pezzati M, Cecchi A, Caviglioli C, Rubaltelli FF. Early extubation and nasal continuous positive airway pressure after surfactant treatment for respiratory distress syndrome among preterm infants <30 weeks' gestation. *Pediatrics* 2004;**113**: 560–3.

18 Bartlett RH. Extracorporeal life support: history and new directions. *Semin Perinatol* 2005;**29**:2–7.

19 Oh W, Poindexter BB, Perritt R, *et al*. Neonatal Research Network. Association between fluid intake and weight loss during the first ten days of life and risk of bronchopulmonary dysplasia in extremely low birth weight infants. *J Pediatr* 2005;**147**:786–90.

20 Gourley GR, Li Z, Kreamer BL, Kosorok MR. A controlled, randomized, double-blind trial of prophylaxis against jaundice among breastfed newborns. *Pediatrics* 2005;**116**:385–91.

21 Bhutani VK, Johnson L. Kernicterus in late preterm infants cared for as term healthy infants. *Semin Perinatol* 2006;**30**:89–97.

22 Bhutani VK, Johnson LH, Shapiro SM. Kernicterus in sick and preterm infants (1999–2002): A need for an effective preventive approach. *Semin Perinatol* 2004;**28**:319–25.

23 Bhutani VK, Johnson L, Sivieri EM. Predictive ability of a predischarge hour-specific serum bilirubin for subsequent significant hyperbilirubinemia in healthy term and near-term newborns. *Pediatrics* 1999;**103**:6–14.

24 Maisels MJ, Kring E. Transcutaneous bilirubin levels in the first 96 hours in a normal newborn population of ≥35 weeks' gestation. *Pediatrics* 2006;**117**:1169–73.

25 Kaplan M, Hoyer JD, Herschel M, *et al*. Glucose-6-phosphate dehydrogenase activity in term and near-term, male African American neonates. *Clin Chim Acta* 2005;**355**:113–7.

26 Vreman HJ, Wong RJ, Stevenson DK. Phototherapy: current methods and future directions. *Semin Perinatol* 2004;**28**:326–33.

27 American Academy of Pediatrics Subcommittee on Hyperbilirubinemia. Management of hyperbilirubinemia in the newborn infant 35 or more weeks of gestation. *Pediatrics* 2004;**114**:297–316.

28 Riordan J, Auerbach KG, eds. *Breastfeeding and Human Lactation*. Boston: Jones & Bartlett, 1993.

29 Gibson RA, Makrides M. Long-chain polyunsaturated fatty acids in breast milk: are they essential? *Adv Exp Med Biol* 2001;**501**:375–83.

30 Fleith M, Clandinin MT. Dietary PUFA for preterm and term infants: review of clinical studies. *Crit Rev Food Sci Nutr* 2005;**45**:205–29.

31 Decsi T, Thiel I, Koletzko B. Essential fatty acids in full term infants fed breast milk or formula. *Arch Dis Child* 1995;**72**:F23–8.

32 Carlson SE, Werkman SH, Rhodes PG, Tolley EA. Visual-acuity development in healthy preterm infants: effect of marine-oil supplementation. *Am J Clin Nutr* 1993;**58**:35–42.

33 Makrides M, Simmer K, Goggin M, Gibson RA. Erythrocyte docosahexaenoic acid correlates with the visual response of healthy, term infants. *Pediatr Res* 1993;**34**:425–7.

34 Birch EE, Birch DG, Hoffman DR, *et al*. Breastfeeding and optimal visual development. *J Pediatr Ophthalmol Strabismus* 1993;**30**:33–8.

35 Paxson CL, Cress CC. Survival of human milk leukocytes. *J Pediatr* 1979;**94**:61–4.

36 Rodriguez NA, Miracle DJ, Meier PP. Sharing the science on human milk feedings with mothers of very-low-birth-weight infants. *J Obstet Gynecol Neonatal Nurs* 2005;**34**:109–19.

37 de Silva A, Jones PW, Spencer SA. Does human milk reduce infection rates in preterm infants? A systematic review. *Arch Dis Child Fetal Neonatal Ed* 2004;**89**:F509–13.

38 Oddy WH. The impact of breastmilk on infant and child health. *Breastfeed Rev* 2002;**10**:5–18.

39 Rubin DH, Leventhal JM, Kraslinikoff PA, *et al*. Relationship between infant feeding and infectious illness: a prospective study of infants during the first year of life. *Pediatrics* 1990;**85**:464–71.

40 Duncan B, Ey J, Molberg CJ, *et al*. Exclusive breast-feeding for at least 4 months protects against otitis media. *Pediatrics* 1993;**91**:867–72.

41 Koletzko S, Sherman P, Corey M, *et al*. Role of infant feeding practices in development of Crohn's disease in childhood. *Br Med J* 1989;**298**:1617–8.

42 Lucas A, Morley R, Cole TJ, *et al*. Breast milk and subsequent intelligence quotient in children born preterm. *Lancet* 1992;**339**:261–4.

43 Morley R, Lucas A. Influence of early diet on outcome in preterm infants. *Acta Paediatr Suppl* 1994;**405**:123–6.

44 Ressel G. AAP updates statement for transfer of drugs and other chemicals into breast milk. American Academy of Pediatrics. *Am Fam Physician* 2002;**65**:979–80.

54 Neonatal encephalopathy and cerebral palsy

Gary D.V. Hankins and Monica Longo

The incidence of cerebral palsy is 1–2 per 1000 births and has remained unchanged over the last 40 years. The occurrence of cerebral palsy is independent of either geographic or economic boundaries. It has also been remarkably resistant to eradication by the introduction of technology such as electronic fetal heart rate monitoring or the increase in cesarean delivery rates. Indeed, the great hope of electronic fetal heart rate monitoring was that intrapartum asphyxia would be promptly identified, delivery rapidly achieved, and neurologic injury of the infant averted. This would in fact parallel the thought processes advanced by the orthopedic surgeon, Little [1], over a century ago, taught that virtually all cerebral palsy was caused by intrapartum events, whether deprivation of oxygen, trauma, or the combination of the two. Unfortunately, despite an escalation of the cesarean delivery rate from approximately 6% in 1970 to a rate approaching 30% nationally today [2], the incidence of cerebral palsy in the USA has remained constant [3]. These facts then would seem to support the evolving concept that cerebral palsy results from the combination of the genetic make-up of the individual and the subsequent collision of that individual during development with the environment that they are exposed to, both intrauterine as well as extrauterine for the first several days, months, or years of life. As examples, the South Australian Cerebral Palsy Research Group has recently reported that inheritance of MTHFR C677T approximately doubles the risk of cerebral palsy in preterm infants. A combination of homozygous MTHFR C677T and heterozygous prothrombin gene mutation increased the risk of quadriplegia fivefold in all gestational ages [4]. This is clearly an example of genetic inheritance leading to cerebral palsy. The same group also demonstrated that perinatal exposure to the neurotropic herpes group B viruses nearly doubled the risk of cerebral palsy relative to the control group [5].

Neonatal encephalopathy

Neonatal encephalopathy is a condition defined in and described for term (more than 37 completed weeks' gestation) and near term (more than 34 completed weeks' gestation) infants. It is a clinically defined syndrome of disturbed neurologic function manifest by difficulty with initiating and maintaining respiration, depression of tone and reflexes, altered level of consciousness, and often seizures. Additionally, it must manifest within the first week of life. The differential diagnosis for neonatal encephalopathy is shown in Table 54.1.

Hypoxia sufficient to result in hypoxic ischemic encephalopathy (HIE) is only one subset of the larger category of neonatal encephalopathy. If there has been intrapartum asphyxia sufficient to result in long-term neurologic injury manifest as cerebral palsy, then the neonate will manifest the injury as encephalopathy during labor. It is biologically implausible to suggest that one can have sufficient intrapartum asphyxia to result in cerebral palsy, yet the newborn would have a completely normal hospital course during labor that was in fact void of encephalopathy.

Cerebral palsy

Cerebral palsy is defined as a chronic neuromuscular disability characterized by abnormal control of movement or posture appearing early in life and not the result of recognized progressive disease [6]. The causes of cerebral palsy are in large part the same as the antecedents of neonatal encephalopathy (Table 54.1). In a sentinel publication, MacLennan [7] notes that epidemiologic studies suggest that in approximately 90%

of cases of cerebral palsy, intrapartum hypoxia could not be the cause and in the remaining 10% intrapartum signs compatible with damaging hypoxia may have had antenatal or intrapartum origins.

A group of investigators led by Badawi [8] reported on the antecedents of moderate to severe neonatal encephalopathy from their patient population in metropolitan Western Australia. This study involved 164 term infants with moderate or severe neonatal encephalopathy and 400 randomly selected appropriate controls. Within their population, the prevalence of moderate or severe newborn encephalopathy was 3.8 in 1000 term live births. The diagnosis of either moderate or severe newborn encephalopathy was associated with a neonatal fatality rate of 9.1%. In Fig. 54.1, the risk factors for newborn encephalopathy in their population that achieved statistical significance are shown and substratified according to whether they occurred preconceptionally, intrapartum, or in the antepartum period. Data shown are the increase in adjusted

Table 54.1 Differential diagnosis of neonatal encephalopathy.

Developmental abnormalities
Metabolic abnormalities
Autoimmune disorders
Coagulation disorders
Infections
Trauma
Hypoxia
Intrauterine growth restriction (IUGR)
Multiple gestations
Antepartum hemorrhage
Chromosomal abnormalities
Persistent breech/transverse lie

odds ratio. Badawi *et al.*'s data are striking inasmuch as the traditional risk factors, including abnormal histopathology of the placenta, the need for emergency cesarean section, or the use of vacuum or forceps to achieve vaginal delivery, were among the lowest, although statistically significant, risk factors identified. In contrast, family history of seizure disorder or neurologic disorder and maternal thyroid disease were much more highly associated with moderate to severe encephalopathy than the traditional risk factors. This again emphasizes the potential role of genetics in causing both encephalopathy as well as cerebral palsy. The role of environment is also demonstrated from Badawi *et al.*'s data, with factors such as viral illness during the index pregnancy, moderate or severe antepartum bleeding, intrapartum fever, and severe preeclampsia being significant increased risk factors for development of these disorders. Thus, we return to the role of genetics and the impact of environment on causation of this neurologic injury. This is repeatedly being affirmed by clinical studies employing a variety of rapidly advancing technologies [4,5].

When Badawi *et al.* analyzed their data as regards the distribution of risk factors for newborn encephalopathy, they concluded that in 69% of the population there were only antepartum risk factors. In 25%, there were antepartum risk factors and potential impact of intrapartum hypoxia, but in only 4% did intrapartum hypoxia seem to be the logical cause (Fig. 54.2). This team of investigators' overall conclusions were that the causes of newborn encephalopathy are heterogeneous and that many of the causal pathways start before birth. A much earlier study by Blair and Stanley [9] had similarly concluded that in only 8% of all children with spastic cerebral palsy was intrapartum asphyxia the possible cause of their brain damage.

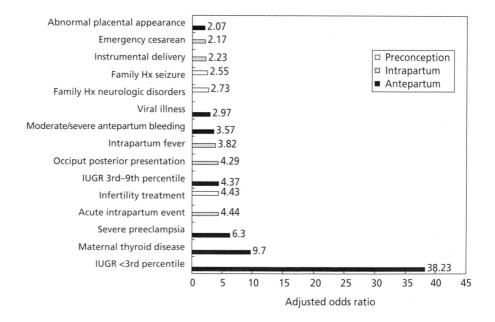

Fig. 54.1 Risk factors for newborn encephalopathy. After Badawi *et al.* [8]. Hx, history; IUGR, intrauterine growth restriction.

The importance of intrauterine growth restriction (IUGR) as a risk factor for newborn encephalopathy deserves special emphasis. In Badawi *et al.*'s study, growth restriction between the 3rd and 9th percentile carried an adjusted odds ratio of 4.37 for moderate or severe neonatal encephalopathy. When the growth restriction was severe, defined as less than the 3rd percentile, the adjusted odds ratio increased to a staggering 38.23. In a series reported by Cowan *et al.* [10], 11–15% of the population with encephalopathy were at the 3–10th percentile, compared with 13–16% when the growth restriction was less than the 3rd percentile. Their study population was recruited from the Wilhelmina Children's Hospital, Utrecht, the Netherlands and Hammersmith and Queen Charlotte's Hospitals, London, UK. Substantially similar results were reported from the University of California, San Francisco, and Loma Linda Children's Hospital, where newborns with either a watershed predominant or a total brain/basal ganglia/thalamus predominant injury had a higher incidence of intrauterine growth restriction than did those infants having a normal scan [11].

The clinician is thus cautioned that while all growth restricted babies are at increased risk for newborn encephalopathy, the risk is extraordinarily high for those infants with growth restriction at less than the 3rd percentile. Accordingly, great care in the timing and route of delivery of these fetuses is encouraged so that they might be delivered in an optimal metabolic condition. It would also seem prudent to have a neonatologist present at the birth and to provide immediate care of the newborn. Induction of anesthesia may be a very high-risk period, as many of these fetuses are marginally compensated and will be poorly tolerant of epidural-induced hypotension. Fetal monitoring is necessary in the operating or delivery room. In cases of cesarean delivery, the interval from fetal monitoring to delivery should be as short as possible.

Task force on neonatal encephalopathy and cerebral palsy

In January 2003, a monograph summarizing the state of the science on neonatal encephalopathy and cerebral palsy was copublished by the American College of Obstetricians and Gynecologists and the American Academy of Pediatrics. At the time of publication it was recognized that the topic would require updating as the scientific database and knowledge on the topic expanded. In that monograph, the criteria to define an acute event sufficient to cause cerebral palsy were listed, as modified by the Task Force from the template provided by the International Cerebral Palsy Task Force (Table 54.2). It was emphasized that all four criteria must be met in order to make this association. Additionally, criteria were also listed that collectively suggest an intrapartum timing, defined as within close proximity to labor and delivery (e.g., 0–48 hours), but which were non-specific to asphyxia insults (Table 54.3). Among the criteria for elucidating timing was early imaging studies showing evidence of acute nonfocal cerebral abnormalities.

Table 54.2 Essential criteria to define an acute intrapartum event sufficient to cause cerebral palsy (must meet all four).

1 Evidence of a metabolic acidosis in fetal umbilical cord arterial blood obtained at delivery (pH <7 and base deficit of ≥12 mmol/L)
2 Early onset of severe or moderate neonatal encephalopathy in infants born at ≥34 weeks' gestation
3 Cerebral palsy of the spastic quadriplegic or dyskinetic type
4 Exclusion of other identifiable etiologies, such as trauma, coagulation disorders, infectious conditions, or genetic disorders

Table 54.3 Criteria that collectively suggest an intrapartum timing (within close proximity to labor and delivery, e.g., 0–48 hours) but that are nonspecific for an asphyxial insult.

1 A sentinel (signal) hypoxic event occurring immediately before or during labor
2 A sudden and sustained fetal bradycardia or the absence of fetal heart rate variability in the presence of persistent late or persistent variable decelerations, usually after a hypoxic sentinel event when the pattern was previously normal
3 Apgar scores of 0–3 beyond 5 minutes
4 Onset of multisystem involvement within 72 hours of birth
5 Early imaging study showing evidence of acute nonfocal cerebral abnormality

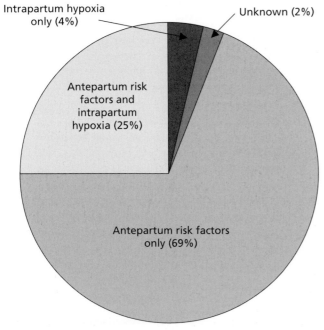

Fig. 54.2 Distribution of risk factors for newborn encephalopathy. After Badawi *et al.* [8]

Subsequent to the publication of this monograph, three important papers on neuroimaging have been published. The first of these publications was by Graham *et al.* [12] and dealt with an earlier gestation than covered by the Task Force, which was restricted to the term and near term infant. In contrast, Graham *et al.*'s study was of the preterm infant of 23–34 weeks' gestation. The significant findings by these authors included that in this specific population, intrapartum hypoxia ischemia as manifested by metabolic acidosis was rarely associating with white matter injury, and was not different from that seen in premature neonates without injury.

The second study was by Cowen *et al.* [10]. These investigators divided their population into two groups. Group 1 was defined as those with neonatal encephalopathy with or without seizures, and evidence of perinatal asphyxia. This group consisted of infants with neonatal encephalopathy, defined by abnormal tone pattern, feeding difficulties, altered alertness, and at least three of the following criteria:

1 Late decelerations on fetal monitoring or meconium staining;
2 Delayed onset of respiration;
3 Arterial cord blood pH <7.14;
4 Apgar score <7 at 5 minutes;
5 Multiorgan failure.

Their second group consisted of infants who had seizures within 72 hours of birth but who did not meet the criteria for neonatal encephalopathy. In the first group, brain imaging studies showed evidence of an acute insult without established injury or atrophy in 80% of infants. Magnetic resonance imaging (MRI) showed evidence of established injury in only two infants (<1%), although tiny foci of established white matter gliosis, in addition to acute injury, were seen in 3/21 on postmortem examination. In group 2, acute focal damage was noted in 62 (69%) infants. Two (3%) also had evidence of antenatal injury. Cowen *et al.* [10] concluded that although their results could not exclude the possibility that antenatal or genetic factors might predispose some infants to perinatal brain injury, their data strongly suggested that events in the immediate perinatal period were most important in neonatal brain injury. A valid criticism of this study is the criteria selected for inclusion into their group 1. Either late decelerations on fetal monitoring or meconium staining are notoriously poor predictors of intrapartum asphyxia. Delayed onset of respirations can be for numerous reasons, and a large number of babies will be born with blood pH <7.1 and almost all will be neurologically intact. What these authors fail to tell us is how many of their total population would have met at least three of the five criteria that they listed for inclusion in the acute injury group.

The study by Miller *et al.* [11] reported that the watershed pattern of injury was seen in 78 newborns (45%), the basal ganglia/thalamus pattern was seen in 44 newborns (25%), and normal MRI studies were seen in 51 newborns (30%). Antenatal conditions such as maternal substance abuse, gestational diabetes, premature ruptured membranes, preeclampsia, and intrauterine growth restriction did not differ between the injury patterns. The basal ganglia/thalamus pattern was associated with more severe neonatal signs, including more intensive resuscitation at birth, more severe encephalopathy, and more severe seizures. The basal ganglia/thalamus pattern was most highly associated with impaired motor and cognitive outcome at 30 months. These authors concluded that the patterns of brain injury in term neonatal encephalopathy are associated with different clinical presentation and different neurodevelopmental outcomes. Further and contrary to prior epidemiologic studies, they noted that measured prenatal factors did not predict the pattern of brain injury. Like Cowan *et al.*, they noted that the MRI findings in their cohort were consistent with the recent, rather than chronic brain injury in the majority of patients and the antenatal conditions measured were remarkably similar between newborns with normal and abnormal MRI scan results. They felt that these observations highlighted the potential of interventions to ameliorate brain injury in the newborn. They remarked that the dissociation of antenatal risk factors from the severity of the clinical presentations supports the hypothesis that the etiology of brain injury in neonatal encephalopathy is distinct from these antenatal risk factors. They further noted that the watershed pattern had predominantly cognitive impairments at 30 months that were not detected at 12 months of age. The cognitive deficits in this group often occurred without functional motor deficits. They hypothesized that abnormal outcome after neonatal encephalopathy may not be limited to cerebral palsy and often requires follow-up beyond 12 months of age to be detected.

Conclusions

How are we to resolve the epidemiologic studies with the more recent conclusions from imaging studies? Because newborns with severe encephalopathy are more likely to be identified for research studies in the intensive care nursery and these newborns are more likely to have the basal ganglia/thalamus injury pattern, it is that possible that the prospective MRI studies of neonatal encephalopathy will over-represent perinatally acquired injury compared with population-based epidemiologic surveys. Because population-based retrospective studies identify a preponderance of antenatal risk factors and smaller prospective cohort studies identify the perinatal occurrence of brain injury, there is a pressing need to establish the mechanistic link between prenatal risk factors and etiology of brain injury. This is critical to the prevention of acquired neonatal brain injury and may be achieved with the development and application of more accurate *in utero* measures of brain injury, such as fetal MRI.

Both the American College of Obstetricians and Gynecologists and the American Academy of Pediatrics acknowledged that their 2003 summary would require updating as the scientific database and knowledge on the topic expanded. They went on to state that only with more complete understanding of the precise origins of the pathophysiology of neonatal encephalopathy and cerebral palsy could logical hypotheses be designed and tested to reduce this occurrence. Finally, they recommended several important areas of research and for research funding. We would again emphasize the need for funding and studies to address this very important issue in neurodevelopment, neuroimaging, and potential improvements in outcomes for populations worldwide.

Case presentation

A 27-year-old G2 P0100 was accepted for maternal transport with diagnoses of 28 weeks estimated gestational age and severe preeclampsia. Her past medical history was significant for a prior intrauterine fetal demise at 31 weeks' gestation, that pregnancy was also complicated by severe preeclampsia. Following successful aeromedical transport, she was received in Labor and Delivery where standard treatment for severe preeclampsia was instituted, including magnesium sulfate for prevention of eclamptic seizures and betamethasone for fetal lung maturation. Because of the severity of her disease process, labor induction with oxytocin was also instituted. Hydralazine was given in 5-mg incremental doses to control and reduce systolic blood pressure to less than 180 mmHg and diastolic blood pressure to less than 110 mmHg. Ten hours into the labor induction, a series of eight repetitive late decelerations was noted. The oxytocin was discontinued, the woman placed in left lateral position, and oxygen was administered at 10 L/min by face mask. The fetal heart rate promptly normalized; however, beat–beat variability was judged to be reduced consistent with the estimated gestational age as well as the administration of magnesium sulfate.

As vaginal delivery was remote, the alternative of cesarean section was discussed because of fetal intolerance of labor. Following informed consent, the patient was taken to the operating room for cesarean delivery. General endotracheal anesthesia was necessitated by maternal thrombocytopenia. A low vertical uterine incision was employed as the lower uterine segment was poorly developed and thick and a vertical incision would allow the most atraumatic delivery. A 970-g infant was delivered and passed to a neonatologist who assigned Apgar scores of 1/0/0/0/0. The fetus/infant was pronounced dead at 20 minutes of age. The admission cover sheet for this infant by the pediatricians recorded a 26–29 weeks' estimated gestational age, male infant with severe birth asphyxia. In the diagnostic codes listed for discharge was included acute respiratory failure with inability to resuscitate the infant in the delivery room and birth asphyxia. The autopsy report also returned findings consistent with chronic intrauterine anoxia, as well as possible acute anoxia secondary to prolonged labor and difficult delivery. These diagnoses were

rendered by the pathologist despite the fact that "gross and microscopic examinations were normal." Cord gases were obtained at delivery and showed for the umbilical arterial blood a pH of 7.273, P_{CO_2} of 57.6, P_{O_2} of 17.4, HCO_3 of 25.9, and base excess of –4.0. A cord venous blood gas showed a pH of 7.30, P_{CO_2} of 50.0, P_{O_2} of 18.6, HCO_3 of 24.1, and base excess of –1.6. Conclusively then, the cord gases rule out "birth asphyxia" and the fetus was additionally delivered in an atraumatic fashion. Fortunately, when neuropathology results were finalized they demonstrated lesions within the brain that dated at least 96 hours of age, placing the injury well before the woman presented to the outlying hospital or before transport to the medical center.

This case demonstrates several critical points. Perhaps the most important is the need to be precise in the terminology that we employ and to diagnose birth asphyxia on objective rather than subjective criteria. Secondly, the value of cord blood studies obtained at delivery and of continuous electronic monitoring to exclude intrapartum asphyxia is well demonstrated. Finally, while the pathologist initially listed several erroneous diagnoses, largely based upon erroneous diagnoses contained in the pediatric chart, the record was eventually corrected with the neuropathology results. This would then point out the importance of a pathologic diagnosis of the intrauterine fetal demise and additionally also supplying the pathologist with accurate information upon which to base their conclusions. This case would beg for the establishment of set criteria for the evaluation of a newborn with suspected intrapartum asphyxia to include set times for neuroimaging studies as well as evaluation of the newborn for multiorgan system injury or insult.

References

1 Little WJ. On the influence of abnormal parturition, difficult labours, premature births, and asphyxia neonatorum, on the mental and physical condition of the child, especially in relation to deformities. *Trans Obstet Soc Lond* 1862;**3**:293–344.
2 Martin JA, Hamilton BE, Sutton PD, Ventura SJ, Menacker F, Munson ML. Births: final data for 2003. *Natl Vital Stat Rep* 2005;**54**:1–116.
3 Clark SL, Hankins GDV. Temporal and demographic trends in cerebral palsy: fact and fiction. *Am J Obstet Gynecol* 2003;**188**:628–33.
4 Gibson CS, MacLennan AH, Hague WM, *et al.* Associations between inherited thrombophilias, gestational age, and cerebral palsy. *Am J Obstet Gynecol* 2005;**193**:1437.
5 Gibson CS, MacLennan AH, Goldwater PN, *et al.* Neurotropic viruses and cerebral palsy: population based case–control study. *Br Med J* 2006;**332**:76–80.
6 Ruth VJ, Raivio KO. Perinatal brain damage: predictive value of metabolic acidosis in the Apgar score. *Br Med J* 1988;**297**:24–7.
7 MacLennan A. A template for defining a causal relation between

acute intrapartum events and cerebral palsy: international consensus statement. *Br Med J* 1999;**319**:1054–9.

8 Badawi N, Kurinczuk JJ, Keogh JM, *et al*. Intrapartum risk factors for newborn encephalopathy: the Western Australian case–control study. *Br Med J* 1998;**317**:1554–8.

9 Blair E, Stanley FJ. Intrapartum asphyxia: a rare cause of cerebral palsy. *J Pediatr* 1988;**112**:515–9.

10 Cowan FM, Rutherford M, Groenendaal F, *et al*. Origin and timing of brain lesions in term infants with neonatal encephalopathy. *Lancet* 2003;**361**:736–42.

11 Miller SP, Ramaswamy V, Michelson D, *et al*. Patterns of brain injury in term neonatal encephalopathy. *J Pediatr* 2005;**146**:453–60.

12 Graham E, Holcroft CJ, Rai KK, Donohue PK, Allen MC. Neonatal cerebral white matter injury in preterm infants is associated with culture positive infections and only rarely with metabolic acidosis. *Am J Obstet Gynecol* 2004;**191**:1305–10.

Index

Protocols
for High-Risk Pregnancies

FOURTH EDITION

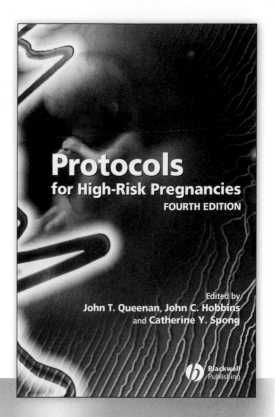

Edited by:

John T. Queenan, MD, Department of Obstetrics & Gynecology, Georgetown University School of Medicine, Washington, DC

John C. Hobbins, MD, University of Colorado Health Sciences Center, Denver

Catherine Y. Spong, MD, Bethesda, Maryland

Now in its Fourth Edition, **Protocols for High-Risk Pregnancies** is an international standard for diagnosing and managing high-risk pregnancies. You can depend on it for procedures and protocols that are not only carefully constructed and easy to follow, but are also solidly based on best evidence practice. The book's seven sections cover all aspects of high-risk pregnancy that you encounter in clinical practice:

Published September 2005
768 pages, illustrated
Paperback
ISBN: 978-1-4051-2579-6

◆ Hazards to pregnancy
◆ Antenatal testing
◆ Special procedures
◆ Maternal disease
◆ Obstetrical problems
◆ Labor and delivery
◆ Clinical reference tables

This book's problem-solving approach gives you a quick summary of the critical issues surrounding each risk factor and then guides you to the optimal choices for your patient. Each chapter has been carefully revised and updated to reflect the latest evidence to manage patients with risk factors such as tuberculosis, STDs, bleeding, and smoking. New chapters present the latest findings and protocols for Doppler ultrasound, nuchal translucency, and AIDS. In addition, the Fourth Edition features expanded sections on intrauterine growth restriction, pre-eclampsia, teratology, and genetics.

www.blackwellobgyn.com

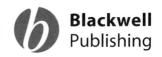

Blackwell
Publishing

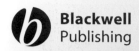
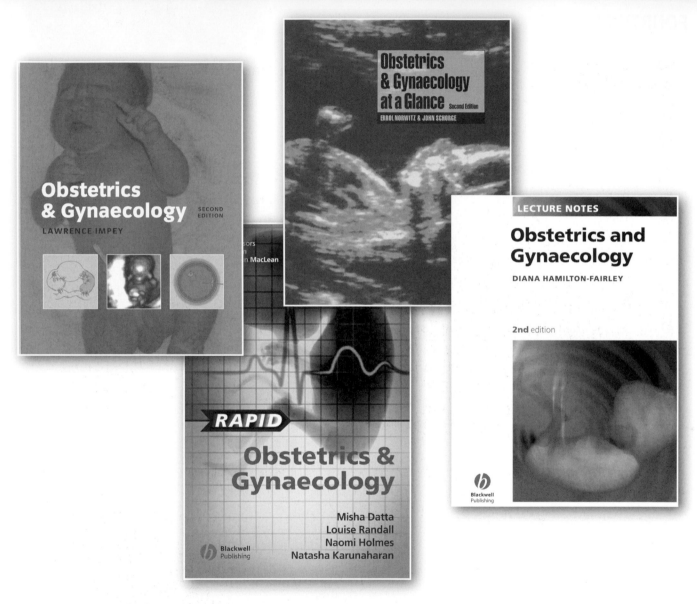

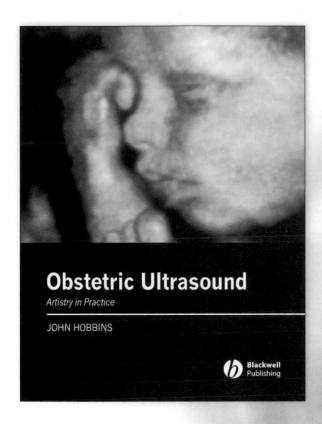